PRACTICE MANAGEMENT FOR UROLOGY GROUPS

LUGPA's Guidebook

SECOND EDITION

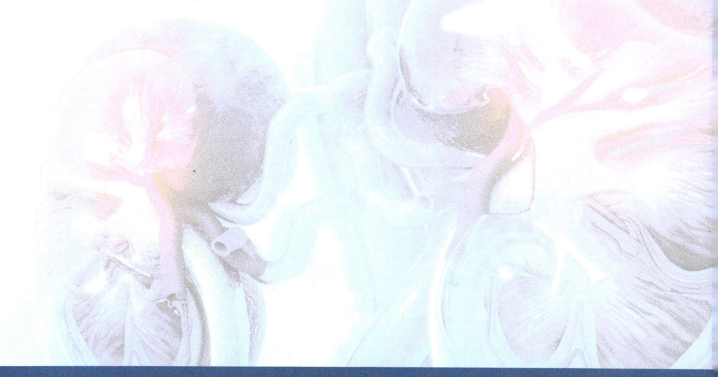

EDITORS:

Evan R. Goldfischer, MD, MBA Editor in Chief | David C. Chaikin, MD
Jonathan Henderson, MD | Celeste G. Kirschner, MHSA | Alec S. Koo, MD
Bryan A. Mehlhaff, MD | Scott B. Sellinger, MD | Alan D. Winkler, MHSA, FACMPE

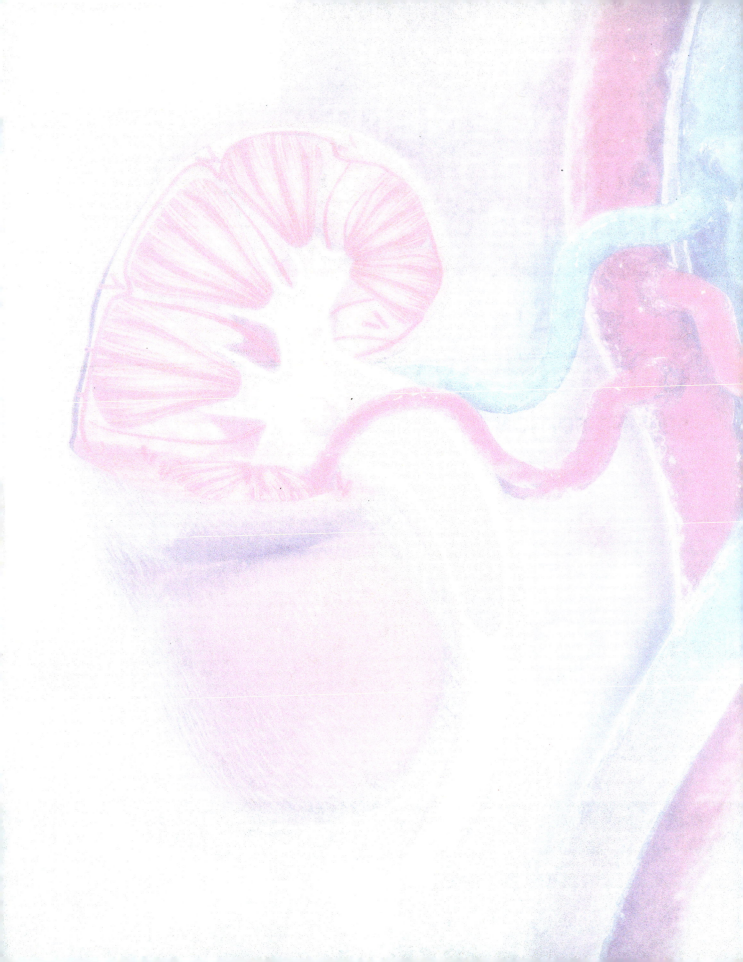

Copyright © 2020

All rights reserved. No part of this publication may be reproduced, distributed, or transmitted in any form or by any means, including photocopying, recording, digital scanning, or other electronic or mechanical methods, without prior written permission of LUGPA, except in the case of brief quotations embodied in critical reviews and certain other noncommercial uses permitted by copyright law. For permission requests, please contact LUGPA.

The information in this book is provided as an educational and informational service by LUGPA. It represents the opinions of the authors but does not necessarily represent the opinions of LUGPA. References to individual drugs or products do not represent an endorsement by LUGPA, nor does the absence of such reference indicate any form of disapproval. The information in this book is provided "as is" and is not intended as a substitute for competent legal or financial advice based on the user's individual facts and circumstances. The user of the book acknowledges that LUGPA accepts no responsibility or liability for consequences arising from the use of the information in the book.

Published by LUGPA, Chicago, Illinois, 2020
Printed in the United States of America by MidAmerican Printing Systems, Inc.

Second Edition
ISBN: 978-0-9988498-2-9
Electronic (PDF) book: 978-0-9988498-3-6
Library of Congress Control Number: 2020918465

Book design by Betsy Gold Designs
Copy edited by Tracie Gipson

For more information about LUGPA go to **www.LUGPA.org**

TABLE OF CONTENTS

IV	Foreword
VI	Preface
VIII	About the Editors
X	Acknowledgments
IX	Online Bonus Materials

1 CHAPTER 1
Legal and Economic Issues in Forming a Group Practice
Robert A. Wild, Esq., Hayden S. Wool, Esq., Gregory R. Smith, Esq., and Nicole F. Gade, Esq.

18 CHAPTER 2
Financial Structures and Risk Management Issues for Urology Groups
J. Jason Shelnutt, CPA

30 CHAPTER 3
Operational and Governance Structure of Urology Groups
Evan R. Goldfischer, MD, MBA

48 CHAPTER 4
Physician Compensation
Steven R. Flageol

64 CHAPTER 5
Urology Practice Mergers and Acquisitions
Peter M. Knapp, MD, FACS

82 CHAPTER 6
Private Equity's Increasing Investment Partnerships in Urology: Current State and Key Considerations
Hector M. Torres, Gary W. Hirschmann and Aaron T. Newman

96 CHAPTER 7
Electronic Health Records: Moving Forward
Robert DiLoreto, MD

116 CHAPTER 8
Managing Human Resources in a Changing Health Care Environment
Laine Belmonte, MBA, PHR

138 CHAPTER 9
Diagnose and Manage Your Marketing Needs for Outcomes-Oriented Tactics
Jennifer L. Dally, MBA and Neil Baum, MD

162 CHAPTER 10
Credentialing
Mia Frausto, BSB, CPCS

178 CHAPTER 11
Negotiating Third-Party Payments: A Never-Ending Challenge
Jerri Wilson-Durbin

198 **CHAPTER 12**
Service Line Agreements with Hospitals
Alan J. Beason, MS, FACMPE

216 **CHAPTER 13**
Urology Coding
Mark N. Painter and M. Ray Painter, MD

244 **CHAPTER 14**
Billing and Revenue Cycle Management
Twila J. Puritty, MBA

264 **CHAPTER 15**
Maximizing Productivity: APPs and Scribes in the Urology Practice
Diane Bonsall, MSN, APRN, ACNS-BC, Evelina Kaminski, MSN, APRN, AGCNS-BC
Gordon Lang, MSN, APRN, FNP-C, Amanda Licea, MPAS, PA-C,
Marcia O'Brien, MSN, APRN, FNP-C

284 **CHAPTER 16**
Medical Imaging
Benjamin Lowentritt, MD, FACS

300 **CHAPTER 17**
Establishing a Urology-Specific Laboratory
Nicholas A. Maruniak, MD, Candy M.H. Willets, MT, E. E. Scot Davis, BA, MPA, MBA, CMPE,
Adam J. Cole, MD and Stephanie J. Evans

324 **CHAPTER 18**
Genomic and Hereditary Testing in Prostate Cancer:
Implications for the Urology Practice
Christopher J.D. Wallis, MD, PhD, FRCSC and Raul S. Concepcion, MD, FACS

344 **CHAPTER 19**
The Basics of Developing an Ambulatory Surgery Center (ASC)
Michael W. Holder, MBA

358 **CHAPTER 20**
In-Office Dispensing (IOD)
Christopher Setzler, MBA, CMPE and Simi Banipal, BS, RHIT

372 **CHAPTER 21**
Durable Medical Equipment: Operationalizing an In-House Catheter Service
Alan D. Winkler, MHSA, FACMPE

386 **CHAPTER 22**
Developing a Radiation Oncology Center
Patrick R. Aldinger, RT, Stephen M. Beach, PhD, DABR and Terry FitzPatrick, MPA

406 **CHAPTER 23**
Establishing a Prostate Cancer Clinic in the Urology Office
Bryan A. Mehlhaff, MD and Christopher Pieczonka, MD

430 CHAPTER 24
The Next Advance In Comprehensive Urologic Oncology Care: Establishing a Comprehensive Bladder Cancer Clinic (CBCC))
Sandip M. Prasad, MD, MPhil

452 CHAPTER 25
Establishing a Women's Pelvic Health Clinic
David C. Chaikin, MD and Michael Ingber, MD

468 CHAPTER 26
Establishing a Medical Spa
David C. Chaikin, MD, Michael Ingber, MD and Anika Akerman, MD

482 CHAPTER 27
Men's Health Clinics
Steven A. Kaplan, MD and Gregory R. Mullen, MD

494 CHAPTER 28
Urology Leadership In Erectile Dysfunction: Emerging Technologies
Judson Brandeis, MD

516 CHAPTER 29
Telemedicine: Implications for the Urology Group Practice
Eugen Rhee, MD, MBA, Matthew Gettman, MD, Eric Kirshenbaum, MD and Aaron Spitz, MD

540 CHAPTER 30
Building a Robust and Sustainable Research Enterprise in the Tertiary Community Urology Setting
Neal D. Shore, MD, FACS, CPI, Raoul S. Concepcion, MD, FACS, Daniel R. Saltzstein, MD, Aretta vanBreda, RN, MS, CRCC, CIP and Thomas A. Paivanas, MHSA,

564 CHAPTER 31
The Future of Value-Based Payment in the US
Alec S. Koo, MD, FACS and John McManus

576 CHAPTER 32
Medicare Quality Payment Program: Updates for Urology
Bob Dowling, MD and Alec S. Koo, MD, FACS

588 CHAPTER 33
Political Advocacy
Deepak A. Kapoor, MD

602 Editors' Disclosures

603 Authors' Disclosures

The LUGPA Board of Directors recognizes the dedication and efforts of the editorial team and authors who have revised our notable publication, Practice Management for urology Groups: LUGPA's Guidebook. This book represents a unique voice in the medical practice management literature, with practical information to enhance the ability of urology group practices to navigate existing and future challenges in urology practice. The variety of subjects covered as well as the respective in-depth analyses and recommendations for corrective adjustments or new initiatives will provide real world value to our member physicians and administrative leaders. We look forward to feedback and suggestions from our readers and LUGPA members.

Richard Harris, MD
President, LUGPA

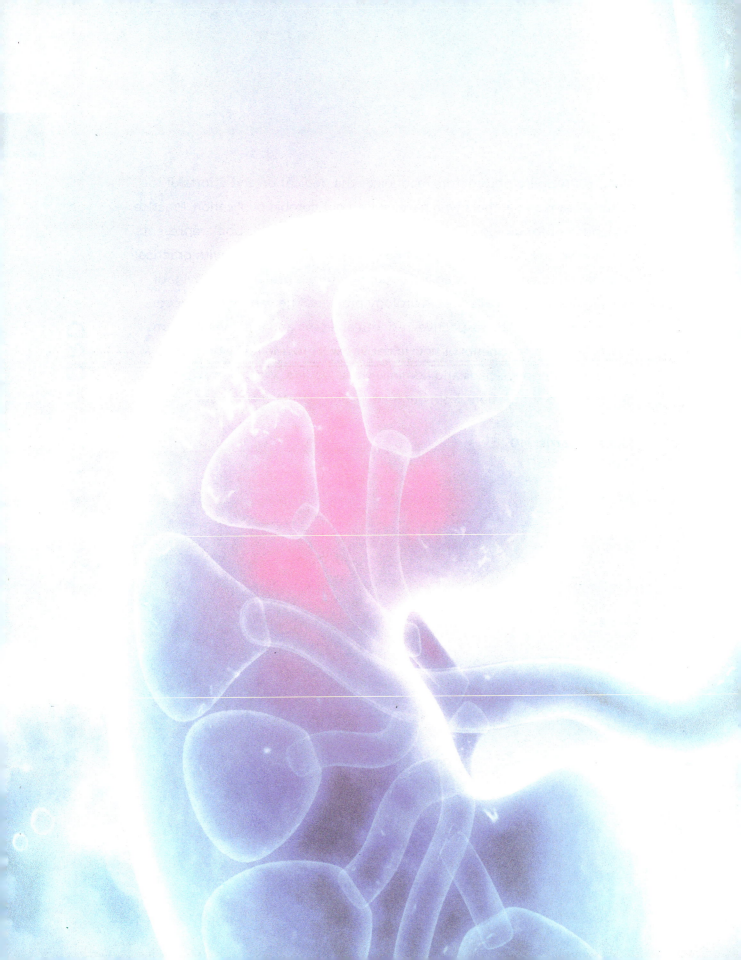

In the three years since the first edition of this book, much has changed in medicine, in general and urology, in particular. We have been fortunate to have new groundbreaking medical advancements in genitourinary cancer, new diagnostic testing for the detection of urinary pathogens, and new imaging modalities amongst other advances care. On the business side of medicine, we have seen the transition to value – based care, investment from private equity firms, and increased regulatory oversight. As such, the need for high levels of performance from independent urology groups has never been more critical. Of course, the focus of LUGPA groups has to be providing excellent care to our patients, while meeting their increased expectations including same day appointments and offering telemedicine visits since the outbreak of the COVID-19 pandemic. Our groups have, also, learned to share ideas through virtual meetings and webinars, as it has become more difficult to have large in-person meetings. LUGPA group must continue to evolve, if they are to not only survive, but continue to thrive.

The second edition of this book represents the work of an outstanding group of authors and editors. Included are thirteen new chapters, including the hot topics of compensation models, developing a MedSpa, genetic testing and more. This edition has never been more relevant to the independent urology group.

Our dedication to sustaining the independent practice of urology remains at the forefront of our organization. LUGPA remains the ONLY national urology organization that advocates for, and provides unique resources to the independent urology group practice. For more information about LUGPA, visit our website at **www.lugpa.org**.

As the ink is drying on this second edition, we have already started to plan for the third edition. The editorial team wants future editions to be both timely and relevant, so please send your ideas to us at ckirschner@lugpa.org. Feel free to tell us how to make the current chapters better and what topics you would like to see in future editions. Thank you, for your membership in LUGPA, and on behalf of the editors and the entire LUGPA Board of Directors, we look forward seeing you at future LUGPA events.

Evan R. Goldfischer, MD, MBA
Editor in Chief
Secretary, LUGPA

ABOUT THE EDITORS

Evan R. Goldfischer, MD, MBA

Dr. Goldfischer received his BA from Tufts University and his MD from Cornell University Medical College. He completed his internship and residency in Surgery/Urology at the University of Chicago. He completed a fellowship in Endourology under the direction of Arthur Smith at Long Island Jewish Medical Center. Dr. Goldfischer received his MBA from the University of Massachusetts and is a Certified Physician Executive. He served as the co-founding CEO of Premier Medical Group of the Hudson Valley as well as founding Director of Research. He has written over 100 peer-reviewed abstracts and publications and has lectured on six continents. He was elected to the LUGPA Board of Directors in 2014. He has served as Secretary of LUGPA since 2019 and will begin his term as President Elect beginning in 2021. He is the author of *Even Urologists Get Kidney Stones – A Guide to Prevention and Treatment*, published in 2018.

David C. Chaikin, MD

Dr. David C. Chaikin received his bachelor's degree in biology for the University of Illinois in Champaign, Illinois, earning his MD at Albert Einstein College of Medicine in Bronx, New York. Dr. Chaikin performed his internship and residency in Urology at the Hospital of the University of Pennsylvania. He completed a fellowship in Female Pelvic Medicine and reconstructive surgery under the direction of Dr. Jerry Blaivas. Dr. Chaikin is board certified in Urology and Female Pelvic Medicine and Reconstructive Surgery. He serves as the Vice President of Garden State Urology in Morristown, New Jersey. He also serves as urology medical director of Morristown memorial hospital of Atlantic health system, and is a former member of the LUGPA Board of Directors.

Jonathan Henderson, MD

Dr. Henderson earned his BS in microbiology at LSU in Baton Rouge. After receiving his MD at LSU Medical Center in Shreveport, he completed his internship and residency in Urology at LSUMC Hospital. Dr. Henderson spent the next six years in practice in Alabama where he pioneered urologic laparoscopy. In 2002, Dr. Henderson returned to Shreveport to join Regional Urology. Currently, he serves Regional Urology as their Chief Executive Officer.Dr. Henderson is certified by the American Board of Urology. He has served on the LUGPA Board of Directors since 2011.

Celeste G. Kirschner, MHSA

Celeste G. Kirschner's career spans nearly 40 years in association management. Since 2015 she has served as the chief executive officer of LUGPA. Farning her BS from Loyola University in Chicago and a master's in health services administration from the University of St. Francis, Ms. Kirschner has authored and edited many books throughout her career. Ms. Kirschner is a Certified Association Executive (CAE).

Alec S. Koo, MD

Dr. Alec S. Koo received his bachelor's Degree and MD from UCLA. He completed his residency in Surgery/Urology at UCLA in 1992, and is a Diplomate of the American Board of Urology. Dr. Koo is well known for his expertise in group management as well as value-based care and health economics outcomes. He is respected for his knowledge in areas including data integration and analytics in medicine, medical group dynamics and provider/pharmaceutical relations. Dr. Koo was the founding managing partner of Skyline Urology in Southern California. Dr. Koo is a former member of the LUGPA Board of Directors.

Bryan A. Mehlhaff, MD

A native of Oregon, Dr. Mehlhaff attended Beloit College in Wisconsin followed by medical school at Oregon Health Sciences University. After completing a general surgery and urology residency at Albany Medical Center he joined the Department of Urology as an Assistant Professor. He practices in Eugene, Oregon. As the Oregon Urology Institute (OUI) Medical Director of Research, he oversees numerous clinical trials in advanced prostate cancer and benign prostate conditions and has developed a comprehensive bone health and advanced prostate cancer clinic. Dr. Mehlhaff is also a managing partner of OUI, and is a former LUGPA Board member.

Scott B. Sellinger, MD

Dr. Scott B. Sellinger completed his Urology residency at the University of Florida and has been practicing in Tallahassee since 1991. He is a Past President of the Florida Urological Society, Past President of the Southeast Section of the AUA, and current President of the American Association of Clinical Urologists. Since his practice merger in 2014, he has developed a special interest in large group practice development and management. As President of Advanced Urology Institute (AUI) Tallahassee Division, he serves on the Board of AUI, representing his care center in one of the largest independent urology practices in the US. He is Chairman of the Advanced Prostate Cancer (APC) Committee and oversees several APC clinics. Since 2015, Dr. Sellinger has served on the LUGPA Board of Directors.

Alan D. Winkler, MHSA, FACMPE

With thirty-nine years of experience in health care, Alan D. Winkler has served as the Executive Director of Urology San Antonio, P.A. since October 2012. Alan holds a master's degree in Health Services from the University of Arkansas for Medical Sciences and has worked in private and corporate settings with physicians of many specialties. Alan is a Fellow in the American College of Medical Practice Executives (MGMA ACMPE) and served on its board of directors for nine years, concluding as its chair. Mr. Winkler currently serves on the LUGPA Board of Directors.

ONLINE BONUS MATERIALS

A new feature of the second edition of Practice Management for Urology Groups: LUGPA's Guidebook, is the addition of online downloadable forms, letters, and other resources that you can use and adapt for your practice.

An icon appears in the following chapters to alert you to the bonus material available online. Go to www.lugpa.org/2020editionsupplementals to view and download the documents.

Chapter 8 Contains:

1. 30-day New Employee Survey – Sample 1
2. 30-day New Employee Survey – Sample 2
3. Performance Evaluation Form – Sample 1
4. Performance Evaluation Form – Sample 2
5. Performance Rating Guide
6. Employee Satisfaction Survey – Sample 1
7. Employee Satisfaction Survey – Sample 2
8. Physician Satisfaction Survey – Sample 1
9. Physician Satisfaction Survey – Sample 1
10. Peer-to-Peer Recognition Form
11. Stay Interview Survey

Chapter 10 Contains:

Figure 1 New Provider Onboarding Checklist
Figure 2 Credentialing Checklist
Figure 3 Practitioner Credentialing and Privileging Checklist
Figure 4 Activity Calendar
Figure 5 Link Tax ID Letter
Figure 6 Status Sheet
Figure 7 Term Notice Letter
Figure 8 Termination Inactive Process Checklist
Figure 8 Provider Demographic Update Letter

LUGPA thanks our valued industry sponsors whose support helped produce the Second Edition of *Practice Management for Urology Groups: LUGPA's Guidebook.*

Platinum Level Sponsors:

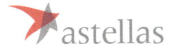
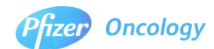
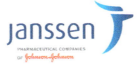

Gold Level Sponsors:

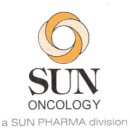

Thanks are also due to the editorial design and publication management team:.

- Celeste G. Kirschner, *CAE, Chief Executive Officer, LUGPA*
- Tracie Gipson, *Editor*
- Betsy Gold, Betsy Gold Design, *Graphic Designer*

CHAPTER 1

Legal and Economic Issues in Forming a Group Practice

Robert A. Wild, Esq.
Hayden S. Wool, Esq.
Gregory R. Smith, Esq.
Nicole F. Gade, Esq.

The information contained in this chapter is not intended and may not be relied upon as legal advice. Readers are strongly encouraged to consult with licensed attorneys and accountants prior to forming any business and entering into any agreements or other arrangements.

I. INTRODUCTION

Physicians contemplating the formation of a group practice must consider a variety of legal and economic issues. One of the first and most important decisions is choosing the most appropriate legal structure for the intended size and function of the practice. This decision requires consideration of a variety of factors, including tax treatment, liability protections, the desired governance and economic structure, the services to be provided and the federal and state regulatory environment. In the first part of this chapter, we will briefly discuss the types of entities most commonly used by physicians to practice medicine. In the second part, we will discuss certain federal and state regulatory considerations that are particularly relevant to the practice's structure, as well as its financial arrangements with referral sources. We strongly recommend that you consult your attorneys and accountants before proceeding with the formation and operation of a medical practice.

II. CORPORATE FORMATION AND STRUCTURE

Determining the most appropriate legal structure for a physician practice will depend significantly on the type of services the practice intends to provide. For example, if the entity being formed will provide ancillary services (e.g., laboratory, imaging, physical therapy) in addition to direct physician services, there are various federal and state "fraud and abuse" laws that must also be addressed. Moreover, if a practice will have financial relationships with individuals or entities that refer to the practice, or vice versa, additional safeguards must be followed.

Financial relationships among the practice and its owners, employees, and independent contractors, as well as financial relationships with third parties in the form of leases, license agreements and/or professional service agreements, all must be carefully structured. The failure to structure these financial arrangements properly can create significant legal risks, and in certain cases, could potentially lead to civil and criminal liability. These issues are discussed in greater detail later in this chapter.

Before discussing the various practice structures available to physicians, it is important to understand a legal doctrine known as the "corporate practice of medicine" doctrine (the "CPM Doctrine"). The CPM Doctrine, which has been adopted by some, but not all, states, was established to protect the public by ensuring that only physicians—as opposed to business corporations or other unlicensed individuals or entities—have the authority and discretion to offer medical services and make medical decisions. In general, the CPM Doctrine prohibits entities from practicing medicine or employing a physician to provide medical services unless the entity is: (i) fully owned by licensed providers (in this case, physicians); and (ii) formed under applicable state law for the specific purpose of practicing medicine.[1] In practice, this effectively means that in states where the CPM Doctrine applies and unless an exception can be satisfied, only physicians may own an interest in an entity that is formed for the purpose of providing medical care. We strongly encourage physicians to consult local attorneys in the state where the practice is being formed in order to ensure that the CPM Doctrine, to the extent it applies, would not be violated by a proposed structure.

The most common corporate structures for physicians include: (a) sole proprietorships; (b) general partnerships ("GPs"); (c) limited partnerships ("LPs"); (d) limited liability companies ("LLCs") and professional limited liability companies ("PLLCs"); and (e) professional corporations ("PCs") and professional associations ("PAs").[2] Each type of entity has specific legal and tax attributes that must be considered.[3] In states that have not adopted the CPM Doctrine, the owners of the practice entity may generally be individuals or entities. In states that have adopted the CPM Doctrine, only licensed professionals, or entities[4] owned by licensed professionals, may be owners of the practice entity. Following is a brief overview of each type of entity.

Common corporate structures for physician practices

1. Sole Proprietorships

Formation: A sole proprietorship is formed when an individual begins conducting business—no formal documentation is needed. Unlike other corporate forms, a sole proprietorship is not distinct from its owner for legal or tax purposes.

Management: Sole proprietorships are managed by the sole proprietor.

Liability Protection: A sole proprietorship is not distinct from its owner, and as a result does not offer any protection from personal liability. As a result, sole proprietorships are generally not recommended for physicians, given the potential liability that can arise from the practice of medicine. While other corporate forms will not protect the owners from professional liability, they will protect against non-professional service liability exposure.

2. General Partnerships

Formation: A GP is formed when two or more individuals or entities agree to associate for the purpose of conducting a business enterprise. Unlike sole proprietorships, a GP is treated as a separate legal entity from its owners. While GPs may be formed by oral agreement of the partners, it is more common to form a GP through a written partnership agreement.

Management: Typically, all partners participate in the management of the GP. However, the partners are free to delegate management to one or more of the partners if they wish.

Liability Protection: Despite status as distinct legal entities, GPs do not offer their owners protection from personal liability. Rather, they expand it. Each owner is jointly and severally liable for the acts and omissions of the GP, whether through its owners, officers, employees, or agents. For this reason, GPs are generally not recommended (unless registered, as provided below) for physicians, given the potential for significant personal liability.

Registered Limited Liability Partnership: Some states, such as New York,[5] will allow a GP to "register" with the state as a limited liability partnership. This registration provides the owner of the GP with protection for the acts and omissions of the other partners and the GP itself, similar to a professional corporation (discussed below). As with a professional corporation, however, the physician-owner(s) will remain liable for their own acts and omissions.

3. Limited Partnerships

Formation: A limited partnership is a partnership of two or more individuals or entities formed for the purpose of conducting a business. In contrast to a GP, an LP may only be formed by filing a Certificate of Limited Partnership (or equivalent document) with the appropriate state governmental authority. One of the LP partners must be designated as the general partner of the LP, and the remaining partners are usually considered limited partners. LPs may be formed by oral or written agreement. This form of entity may not be available in many states for a medical practice.

Management: LPs are managed by the general partner, with certain limited voting rights for major decisions reserved to the limited partners.

Profits and Losses: Allocations of profits and losses are typically governed by the LP agreement, if any. If not, the allocation of profits and losses are governed by statute which generally provides that in the absence of an agreement, profits and losses will be shared pro-rata in proportion to each partner's capital contribution.

Personal Liability: Personal liability is joint and individual for the general partner who is responsible for the obligations of the partnership. Limited partner(s) are liable only to the extent of their capital contributions to the partnership.

4. LLCs and PLLCs

Formation: A limited liability company or a professional limited liability company is formed by filing Articles of Organization with the relevant state authority. Both entities are legally distinct from their owners, known as "members." Depending upon state law, an LLC or PLLC may be required to enter into a formal, written governing document among its members called an "operating agreement." Whether or not it is legally required, an operating agreement is advisable in order to ensure that the rights and responsibilities of the members, as well as the governance structure, are clearly understood by all members. In addition, employment agreements for all professionals are highly recommended.

Management: One advantage of an LLC/PLLC is the flexibility afforded to governance issues. The entity may be managed by all members collectively or may be delegated to one or more specific members who are known as the "managing member(s)." If management is not delegated to one or more specific managing members, all members have equal management rights regardless of their equity ownership. Even if the entity is governed by managing members who are elected or appointed by all members, unless otherwise set forth in the operating agreement of an LLC or PLLC, most states reserve certain specified actions to be decided by the members (e.g., the admission of new members and issuance of membership interest(s); the adoption, amendment, or restating of the articles of organization or operating agreement; the dissolution of the LLC/PLLC; the sale, exchange, lease, mortgage, pledge or other transfer of all or substantially all of the assets of the LLC/PLLC; or the merger or consolidation of the LLC/PLLC).

Liability Protection. One of the advantages of an LLC/PLLC is the degree of personal liability protection it provides to its members. While a member will always be liable for his or her own professional medical negligence or misconduct, the LLC/PLLC will—unless otherwise agreed to by a member (e.g., through a personal guarantee)—protect the members from most other liabilities of the entity.[1]

5. Corporations, Professional Corporations, and Professional Associations

Formation: Business corporations, professional corporations, and professional associations are typically formed by filing a certificate of incorporation or articles of association with the state.

Management: PCs/PAs are required to have bylaws that set forth the entity's governing and operating structure, including the process for electing or appointing officers and directors. Bylaws are typically adopted by the Board of Directors and shareholders. Corporations are typically managed by a President and/or Chief Executive Officer, with oversight provided by the Board of Directors and various committees tasked with more specific oversight responsibilities. Often, depending on the state in which the entity is organized, all the officers of a PC or PA must be physicians.

Liability Protection: Similar to an LLC/PLLC, a corporation provides personal liability protection to its shareholders (other than for his or her own professional medical negligence or misconduct, for which each shareholder remains individually liable).

Regardless of the type of entity selected, it is strongly recommended (whether required by state law) that participants in the practice entity enter into a written agreement that details their respective rights and obligations. This agreement (often referred to as a "Partnership Agreement," "Operating Agreement," or "Shareholders' Agreement," depending on the form of entity selected), together with separate employment agreements, if utilized, will detail the obligations of the parties vis-à-vis each other. They will address important issues such as compensation, restrictions (both while in the practice and after withdrawal), withdrawal payments, management and voting (subject to state law requirements), as well as other key issues and responsibilities. In addition, employment agreements for all professionals are highly recommended.

III. REGULATORY AND COMPLIANCE ISSUES

State law considerations and the needs and desires of the participants largely influence the type of legal structure that is most appropriate for a newly formed physician group. However, there are several federal laws that significantly impact the economic structure of a group practicing together in a single legal entity, particularly the group's financial arrangements with its physicians. In addition, these laws often impact the group's transactions with third parties. The most significant of these laws are the federal physician self-referral law (the "Stark Law") and the federal anti-kickback statute ("Anti-Kickback Statute").[10] It is incumbent upon all physicians to understand how these laws may be implicated when forming a group practice, and to protect themselves accordingly.

The Stark Law

The Statutory Prohibition on Referrals for Designated Health Services (DHS)

The Stark Law was originally created in response to a concern that physicians were more likely to refer business to entities with which they had a financial relationship, thereby profiting from their own referrals. In short, the Stark Law prohibits a physician from making a referral for certain "designated health services" ("DHS")[11] that are paid by Medicare[12] to an entity with which the physician (or his or her immediate family member) has a "financial relationship" *unless* an exception to the Stark Law is met.[13] If an applicable Stark exception is not met—and the burden of proof is on the person or entity seeking the protection of the exception—then the physician's referral is prohibited, and a bill may not be submitted by the person or entity that receives the prohibited referral. The Stark Law would prohibit a physician for referring any DHS (e.g., a simple x-ray, lab test) within their own practice unless the practice is structured to meet an applicable exception. In addition, the law would similarly prohibit referrals outside of the practice to entities with which the physician or the group has a financial relationship (e.g., a lease between referring providers), unless an applicable exception can be satisfied.

While the basic Stark Law prohibition is simple enough, the Centers for Medicare and Medicaid Services ("CMS") has since published thousands of pages of commentary and regulations intended to clarify and expound upon the basic prohibition and its various exceptions. The resulting regulatory paradigm is, to put it mildly, difficult to navigate even for experienced health care attorneys. Therefore, it is strongly recommended that any transactions or arrangements between a physician and entities with which the physician (or his or her immediate family members) has a financial relationship be fully reviewed and structured by legal counsel.

As a threshold issue, one of the most important factors in determining if the Stark Law may be implicated by a particular arrangement is understanding when a physician has a "financial relationship" with an entity to which he or she refers.

There Are Four Basic Types Of Financial Relationships That Implicate The Stark Law:

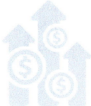

- Direct ownership/investment interests
- Indirect ownership/investment interests
- Direct compensation arrangements
- Indirect compensation arrangements

It is beyond the scope of this chapter to analyze the different types of financial relationships, but it is important to note that financial relationships may be formed—and thus implicate the Stark Law—in ways that are not always obvious. For example, if a physician is employed by an entity to which he refers, he will quite obviously have a direct financial relationship with that entity. However, if a physician is employed by Entity A, and Entity A has a contract with Entity B, then the physician will (1) have a direct financial relationship with Entity A, ***and*** (2) also have an indirect financial relationship with Entity B. As a result, the physician's referrals to Entity A and Entity B must each satisfy a Stark Law exception.

Unlike the Anti-Kickback Statute (discussed below in Section B), no specific intent or mental state is required to violate the Stark Law. The Stark Law is a strict liability law, under which it is illegal—regardless of the parties' intent—to: (1) make a prohibited referral or order; or (2) submit a claim for payment based upon a prohibited referral or order. Therefore, although both the Anti-Kickback Statute and the Stark Law were intended to address the same basic problem—i.e., health care providers acting out of financial self-interest—they have different requirements, and providers can violate the Stark Law without violating the Anti- Kickback Statute, and vice versa.

The penalties for violating the Stark Law are severe, and include: (i) the denial of, or the requirement to refund, any payments for services that resulted from an unlawful referral; (ii) civil monetary penalties of up to $15,000[14] for each service for which a person presents or causes to be presented a bill or claim that they know or should know results from a prohibited referral, or for which a required refund has not been made, plus an assessment of up to three times the amount claimed in lieu of damages; and (iii) exclusion from the Medicare and Medicaid programs as well as other federal health care programs. For "circumvention schemes" (i.e., those arrangements that are designed to obtain referrals indirectly that cannot be made directly), a civil monetary penalty of up to $100,000[15] for each such arrangement or scheme may be imposed on any physician or entity that knows or should know that the scheme/arrangement has a principal purpose of assuring referrals by the physician to a particular entity that could not be directly made under the law.[16] In addition, a Stark Law violation can also serve as the basis for a federal False Claims Act (FCA) action or litigation.[17] Under the FCA, a party can now be subjected to fines of up to $22,363 for every false claim submitted to the United Sates (or a contractor of the United States, such as a Medicare Administrative Contractor) as a result of an arrangement that violates the Stark Law, as well as an additional fine of treble damages (i.e., three times the amount of the (i.e., three damages times the amount of the underlying claim).[18]

The Stark Law prohibits referrals by a physician to an entity for the provision of "designated health services" if:

- The entity has a direct or indirect financial relationship with the physician, and
- The financial relationship does not satisfy a statutory or regulatory exception to the Stark Law. (Note: To avoid a Stark violation, the arrangement must meet every requirement of the applicable exception.)

Stark Law Exceptions

If an arrangement implicates the Stark Law, the parties must satisfy an exception in order to avoid a violation. There are a number of Stark Law exceptions that permit a variety of legitimate arrangements, most of which are outside the scope of this chapter. The most common Stark Law exceptions relied on by urology groups to be able to provide ancillary services within the group are the "in-office ancillary services exception" and the "physician services exception," each of which are discussed on the next page. Note that both exceptions are "all-purpose" exceptions, meaning they can be used for both direct and indirect financial relationships. In order to utilize either of these important exceptions, the group must meet the definition of a "group practice" under the Stark Law. The requirements of the "group practice" definition are designed to ensure that physicians are truly practicing together in an integrated manner, as opposed to a loosely affiliated physician group that has only been formed to share ancillary revenues and profit from their own referrals.

PENALTIES:

1) Denial of Payment

2) Refunds of Collected Amount

3) Penalty up to $15,000 for Each Bill

4) Penalty up to $100,000 for Each Arrangement

5) Fine of 3X the Amount Improperly Collected

Definition of a "Group Practice": In order to qualify as a "group practice" for purposes of the Stark Law, a group must satisfy *all* the following criteria:[19]

- The group must be a single legal entity organized for the purpose of being a group practice;

- The group must have at least two physicians who are members of the group (whether full or part-time employees, locum tenens physicians, physicians with a direct or indirect ownership interest in the practice, or a physician who provides on-call services for other members of the group practice);[20]

- Each physician who is a member of the group must furnish substantially the full range of patient care services that the physician routinely furnishes, including medical care, consultation, diagnosis, and treatment, through the joint use of shared office space, facilities, equipment, and personnel;

- With limited exceptions, substantially all of the patient care services of the physicians who are members of the group (that is, at least 75% of the total patient care services of the group practice members) must be furnished through the group and billed under a billing number assigned to the group, and the amounts received must be treated as receipts of the group;

- Members of the group must personally conduct no less than 75% of the physician-patient encounters of the group practice (i.e., no more than 25% of the physician-patient encounters may be done by independent contractors);

- The overhead expenses of, and income from, the practice must be distributed according to methods that are determined before the receipt of payment for the services giving rise to the overhead expense or producing the income;

- The group practice must be a unified business consisting of (a) centralized decision-making by a body representative of the group practice that maintains effective control over the group's assets and liabilities (including, but not limited to, budgets, compensation, and salaries); and (b) consolidated billing, accounting, and financial reporting; and

- No physician who is a member of the group practice directly or indirectly receives compensation based on the volume or value of his or her referrals, subject to special rules for productivity bonuses and profit shares.

The In-Office Ancillary Services Exception (IOAS)

The IOAS exception[21] allows a group practice to make referrals of DHS (e.g., radiation therapy, diagnostic imaging and pathology services, etc.) to other physicians that are part of the same "group practice" (as noted and defined above).

If the "group practice" definition is met, three additional and distinct tests must be satisfied in order to satisfy the IOAS exception: (1) the group must ensure that certain performance or supervision requirements applicable to the referred DHS are satisfied; (2) the services must be performed in either (A) the "same building" where the referring physician (or another physician who is a member of the same group practice) furnishes services unrelated to the furnishing of DHS, or (B) a "centralized building;" and (3) the DHS must meet certain billing requirements.

Each of these tests are briefly summarized below.

(ii) Performance/Supervision Requirements. The DHS itself must be furnished personally by one of the following individuals: (i) the referring physician; (ii) a physician who is a member of the same group practice as the referring physician; or (iii) an individual who is supervised by the referring physician or, if the referring physician is in a group practice, by another physician in the group practice, provided that the supervision complies with all other applicable Medicare payment and coverage rules for the services.

Location Requirements. The IOAS exception also requires that the DHS be provided in one of two locations—the "same building" or (for groups only, not for solo practitioners) a "centralized location," each of which have detailed requirements that must be analyzed on a case-by-case basis.

Billing Requirements. The DHS must be billed by one of the following: (A) the physician who performs or supervises the services; (B) a group practice of which the performing or supervising physician is a member under a billing number assigned to the group practice; or (C) an entity that is wholly owned by the physician or group practice.

Physician Services Exception. The physician services exception allows physicians to make referrals to other physicians for "physician services" that constitute DHS in the same "group practice."

- The physician to whom the referral is made must be either (A) a "member" of the referring physician's group practice, or (B) a physician in the same group practice as the referring physician; and

- The physician services must be furnished either (A) personally by the physician to whom the referral was made, or (B) by an individual under the supervision of a physician who is either a member of the referring physician's group practice or a physician in the same group as the referring physician.

Again, the Stark Law is extraordinarily complex, and the foregoing is not intended as an exhaustive review of all its requirements. We strongly urge all physicians to engage experienced counsel to ensure that all arrangements are in compliance with the Stark Law.

The Federal Anti-Kickback Statute

The Basic Prohibition. The federal Anti-Kickback Statute makes it a criminal offense to knowingly and willfully offer, pay, solicit or receive any "remuneration" to induce or reward referrals of items or services reimbursable by a federal health care program.[22] A "federal health care program" generally includes any health care program[22] that receives funding from the United States government (e.g., Medicare, Medicaid, Tricare, etc.), as well as any state health care program.[23] At its core, the Anti-Kickback Statute is designed to ensure that referrals for health care items or services are made based on medical necessity, as opposed to financial motives. Despite its relative simplicity, the Anti-Kickback Statute is exceptionally—and often counter intuitively—broad. For example, the Anti-Kickback Statute defines the of value given "directly or indirectly, overtly or covertly, in cash or in kind."[24] This means that actions that in any other industry would be considered common cour tesies—for example, sending a holiday gift basket to a referral source, if done with improper intent—potentially implicates the statute.[25] The key to understanding the Anti- Kickback Statute is recognizing that violations turn on a specific intent or state of mind—"knowingly or willfully." Without the intent to induce or reward a referral, a violation generally cannot occur. However, if the intent to induce or reward referrals is present—despite the presence of other legitimate reasons for the arrangement—it can still result in a violation of the Anti-Kickback Statute.[25]

It must be noted that the Anti-Kickback Statute is a criminal law; indeed, violations are felonies that can result in significant fines (up to $100,000) and/or imprisonment for up to ten years for both partiesto an illegal kickback arrangement. In addition, substantial civil monetary penalties and exclusion from federal and state health care programs may also result from violations of the Anti-Kickback Statute.[26] In fact, the law is clear that a violation of the Anti-Kickback Statute can be a basis for imposing penalties under the FCA.[27] Under the FCA, a party can now be subjected to fines of up to $22,363 for each false claim submitted to the United States or one of its contractors as a result of an arrangement that violates the Anti-Kickback Statute, as well as an additional fine of treble damages (i.e., three times the amount of the underlying claim).[28]

	ANTI-KICKBACK STATUTE
TARGET	Medicare/Medicaid Service Providers
FOCUS	Hidden Remuneration
SERVICE	Any Type
CRIMINAL PENALTY	5-Year Max Sentence
CIVIL PENALTY	Could be Trebled
USUAL PENALTY AMOUNT	Jail with <$25,000 or $50,000 for Each Violation, Plus <3x Fine
OTHER PENALTIES	Exclusion from Medicare/Medicaid
PRIVATE RIGHT OF ACTION	No (some exceptions)
INTENT/DEFINITION	Intent Must be Proven Knowing and Willful Manner

Anti-Kickback Statue

The Anti-Kickback Safe Harbors. The Anti-Kickback Statute and its regulations provide for a number of limited "safe harbors" to protect certain arrangements that are not considered fraudulent or otherwise abusive. The safe harbors cover a range of common arrangements, including employment, space and equipment leases, investment/ownership interests in public and private entities, personal services, sales of practices, discounts and rebates, recruitment, and investments in ambulatory surgery centers.

Each safe harbor has its own unique requirements. Any arrangement that fits squarely within the four corners of a "safe harbor" exemption is presumptively protected from prosecution and the imposition of applicable penalties. It is therefore always advisable to be within a safe harbor—or to meet as many of the requirements of a safe harbor as possible, which can help mitigate the risk of an Anti-Kickback violation. The fact that an arrangement does not qualify for one of the safe harbors does not render it illegal per se. Rather, the arrangement simply will not receive presumptive protection and, if scrutinized by the government, will be evaluated for its relative potential for fraud and abuse.

Even if the government declines to prosecute a potentially illegal arrangement, the legal and emotional costs of an investigation are considerable. Being outside of safe harbor inevitably creates risk, which should be considered and weighed against the business objectives involved.

STARK LAW	ANTI-KICKBACK STATUTE
Prevent physicians from referring patients to entities providing designated health services if the physician or an immediate family member has a financial relationship that entity	Prohibits offering, paying, soliciting or receiving financial incentives to induce referrals of items or services covered by Medicare, Medicaid and other federally funded programs

Other Requirements Involving Referral Arrangements

Although it is beyond the scope of this chapter to discuss every type of arrangement that may implicate the Stark Law or the Anti-Kickback Statute, it is important to note that any arrangement between parties who have a direct or indirect financial relationship and refer to one another (e.g., a space or equipment lease arrangement, a professional services arrangement, an employment arrangement, etc.) must be structured to meet an applicable Stark Law exception if there are any DHS referrals between the parties,[29] and should be structured to meet a safe harbor (or as many elements of a safe harbor as possible) under the Anti-Kickback Statute. In general, all agreements should be in writing and clearly delineate the covered duties; the compensation must be fair market value without giving effect to the volume or value of referrals or other business generated between the parties; and the arrangement must be commercially reasonable even in the absence of referrals between the parties. Given the complexity of these laws and the often counter-intuitive nature of their application, is strongly recommended that all arrangements between parties who refer to one another be reviewed by experienced health care counsel before they are implemented.

State Professional Misconduct Laws

Many states have also enacted professional misconduct laws that, in addition to delineating practice standards, impact financial relationships with other parties. For example, these types of laws often prohibit payments of any kind to induce referrals and acting in ways that may unduly influence patient choice. In addition, many states have adopted other laws that prohibit physicians from sharing their professional fees with non-physicians, commonly referred to as "fee splitting." For example, the New York State Education Law provides that it is professional misconduct for a physician to "fee-split" his or her professional fees with any person, other than a partner, employee, associate in a professional corporation, professional subcontractor or consultant authorized to practice medicine, or a legally authorized trainee practicing under the supervision of a licensee.[31] In New York, this prohibition includes any arrangement whereby the amount received in payment "constitutes a percentage of, or is otherwise dependent upon, the income or receipts of a licensee."[31] For example, rental arrangements that provide for rental fees based on a percentage of the revenue generated would be prohibited by this limitation.

Physicians are faced with an ever-increasing web of complex laws and regulations affecting the practice of medicine. Now more than ever, physicians are strongly encouraged to ensure that their legal and economic structure is thoroughly reviewed and discussed with experienced health care counsel prior to forming a practice. As with one's health, an ounce of prevention is worth a pound of cure.

REFERENCES

1. Many states have enacted exceptions to the CPM Doctrine. While the exceptions vary from state-to-state, some of the more common exceptions include: (a) employment by a licensed facility (e.g., a hospital), (b) independent contractor arrangements with licensed facilities, (c) employment by a school of medicine or other health education institute, (d) employment by health insurers for quality assurance purposes, and (e) employment by a governmental authority or governmental entity.

2. Please note that, while certain states may permit the provision of medical services through other corporate forms, such as business trusts, we have limited our discussion to the most commonly utilized corporate forms.

3. Tax issues are outside the scope of this chapter. Physicians are encouraged to consultant tax attorneys and/or accountants prior to organizing.

4. Note that certain states only permit natural persons – not entities - to be owners.

5. *See* N.Y. Partnership Law § 121-1500(a).

6. A registered limited liability partnership is not the same as a limited partnership, which is discussed separately.

7. A general exception to the limitation on personal liability is a failure to pay wages or benefits which have been agreed upon, as well as the failure to pay taxes.

8. Although the nomenclature varies by state, the essence of this type of entity is a corporation.

9. For example, in Section 1508(a) of the New York Business Corporation Law provides that all directors and officers of a professional corporation be physicians licensed to practice in New York State. However, the definition of an "officer" specifically excludes the Secretary if there is only one shareholder. See N.Y. Business Corporation Law § 1501(e).

10. See 42 U.S.C. § 1395nn and 42 U.S.C. § 1320a-7b, respectively. Many states have also enacted their own versions of these laws with many of the same - or in some cases, more stringent – prohibitions as their federal counterparts.

11. The term "designated health services" means any of the following services: (i) clinical laboratory services; (ii) physical therapy, occupational therapy, and outpatient speech – language pathology services; (iii) radiology and certain other imaging services; (iv) radiation therapy services and supplies; (v) durable medical equipment and supplies; (vi) parenteral and enteral nutrients, equipment, and supplies; (vii) prosthetics, orthotics, and prosthetic devices and supplies; (viii) home health services; (ix) outpatient prescription drugs; and (x) inpatient and outpatient hospital services. See 42 C.F.R. § 411.351.

12. On its face, the Stark Law only prohibits referrals for "designated health services" that are paid for by Medicare. However, the Social Security Act prohibits any federal financial participation payment to a state under the state's Medicaid plan for "designated health services" furnished on the basis of a referral that would result in a denial of payment under Medicare if Medicare covered the services in the same way as the state plan. See 42 U.S.C. § 1396b(s). In other words, arrangements that would be improper under the federal Stark Law may prevent the relevant state from receiving federal matching funds for those services provided under its Medicaid Program.

13. See 42 U.S.C. § 1395nn.

14. This maximum penalty is subject to annual adjustments for inflation and has been increased to $25,820 for each service as of January 17, 2020. See 45 C.F.R. § 102.3.

15. The penalty for circumvention schemes has also been increased as of January 17, 2020, up to a maximum of $172,137. Id.

16. See 42 USC § 1395nn(g).

17. There have been numerous litigations involving allegations of Stark Law violations that form the basis of False Claims Act cases. For example, in 2018, a Tennessee physician agreed to pay $200,000 to the United States government to settle allegations that involved a scheme with laboratories that caused the submission of false claims to Medicare. The laboratory allegedly induced the physician and others to enter into a sham "investment" that provided her with a guaranteed "dividend" of $5,000 for each month provided she continued to refer the same level of urine drug screens to the lab. See Settlement Agreement Between the United States and Brenna Green, D.O. (announced April 26, 2018). In another case, U.S. ex rel., Drakeford v. Tuomey Health Care System, Inc., 792 F.3d 364 (4th Cir. 2015), the Court of Appeals affirmed a jury verdict in which the defendant health system was held to have violated the Stark law by entering into part-time employment contracts with physicians that compensated them above fair market value and varied with the volume or value of their referrals. Based on these illegal referrals, the jury also found that the defendant knowingly submitted 21,730 false claims to Medicare. The Court also affirmed the jury's award of civil penalties and treble damages amounting to $237,454,195.

18. See 31 U.S.C. § 3729(a); 28 C.F.R. § 85.5.

19. See 42 C.F.R. § 411.352.

20. Note that independent contractors and leased physicians (unless the leased physicians meet the definition of an "employee" under IRS rules) are not considered "members" of a group practice under the Stark Law.

21. See 42 C.F.R. § 411.355(b).

22. 42 USC §1320a-7b(b).

23. 42 U.S.C. § 1320a-7b(f).

24. Id. at (b).

25. See *United States v. Nagelvoort*, 856 F.3d 1117 (7th Cir.), cert. denied, 138 S.Ct. 556 (2017); *United States v. Borrasi*, 639 F.3d 774 (7th Cir., 2011); *United States v. Katz*, 871 F.2d 105 (9th Cir., 1989); *United States v. Greber*, 760 F.2d 68 (3rd Cir.), cert. denied, 476 U.S. 988 (1985).

26. See 42 U.S.C. § 1320a-7a(a)(7).

27. See 42 U.S.C. § 1320a-7b(g).

28. See 31 U.S.C. § 3729(a); 28 C.F.R. § 85.5.

29. An exception must be met even if the transaction itself does not involve DHS if there are other DHS referrals between the parties.

30. See N.Y. Ed. Law § 6530(19).

31. Id.

KEY POINTS

- **Financial relationships** among the practice and its owners, employees, and independent contractors, as well as financial relationships with third parties (e.g., leases, license agreements, professional service agreements, or otherwise) all must be carefully constructed.

- **The most common corporate structures** for physician practices include: (a) sole proprietorships; (b) general partnerships ("GPs"); (c) limited partnerships ("LPs"); (d) limited liability companies ("LLCs"); (e) professional limited liability companies ("PLLCs"); (f) professional corporations ("PC"); and (g) professional associations ("PAs"). Choice of entity should be discussed with legal, accounting and tax advisors.

- **Regardless of the type of entity selected,** it is strongly recommended (whether required by law or not) that participants in the practice entity each enter into a written agreement that details their respective rights and obligations.

- **Adhere to the Stark Law,** which is the statutory prohibition on Physician (as defined in such provisions) referrals for designated health services (also as defined in such provisions).

  - Among the most common Stark Law exceptions relied on by urology group practices to be able to provide ancillary services with the group are the "in-office ancillary services exception" and the "physician services exception." The group must meet the definition of a "group practice" under the statutes and regulations to utilize these exceptions.

- **Adhere to the federal Anti-Kickback Statute,** which makes it a criminal offense to knowingly and willfully offer, pay solicit or receive any "remuneration" to induce or reward referrals of items or services reimbursable by a federal healthcare program.

  - The Anti-Kickback Statute and its regulations provide for several limited "safe harbors" to protect certain arrangements that are not considered fraudulent or otherwise abusive.

- **Adhere to any state professional misconduct laws that**, in addition to delineating practice standards, impact financial relationships with other parties.

Robert A. Wild, Esq.

Mr. Wild is a founding member of Garfunkel Wild, P.C., and has served as the firm's Chairman since its inception. Mr. Wild's practice primarily focuses on complex transactions for health care providers. Mr. Wild is a frequent lecturer and author in the field of health law, and has addressed a broad variety of groups, organizations and health care providers. Mr. Wild received his B.A. in 1964 from the State University of New York at Buffalo, and his J.D. in 1967 from St. John's University School of Law.

Hayden S. Wool, Esq.

Mr. Wool is a Partner/Director of Garfunkel Wild, P.C., which he joined in 1992. Mr. Wool advises clients on a variety of business, regulatory and transactional issues, with a particular expertise in the application of the Federal and New York State self-referral (Stark) laws and Anti-Kickback laws. Mr. Wool received his B.S. in Health Care Administration and Management, With Honors, from Alfred University in 1982, and his J.D., With Honors, from Albany Law School of Union University in 1985.

Gregory R. Smith, Esq.

Mr. Smith is a Partner at Garfunkel Wild, P.C., which he joined in 2002. Mr. Smith advises clients on a wide range of compliance matters, including Medicare and Medicaid audits, application of the Federal and New York State self-referral (Stark) laws, Anti-Kickback laws, and other fraud and abuse issues. Mr. Smith received his J.D., With Distinction, from the Hofstra University School of Law in 1999, and his B.A. from the State University of New York at Plattsburgh in 1993.

Nicole F. Gade, Esq.

Ms. Gade is a Senior Attorney at Garfunkel Wild, P.C., which she joined in 2015. Ms. Gade advises clients on a variety of health care and general commercial matters, including business structuring, Federal and State law regulatory compliance, mergers, sales and acquisitions, and other corporate matters. Ms. Gade received her B.A. from the University of Michigan in 1998, an M.P.A. with a concentration in Health Care Financial Management from New York University's Wagner School of Public Service in 2000, and a J.D. from St. John's University School of Law in 2004.

CHAPTER

Financial Structure and Risk Management

J. Jason Shelnutt, CPA

Successful independent groups are structured in many ways, which in turn impacts the sources and availability of capital as well as the options the group will have to minimize risk within the organization. Additionally, economic and environmental circumstances may change and change rapidly. It is important that an organization's leadership evaluate all the options for capital access and risk reduction and develop the relationships that will support the ability to adapt to specific circumstances as they arise. These relationships include banking, leasing/rental organizations, shareholders/owners and potentially, private equity.

BANKING

A banking partner who has the expertise and resources that match the needs of your organization is critical. In selecting that banking partner, you want to make sure that they have experience, stability, and focus in your field that will allow them to quickly understand and respond to the needs of your organization. You may be able to find this in a community bank who is willing to commit the time to understand your business. An alternative is a regional or national bank with a division and dedicated personnel that focuses on health care and physician practices in particular.

Historically when margins were significant in health care, banks thought of physician practices as golden and were willing to lend on a signature. It is much different today where health care margins are thin, physician practices more transient and banks are more focused on their own stability and sustainability.

When applying for a loan, groups will be asked to provide their banking partner with specific information about the practice and its operations, historical financial results, corporate tax returns, and projected operating results indicating the need for the loan. The bank will want to review and update this information at least annually, perhaps more often if circumstances change significantly. Be prepared to pledge corporate assets, which are mostly accounts receivable, and equipment as surety for the loan. If that is insufficient or the organization has a short operating history, a personal guarantee is often requested.

Even good banking partners are trained to get as much collateral as they can to lower their risk. You will need to test the relationship between the amount of lending the banking partner will make available and the need for more collateral. In most cases loans are limited to between 60% and 80% of the value of the collateral depending on the quality of the assets being pledged. That can be affected by the length of the relationship as well as the size and stability of the organization.

When the amount of collateral requested exceeds that available at the corporate level you will need to determine if the need for capital is worth risking personal assets. To the extent possible, try to limit that risk to the Group's owners. One way to limit risk is to specify the amount of guarantee provided by each owner. Another method is to limit the time over which it will be required or negotiate metrics that will release the guarantee.

Banking partners will usually provide debt funding for working capital with accounts receivable pledged, as well as real estate loans secured by the property purchased or constructed. Most loans provided in the recent past are variable interest rate loans due primarily to low short-term interest rates. Longer-term loans are available at a fixed rate. In addition, interest rate swaps can effectively fix the interest rate for a specified period on an underlying variable-rate loan. This usually occurs on loans exceeding a dollar threshold, but for a larger loan it can be worth the trouble. Variable interest rates are usually pegged to an index with the LIBOR (London Interbank Offered Rate) Index being the most common. Some banks will index on the prime rate, which changes much less frequently.

EQUIPMENT LEASING/RENTAL ARRANGEMENTS

Rental and leasing agreements can be a means to finance equipment for the practice. Short-term rentals are appropriate for equipment for which you have an infrequent need, are evaluating or that has a rapid obsolescence. In these cases, you should evaluate the potential revenue stream against the cost of having the equipment. The occasional need for an expensive laser, or a new benign prostatic hyperplasia (BPH) technology often fall into this category. These arrangements can also be useful when you are uncertain how much volume a new service will produce.

Equipment for which you have higher confidence about the length of time it will be needed can be considered for a three-to five-year lease, depending on the life of the asset. This type of lease is merely an alternative to a loan. Caution should be taken to understand all the inherent terms of a lease, including actual or imputed purchase price of the equipment, effective interest rate, payment terms, and buyout provisions. Leases often have usage factors that can result in additional payments. Leases provided by a vendor of the equipment may be designed to promote sales and have favorable terms. More often, it is designed with convenience in mind for the equipment purchaser at a potentially higher

> **UNDERSTANDING LEASE TERMS**
>
> I. Actual or imputed purchase price
> II. Effective interest rate
> III. Payment terms, buyout provisions
> IV. Usage factors

lending risk. These costs are included in the effective interest rate of the lease. The lease should be broken into its component parts of interest, principal, and sometimes maintenance in order to compare it with other financing alternatives. This can be done using a known interest rate and finding the net present value of the asset, or by using the cash purchase price and imputing the interest rate.

COST OF FACILITIES

One of the largest assets of a physician organization as well as the largest capital need are their facilities. This is true whether there is an opportunity to own or lease. The cost of this asset is dependent upon location, size, and the length of occupancy time. The type of structure, along with the complexity of its design, also impact cost. These factors may not be within control in a market unless the practice builds and owns the facility. In a saturated market, this may not be possible. In other newer markets with more land available at a reasonable cost, it may be a good option. An organization should evaluate the stability of the market and the risk of the changing needs of the practice when making the lease or own decision.

Whether you decide to lease or own, it is important to evaluate the cost of the underlying building structure, the cost of improvements, and the cost of the operating of the space over a comparable period. In the case of ownership, evaluate the cost or benefit of selling the property. You may have to impute or estimate some of these components depending on how a lease proposal is structured and your knowledge of the building's history. Triple net leases include only the cost of the basic structure and a portion of improvements in excess of a specified allowance, taxes, insurance, and operating costs. Care should be taken to define limits on pass through of these costs, either by getting hard estimates or contractually limiting increases. What looks like a low-cost lease can turn into an inordinately high total occupancy cost. Time value of money—which states that money available today is worth more than the identical sum in the future due to its potential earning capacity—should also be considered in this calculation. As more of the cost components are included in a fixed lease payment, it may be easier to look at discounted cash flow.

Remember that office space leases are subject to market conditions and competition and are negotiable. Quality of the space, the other tenants in the building, convenience to the hospital, and convenience for your patients are additional considerations. Low space cost does not always mean greater profits.

Accounting standards have changed for leases, and longer-term leases are usually reflected as an asset with a corresponding liability. The asset is amortized over the period of the lease as payments are made against the liability.

PRIVATE EQUITY

Private equity can be available either internally from existing or new owners or from external sources. Internal sources usually have a vested interest in the success of the practice and so the rate of return expected may be slightly lower than external sources. However, you should question the wisdom of the investment if you cannot come close to market rate returns even when requesting capital from existing ownership. Capital from this source can be funneled into the existing organization or structured as a separate specific purpose organization with a more limited and flexible horizon. Real estate is often funded in this nature and it allows for divestiture when market conditions are right. Ability for investment by future owners of the organization as well as circumstances under which ownership may be redeemed should be addressed as you form these organizations.

External private equity is a fast-evolving field of opportunity which can be a good source of capital. A full exploration of this area is beyond the scope of this chapter. However, you should expect that private equity firms will want a return on their money usually paired with growth targets and an exit strategy after three to five years. For additional discussion of private equity issues, refer to Chapter 6.

RISK MANAGEMENT AND INSURANCE

Risk is inherent in the practice of medicine and the conduct of business. The question then becomes how to minimize risk to our patients, guests, employees, and the organization. The risk can come from the clinical decisions providers make, the people and processes supporting patient care, as well as the patients themselves. The chance for risk can be minimized, but rarely can it be eliminated. When untoward events happen, the question is how to minimize the impact and provide funding for the expense. Key areas to fund risk are health insurance claims, malpractice claims, and general liability, including accidents, business interruption, and intrusion into data systems.

Health insurance claims are the most frequent and over time more predictable. The options for paying these claims range from full insurance to a completely self-insured program. Full insurance through an outside party, may bring a more predictable spend in the short-term, but gives little opportunity to control or change the trajectory of your health costs. Smaller physician organizations have little choice but to accept this reality. The result is substantially increased costs the year following a bad claims year and a little relief following a good claims year.

As practices increase in size, they may move across the continuum toward being self-insured and having more control of plan design, incentives, and strategies to reduce cost. Along that continuum are "partially" self-insured products in which all the components (claims processing, network costs and reinsurance) are provided by a single

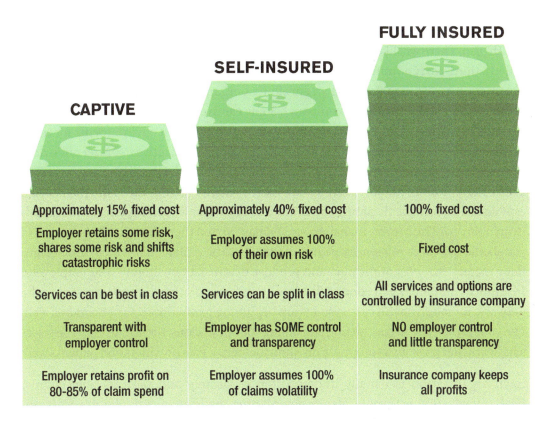

source and is like full insurance in many respects. However, if claims experience is better than expected you may benefit from at least some of the savings. There is usually a cap on claims liability giving a maximum spend as well. There are many flavors of this type of product and some flexibility in plan design, however, most of the control over information and plan design still rests with the insurance organization.

The next step along the continuum is a captive insurance company. Captive insurance companies are a collection of like-minded organizations who band together to have a cooperative insurance company. They do not have to all be from the same industry, in fact it is sometimes better if they are not. However, they should all be willing to take a more active role in managing their health plan. Captives offer a lot of flexibility in plan design and much more control in managing costs. Group sizes of 75 to 1,000 are common for captives.

This may be a point where you must evaluate the skills and perspective of your insurance broker. This is a very different task for them, and they are likely paid differently as well. If your broker serves a lot of mid-market companies, he may have followed the trend toward captives and self-insurance and be skilled in helping you with the process. If they have not, you may want to consult with a broker who has that type of experience. It is possible to work directly with some captives, but it will increase the time required from management.

When working with a captive, you will need to evaluate all the components involved in a health plan. There will likely be a captive manager, a claims processing organization (often called a third-party administrator), a network providing the contracts with providers, a pharmacy benefits manager, and an enrollment organization (if this isn't done by you or your broker and reinsurance company). Some captives also have a wellness program, perhaps through a vendor that provides steerage to lower-cost environments for more expensive services ranging from transplants to imaging. The captive manager often does the underwriting of the various organizations participating along with the reinsurer. The Third-Party Administrator (TPA) receives and evaluates claims under the plan design established by each participating entity. You need to evaluate their experience in reliability in doing so. The captive managers should have vetted them, but that does not mean you should not check references. Failure of the TPA to be vigilant in this area can substantially increase the cost of the plan and produce dissatisfaction among your employees. Insurance companies you conduct business with are among options for providing the network, although health care systems are beginning to offer narrow networks as well. Use your experience in contracting and billing your physicians' services to help you select a network that gives an appropriate discount, but also treats providers and patients well.

Each organization is usually underwritten separately and pays its own claims. Each organization is responsible for determining the level of variation in cost it can tolerate and set its reinsurance points accordingly. You will need to select the large claim reinsurance point and the total claims reinsurance point. The lower your reinsurance points, the more consistent your claim costs will be from period to period. However, this may reduce the opportunity to benefit from good claims experience, and in the long run, your costs may be higher. Your reinsurance costs will be determined by these decisions.

The captive will keep a layer of the reinsurance within the captive and get external reinsurance for a portion of the risk. This layer of reinsurance retained by the captive is a shared expense among the captive members, and when you boil it all down, it is the real business of the captive. If an individual organization has a reinsurance point for claims of a specific individual of $50,000 per year, the captive may reinsure another $250,000 on that individual before turning it over to the larger reinsurer. The captive will also retain a significant portion of the reinsurance premium matching the risk that it retains. If the captive's overall loss experience is good, members participate in return of profits from the captive's reinsurance activity as profits of the captive. Claims experience for each company below the specific and aggregate reinsurance points can be better or worse than expected, but that cost, or benefit accrues directly to that company. Network, TPA, commissions and management fees are passed through to each company based on initial contract agreements.

The last stop along the continuum is a stand-alone self-insurance plan. This is usually not advised for groups of less than 500. Health plans depend on the law of large numbers to smooth out claims experience and make reinsurers more comfortable in funding their layer of costs. It works much like the captive and may in fact be organized in that way, but with a single participant.

Underpinning all these risk management tools should be a risk management program. Programs that promote the health of employees, safe and effective clinical practices, as well as, safer facilities will help to deter claims and costs to the organization. Consult the professionals working with you in each area discussed above for help in implementing these programs.

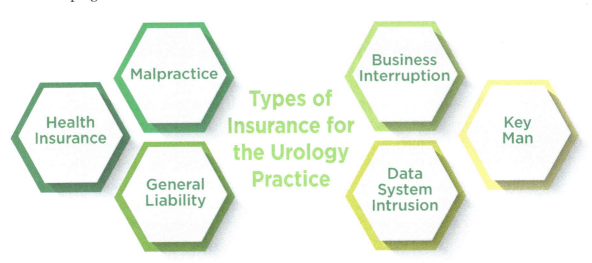

Malpractice claims are much less frequent, but much more costly when they do occur. Most private practice physicians pay for a fully insured product and then hope they never have to use it. Sometimes they negotiate together through a medical association who provides some basic risk management support. Larger organizations in urology have banded together to form a risk retention group (RRG), which functions much like a captive as described in the individual health insurance companies. Physician groups that participate in that organization commit to following risk management protocols recommended by the group, participate in clinical education designed to reduce risk of claims, and potentially profit from the reduction of costs on a long-term basis.

Because of the long-term nature of malpractice claims, the insured physicians pay into the RRG each year to fund administrative, defense, reinsurance costs, and payments to claimants. To provide more stability for the RRG, regulating authorities will require capital contributions by participants to establish reserve funds. This capital is usually returnable depending on the RRG bylaws and structure; however, it may be years after a member withdraws from the RRG.

An RRG usually sets annual contributions at levels approximating market rates for fully insured products. Profits are returned to the insured owners of the RRG as the opportunity presents, given the need for capital reserves and the ongoing claims experience. Full self-insurance is not a viable option for urology groups as they exist today.

General liability or what is often known as "Property and Casualty" insurance is the type of risk most often covered by a fully insured product. Deductibles can be raised to significant levels in order to retain a portion of the risk. This area tends to have the least number of claims and while they can be substantial, often are not. The result is low cost for full insurance and little benefit of pursuing anything along the self-insured continuum. There are provisions in the IRS code for establishing 831b micro captives for liabilities where you can deduct up to $1.2 million set aside to insure property and casualty risks. This is an aggressive strategy for a physician organization and beyond the scope of this discussion. If you have an interest, seek professional counsel.

Another area of risk to insure is the disability or loss of a physician. You may jointly provide life insurance or disability insurance, which would pay the physician or his family in the case of the death or disability of a physician. However, this is a severe loss for the organization as well. The organization is facing both the loss of productivity, which covers the overhead related to the lost physician, but perhaps a buyout of that physicians' interest as well. The smaller the organization, the most catastrophic and disruptive this can be. A larger organization may be able to withstand this loss and self-insure the risk, however, a smaller organization cannot. What is frequently known as "Key Man" insurance is available from many brokers, and the benefits are retained by the organization to bridge the gap until the physician returns or is replaced.

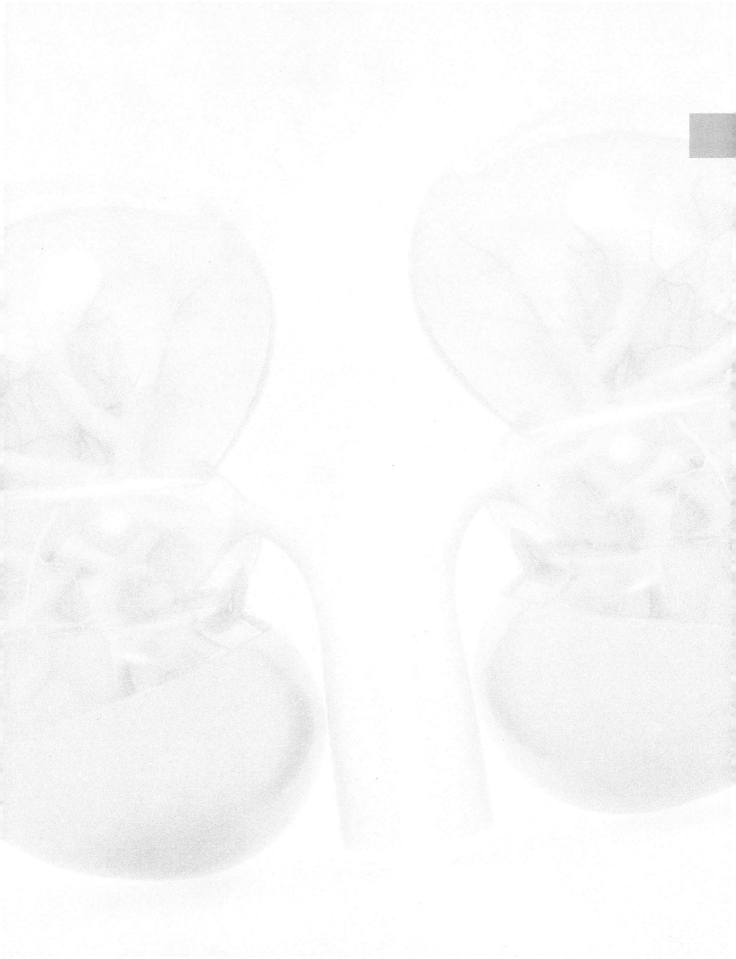

KEY POINTS

- **Banking partners** can provide debt funding for working capital with accounts receivable pledged, as well as real estate loans secured by the property purchased or constructed.

- **Whether leasing or owning,** it is important to evaluate the cost of the underlying building structure, the cost of improvements, and the cost of operating the space over a comparable period.

- **Rental and leasing agreements** can be a means to finance equipment for the practice.

- **Key areas** in which to evaluate and fund risk are health insurance claims, malpractice claims, and general liability, including accidents, business interruption, and intrusion into data systems.

- **Captive insurance companies** are a collection of like-minded organizations who band together to have a cooperative insurance company.

- **A risk management** program that promotes its employees' health, safe and effective clinical practices, and safer facilities will help deter claims and costs to the organization.

- **Because of the long-term** nature of malpractice claims, the insured physicians pay into the RRG each year to fund administrative, defense, reinsurance costs, and payments to claimants.

- **General liability** or what is often known as "Property and Casualty" insurance is the type of risk most often covered by a fully insured product.

J. Jason Shelnutt, CPA

J. Jason Shelnutt has served as the CEO of Georgia Urology for the last 18 years. Prior to that he served as a COO and CFO in the hospital setting and consulted with a variety of health care organizations and worked for a national CPA firm. In addition, he was a founding board member of LUGPA and continues to serve as a board member of SCRUBS, a national risk retention group for Urology practices. He has expertise in health care business development, real estate, and risk management.

CHAPTER 3

Operational and Governance Structure of Urology Groups

Evan R. Goldfischer, MD, MBA

INTRODUCTION

Health care constitutes about 18% of the Gross Domestic Product of the United States making it a 3.3 trillion-dollar industry. Businesses and consumers constitute almost half of that amount. In an effort to contain costs over the last five years, an increased emphasis has been placed on value-based health care in addition to new regulations on medical practices. Many physicians and physician groups have found the new regulations too burdensome and have joined large health care systems. The early 2000s saw the first wave of consolidation of urology practices. There is now a second wave of consolidation as urologists try to preserve independent practice. As a result, the management and structure of large urology group practices has become more complex. Today's integrated, private urology group practice is an extremely sophisticated, multilayered business machine. Each practice typically involves several business units, companies, and operational units that follow local, state, and federal regulations. The operational variations between practices are as expansive and varied as medicine itself—and often prove themselves just as complicated.

This chapter is not an attempt to provide a detailed plan as to the "perfect" way to implement operations and structure, but rather offers a 50,000-foot view of different options and methods to achieve the shared goal of an efficient, financially vibrant and healthy urology group practice. There are innumerable components of a successful urology practice. We will address only a few key points to provide a starting point in which to create or fine tune individual practice operations. These include the following: physician—administrator dyad, Board of Directors composition, practice committees, the role of the practice administrator, senior management team, standardization of care, providing specialized care, alignment to health care transformation, corporate culture, practice benchmarking, and internal education and continuum of care.

PHYSICIAN-ADMINISTRATOR DYAD MODEL

The most successfully integrated practices have embraced this dyad relationship. It is extremely rare to find a physician with the time and business experience to be able to solely manage a large urology practice, and it is even rarer to find a businessman who truly understands the intricacies of urology practice. A successful model has a physician Chief Executive Officer (CEO) lead the group, who understands the fundamentals of patient care, but allows an experienced administrator to operationalize the vision and provide detailed financial reports. Depending on the size of the group, the administrator may function as both the chief operating officer and chief financial officer. Hence, it's important to find someone with the right skill set, personality, and chemistry. The individual also needs a competitive salary and bonus.

Table 1.0 from the 2019 LUGPA salary survey should provide a basis for discussion in hiring an administrator. However, understand that every market is different, and these

Shared	Physician Member	Administrative Member
Developing or implementing strategy and associated action plans	Providing "medical staff" supervision • Performance review • Discipline • Recruiting onboarding	Developing operational goals, priorities, responsibilities
Fostering group culture		Monitoring group financial functions – budgeting, accounting, reporting
Promoting, monitoring, and reporting group and individual performances • Quality of care • Patient safety • Patient experience • Operational effciency • Operating budget	Creating, implementing, and monitoring clinical practice guidelines	Managing and developing human resources consistent with organizational guidelines, established contracts, and legal requirements
	Driving population health management Initiatives	
Developing internal and external organizational relationships	Evaluating clinical outcomes (effectiveness and efficiency)	Coordinating necessary support function – marketing, IT, financial
Optimizing clinical informatics and data analytics systems	Supporting Administrative Member	Supporting Physician Member

numbers should only serve as a guideline. The chemistry and trust between the CEO and the administrator in the dyad model is crucial to making the model work. The employees must view them as having equal status, and both should have equal accountability to the governing board and shareholders.

BOARD OF DIRECTORS COMPOSITION

Most, but not all, urology practices have a Board of Directors. Members are typically nominated and then elected for a specific term, with or without additional financial compensation. Some boards have term limits to allow other practice members to have a say in governance, while other practices find their physicians don't want to take on additional responsibility. Some groups are autocratic and run by an all-powerful respected leader. However, most groups will not have someone with this skill set. More commonly, they develop a culture where the thoughts and feelings of all members are heard and respected, and where everyone ultimately submits to the will of the democratic process. This model also encourages participation and helps with succession planning. The board should consist of members who have an interest in the business of the practice and a desire to take an active role in making improvements. Understanding the business of a urology practice is also a necessary skillset. Meetings are typically held biweekly or monthly, often after hours, with the board making decisions as guided by the partners of the group. A typical board task is to research and vet various approaches to a particular matter, then present a summary to the partnership at large for final disposition. It is important that the Board represent the practice's various geographies and age groups, and the administrator should be either a full voting member or ex-officio board member who attends all meetings. The board should also provide a mechanism to resolve disagreements and problems prior to presenting the matter to the group at large.

A well-functioning board will conduct the business in the actual board meeting, not in the hallway or exam room within earshot of listening employees, partners, and other physicians. Inappropriate discussions in public spaces can be taken out of context very quickly—and create rifts between physicians, employees, and various stakeholders of the practice.

Also, a word of caution: The number of members should be manageable—having a very large board can be cumbersome at best, and a painful waste of time in the worst case.

PRACTICE COMMITTEES

An effective practice committee is one in which a small number of members are very engaged in specific practice issues. They can provide insight, in-depth understanding of the subject matter, and effective solutions. Practice committees are typically nominated positions that may or may not require an election process. In most cases, they are not granted any special powers or abilities outside of the normal methods of carrying out the business of the group. Some practices compensate employees who are involved in committees with payment or time off. However, members typically do not receive any additional compensation for their work, as it is typically not extremely burdensome or time intensive. Rather, committees exist to carry out a narrow scope of review or action

TABLE 1.0 CHIEF EXECUTIVE OFFICER (CEO) LUGPA 2019 Salary Survey

	TOTAL COMPENSATION (excluding bonuses)					TOTAL BONUSES				
	base	mean	25th percentile	50th percentile (median)	75th percentile	base	mean	25th percentile	50th percentile (median)	75th percentile
Total	27	$191,000	$142,800	$187,300	$250,000	25	$50,300	$0	$20,000	$51,500
Number of Practice Locations										
5+	17	$202,500	$131,400	$215,000	$250,000	15	$70,600	$0	$22,000	$66,800
<5	10	$171,500	$136,900	$176,500	$208,700	10	$19,800	$0	$13,800	$34,000
Number of Physicians										
10+	18	$220,100	$185,500	$222,500	$250,000	16	$68,300	$0	$20,000	$65,300
<10	9	$132,800	$98,800	$142,800	$161,400	9	$18,300	$0	$20,000	$24,500
Number of Total Employees										
100+	16	$221,200	$181,800	$220,000	$250,000	14	$78,400	$0	$32,500	$71,300
<100	11	$147,000	$100,000	$142,800	$180,000	11	$14,600	$0	$11,000	$22,000
Region										
Northeast	3	-	-	-	-	3	-	-	-	-
Midwest	10	$184,300	$109,500	$177,600	$251,700	9	$34,800	$5,500	$40,000	$62,900
South	8	$224,000	$185,000	$220,000	$247,500	7	$124,400	$0	$20,000	$270,400
West	6	$162,100	$96,100	$164,000	$216,300	6	$12,400	$0	$13,800	$22,800
Is CEO a physician?										
yes	6	$178,300	$104,000	$185,000	$250,000	5	$96,000	$0	$0	$240,100
no	21	$194,600	$152,500	$187,300	$232,500	20	$38,900	$1,900	$21,000	$56,200
Is CEO position full time?										
yes	24	$189,000	$144,600	$183,700	$236,300	22	$35,400	$0	$20,000	$46,900
no	3	-	-	-	-	3	-	-	-	-

NOTE: results not shown if fewer than 5 valid values

in a short period of time—often for just a few weeks. Committees that do have long-term goals and processes may require additional time and resources to fulfill their mission.

Most committees assemble their findings and prepare materials to report their action or findings to the group at large. Smaller practices may only have an executive committee that reports to the board and oversees the senior management team, while larger practices may have committees and subcommittees to utilize the expertise of the various shareholders. These committees may include a finance committee, medical guideline committee, real estate committee, new technology committee, compensation committee, data management/benchmarking committee, and disciplinary committee to name just a few. The most important committee is the executive committee. Convening a board meeting with all members present is often difficult due to busy schedules, vacations, conferences, and in large practices geography is often an issue. A high functioning empowered executive committee should meet on a regular basis to act on matters to keep the practice functioning and should provide an additional layer of oversight and a resource for the practice CEO and administrator.

SENIOR MANAGEMENT TEAM

Most practices are too small to hire separate individuals for each of these positions, but the bottom-line is they need to get done, even if one person holds several positions. If it is a small group and every partner contributes to the management of the group, financial compensation is rarely required. However, in larger groups when few individuals shoulder the management burden, compensation is needed, either financially, or with allotted time during the work week so they can perform their jobs. The senior management team is often under appreciated by physicians who work "in the trenches" seeing patients as they often do not understand the important role administrators play behind their desks. It is necessary to remember that a well-run practice can make a physician's workflow much easier and more pleasant while maximizing financial returns.

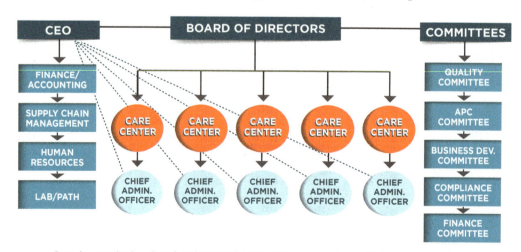

Sample organization chart for a large urology practice. Source: Advanced Urology Institute of Florida

THE ROLE OF PRACTICE ADMINISTRATOR

In short, a Practice Administrator ensures that the office runs smoothly. It sounds simple, but Practice Administrators must have layers of knowledge, skills and abilities to understand the practice from the perspective of physicians and patients. Providing both groups with what they need and expect is key to success in this role.

A Practice Administrator's role varies in small versus large groups. In a small group, the Practice Administrator will wear many hats, with tasks that overlap with the C-Suite officers. As a jack-of-all-trades, the role may include:

- Ensuring the practice follows current federal, state and local laws and regulations.

- Taking on a Human Resources (HR) role to recruit, hire, train and onboard new staff members.

- Prioritizing patient care by training staff, reviewing patient feedback, and implementing customer-preferred electronic systems to communicate appointment reminders, etc.

- Possessing the knowledge to have a direct impact on the revenue cycle by controlling expenses and budgeting.

In a large group, the role of a Practice Administrator is more defined. The work entails:

- Anticipating and preparing for providers' needs to deliver excellent patient care, such as staffing appropriately, maintaining a high-quality facility and adequately stocking and cleaning exam rooms and other office areas. Maintaining adequate par levels for supplies and medications, but being careful not to keep too much inventory on the shelves.

- Communicating with physicians on a regular basis to follow through with, or delegate, tasks the doctors request. Examples include contacting patients to schedule follow-up appointments or to remind them of upcoming ones; following up on prior lab requests, obtaining hospital records, and communicating with referring providers.

- Ensuring patient information, such as demographic and insurance data is current in the electronic systems.

- Maintaining appropriate levels of pharmaceuticals and devices needed for treating patients, and updating an inventory tracking system for internal control and budgeting.

It is important to note that some practices opt to have managers in different departments in lieu of a Practice Administrator. Understand that the Practice Administrator is one of the most important jobs in the practice. This person ensures the patient has an optimal experience, physicians are not overburdened with administrative functions and can practice good urology, and that the staff feels there is a solid leadership and resource they can turn to for help, which will decrease employee turnover. To facilitate succession planning, or in case this key administrator leaves, consider having this person maintain a diary of all of the daily/weekly/monthly/quarterly/yearly tasks they perform, which can be given to future managers as a road map of practice functions.

STANDARDIZATION OF CARE

Essential to the operational success of a urology practice is the standardization of care. While this has several different connotations, one of the most important is ensuring that patients consistently receive top quality care from every physician. A practice that lacks clear standardization of care guidelines is at risk of failing. It is unfair to patients whose care pathways differ greatly depending on the practitioner they are assigned to see.

What's worse, the standard of care could be very different on nights and weekends depending upon which physician takes the call. From a data mining and cost projecting perspective, standardizing care paths is critical to running an efficient practice.

While medicine is certainly an art, the practice should develop and enforce guidelines that address standard of care for most of the urologic disease states. These guidelines must take into consideration the local standard of care (and this standard may need to be elevated to provide for better patient care), local and state regulations, and of course, local payer considerations.

While every practice has admirable goals to improve patient care, the unfortunate modern reality is that "occasionally" the payers' (commercial and governmental) goals and policies simply do not align. Dealing with this misalignment of care continuum is something the practice must address to effect change.

Standards for patient care regarding different disease states exist in multiple different forms.

Standard Members of the C-suite

- **Chief Executive Officer –** Leads the development and execution of the strategic direction, including growth initiatives, budget proposals, policies and procedures, and acquiring new services and technology.

- **Chief Medical Officer –** Provides clinical direction, develops standardization of care guidelines, and implements innovative clinical programs.

- **Chief Operating Officer –** Oversees daily operations of the urology group and is available to human resources for questions or concerns.

- **Chief Financial Officer –** Tasked with the urology group's financial planning, accounting practices, and relationship with financial institutions, including pay sources.

- **Chief Information Technology Officer –** Stays up to date on technology needs for the urology group and ensures the information technology is working effectively.

- **Chief Compliance Officer –** Charged with ensuring the Board of Directors, physicians and staff are in compliance with rules, regulations and the urology group's policies and procedures.

In the simplest form, they are unwritten guidelines that exist in the heads of the provider team, typically shared with new providers as they enter the practice. More officially, they are deeply detailed documents that exist as a "go to" resource to provide for better patient care. These more formally written guidelines provide the basis for high-level patient care as they integrate both clinical and technological advances and changes in payer policies. The guidelines are an efficient means to continually improve the service delivered to the patient. The Chief Medical Officer of the practice is responsible for developing the practice guidelines and will often chair the practice guidelines committee.

PROVIDING SPECIALIZED CARE

Consideration must be given to creating a robust process to shift the advanced disease state patient to the best-suited provider. This physician should have the expertise, mindset, and desire to care for a complicated, advanced disease—especially when considering the individual practice mode and compensation formula. Specialty services for prostate cancer and overactive bladder can be two of many areas that may benefit from specialized care.

> **For example,** the patient with advanced prostate cancer should have an opportunity to have the resources of a provider who has a special interest in this area. This provider should devote significant time to stay up to date on new treatment modalities and trends to provide the most-up-to date, technologically advanced, and efficient care for the patient. The same can be said for patients diagnosed with advanced incontinence, stone disease, infertility, bladder cancer, and kidney cancer, as well as other subspecialties. Shifting them to a subspecialized provider is critical to improve patient outcomes and provide top quality standardized care in the urology practice.

The MUSIC (Michigan Urological Surgery Improvement Collaborative) initiative demonstrates improved quality and the development of evidence-based pathways for the treatment of patients with prostate cancer. Quality is defined, reported, and analyzed by a leadership team that has resulted in better outcomes and lower costs for patients and better remuneration for physicians who participate in the program. The initiative is expanding to include management of patients with urolithiasis.

Standardizing care helps ensure that no matter who the patient sees, he or she will receive efficient and effective care, vetted by numerous providers. If a provider is unavailable, standardization allows another physician to provide care without guesswork as to the next steps in the patient's treatment and goals to be achieved. The most effective practices will waste no time in determining a plan of action for a patient with a common disease state since the general care plan will have already been reviewed, written, and understood by all providers.

ALIGNING TO HEALTH CARE TRANSFORMATION

While we are certainly in a transitional phase in health care payment models, the stark reality is that change is already here, more change is coming, and it is coming very quickly. Physicians within a practice must undertake the necessary steps to align themselves with changes in payment structures. While many disagree with or dislike changes already present and those coming, the reality is that carriers that reimburse our practices for services rendered are changing the model. Therefore, practice physicians and management must simply adapt to survive and stay profitable. The successful practice will adopt a culture of accountability and openness to change that encourages vibrant discussion and ideas about how to adapt to upcoming requirements.

At the same time, the practice must make sure all providers align patient treatment with the payer's goals and policies of change. As has been often stated, there is opportunity in change—the key is to embrace change and position the practice to achieve, not fail. Simply "riding it out" or "doing things the way I always have" because a provider may only have a couple of years left prior to exiting the practice is not an option. That method will not align with payer requirements and will lead to great issues—both with payers and other members of the group. Every provider must be engaged and on the same page as to how the practice adapts to change.

Part of this change and alignment requires providers to be educated in new operation structures. Providers must fundamentally understand the foundation of what is changing and why; how they are reimbursed for services rendered; and about new systems they need to understand and support. Creating buy in with providers, one small win at a time, is critical to the overall goal of adapting to the large, sweeping changes urology practices will face in the coming years. Understanding where health care in the United States is likely to go in the next five years and planning for multiple contingencies is one of the most important responsibilities of the dyad leadership and senior management team. While their planning may seem to many shareholders who focus solely on seeing patients as an unproductive use of time, having contingency plans is crucial. They can allow a practice to react quickly to forces in the local, regional, and national markets that can lead a group to realize new opportunities, or reconfigure operations to quickly result in increased profitability.

CORPORATE CULTURE

In order to support change, the practice's leadership must establish a functional culture that allows for robust discussion; accountability for diverging from practice guidelines; respectful disagreement; and ultimately support for majority decisions. The most important job of the CEO is to define the corporate culture—in mission, vision and value statements. These documents should be posted in conspicuous places throughout the practice, and new hires should be instructed as to how these principles guide the operations. The documents should be revised regularly, as the practice evolves, and long-term employees should be given an opportunity to provide their input as representatives of the rank and file. The practice culture must also embrace the fact that some providers may simply not be able to adapt to the requirements of a changing environment. Depending on the group culture of the practice, providers must either be incentivized to provide quality guideline-based care or face negative consequences for not providing this type of care.

Some practices have instituted a hybrid approach that embraces both incentives and negative consequences, and there seems to be some validity to that method. The best approach depends on the overall culture and appetite for change within the practice.

Everyone wants to live in a world where every provider exists in perfect harmony with the rest of the group. The reality is, divergence occurs regarding what the group and management tolerates and allows, the quality of patient care that is provided, how behavioral issues are dealt with, and generally, how individuals support the attitude and culture of the group. The group must deal with this divergence before it creates a bigger chasm in the group and has significant, long lasting effects. The larger group cannot allow the actions, or lack, thereof, of one or a few physicians to control the entire group and essentially hold it hostage. On the other hand, urologists are extremely hard to recruit. Losing a provider can result in the loss of revenue, increased on-call burden, and signal the rest of the medical community that the practice is running poorly, could be breaking up or become a prime target for a takeover. In short, forces within a group can be more destructive than external forces. Therefore, it is important to cultivate buy-in from stakeholders before making bold sweeping changes to a practice. If there is significant reservation, it is necessary to understand the stakeholders' concerns, as there may be merit to the objections, and they may represent a perspective that had not otherwise been considered.

Collaborative efforts overlap in a successful practice to create a strong corporate culture

Agreeing on practice standards for taking care of patients is only one step to developing a positive corporate culture. Physicians must also commit to staying up to date on medical education and changing treatments, attending meetings, engaging in the practice and accepting overall behavioral standards.

In addition, providers must engage with staff, support a never-ending desire to improve the business, and provide a better delivered patient care product. Not everyone at all levels possesses these goals, but strong support from the management team forms a solid basis for a healthy cultural environment that allows for expansion, change, and improvement without disparaging new ideas or specific personalities in the group. By agreeing to this level of professionalism, performance, and structure from the top down, subpar performers cannot remain in comfort while others are raising the bar of the practice to yet another higher level. Maintaining a high performing practice is a critical part of the current transformation of health care and is one part of the many building blocks of a successful practice.

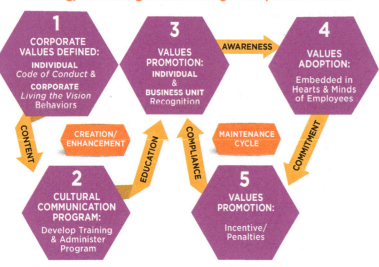

A positive corporate culture includes a clear and consistent vision of how everyone—staff and patients—view the company Source: blogs.sas.com

Promotion of a positive culture is as varied as the number of individual urology practices. The group meeting, the dinner presentation, and event attendance all play a role in creating and fostering the group's ability to function as a cohesive unit, to provide for the best possible patient and provider experience—and to have a basis of common ground in which to stand on when conflict does arise (and it will).

PRACTICE BENCHMARKING DATA

Practices must define, measure and improve quality through benchmarking. Various methods of benchmarking data currently exist, either by informal, like-minded groups comparing isolated datasets; regional initiatives that provide a more varied dataset; or national organizational datasets that seek to provide a national data perspective. All play a role in a successful practice.

Practices should seriously consider obtaining objective third-party data to help them develop a better understanding of their performance and to measure comparative data locally, regionally, or nationally. Several leaders have emerged in the field, including PPS analytics and Infodive.® (Read more about Infodive® in this chapter).

Practices can use the data to identify improvement activities and to help the senior management team instill accountability for organizational performance. Also, when negotiating third party payments, insurance companies maintain data on practices that they will rarely reveal. Understanding your own data and how you compare to other

LUGPA practices will allow the group to be in a better position to negotiate contracts. This can be especially important in capitated arrangements when understanding utilization of practice resources can help decide if a contract will be profitable.

It is imperative to know and report this information. Competitors are measuring this data; practices who don't are at a disadvantage. In evaluating methods to benchmark data, it is valuable to note a specific point: With larger datasets that involve more practices and larger data pools, there is a tendency for data to become less relevant to one's practice since the dataset may not compare exactly.

Also, other practices may have interpreted the data request differently, resulting in statistically significant differences that can skew the resulting data. It is always best to note that when using comparative data, one may not be directly comparing "apples to apples."

With that being said, comparing data is immensely valuable in that one can determine trends, areas of lack in one's own practice, and areas in which one's own practice is performing very well.

Regarding internal data benchmarking, there is no substitute for having a firm grasp of one's own individual practice numbers, knowing why and when they begin to vary and diverge.

> **Internal data benchmarking** is extremely effective in determining outliers and providers who may need additional training. As a very simple example, if internal data benchmarking revealed that 60% of Dr. A's office visits are level 5 visits, while the practice average is 15%, this discrepancy must be addressed. Further review could show that Dr. A only sees complex, sub-specialized, and advanced disease state patients that justify the coding delta. Therefore, this benchmarking effort may also reveal an opportunity ders understand and can justify the higher coding levels.

Equally valuable is an in-depth understanding of the datasets being pulled before making any assumptions. It is extremely important to understand exactly the parameters of the data requested, the time period for the dataset, and any other contributing factors that could cause skewing, misalignment, or questionable results. A terrible mistake, yet one most people have made, is to make decisions or directional changes based on datasets we thought we understood.

Data benchmarking is a critical part of today's practice. LUGPA offers a unique program of practice benchmarking and presents a summary of this data at the annual Fall meeting. LUGPA has partnered with Infodive® to allow practices to do their own internal benchmarking, but also for each group to compare itself to the other LUGPA groups in the database. Infodive is being used by many groups and has garnered very positive reviews. For more information, visit the LUGPA website at **lugpa.org**.

INTERNAL EDUCATION AND THE CONTINUUM OF CARE

Corporate education is a mechanism for organizations to convey their corporate culture and engage employees in the company's mission, vision, and practices. Successful corporate education provides a defined curriculum about the history of the practice, its philosophy, operating procedures, and policies. It differs from corporate training, which outlines skills an employee needs to perform a specific task.

Corporate education can be offered by a company's HR department and should be overseen by the Chief Operating Officer (COO) or a practice committee. If the HR department does not have enough resources to perform this function, corporate education can be outsourced to professional companies. Large payroll companies often offer this service, but better results are achieved if the education curriculum is developed by the practice, so it reflects the culture and actual procedures of the company.

Upon hire, every employee, including providers, should receive a comprehensive company handbook including all policies and standard operating procedures. The employee should be allowed ample time to read it and subsequently sign an official form, acknowledging he or she has received and read the manual and agrees to abide by it. The manual should be supplemented with in-person training by a member of the HR department to reinforce certain policies. There are many videos available online that employees can watch to reinforce sensitive topics such as bullying, sexual harassment, and cultural sensitivity. The manual should be updated on a regular basis, usually yearly, and employees need to be re-educated as updates are made. It is a mistake to buy a generic employee manual and simply brand it with the practice's logo. This is an important tool to differentiate an individual practice's policies and culture.

During the year, departmental meetings should be scheduled at regular intervals to update employees about policy and procedural changes. These meetings also provide an opportunity to reinforce corporate culture and to educate employees on national, regional, and local updates in medicine that might affect practice policies and procedures, such as the Affordable Care Act, ICD 10, and the Medicare Access and CHIP Reauthorization Act. Supervisors should schedule regular meetings with the CEO and/or COO, so they can take the lead in educating employees about changes that affect their jobs. Subsequently, supervisors should incorporate those changes into company operations.

Some practices plan employee retreats that provide educational initiatives and workshops, opportunity to engage in the company mission and vision. In addition, retreats allow employees to provide feedback and be involved in the company problem-solving process.

Finally, it is important for providers to attend employee education conferences to set a positive tone for meetings and reinforce their importance. Attendance by the partners gives meetings credibility and helps support supervisors and administrators who formulate the curriculum.

Gaining Insights with InfoDive® and LUGPA Benchmarking Data

Below is one of several reports your practice can utilize to identify gaps in performance. The physician used in this sample is a senior partner (30 years in practice) and appears to be slowing down on the number of new patients he sees, however, he remains highly productive as he is above the 75th percentile in relative value units (RVUs) produced. While he has a typical volume of surgical cases, the case complexity is high with the typical surgery generating 13.4 work RVUs (90th percentile). Because complex surgeries often involve multiple procedures, he also is in the 90th percentile for the reduction in work RVUs due to multiple procedure payment rules. Reimbursement for services he generates are being paid at 115% of Medicare, slightly below the 75th percentile. While his compensation is just below the 90th percentile, he is at the median for compensation per work RVU. A quick scan of the evaluation and management (E&M) coding bell curves shows this physician tends to code higher on new patients and code lower on established patients.

2018 LUGPA Benchmarks

COMPENSATION	YOUR EXPERIENCE	10TH %	25TH %	50TH %	75TH %	90TH %
Years in Practice	30	5	10	18	26	32
Compensation	$622,564	$262,945	$358,000	$434,837	$591,066	$638,123
Comp per wRVU	$56.72	$31.47	$40.1	$48.59	$59.51	$78.27
% Comp of Payments	45%	28%	37%	46%	55%	72%
PRODUCTION						
New Patients	447	353	501	678	880	1,089
Est Patients	1,883	1,205	1,674	2,190	2,846	3,709
Visits - Face to Face	4,288	3,177	4,011	5,233	6,574	7,833
Surgical Cases - Global 90	140	57	112	169	232	298
tRVU	24,696	12,172	15,239	18,808	23,291	29,241
wRVU	10,977	5,791	7,296	9,011	10,967	13,747
% wRVU Adj	12%	1%	2%	3%	5%	9%
wRVU per Facility Surg Case	13.4	4.5	5.4	7.4	9.1	11
REVENUE						
Payments	$1,390,388	$602,787	$758,277	$934,326	$1,268,717	$1,621,637
% of Medicare	115%	99%	102%	108%	118%	129%
Payments - EM	$286,593	$203,334	$251,184	$308,560	$393,077	$504,202
Payments - Surg	$525,540	$196,714	$276,167	$361,427	$488,456	$599,927
Payments - Med	$6,834	$1,817	$3,054	$5,812	$11,650	$17,959
Payments - Lab/Path	$144,870	$3,784	$6,921	$19,869	$43,319	$70,420
Payments - Rad	$99,404	$4,292	$9,226	$25,551	$57,380	$89,842
Payments - HCPCS	$318,844	$33,797	$59,148	$108,255	$234,395	$566,865
Payments - Other	$8,303	$0	$20	$510	$20,992	$99,369

Statistics for providers working part-time or partial year have been adjusted to reflect full-time effort for entire calendar year

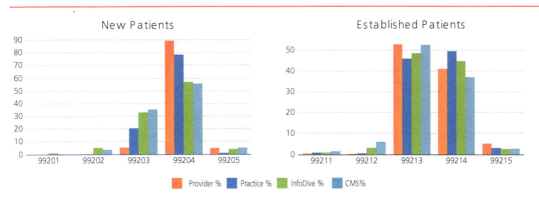

Provider %, and Practice % reflect data as of the latest practice extract | InfoDive % reflects data as of the latest benchmark (R12) | CMS % reflects latest CMS report (2017)

CHAPTER 3 | 43

▶ PROVIDER EDUCATION

As residents and fellows, all urologists should be involved in formalized conferences and clearly define their educational curriculum. In private practice, hospitals and third-party payers usually require a minimum number of annual CMEs to remain credentialed, but the pressures of clinical practice can force education to take a back seat. This is unacceptable in a value-based model of medicine.

Urology is a rapidly changing field, and it is important that physicians continue to understand advances in the field in order to provide the best options and outcomes for patients. Some practices carve out time during the week or month for formal conferences, while others schedule meetings after clinical hours. Some groups require onsite attendance, while others allow doctors to call in using a conference line. Some groups even pay doctors to attend the meetings to ensure attendance, while others fine doctors who routinely skip meetings. It is important to conduct regular educational meetings and require doctors to attend. New physician employees must understand that attendance at these meetings is an obligation of employment by the group. These conferences also serve as an opportunity to review practice guidelines, which should be regularly updated by the guidelines committee.

▶ PARTNERS MEETINGS

Partner meetings often focus on the the business of medicine. These meeting, often scheduled during evenings or on weekends, are an ideal forum to feature lectures about new procedures or pharmaceutical agents. Typically, lectures are scheduled at the beginning of a meeting, so that an invited speaker can exit while the business meeting proceeds.

▶ TUMOR BOARD

A multispecialty Tumor Board with attendance by urology, radiation therapy, oncology, pathology, and radiology representatives is vital to ensure top care of the cancer patient. Tumor Boards offer attendingphysicians the opportunity to discuss the need to formally present and review pathology slides and radiological film with patients, and subsequently provide the best and most appropriate treatment recommendations to them.

▶ MORBIDITY AND MORTALITY

Everyone can make mistakes in judgment or execution. Morbidity and Mortality meetings offer an opportunity to examine common errors and institute corrective actions to prevent them from recurring. Morbidity and Mortality meetings should not be punitive in nature, but should be educational and led by well-respected clinical staff members who are both knowledgeable and skillful in providing insight into erroneous actions in patient care.

▶ JOURNAL CLUB

Journal Club provides a great opportunity to educate a group about new developments in urology. Journal Club meetings can entertain a specific theme (prostate, infertility, stone disease, etc.), and should feature a variety of journals. Journal Club can provide an excellent opportunity for new physicians to actively participate in a leadership role.

▶ CASE CONFERENCE

Urology groups see a plethora of pathology, and case conferences provide an opportunity to discuss unusual non-oncology cases. These conferences also provide an opportunity for new providers to take an active leadership role in their industry.

▶ EDUCATION DAYS/RETREATS

While more time consuming, these day or weekend educational retreats should be conducted off site. If planned well in advance with a robust agenda, practice business and education can both be incorporated to provide an enriching and transformative experience. Retreats also provide an environment to build the group's culture, rapport and internal working dynamics.

These operational elements are only a few of the components that make for a successful practice. While no practice can perfectly operationalize every aspect of running a practice, opportunity certainly exists to innovate, improve, and transform it to a higher performing enterprise to capture the one aspect of a urology practice all providers agree on—improving the quality of patient care. LUGPA has offered seminars at its annual meeting on the value of a retreat and how to properly run one.

KEY POINTS

- **Consider** forming a urology practice Board of Directors—it is not required, but can help make improvements to the organization.

- **Identify** a senior management team.

- **Form** a practice committee that can provide in-depth understanding of specific practice issues.

- **Create** guidelines outlining the practice's standard of care to ensure patients receive consistent top-quality care from every physician.

- **Be open** to adapting to health care transformation, including changes in requirements and payment structures.

- **Promote** a positive corporate culture by establishing a mission, vision and value statements that provide for robust discussion, accountability for diverging from practice guidelines, and support for majority decisions.

- **Benchmark** your practice to determine trends and whether specific areas are lacking or performing well.

- **Offer** internal education for all employees and physicians that includes a defined curriculum about the company's history, its philosophy, operating procedures, and policies.

- **Ensure** physicians maintain the required number of CME credits by conducting regular educational meetings and require doctors to attend.

Evan R. Goldfischer, MD, MBA

Dr. Goldfischer received his BA from Tufts University and his MD from Cornell University Medical College. He completed his internship and residency in Surgery/Urology at the University of Chicago. He completed a fellowship in Endourology under the direction of Arthur Smith at Long Island Jewish Medical Center. Dr. Goldfischer received his MBA from the University of Massachusetts and is a Certified Physician Executive. He served as the co-founding CEO of Premier Medical Group of the Hudson Valley as well as founding Director of Research. He has written over 100 peer-reviewed abstracts and publications and has lectured on six continents. He was elected to the LUGPA Board of Directors in 2014. He has served as Secretary of LUGPA since 2019 and will begin his term as President Elect beginning in 2021. He is the author of *Even Urologists Get Kidney Stones – A Guide to Prevention and Treatment*, published in 2018.

CHAPTER 4

Physician Compensation

Steven R. Flageol

Providing positive outcomes for patients in need of urologic care is a complex profession led by physician specialists in a field that is challenged by physician recruitment difficulties. The increased complexities of modern medicine, regulatory requirements from countless agencies, and the extreme cost of education are driving individuals away from the practice of urology at a time of increased needs. Providing equitable compensation to urologists that reflects the increased patient demand is paramount to the survival of the specialty.

In the setting of a large medical practice, the infrastructure has numerous business components that must be understood before addressing physician compensation. The components of revenue (incoming cash) and expenses (outgoing cash) combine to dictate the dollars available for compensation.

REVENUE

Revenue in a medical practice is one of the rare instances in the United States where the business is told what they will be paid for providing services. When costs of a physician's business increases 2%, the physician cannot demand a corresponding 2% increase in reimbursement from insurance carriers or governmental agencies like Medicare. Reimbursements have faced decreases for clinical and surgical care over the last few decades and the trends are continuing for further reductions.

EXPENSES

Expenses in any business represent numerous other entities that demand payments before a medical practice can attempt to divide remaining funds for physician compensation. The charts on pages 50 and 51 are examples of costs of a large medical practice. Almost all the expenses listed above increase annually through market forces and external vendors. When expenses increase, most business simply raise their costs to other businesses and consumers for net income to remain the same or even increase. Medical practices cannot demand more money from insurance carriers or the government. Contracts with insurance carriers can be negotiated; however, this often requires physicians to stop providing services to carriers for a long length of time during negotiations. Reimbursement negotiations are not good for patients as they limit access to care.

EXPENSES

Salaries – Base/Regular
Salaries – Bereavement
Salaries – Bonus
Salaries – Holiday
Salaries – Jury Duty
Salaries – Miscellaneous
Salaries – On Call
Salaries – Overtime
Salaries – Paid Time Off (PTO)
Salaries – Independent Contractor
Salaries – Payroll Taxes
Salaries – Workers Compensation
Benefits – Automobile
Benefits – Dental
Benefits – Health
Benefits – COBRA
Benefits – Life/AD&D/LTD
Benefits – Other
Benefits – 401(k) Match
Benefits – 401(k) Profit Sharing
Professional Fees – Administrative
Professional Fees – Audit/Tax/Accounting
Professional Fees – Compliance
Professional Fees – Consulting
Professional Fees – HR/Benefits
Professional Fees – IT
Professional – Legal
Professional Fees – Payroll Processing
Professional Fees – Other
Medical Contract – Courier
Medical Contract – EMR

Medical Contract – Fellows
Medical Contract – Imaging (XRay/Ultrasound/CT)
Medical Contract – Lab
Medical Contract – Laundry/Uniforms
Medical Contract – Patient Incentives/Reimbursement
Medical Contract – Physicians
Medical Contract – Medical/Biohazard Waste
Medical Contract – NP/PA/RN/RVN
Medical Contract – On Call
Medical Contract – Record Archive Retrieval
Medical Contract – Record Shredding
Medical Contract – Surgical Technician
Medical Contract – Transcription
Medical Contract – Other
Billing/Collections – External Fees
Medical Contract – Collection Agency
Medical Contract – Bank/Credit Card Fees
Medical Contract – Managed Care/Credentialing
Medical Contract – CPT Coding
Medical Contract – Other
Insurance – General Business Liability
Insurance – Malpractice
Insurance – Officer/Board
Insurance – Owned Automobile
Communications – Answering/Reminder Services
Communications – Long Distance
Communications – Patient Education
Communications – Telephone/Internet
Communications – Web Design/Consult
Communications – Wireless
Communications – Other

EXPENSES

- Occupancy – Clinic/Office Lease
- Occupancy – Electricity/Gas
- Occupancy – Moving
- Occupancy – Offsite Storage Rental
- Occupancy – Parking Lease
- Occupancy – Plants/Landscaping
- Occupancy – Property Insurance
- Occupancy – Property Tax
- Occupancy – Repairs/Maintenance/Janitorial/CAM
- Occupancy – Security
- Occupancy – Waste Removal
- Occupancy – Water/Sewer
- Occupancy – Other
- Supplies – Office
- Supplies – Rebates
- Supplies – Clinics
- Supplies – Imaging (XRay/Ultrasound/CT)
- Supplies – Lab
- Supplies – Physical Therapy
- Supplies – Medication/Drugs/Injections
- Supplies – Durable Medical Equipment (DME)
- Supplies – Implants
- Supplies – Non-Billable
- Supplies – Other
- Travel – Airfare
- Travel – Leased Auto Expense
- Travel – Auto Rental
- Travel – Mileage/Tolls/Parking
- Travel – Lodging
- Travel – Meals/Entertainment (50% Rule-Offsite)
- Conference – Meals/Entertainment (100% Rule-Onsite)
- Conference – Fees/Seminars/Training
- Equipment/Software – Minor Purchases
- Equipment/Software – Repair
- Equipment/Software – Contract Maintenance Fees
- Equipment/Software – Lease – Auto
- Equipment/Software – Lease – Equipment
- Equipment/Software – Lease – Medical
- Equipment/Software – Copier/Printers
- Equipment/Software – Phone
- Equipment/Software – Lease – Postage Meter
- Employee Recruitment/Advertising/Fees
- Advertising/Marketing
- Bad Debt on Accounts Receivable
- Donations/Contributions/Charity Care
- Employee Recognition/Gifts/Awards
- License/Dues/Membership/Sub (Deductible)
- License/Dues/Membership/Sub (Nondeductible)
- Postage/Meter Supplies
- Printing/Publications
- Penalties Levied on MDs
- Late Charges/Lost Discounts
- Loss on Sale of Assets
- Miscellaneous
- Interest Expense
- Income Tax
- Sales and Use Tax
- Depreciation

ANCILLARY SERVICES

A vital attribute of a large medical practice is the ability to incorporate ancillary services. Ancillary services are the business segments added within the practice that enhance patient care. Ancillary services are required care that would normally be obtained externally from the business if there were only one or two physicians in a practice. When a large medical practice is formed, internal ancillaries are needed for continuum and control of excellent care for successful patient outcomes. Large groups have the patient volumes and financial means to bring ancillary services into the practice under one umbrella to improve patient care.

ANCILLARIES INCLUDE:

Clinical Procedures	Physical Therapy
Laboratory, Pathology	Shockwave Therapy
Ultrasound, CT images,	Urodynamic Study (USD)
Advanced Therapeutics	Lithotripsy
Research	Pharmacy
Clinical Trials	Durable Medical Equipment (DME)
Intensity-Modulated Radiation Therapy (IMRT)	Ambulatory Surgical Center (ASC)
	Advanced Practice Providers (APPS)

Ancillaries are vital to the survival of private physician practices. Revenue from professional fees are held static or reduced while all expenses increase annually. Ancillaries are not only important for patient care; they bridge the financial loss of lower revenue and increased expenses. Continued financial downward pressures of a practice must be offset by growth in ancillary services and the growth of the number of providers in the practice. An increase in providers has the potential to generate more ancillaries; it also dilutes numerous indirect overhead costs. Dilution of indirect overhead occurs when internal and external costs remain the same as more providers are added to the practice. Indirect overhead includes full department costs containing administration, accounting, human resources, information management, marketing, management, and general, call center, scheduling and clinic management. Full department costs include staff, benefits, occupancy, equipment, and supplies. Favorable utilization of occupancy occurs with additional providers who use vacant gaps in clinic space without further costs.

NET INCOME

Physician compensation is calculated after determining revenue and expenses of the entire group, including all business segments such as ancillaries. Revenue minus expenses represents net income before distributions in a medical practice. Distributions to physicians for compensation (further expenses) are then calculated and released, resulting in the final net income or loss to the practice after distributions to physicians have occurred. Net income after distributions in a medical practice should, in simple theory, be near zero. The goal of a practice is to have no income per book and especially no income per tax.

Balance sheet expenses, such as partner buy-outs greater than buy-ins, create unavoidable tax consequences to a practice. As an example, $500,000 in capital buy-outs greater than the buy-ins paid out by the practice amount cannot be expensed, resulting in net income per book and taxes of $500,000, and $105,000 paid in federal taxes by the practice. In turn, this causes another $105,000 that cannot be distributed as compensation.

Other significant items affecting compensation and the timing of funds available for use in calculating compensation are working capital, fixed assets, loans, and other cash inflows and outflows that are reported on the balance sheet instead of the income statement. There are also items not reportable as expenses on the tax return such as meals, entertainment, and political lobbying.

PHYSICIAN CATEGORIES

Medical groups often have several physician categories, such as voting partner, non-voting partner, and employed physician. New physicians entering a group are often brought on as employed physicians for a set period, usually one to three years, called a discovery period. During this time, the existing physician partners determine if the new physician will be an ideal addition and work well with the group. Employed physicians in a group can also be comprised of physicians who do not want to accept all the requirements of a partner, such as working part-time, not taking call, reduced clinic schedule, not performing surgeries, near retirement, or not wanting to be an owner (Partner) in the business.

Employed physicians in a salaried or equal compensation setting are usually salaried and might also receive additional compensation for productivity and/or value-based goals. New physicians joining a large production-based group may have the ability to set their own compensation during their discovery period with loans based on their own future productivity. Large groups have historical trends on what a physician produces and have the ability to temporarily subsidize the discovery period with a contractual loan with the new physician. Temporary payback subsidies along with new hire and relocation bonuses aides in new physician recruitment.

The understanding of medical practice revenue, expenses and net income provides a starting point for understanding physician compensation. Methods used in most practices are often an evolution over many years, several modifications, and numerous leadership changes. Drastic or complete changes to suit the current needs of a practice are often unattainable due to the dynamics and of a large group. A group should examine and modify physician compensation periodically as it should for any business component to keep it top of mind and compete in the market. Competition for physician recruitment includes other groups, hospitals, universities and several governmental agencies including the military. Competition is not merely local, but across the country.

Methodologies for physician compensation are as numerous as the number of large practices that exist when specific details are involved. All methods of physician compensation have a core focus that can be placed in one of the following general categories.

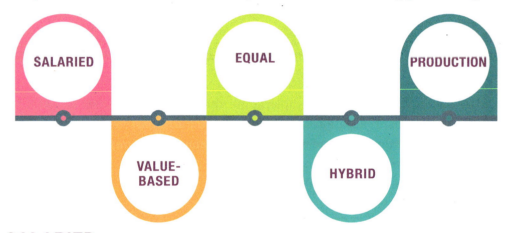

SALARIED

Salaried or fixed compensation is the simplest way to pay a physician. It is often used by hospitals, academic, and governmental agencies. The salary could sometimes be negotiated by the physician but is more often dictated by the entity. Salaries should be benchmarked and reflect regional averages for any group to attract physicians.

The advantage of a salary is that both parties know the exact amount and can easily budget for the future.

The disadvantages of a salary for physicians, is the absence of increased compensation when they are highly productive and efficient, and they will not benefit from the net income of the group. Salaries have no correlation with productivity, the business financial statements, or cash flow.

EQUAL

In a group, physicians can elect to split business net income equally between all partners. The amount of compensation remains unknown until all revenue and expenses are accounted for each period. A minimum periodic salary can be released, bi-weekly, for example, based on historic trends. Then, any remaining amount of available net income is divided equally at other intervals, such as quarterly.

An advantage of equal pay for all partners can incentivize better care for patients. Physicians in an equal compensation setting freely refer patients to colleagues who are best suited to handle patient needs. In urology, there are numerous clinical and surgical procedures and innovative treatments. Physicians focus their skills and become experts in areas, such as robotic surgery, advanced therapeutics, research and clinical trials, Rezūm™, UroLift®, penile reconstruction, vasectomies, female pelvic medicine, pediatrics, and other procedures. Equal pay models remove the physicians' fear of sharing patients as there is no monetary penalty. Other pay models may incentivize physicians to perform procedures and surgeries where they do not have extensive experience. Patients often benefit by receiving appointments sooner and have longer one-on-one interaction with the physician or advanced practice provider (APP) that is supervised by a physician.

Equal pay also allows physicians to share APPs, medical assistants, and other indirect overhead infrastructure expenses. Equal pay often affords the physician, and the entire medical practice, more attention to patient care and less on how to achieve higher pay. Quality of life is sometimes enjoyed by equal compensation models as it allows for equal and possibly increased amounts of time away from the practice in the form of vacations and paid time off. More time off is one solution to the increasing trend of physician burnout. Burnout results in individuals in any profession to leave an industry and is a deterrent to others on entering stressful career paths.

Disadvantages of equal pay can include being paid the same for unequal work performance. In any large medical group there will be physicians, and other staff, working at vastly different productivity rates. Equal pay will not encourage staff who are less productive to become more efficient. Equal pay will also frustrate and potentially drive away highly productive physicians. The dynamics of low and high producers is not unique to physicians and medical practices as it creates emotional tension across all facets of life.

PRODUCTION

Productivity-based compensation plans are paid based on the direct clinic and surgical activity of each individual physician. Production for direct professional services performed can be derived from gross billed charges, net cash collected, Relative Value Units (RVUs) or a combination of these or similar measurements. Less commonly used methods would include the number of patients seen or the number of Current Procedural Terminology® (CPT) codes generated. Production-based compensation is the most prevalent method used to calculate each physician's direct activities.

Production-based compensation can be used as the sole method when no ancillary services exist within a medical group's infrastructure. Other components of revenue that a large medical group may have, such as ancillary services, should not be paid based on each physician's referral. Medical groups need to refer to the Physician Self-Referral Law, commonly referred to as Stark Law when allocating ancillary service net income to physicians within the group. To avoid regulatory non-compliance, the best way to allocate net income from ancillary services, is equally to all physician owners or partners.

Advantages of production-based compensation include an incentive to be productive, pay based on work effort, and an increased patient volume that aids ancillary services. Physicians also become more diverse by broadening their locations and retaining additional types of procedures and surgeries. As individual productivity increases pay, ancillary services also increase. This allows for additional resources for group growth and expansion and distribution of additional compensation.

Disadvantages of production-based compensation can include delayed patient access, reduced peer referrals, less vacations, physician burnout, segmented marketing and community development, competition within the group, and variable pay. Patient access to care could suffer as appointments are scheduled three or more months out and daily encounters are increased in order to retain as many patients as possible to increase production. Intra-group peer-to-peer referral of patients decline in production-based models. Higher compensation goals develop competition within the group for more patients and patients with better insurance contracts. Physicians may work more and take fewer vacations as productivity immediately impacts compensation. Productivity based compensation is an unknown variable. It is difficult to predict and budget for the future as numerous things will impact compensation. Impacts to compensation could occur from infrastructure, administration, EMR systems, billing, collections, verifications, physician and patient referrals, billable days, marketing, staffing, vacations, sickness, and other issues.

VALUE-BASED

Value-based compensation is based on a single or combined metric of patient out comes, patient satisfaction, utilization management, quality of care, and other metrics. Value-based is similar to production-based as there are periodic metrics used to derive pay. Value-based pay is different from production based as it focuses on patient outcome metrics instead of monetary measurements. Valued-based is rarely used as a sole method of physician compensation.

All groups should implement value-based metrics in order to comply with regulatory requirements and to have historical data and trends available for potential changes in physician compensation methodology.

The advantages of value-based compensation plans are; patient outcome is a focus; improvements to patient care is a goal; unnecessary care is monitored; patient referrals to the group increase; physicians with poor patient care or outcomes are weeded out of the group; and data can be provided to patients, regulators, legislators, and insurance carriers in negotiating contracts. Regulatory requirements such as Merit-Based Incentive Payment System (MIPS) are the beginning attempts to track value-based information. The data MIPS presently uses is not useful in truly improving patient care and outcomes or as the sole basis for physician compensation.

The disadvantage in using value-based compensation is the data is extremely difficult and costly to obtain. It is additional information that is not required to conduct basic core business. Collection of data requires an additional layer of resources and expertise in database management, marketing, and patient management that medical groups may not have in place. It also requires high interaction with all patients via electronic means, such as portals and emails, using consistent email reminders or marketing survey tools. Patients often refuse to release emails, opt out of repeated marketing surveys, or do not respond. Lack of data and additional time can adversely skew and delay compensation. Value-based may not correlate to high or low productivity and revenue resulting in the redirection of professional fees based on the group's non-monetary goals. There are arguments that multiple contributors effect positive patient outcomes, not merely one individual physician. There is a lack of regional and national comparative data on value-based benchmarks in order to set goals for a medical practice or an individual physician.

HYBRIDS

The most common type of physician compensation is a hybrid model that includes combinations of Salaried, Equal, Production, and/or Value-based. In production hybrids, direct professional fees identified by the payment management system in billing and collection are credited to each physician and other departments, such as ancillaries. Most practices credit each physician's direct professional fees into the physician's individual income statement and divide ancillaries equally to each physician partner after all direct and indirect expenses have been allocated. Ancillary services are equally distributed to all physician partners to comply with regulatory laws.

Direct expenses include malpractice insurance, dues, memberships, automobile, travel, training/CME, uniforms, office supplies, equipment depreciation, software licenses, EMR systems, and 100% of employee and employer costs of benefits and retirement plans for the physician. Indirect costs have two components: variable and fixed. Variable indirect costs include allocations based on volumes and usage for billing and collection, call center, occupancy, and direct staffing with benefits. Indirect overhead fixed costs include all other expenses, such as administration, accounting, human resources, information management, marketing, management and general, call center, scheduling, and clinic management.

More complex compensation models may split net income before distribution, or split ancillary service net income into two or more categories. Allocation categories could include proportions of direct professional fees and remaining proportions allocated based on other specific goals, for example; 80% direct professional fees and 20% patient satisfaction. Production and production hybrids can calculate most of the available compensation funds no sooner than monthly and the remainder at any other periodic interval of quarterly, semi-annually or annually.

Equal compensation hybrids can split a majority of net income equally before distributing on a weekly, bi-weekly, or monthly basis, and the remainder at any other periodic interval. Compensation not distributed equally can consist of numerous metrics depending on value-based goals of the practice or other predetermined allocation methods.

ILLUSTRATIVE EXAMPLES

Distributions can be derived in endless methods. Below and on the next two pages are hypothetical examples of the most common compensation calculations.

Bonus Allocation Examples

Physician Partner Quarterly Bonus: 100% Equal Distribution;

	Quarter 1	Quarter 2	Quarter 3	Quarter 4
Bonus Pool by Quarter	$1,000,000	$1,200,000	$800,000	$1,100,000
Divided by Total Physician Partners	20	20	20	20
Quarterly Bonus Per Physician Partner	$50,000 A	$60,000 B	$40,000 C	$55,000 D

Physician Partner Quarterly Bonus: 75% Productivity Based and 25% Equal;

Quarter 1 Bonus Pool: $1,000,000   **Bonus Allocation**

Physician Partners	Quarterly Gross Charges*	Percent of Average	Productivity Basis Average	75% Productivity Basis	25% Equal Basis	100% Total Bonus	
Physician 1	885,000	142.0% x	37,500 =	53,249 +	12,500 =	65,749	E
Physician 2	765,000	122.7% x	37,500 =	46,029 +	12,500 =	58,529	F
Physician 3	765,000	122.7% x	37,500 =	46,029 +	12,500 =	58,529	
Physician 4	735,000	117.9% x	37,500 =	44,224 +	12,500 =	56,724	
Physician 5	720,000	115.5% x	37,500 =	43,321 +	12,500 =	55,821	
Physician 6	705,000	113.1% x	37,500 =	42,419 +	12,500 =	54,919	
Physician 7	690,000	110.7% x	37,500 =	41,516 +	12,500 =	54,016	
Physician 8	660,000	105.9% x	37,500 =	39,711 +	12,500 =	52,211	
Physician 9	645,000	103.5% x	37,500 =	38,809 +	12,500 =	51,309	
Physician 10	630,000	101.1% x	37,500 =	37,906 +	12,500 =	50,406	
Physician 11	600,000	96.3% x	37,500 =	36,101 +	12,500 =	48,601	
Physician 12	585,000	93.9% x	37,500 =	35,199 +	12,500 =	47,699	
Physician 13	570,000	91.5% x	37,500 =	34,296 +	12,500 =	46,796	
Physician 14	570,000	91.5% x	37,500 =	34,296 +	12,500 =	46,796	
Physician 15	540,000	86.6% x	37,500 =	32,491 +	12,500 =	44,991	
Physician 16	525,000	84.2% x	37,500 =	31,588 +	12,500 =	44,088	
Physician 17	525,000	84.2% x	37,500 =	31,588 +	12,500 =	44,088	
Physician 18	480,000	77.0% x	37,500 =	28,881 +	12,500 =	41,381	
Physician 19	450,000	72.2% x	37,500 =	27,076 +	12,500 =	39,576	
Physician 20	420,000	67.4% x	37,500 =	25,271 +	12,500 =	37,771	G
Total =	**12,465,000**			**750,000 +**	**250,000 =**	**1,000,000**	
Average =	**623,250**			**37,500 +**	**12,500 =**	**50,000**	

*Ancillary Services Excluded

Total Annual Compensation Examples

Equal Base + Equal Bonus

						Physician 1		Physician 2		....Physician 20
Bi-Weekly Base Salary	Equal	$10,000	x	26	=	260,000		260,000		260,000
Quarter 1 Bonus	Hypothetical example calculated above				A	50,000	A	50,000	A	50,000
Quarter 2 Bonus	Hypothetical example calculated above				B	60,000	B	60,000	B	60,000
Quarter 3 Bonus	Hypothetical example calculated above				C	40,000	C	40,000	C	40,000
Quarter 4 Bonus	Hypothetical example calculated above				D	55,000	D	55,000	D	55,000
	Total Annual Physician Partner Compensation =					465,000		465,000		465,000

Equal Base + 75% Productivity Bonus

						Physician 1		Physician 2		....Physician 20
Bi-Weekly Base Salary	Equal	$10,000	x	26	=	260,000		260,000		260,000
Quarter 1 Bonus	Hypothetical example calculated above				E	65,749	F	58,529	G	37,771
Quarter 2 Bonus	Hypothetical, calculation not shown					54,311		48,880		34,216
Quarter 3 Bonus	Hypothetical, calculation not shown					47,560		42,804		29,963
Quarter 4 Bonus	Hypothetical, calculation not shown					62,144		55,930		39,151
	Total Annual Physician Partner Compensation =					489,764		466,142		401,100

Productivity Base + Equal Bonus

		Physician 1		Physician 2		....Physician 20
Productivity Base Salary	Hypothetical collections less expenses	283,200		244,800		134,400
Quarter 1 Bonus	Hypothetical example calculated above A	50,000	A	50,000	A	50,000
Quarter 2 Bonus	Hypothetical example calculated above B	60,000	B	60,000	B	60,000
Quarter 3 Bonus	Hypothetical example calculated above C	40,000	C	40,000	C	40,000
Quarter 4 Bonus	Hypothetical example calculated above D	55,000	D	55,000	D	55,000
	Total Annual Physician Partner Compensation =	488,200		449,800		339,400

Productivity Base + 75% Productivity Bonus

			Physician 1		Physician 2		....Physician 20
Productivity Base Salary	Hypothetical collections less expenses		283,200		244,800		134,400
Quarter 1 Bonus	Hypothetical example calculated above	E	65,749	F	58,529	G	37,771
Quarter 2 Bonus	Hypothetical, calculation not shown		54,311		48,880		34,216
Quarter 3 Bonus	Hypothetical, calculation not shown		47,560		42,804		29,963
Quarter 4 Bonus	Hypothetical, calculation not shown		62,144		55,930		39,151
	Total Annual Physician Partner Compensation =		512,964		450,942		275,500

CONCLUSION

Physician compensation in large medical groups must achieve several outcomes. Compensation needs to reimburse physicians for their professional services, compete with the market, satisfy new physician recruitment, be successful against competitors, provide benefit to patients and insurers, and induce efficiency to the practice while fairly compensating numerous physicians working at different levels.

Compensation cannot ignore other business needs, regulatory requirements and tax consequences. It must be calculated in an understandable and predictable method and change as the practice evolves. The survival and growth of the undeserved specialty of urology must answer the complexities of physician compensation in order to introduce growth in the specialty as our population demands more care from urologists.

KEY POINTS

- **Providing compensation** to urologists that reflects the increased need is paramount to the survival of the specialty.

- **Continued financial** downward pressures of a practice must be offset by growth in ancillary services and the growth of the number of providers in the practice.

- **Competition for physician recruitment** includes other groups, hospitals, universities and several governmental agencies including the military.

- **Physician compensation** is calculated after determining revenue and expenses of the entire group, including all business segments such as ancillaries.

- **Salaried or fixed compensation** is the simplest way to pay a physician. It could be negotiated by the physician, but more often dictated by the entity and should be benchmarked to reflect regional averages to attract physicians.

- **In the Equal Pay model,** physicians can elect to split business net income equally between all partners. Patients often benefit by booking appointments sooner, receiving specialized care, and longer one-on-one interaction with the physician.

- **Productivity-based compensation** plans are paid based on the direct clinic and surgical activity of each individual physician.

- **Value-based compensation** to physicians is paid based on a single or combined metric of patient outcomes, patient satisfaction, utilization management, quality of care, and other metrics.

- **The most common type of physician compensation** is a hybrid containing combinations of Salaried, Equal, Production, and/or Value-based.

Steven R. Flageol

With twenty-eight years of experience in health care, Steven R. Flageol, has served since 2013 as Director of Finance at Urology San Antonio, a practice of thirty-five providers. Steve holds a BS degree in Accountancy from Bentley University and has attended Champlain College and the American University of Paris. His career started in Houston at DePelchin Children's Center, a large not-for-profit health care organization, where he achieved the position of Controller following ten years of service. Prior to joining Urology San Antonio, he worked ten years as the CFO of The San Antonio Orthopaedic Group, consisting of twenty-five physicians.

CHAPTER

Urology Practice Mergers and Acquisitions

Peter M. Knapp, MD, FACS

INTRODUCTION

Independent urology practices have merged over the past 25 years in response to market pressures threatening their survival. The emergence of managed care insurance plans with narrow provider panels, hospital consolidation, and hospital hiring of primary care physicians (PCP) and specialists threatened historical referral lines and limited patient access to non-aligned specialists. Merged urology practices serving different hospitals, PCP networks and managed care plans were able to retain access to a larger number of patients while expanding urology practice service lines. They are also better positioned to purchase capital equipment and make facility investments to provide traditional facility-based services inside the larger practice. Over time, practices began adding ambulatory surgery centers, clinical and anatomical pathology laboratories, advanced imaging centers, and cancer centers with radiation therapy to their practices to provide higher quality and more efficient care to their patients.

Today, urology practice mergers continue the successes achieved by many established large practices. They have expanded clinical service lines, developed guideline-based clinical pathways, provided improved patient care and service, and are positioned to thrive in future value-based reimbursement models. Drawing on the experience of many large group practice mergers, this chapter will outline **10 Steps to Successful Practice Mergers and Acquisitions** (**Table 1**) and the **5 Keys to Success** (**Table 2**) that can be helpful, whether considering a merger between two or more groups or an acquisition of a smaller practice. Progressing in an organized systematic fashion and putting **first things first** can keep the process moving forward in a timely manner while avoiding time-consuming and costly pitfalls.

TABLE 1

10 Steps to Successful Practice Mergers and Acquisitions: Create a Vision, Assemble a Team, Legal Consideration, Financial Analysis, Term Sheet, Operating Agreement, Management, Transition Team, Practice Approval, Go Live

In keeping with the LUGPA mission of preservation, growth and collaboration of independent practices, this chapter will help practices build a comprehensive integrated independent urology group that provides improved patient care and services to the community.

PRACTICE MERGERS
First things First

01 CREATE A VISION

Practices considering a merger need to create a shared vision. It will provide the motivational impetus to bring physician groups together and the incentive to invest needed resources to complete the merger process. It is important to initiate discussions with "like-minded" urologists, whose goals are centered around advancing patient care.

The vision can be developed by carefully examining the goals, objectives, and opportunities to achieve by completing a practice merger. These common goals and objectives will serve as a guidepost for all subsequent merger discussions.

Ensure the goals and objectives are of significant value to justify the time, effort, and sacrifice necessary to successfully complete a merger. They can include both short-term and long-term goals. Short-term goals should be achievable in a reasonable period of time to demonstrate the merger's value, and provide momentum to keep the merged entity moving forward. The importance of the goals and objectives cannot be over emphasized. If they are meaningfully significant, all other obstacles become insignificant and negotiable.

> **Goals and objectives can take two forms:**
> **Practice Growth and Solving Common Problems.**

Practice Growth

Growth goals can include capturing increased market share through improved geographical coverage, increased PCP referral base, expanded hospital coverage, or additional payer contracts. Growth can also be realized by the merged entity's ability to invest in capital equipment and treatment centers that will provide additional integrated services in the practice. They include specialized centers of excellence, advanced imaging, radiation therapy, clinical and anatomical pathology services, ambulatory surgery centers, and in-house dispensaries or pharmacies. These growth objectives provide significant motivation for practice mergers as they increase top line revenue opportunities that can provide more integrated care and service to a wider range of patients.

Solving Common Problems

The second set of goals and objectives can be built around the merged entity's ability to solve common practice problems better than independent practices. Common problems facing all independent practices include revenue cycle management, clinical operations management, human resources, employee hiring and retention, physician workforce distribution, physician recruiting and hiring, electronic health record (EHR) maintenance, and management of practice overhead. The combined resources of a merged entity often put the practice in a better position to hire experienced and talented managers who can build an adequate infrastructure to support a large number of physicians and address these common problems. In some cases, capturing economies of scale and maximizing operating efficiencies are significant enough to provide the incentive needed to proceed with the merger.

Selecting merger goals and objectives to create a vision is essential at the outset of merger discussions. It is also valuable to draft a preliminary business plan that includes the expanded goals and objectives to help outline the merger's purpose to other group members. The business plan can also serve as a roadmap of targeted goals following completion of the merger. Finally, the business plan should be presented as a draft to allow future changes during the merger process and following its closure.

ASSEMBLE A MERGER TEAM

Successful mergers require active involvement of physician leaders and senior management from each practice in the proposed merger. The physician leadership needs to be motivated by a shared vision and pathway to achieve the agreed upon goals and objectives. Physician leaders also need to have the ability to build consensus within their respective groups to gain the necessary approval for the merger. In many cases, physician leadership can develop a vision understood by other physician leaders but not appreciated or valued by physician members of their own group. Physician leaders must recognize internal obstacles or objections that exist and attempt to reconcile them before proceeding down the merger pathway. It is also essential that physician leadership evaluates their counterparts from the other groups and accesses their ability to garner approval internally. It is in everyone's best interest to be certain that the leaders at the table represent the interests of their respective groups and can lead their group to merger approval before investing resources in the process.

In addition to physician leadership and management, it is also helpful to identify a merger facilitator to help keep the individual physicians, managers, and group entities focused on the goals and objectives as inevitable challenges arise. The facilitator can be a mutually agreed upon accountant, lawyer, or business advisor capable of working constructively to solve problems.

03 LEGAL CONSIDERATIONS

Once satisfactory goals and objectives are identified and the merger discussion team has been assembled, three immediate legal considerations need to be addressed. **First is the execution of a confidentiality agreement.** All practice entities possess important private financial and strategic information that needs to be protected by a nondisclosure agreement (NDA) before information can be exchanged. A carefully created document can protect all parties in the event that the merger does not consummate and practices return to their separate independent status.

The second immediate legal consideration should include an antitrust assessment from outside legal counsel. Practice mergers can cause fear and suspicion in the local health care community by hospitals, payers, and competitors. During the antitrust evaluation, it's important to carefully examine potential issues raised by impacted parties. It is helpful to prepare a white paper in advance to use if objections arise. The antitrust evaluation can be formulated rather quickly and provide an outline of a defense to any antitrust charges. It also provides an opportunity for legal counsel to advise the practice entities on proper behavior to avoid unfair business practice accusations.

The third early legal consideration is to identify and secure a name and corporate identity for the merged entity. The new name needs to be legally secured for a future URL, website address, marketing, and tax identification number. Although agreeing to a new name can be time-consuming and delayed to later in the process, it is an important legal checkpoint to accomplish to avoid a post-merger name change that confuses the market and disrupts the practice.

04 FINANCIAL ANALYSIS AND DUE DILIGENCE

After completion of the NDA, practices need to disclose their financial information for the past several years. Disclosure of 3 to 5 years is adequate to provide appropriate practice trends in areas of billing, receipts, collection percentage, relative values units (RVU) analysis, payer analysis, accounts receivable, accounts receivable aging, and accounts payable. The patient encounter information also needs to be examined carefully. New patients and consult trends over several years are valuable to examine the practice's health. Examining total patient visit trends gives insight into the market share held by each practice. Complete the clinical volume assessment by examining the number of hospital consults, hospital admissions, and surgery volume. Also provide fixed assets, including office and medical equipment inventory.

Other relationships, including ownership in medical office buildings, capital equipment, and integrated service lines should be completely disclosed. It is important for all parties to understand the current structures of each group, as some may have separate Limited Liability Corporations (LLC) for ambulatory surgery centers, mobile lithotripsy, and radiation centers. These various LLCs may or may not be included in the practice merger. Disclosure extends to practice review, including the number of offices, locations, management structure, and manager responsibility. The number of physicians, age, compensation, and years to retirement should also be carefully reviewed.

Close examination of the financial information should provide needed visibility into each of the practice's financial relationships and financial condition. The review can provide additional insight into future business growth and expansion opportunities, as well as opportunities to consolidate staff, offices, and managers.

TERM SHEET

The merger team should create a term sheet after identifying significant achievable goals and objectives and completing the financial analysis and due diligence. The term sheet should include expanded goals and objectives developed during the due diligence process as well as details regarding practice structure, governance, and compensation to include in the operating agreement. The term sheet provides an opportunity for all parties to collectively agree on deal terms and justify further investment of time, energy, and legal cost moving forward. It also provides a useful document to return to each group's membership for approval. As the merger team discusses the term sheet with individual group members, they have the opportunity to learn the internal objections that may persist and resolve any concerns early in the merger process. Approval of the term sheet can be memorialized by executing a mutual letter of intent (LOI) confirming each practice's commitment to move forward.

OPERATING AGREEMENT

Development of the operating agreement will require substantial time and effort on the part of the practice leadership and legal team. Each entity's operating agreement needs to be reviewed and a common one needs to be developed. It will include identification of the practice corporate structure, contributed assets, covenants, compensation, member buy in and buy out, member additions and dissociations, non-compete, member disability, practice dissolution, and wind-up provisions.

The operating agreement also provides an opportunity to determine the degree of practice integration that will occur in the merged group. Some groups will prefer to maintain separate divisions while forming a combined management service organization (MSO). The MSO may also be structured to contain individual practices as members, allowing individual physicians to remain members of their respective practice division. The MSO may include a common governing body, senior management, revenue cycle management and some combined integrated service lines including laboratory, advanced imaging, office dispensary or pharmacy, ambulatory surgery center (ASC), and radiation therapy.

Other practices may prefer more complete practice integration, including governance, management, common compensation formula, office consolidation, common electronic health record (EHR), as well as combined integrated service lines. Development of the operating agreement provides the platform to decide the level of practice integration that meets the goals and objectives of the merger.

The operating agreement serves as the backbone of the new entity. Considerable time must be spent to ensure accuracy and fairness. The process may take several months, with many document revisions; patience is important during this arduous process. Throughout the life of the group, the operating agreement should periodically be reviewed to make any necessary adjustments that result from the ongoing evolution of the group.

Experienced legal advice is essential to achieve a fair and equitable arrangement for all parties and provide a process for the merged entity to conduct business going forward. It's also wise to include incentives to help the merger remain intact, create significant barriers to dissolution, and meet all regulatory requirements.

07 PRACTICE APPROVAL

Following completion of the operating agreement, the merger teams return to their respective practices to receive final approval of all merger documents. This is often a formality if the respective practice leadership teams have followed best practices of regularly updating their practice members and seeking real-time feedback. Prior approval of the term sheet and the LOI will minimize any last-minute objections.

08 MANAGEMENT

An important task in all practice mergers is to assess the future management needs of the merged entity. Most practices have assembled competent management leadership into their practice structure and rely heavily on their expertise and judgment in day-to-day operations, contracting, and personnel decisions. Merged practices need to consolidate management teams as well. This can result in realignment of managerial positions, including assignment of new responsibilities or in some cases eliminating positions and associated overhead. Identifying the best management team for the new entity moving forward is critical and can often be found within the existing collective pool of managers. A new manager can also be identified from outside who is agreeable to all parties. Identifying the management team structure and chain of command is a critical step to achieve proper practice functionality.

Most large practices create a senior management team that includes a Chief Executive Officer, Chief Operating Officer, Chief Financial Officer, Chief Medical Officer, Chief Information Officer, Human Resources Officer, and Supply Chain Manager, depending on specific group needs. While designing the management structure, it is important to avoid unnecessary increases in administrative costs. It is reasonable, however, to expect central administrative costs of 2-3% of practice revenue.

TRANSITION TEAM

Once the practice entities agree to move forward with the merger, they need to establish an appropriate merger timeline and identify a transition team to bring the merger to closure and full operation. The work of the transition team can be initiated upon completion of the LOI and confirmation of the management team and structure. The transition team needs to be led by the practice management team including finance, billing, coding, accounting, human resources, Information Technology (IT), as well as service line directors including laboratory, imaging, radiation, and ambulatory surgery centers. Senior management needs to carefully identify the role of each team member needed to bring everything into alignment prior to the go-live date. Placing emphasis on the revenue cycle management department can ensure needed cash flow for the new entity. Invariably, one or several payers will delay payment to the new entity despite the best efforts to notify them in advance and obtain necessary provider number changes. It is essential that the practice establish a sufficient line of credit with a banking institution to enable cash withdrawals to maintain operations in the event of a delay in payments from insurers. The line of credit may be several million dollars, depending on the size of the new group.

The transition team should also put processes in place to ensure proper patient and specimen flow to utilize the combined integrated services. Coordination of specimen flow to the laboratory and patient scheduling for imaging, subspecialty services, surgical procedures, and radiation therapy need to be in place prior to the go-live date.

10. GO-LIVE

Preparation for go-live is a process that takes several weeks or months. Proper execution requires everyone to be prepared and billing systems to be in place. Senior management will need all hands on deck to manage any unforeseen problems. As transition advisers begin to disengage, the new entity may consider hiring a third party consultant to help with the integration process. Inevitably, challenges will arise and the involvement of a consultant may help overcome them.

5 KEYS TO SUCCESS

Urology practice mergers have met with varying degrees of success. Some have coalesced into high performing health care delivery enterprises while others have failed to achieve their full potential. Upon review of many merged practices with varying degrees of success, **5 Keys to Success** emerge (**Table 2**).

TABLE 2

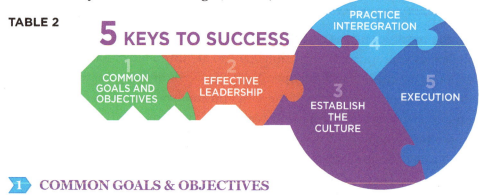

1. COMMON GOALS & OBJECTIVES

The first key to success is to develop a shared vision and meaningfully significant goals and objectives. The shared group vision and objectives serve as the impetus to merge and become the template for future growth and development. The objectives may include some of the same elements of practice growth and solving common problems outlined in Practice Mergers' Step 1 to Create a Vision but may also include other local or regional objectives important to the practices. Most merger goals include a combination of clinical and administrative objectives.

Clinical Goals

Combining practices in the same metropolitan area or geographical region can enhance the market share of the combined group. Increasing the number of hospitals covered, payer contracts, and patients served provides the foundation for growth of expanded service lines and sub specialization. Expanded service lines may include clinical and anatomical pathology laboratory, advanced imaging, an in-house dispensary or pharmacy, radiation therapy, and ambulatory surgery center. The additional service lines can generate significant top line revenue in addition to providing improved patient care and services.

Increased market share can also result in improved negotiating position with commercial insurers. As a provider to a large number of patients and a larger percentage of the payer's members, the group may be in a better position to negotiate professional and facility fees. A discussion centered around optimal patient care and how the larger group can provide a premium product to the payer and their members is most effective. The larger percentage of local patients receiving care also places the practice in a better position to negotiate risk sharing contracts in the future pay-for-value reimbursement models.

Administrative Goals

Another shared goal may include additional capabilities in managing physician and advanced practice providers (APP) workforce needs. The first advantage will be seen in improved geographical coverage. In most cases there is some geographical office overlap that can be eliminated by combining offices and realigning physician and APP workforce distribution. New workforce distributions may provide an opportunity for employing and placing APPs in areas of increased demand. The addition of APPs increase the physician's capability to improve hospital and office coverage by providing an additional professional to accommodate urgent office patients or hospital and emergency room consults. Larger merged practices can also take advantage of more strategic physician hiring. Typically, individual practices have plans in place to hire additional physicians for new coverage areas or to replace retiring physicians. New physician hiring can be competitive between existing groups and often results in duplicate hiring. In the new entity, physician hiring can be more strategically planned and possibly result in hiring fewer physicians by maximizing workforce distribution and increasing the use of APPs.

Merged group practices are also better able to support sub-specialization within the practice. A larger number of physicians seeing a larger number of patients can concentrate patient care in the hands of the practice's physicians who have subspecialized in a particular area. The result is improved patient care provided by the most experienced and specialized physician, which supports the subspecialty infrastructure required to deliver high-quality care.

2 EFFECTIVE LEADERSHIP

A combination of physician and managerial leadership is essential for merger success. Most large group practices create a representative physician Board of Directors who are delegated the responsibility to lead the practice. Most successful practices also identify a physician leader and management leader who will work in tandem to develop and implement approved board directives. The structure and functionality of the board is variable and can be designed to meet the individual practice needs. The extent of delegated board authority can be outlined in the operating agreement as well as the limits of authority.

The physician Board of Directors also need to delegate responsibilities for implementation and some decision making to the senior administrative team in order to achieve practice goals and objectives. It is important for physician leadership to understand the difference between leadership and management. The description of leadership function and managerial function has been described by Prof. John Kotter from the Harvard Business School in his book Leading Change (**Table 3**). Physicians in larger group practices often need to remove themselves from previous managerial roles and delegate managerial functions to professional managers while providing much-needed leadership functions outlined by Kotter.

3. ESTABLISH THE CULTURE

Early establishment of the practice culture sets the stage for future success. The new group needs to adopt a definitive culture that aligns the interest of all parties, delegates authority to selected leadership, and promotes cooperation and compromise to achieve practice goals and objectives. Development of the practice Mission Statement, Vision Statement, and Business Principles is a useful process that builds consensus and serves as an instrument to define the new group culture.

As a health care delivery organization serving patients and the community, it is important to maintain a culture that is focused on delivering exceptional patient care and service. It is also helpful to develop a culture that places group interests above those of any individual physician or manager. A culture that puts patients first, group practice second, and individual interests third, positions the practice for clinical excellence, market acceptance, and future growth. Practice leadership needs to take responsibility to develop and foster the group culture and emphasize it in all internal and external communication. Practice members need to exemplify the group culture in all daily interactions with patients, staff, and referring physicians.

Annual, biannual, or quarterly group meetings away from the office can help promote a positive group culture and enhance practice integration. This is especially helpful for very large practices where partners may not see each other on a daily basis.

4. PRACTICE INTEGRATION

The degree of practice integration can determine the degree of success of the merged practice. Practice integration can occur at many levels and can be detailed in the initial operating agreement or developed overtime. Integration most commonly occurs at the governance and leadership level. This is usually outlined in the operating agreement. Revenue cycle management and accounting is often integrated in the merged entity to capitalize on best practices and personnel to maximize the merger's financial benefit. Governance, leadership, and revenue cycle management can be assembled in a management services organization (MSO) supported by each practice division in a divisional model. Various ancillary services, including laboratory, advanced imaging, ASC, office dispensary or pharmacy, and radiation therapy can also be integrated into the MSO to enhance practice integration and member alignment. In the MSO divisional model, care centers or pods may have more autonomy regarding hiring, firing, capital purchases, local decision making, and individual compensation formulas. This model allows for continuation of legacy policies, but takes advantage of the new economies of scale and central management.

Further integration of compensation formulas, electronic health record (EHR) and clinical subspecialty service lines are another level of practice integration, which can bring further member alignment and enterprise value. Integration of MSO services, ancillary service lines, compensation formulas, EHR, and subspecialty services can bind a group together and enhance the group culture.

5. EXECUTION

The difference between a good and a great practice merger is execution. Realization of the planned goals and objectives is critical to success and can only be achieved through execution of the business plan. The management team and physician leadership need to create a realistic timeline for each goal and work together to achieve them. Fulfillment of goals and objectives through prioritization and execution are essential to realize the merger's promise. However, post-merger integration is not the responsibility of management and leadership alone. The merged practice will be more successful if each member in the organization adopts the practice culture and plays an active role in executing the mission and vision of the group. Active member support of the merger will accelerate practice integration and contribute to building a cohesive team.

Perils and Pitfalls

The risks of practice mergers are centered around the changes that a larger group imposes internally on the practice as well as externally on patient and referring physician customers. These challenges are the downside of practice mergers which will need to be actively managed to prevent them from becoming a significant detriment to ongoing success.

Change of Culture

Merging existing practices will typically require a change of culture both internally and externally. Internally the larger group practice will require additional structure, delegation of authority and physician compromise. A smaller group practice may have all members involved in all decision making which will no longer be practical in a larger group practice. Most large group practices have created a physician board of directors who have been delegated the responsibility of managing the practice by the other member physicians. The structure and functionality of the board is variable and can be designed to meet the individual practice needs. The managing physician board will also find they need to delegate responsibilities for implementation and some decision making to the senior administrative team in order to achieve practice goals and objectives. It is important for physician leadership to understand the difference between leadership and management (**Table 3**). Physicians in larger Group practices often need to remove themselves from previous managerial roles and delegate managerial functions to professional managers while providing much-needed leadership functions.

Physicians in larger practices also need to recognize that increasing the number of physicians also increases the number of agendas. The amount of compromise needed among physicians in small practices is magnified in large practices. A culture of delegation and compromise will go a long way to ensure the success of the merged entity.

Large group mergers can also change the culture of the group externally. A larger group may appear big and impersonal to patient and referring physician customers. Communication can become difficult both internally and externally making access to physicians by outside patient and referring physician customers challenging. Recognition of this potential is the first step in managing the problem. Measures can be employed internally to maintain the personal nature of patient and referring physician communication to ensure that the quality of service remains unaltered or improved.

Increased Overhead

Large group mergers can also present the potential for increased overhead. A larger organization with increased number of employees will typically require additional middle management which can add to the practice overhead. Overhead management with attention to the number and role of employees and managers is essential to control costs.

Increased overhead can also be seen by adding significant profitable service lines with smaller profit margins. Some service lines such as pharmacy generate significant profits but have small percentage profit margins increasing practice overhead percentage. Small profit margin service lines need to be actively managed to realize the profitability and may require separate accounting lines to accurately track historical practice overhead percentage.

TABLE 3
MANAGEMENT vs LEADERSHIP

▸ **Planning and Budgeting:** Establishing detailed steps and timetables for achieving needed results, then allocating the resources necessary to make it happen.

▸ **Organizing and Staffing:** Establishing some structure for accomplishing plan requirements, staffing that structure with individuals, delegating responsibility and authority for carrying out the plan, proficient policies and procedures to help guide people, and creating methods or systems to monitor implementation.

▸ **Controlling and Problem Solving:** Monitoring results, identifying deviations from plan, then planning and organizing to solve these problems.

▸ **Establishing Direction:** Developing a vision of the future — often the distant future — and strategies for producing the changes needed to achieve that vision.

▸ **Aligning People:** Communicating direction in words and deeds to all those whose cooperation may be needed so as to influence the creation of teams and coalitions that understand the vision and strategies and that accept their validity.

▸ **Motivating and Inspiring:** Energizing people to overcome major political, bureaucratic, and resource carriers to change by satisfying basic, but often unfulfilled, human needs.

SOURCE: A Force for Change: How Leadership Differs from Management from John P. Kotter, Copyright 1990 by John P. Kotter, The Free Press, a Division of Simon & Schuster.

Employee Turnover

Practice mergers also inevitably result in employee turnover. The new organization and culture will have a different appearance and feel to some employees who will choose to take their talents elsewhere to the detriment of the group and some individual physicians. It is essential to understand that employee turnover after mergers is inevitable and should be anticipated in advance to minimize the pain associated with change. Some smaller practices merging into larger established practices have reported employee turnover greater than 50% due to the change in structure, culture, and feel of the new entity. Anticipation of attrition and building an initial surplus of key operational personnel may minimize the impact of staff departures.

Practice Consultants

Another challenging aspect of practice mergers is the need to make difficult decisions in the choice of advisors. Typically, separate practices will have their own legal, accounting and benefit manager consultants. The new merged entity is unlikely to need all of them and will need to select which ones to retain or replace. The selection should focus on identifying the best consultants for the combined entity and be made by the new physician leadership and management team.

Managing External Reactions

Fear and uncertainty caused by the merger can influence the outside community. Hospitals, payors, and competitors can become threatened and fearful of the merger causing them to attempt to discredit the merged entity or even attempt to derail it with an antitrust lawsuit. A strategic communication plan including how and when to inform hospitals, payors, and competitors of the impending merger is critical. Some groups may choose to notify other parties in advance of the merger, while some groups have also had success flying under the radar and waiting until the merger is consummated before announcing the new organization. Either approach requires a communication plan for the announcement and promotion of the new entity in a fashion that minimizes threats to impacted parties.

In addition to the hospitals, payors, and competitors the various physician colleagues of each practice can also be fearful of the new merged entity. This may include referring primary care physicians, radiologists, pathologists and radiation oncologists. These relationships also need to be actively managed to emphasize the positive aspects of the practice merger while minimizing the impact the merger may have on other medical colleagues.

It is also important to understand that practice mergers may result in broken long term relationships. These relationships may be with partners, associates, managers, or outside colleagues. Most of these problems can be avoided with positive, proactive communication and explanation. But despite the best efforts some broken relationships may occur. The groups individual physician members need to understand the potential risk, avoid them if possible and accept that the goals and objectives of the merger are most important.

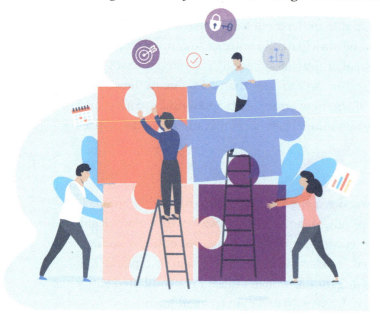

The **Perils and Pitfalls** of practice mergers need to be proactively managed to minimize the negative impact and convert them into opportunities to make the merged practice stronger than any of the original practices. As was emphasized earlier, the goals and objectives need to be significant enough to make the downside aspects worth managing and enduring. Proactive management of these issues will usually allow the merger to achieve success.

SUMMARY

Market forces remain that incentivize large practice formation. The large urology practice has the ability to further develop subspecialty expertise, expand integrated service lines, improve operational efficiencies and provide access to exceptional care and service for a larger number of urology patients. Large urology practices are also better positioned for future pay for value reimbursement plans through their ability to provide comprehensive integrated care. The value of large practices has recently been reinforced by the corporate and private equity acquisition of large urology practices.

Realization of the potential benefits requires attention to many details and continued execution of the business plan after merger closure. Utilization of the **10 Steps to Successful Practice Mergers and Acquisitions** can facilitate the merger process and position the practice for the future. Special attention to the **5 Keys to Success** with emphasis on aligning interests, creating aligned incentives and keeping patients first with a focus on clinical excellence can lead to long-term success and professional gratification for all involved.

KEY POINTS

- **Market forces** remain that incentivize large practice formation. The large urology practice can develop subspecialty expertise, expand integrated service lines, improve operational efficiencies, and provide access to exceptional care and service for a larger number of urology patients.

- **Large urology practices** are also better positioned for future pay-for-value reimbursement plans through their ability to provide comprehensive integrated care.

- **The value of large practices** has recently been reinforced by the corporate and private equity acquisition of large urology practices.

- **Merged practices** should identify clear objectives that define growth goals and problem solving using combined resources.

- **Merger teams** need to address three immediate legal considerations: a confidentiality agreement; an antitrust assessment from outside legal counsel; and the need to secure a name and corporate identity for the merged entity.

- **Practices need** to disclose their financial information for the past several years for review to provide visibility for the merger.

- **Merger teams** need a term sheet for all parties to collectively agree on deal terms, and a common operating agreement needs to be developed by the practice leadership and legal team.

- **Mergers need** to identify a transition team prior to go-live and prepare to consolidate management structure.

- **Practice mergers** can benefit economically and from increased provider manpower and management to improve patient care.

- **Mergers should** be prepared for increased overhead and employee turnover and develop a strategic communication plan that includes how and when to inform hospitals, payers, and competitors of the impending merger.

- **Realization** of the potential benefits requires attention to many details and continued execution of the business plan after merger closure.

- **Utilization** of the 10 Steps to Successful Practice Mergers and Acquisitions can facilitate the merger process and position the practice for the future.

- **Special attention** to the 5 Keys to Success with emphasis on aligning interests, creating aligned incentives, and keeping patients first with a focus on clinical excellence can lead to long-term success and professional gratification for all involved.

ABOUT THE AUTHOR

Peter M. Knapp, MD, FACS

Dr. Peter Knapp is Co-Founder and Past President of Urology of Indiana and is Volunteer Clinical Associate Professor of Urology at Indiana University School of Medicine. He was a founding board member and Past President of LUGPA and Past President of the North Central Section of the AUA. Dr. Knapp has over 30 years of health care experience in medical practice growth, including practice mergers, development of clinical service lines and medical service companies as independent entities and as joint ventures with hospitals, other medical practices and industry partners.

CHAPTER

Private Equity's Increasing Investment Partnerships in Urology
Current State and Key Considerations

Hector M. Torres
Gary W. Herschman
Aaron T. Newman

As the U.S. faces an unprecedented era stemming from the outbreak of COVID-19, we as a nation have been starkly reminded of the critical role health care providers play in the provision of essential services to communities and patients across the country. While many health care providers presently find themselves under immense clinical, operational, and financial pressure, it remains of vital importance for independent physician group leaders to monitor organizational readiness and sustainability in both the current and post-COVID-19 environment.

Despite COVID-19, the urology sector remains an attractive area of investment for private equity because the demand for urological care is at an all-time high, yet the supply of urologists in the U.S. is relatively low. This supply and demand imbalance provides for long-term sustainable growth of urological services within what remains a highly fragmented clinical specialty. With an approximate $1.8 trillion dollars of private equity capital poised and ready to be deployed within the health care services industry, no matter where you stand in the life cycle of your practice, private equity has been, and will continue to be, an increasingly more available option to urology groups. Private equity interest in health care services has been further bolstered by the secular disruption in other industries as a result of COVID-19, contrasted to health care services which, remains a durable and even more essential long-term sector of the economy.

Prior to COVID-19, many independent urology groups were generally considering, or in some instances, actively exploring partnerships with private equity firms to "monetize" the value of their practices, create physician shareholder liquidity, and provide capital for growth. While partnerships among and between urology groups and private equity firms can result in significant benefits, in today's environment, private equity may also serve as an advantageous pathway for independent urology groups to bolster their financial strength and better position themselves to weather the COVID-19 storm. In keeping with the LUGPA mission of preservation, growth, and collaboration of urology practices, in this chapter, we will explore the key trends and considerations of private equity partnerships with urology groups.

Current Climate of the U.S. Physician Group Industry

Over the past several years, M&A transaction activity within the U.S. physician group sector has accelerated in large part due to the proliferation of new market entrants—namely, private equity groups and vertically integrated health care companies. As a result, physician group M&A transactions have been occurring at a rapid pace, with **219** transactions announced in 2019, up **21.7%** from **180** transactions in 2018; and growing at a compounded annual growth rate of approximately **29.6%** since 2014 (see **Figure 1**).

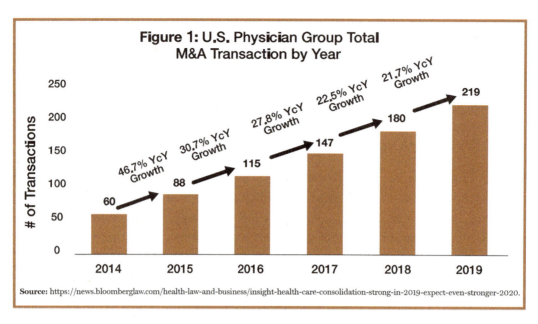

Figure 1: U.S. Physician Group Total M&A Transaction by Year

Source: https://news.bloomberglaw.com/health-law-and-business/insight-health-care-consolidation-strong-in-2019-expect-even-stronger-2020.

Many industry experts believe the immense financial and operational pressures facing independent physician groups as a result COVID-19 will ultimately catalyze increased levels of transaction activity in the second half of 2020, and beyond. Physician group transaction activity is forecasted to increase due to the vast array of operational challenges facing independent practices, as summarized in **Figure 2** below:

Figure 2: Key Operational Challenges Facing Independent Physician Groups
✔ Uncertain reimbursement environment and future regulatory changes
✔ Continued consolidation by new market entrants (i.e. private equity) resulting in larger and more well-capitalized competitors
✔ Acquisition of independent primary care referral sources by local hospitals, regional multispecialty groups and national companies (e.g., Optum) which also employ specialists (including urologists)
✔ Shift from fee-for-service to value-based payment structure and risk programs
✔ Greater need for strategic working capital to invest in information technology, advanced data analytics, EMR and new/expanded ancillary services
✔ Shift from legacy hospital-based/inpatient setting of care to ambulatory/outpatient setting
✔ Lack of liquidity and working capital to fund ongoing clinical and non-clinical practice operations in the COVID-19 environment

Concurrently, private equity's growing interest in the physician group sector stems from an investment thesis driven by themes highlighted in **Figure 3**. Despite the recent economic upheaval, the demand for physician group investments by private equity will remain robust, as most, if not all the core investment thesis elements will remain intact. Conversely, the many secular challenges faced by independent physician groups will be amplified due to diminished, or in some instances temporarily non-existing, clinical revenues resulting from COVID-19's shelter-in-place protocols. These converging factors are projected to sustain, or potentially accelerate the level of private equity investment in physician groups, as independent practices seek a partner to mitigate the core challenges resulting from COVID-19, and strengthen practice infrastructure to more effectively compete in the continually changing landscape.

Figure 3: Drivers of Private Equity Physician Group Investment Thesis

- ✔ Highly fragmented industry ripe for consolidation resulting in opportunity to quickly realize sizeable investment returns from a growth-oriented strategy
- ✔ Supply/demand imbalance from an aging population and associated growing demand for clinical services relative to the number of clinical providers available and/or coming online
- ✔ Growth in health care spending and the associated essential service nature of clinical services result in the sector economic sustainability
- ✔ Shift to outpatient/ambulatory setting of care leading to increased opportunities to participate in high-margin procedures and other ancillary services with strong reimbursement trends

The Anatomy of a Private Equity Partnership

While variability exists from one partnership transaction to another, private equity firms usually seek to acquire a controlling interest in a urology group by essentially "buying out" a majority interest from the existing physician shareholders. As compensation, the firm offers a guaranteed percentage of personal productivity collections to the physician partners. Physician partners often continue to own a minority ownership interest via "roll-over equity" in the partnership investment platform. Thus, they share with the private equity investor in upside value appreciation post-transaction (e.g., upon the investor's eventual "exit"). This typically results in physician shareholders receiving a large upfront tax-advantaged payment (i.e. long-term capital gains), in exchange for yielding control of the operations of their practice, but not the medical or clinical aspects.

There are essentially two types of investments that private equity firms make in physician groups. The first is called a platform investment, and this is typically the firm's initial investment in a large single-specialty independent physician group that has a very well-functioning infrastructure in place. For example, a private equity firm will go out in the market and find a larger, well-operating independent urology group and make that acquisition its first investment in the urology sector. The private equity firm will then use this platform—with a professional business infrastructure (including senior management team, effective revenue cycle, EMR/IT systems, human resources function, managed care expertise, compliance program, etc.)—as the vehicle to make the second type of investment, called a bolt-on, or add-on investment. These usually involve acquisitions of smaller, independent urology practices either in the same geographic region, or elsewhere, which can efficiently and seamlessly benefit from the platform's professional business infrastructure. This general deal structure is unlikely to change in a post-COVID-19 environment, and as previously indicated, may even accelerate as smaller groups seek to partner with well-capitalized and professionally managed organizations.

What Does Private Equity Bring to the Table?

At the highest level, private equity firms provide physician shareholder liquidity, working capital and management expertise to partnerships with urology groups. Many urology groups can greatly benefit from private equity firms by:

- Monetizing the value of the medical practice versus the status quo, which usually means that upon retirement, relocation, death or disability, shareholder physicians receive a nominal payment under their existing buy-sell agreements. Monetization in a private equity partnership includes all three of the following:

  - an initial upfront purchase price based on the "market value" of the practice;

  - a buy-out of physician shareholder rollover equity at fair market value upon retirement (after a certain minimum time period, such as 5 years), disability, etc.; and

  - additional purchase price for all or part of their rollover equity when the investor "exits" via a sale of its interest in the practice

- Helping realize cost savings through the consolidation and optimization of back-office functions and ongoing investment in areas, such as EMR, data analytics, value-based reimbursement programs, and practice infrastructure;

- Providing capital and resources to support growth (new offices and ancillary services), improve infrastructure, and optimally manage the burden of administrative functions.

Strategic Options – The Pros and Cons of Private Equity Partnership

It is of critical importance for independent urology groups operating in today's environment to consider the benefits and potential risks of a private equity partnership. **Figure 4** below provides a framework for urology groups considering their strategic options in relation to a potential private equity partnership.

A partnership with private equity can be appealing option for urology groups, but physicians must also understand the overall goals of private equity. While all the clinical

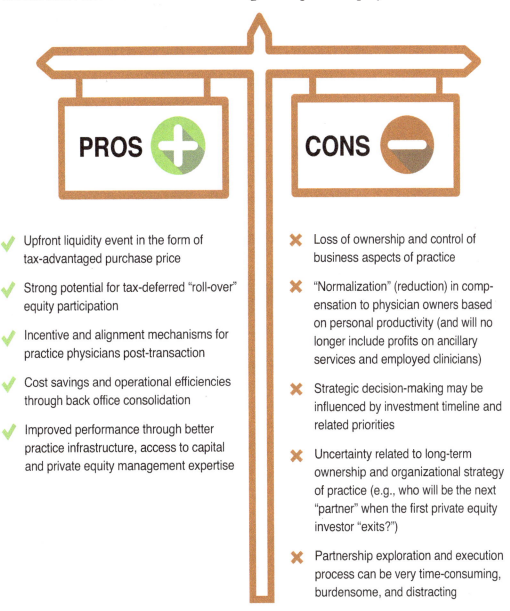

PROS
- Upfront liquidity event in the form of tax-advantaged purchase price
- Strong potential for tax-deferred "roll-over" equity participation
- Incentive and alignment mechanisms for practice physicians post-transaction
- Cost savings and operational efficiencies through back office consolidation
- Improved performance through better practice infrastructure, access to capital and private equity management expertise

CONS
- Loss of ownership and control of business aspects of practice
- "Normalization" (reduction) in compensation to physician owners based on personal productivity (and will no longer include profits on ancillary services and employed clinicians)
- Strategic decision-making may be influenced by investment timeline and related priorities
- Uncertainty related to long-term ownership and organizational strategy of practice (e.g., who will be the next "partner" when the first private equity investor "exits?")
- Partnership exploration and execution process can be very time-consuming, burdensome, and distracting

Figure 4 – Private Equity/Urology Group Partnerships Pros and Cons

aspects of the practice will remain within the sphere of influence of the physicians in a private equity partnership, physicians may have very little influence on the business aspects of the practice. Initiatives such as the streamlining of administrative tasks, pursuit of economies of scale for purchasing, onboarding of new vendors, and installing new leadership teams within the practice are all examples of areas in which private equity will reserve unilateral decision-making.

Further, understanding the transactional nature of private equity is an important consideration. Physicians that enter partnerships with private equity will typically receive a large upfront tax-advantaged purchase price and retain only a minority equity ownership interest in the practice post-transaction. As a result, if the private equity firm is successful and the practice is sold several years later, the physicians will have limited input regarding how and when this secondary transaction is structured and to whom the practice is ultimately sold. Buyers of the practice may include hospitals, health systems, strategic practice consolidator organizations or even another private equity firm, yet the final decision as to whom the practice is sold will be made by the private equity firm.

Lastly, gaining comfort with private equity's motivations for the pursuit of urology group partnerships is paramount. Private equity firms are profit-minded investors that deploy a "bottom line" financial performance approach to the management of their investment in a urology group. Private equity is not as concerned with maintaining access to a clinical specialty or with the pursuit of a charitable mission like a non-profit hospital or health system would be, for example. Private equity firms are typically seeking to rapidly develop scale within a clinical specialty, in order to build a larger, more valuable clinical enterprise which can then later be sold at an outsized profit.

Private Equity Due Diligence of Urology Groups

Urology groups should understand that before a private equity firm invests tens of millions of dollars (or more) in a partnership with a urology group, it will conduct comprehensive—upside down, inside out—due diligence on the group, and will incur an average of $3-4 million on due diligence and other transaction expenses. This extensive diligence is time-consuming and can at times be distracting to the group's physicians and management team. The top 12 areas that a private equity will scrutinize include:

 All financial books and records, and in considering "value," investors will have their accountants assess the practice's "EBITDA" (or free cash flow) on a "GAAP" basis, which entails an extensive process of recasting financial figures from cash basis to accrual basis accounting;

02. Coding, medical record documentation, and billing & collection practices of the group, with a careful eye towards identifying any aggressive billing or coding trends that could later be challenged by Medicare or commercial payors and result in demands for recoupment;

03. Human resources and benefit programs, policies, and procedures to assess any potential employment and benefits-related exposure;

04. Any existing or past governmental or payor investigations and audits;

05. Any existing or prior litigation or disputes (commercial, employment-related, or otherwise) that could result in exposure;

06. Diversity of payor mix, the preference being in-network participation with multiple payors (and non-reliance on any one managed care entity);

07. All professional services agreements that provide revenue to the group (e.g., on call, medical directorships, clinical coverage, etc.), and related federal and state fraud and abuse compliance;

08. All debt and financing arrangements, including capital leases, and the terms of key real estate leases;

09. The group's corporate documents and shareholder and operating agreements reflecting governance, distribution, and buy-sell terms, as well as ownership structure of ASCs and other ancillary services;

10. Employment agreements for clinicians, including compensation and restrictive covenant provisions;

11. The practice's information systems, and any related cybersecurity and HIPAA/privacy breaches; and

12. Whether the group has a robust and documented corporate compliance program.

Urology groups exploring private equity partnerships also need to conduct their own diligence on the private equity firms making partnership proposals (commonly referred to as "reverse diligence"). Investment bankers typically assist groups in this reverse diligence by investigating each investor's prior experience with other physician groups, and its track record of financial success. It is also imperative for a group's physicians to meet (preferably in-person or virtually) with other physicians who have partnered with a particular private equity firm, in order to obtain a first-hand account of what it's like to partner with the investor, whether the firm is viewed as being "physician-friendly," and attain a feel for the overall culture of the investor organization.

Key Protective Provisions for Physicians in Private Equity Agreements

In a partnership transaction with private equity, there are many contractual terms that are important to focus on to protect the interests of physicians both in the short-and long-term. The top 12 contractual protections that are most important include:

1| Structuring the purchase price to maximize long-term capital gains treatment;

2| Other terms that materially impact purchase price, include understanding that most valuations (offers) from investors are based on the "enterprise value" of the entire group not just the percentage being purchased, after (a) paying off all debts, and (b) is subject to having normalized "net working capital" at closing (cash and collectible accounts receivable), and to the extent of deficiency having a corresponding deduction from net proceeds at closing;

3| Whether "tail policies" for professional liability insurance and directors and officer's liability insurance are required at closing, and how the cost is apportioned;

4| Ensuring that the rollover equity component of the purchase price consists of the same class of security as the investor, with customary dilution protections, and with board representation for "platform" and other large groups;

5| Post-closing employment agreements, including the term (e.g., 5 years), the specifics of compensation and bonuses (mostly based on personal productivity), and having fair (and narrow) termination provisions;

6| Reasonable restrictive covenants, including: (a) geographically, preferably based only on a physician's primary office location, or two; (b) customary carve-outs for teaching, consulting, inventions, books, expert witness work, directorships and other outside positions; and (c) a timeframe, which usually is 5 years from the closing (under the purchase agreement), plus during the term of employment and 1-2 years thereafter;

7| Indemnification terms, including how long representations and warranties "survive" beyond the closing, the maximum (or "cap") on exposure, and potentially having the investor obtain "representation & warranty" insurance to substantially limit this potential exposure;

8| How much of the purchase price is "escrowed," which depends on various factors and for how long (usually 12-24 months) to collateralize the indemnity obligations, and staggering the terms of the release of such escrowed funds (e.g., 1/3 every 6 months, etc.);

9| What decisions require consent of the group's "local leader" or relevant physician, such as: hiring new physicians, terminating physicians, opening new offices, changing a physician's primary office, terminating a key office lease, changing clinical protocols, etc.;

10| Triggers for buyouts of a physician's rollover equity, and calculation of the purchase price (which could vary depending on the trigger);

11| The terms pursuant to which senior management (executives) of the group at closing, and current and future associate physicians thereafter, obtain equity in the platform entity; and

12| The management and advisory fees (if any) that the investor is paid at closing, and more importantly, on an ongoing basis for management, entering subsequent add-on transactions, or otherwise.

Key Questions for Urology Groups Considering Private Equity

With the spectrum of private equity options available to urology groups today, physicians should develop guiding principles upon which the merits of a potential partnership can be measured. This approach helps validate whether private equity may be a good fit for your group, defines the characteristics of the optimal partner, and identifies the most important partnership terms.

Key Questions to Consider When Contemplating a Private Equity Partnership Include:

What are my practice's goals and objectives?

Knowing what goals and objectives are most important to you and your physician partners will validate whether private equity is a strong fit. For example: (a) is monetizing the value of physician ownership in the practice important? (b) is the growth of the practice a strategic imperative? and (c) is access to working capital, resources, and related support an absolute necessity for the group's long-term survival and success?

What are the nuances and imperatives related to my specific local/regional market?

Local market trends and priorities inform the need or desire for urology groups to partner with private equity. For instance, a private equity partnership may be the right vehicle to provide the capital needed to achieve: (a) the ability to effectively compete with a large hospital system or multi-specialty group (especially if due to PCP acquisitions, there are less and less independent primary care referral sources in the community);

(b) the need to lower operating costs; and (c) the need for substantial investment to improve practice infrastructure and expand to more effectively compete with other urology groups.

How much non-clinical autonomy is my practice willing to give up?

While physicians who partner with private equity will always continue to have the authority and responsibility to engage in the professional practice of medicine, how willing and to what degree is your practice able to surrender non-clinical and operational control of the practice? Many urologists today want to be freed from the administrative burdens of operating their practice to focus entirely on the delivery of clinical care. Business-related changes, such as consolidation of back-office operations and related infrastructure, are just a few examples of areas in the private equity firm's sphere of influence. Knowing upfront how much non-clinical autonomy your practice can live with is an important factor in the overall suitability of a private equity partnership.

What are the potential risks and areas of exposure within my practice that could impact its value in a possible transaction?

Prior to considering a partnership with private equity, be sure to undertake a thorough review of the operational, financial, clinical, legal, and regulatory aspects of your practice. Any areas of risk or exposure could result in a material negative impact on the valuation of your practice, the structure of the partnership and/or the likelihood of the partnership transaction closing. Taking time up front to ensure your "house is in order" will avoid a reduction in the value of your practice and pay dividends if/when you decide to explore a private equity partnership.

What is the current and future impact of COVID-19 on my practice?

While private equity partnerships with urology groups will remain buoyant, practice leadership teams and physician shareholders alike should prepare to address COVID-19's impact on both historical and projected financial performance, as well as on the overall solvency of the enterprise. While having been severely impacted by the COVID-19 crisis will not necessarily rule out the possibility of a private equity partnership, having undertaken measures, such as securing Federal relief aid funding and rapidly deploying telehealth medicine capabilities are just two examples of important elements that private equity investors will analyze when measuring the strength of your practice. Most importantly, investors will want to understand your practice's ability to recapture lost patient volume and revenue resulting from COVID-19.

Is private equity the right choice for my urology group?

Whether your practice has already been approached by one or more private equity firms, is contemplating a partnership with private equity, or is simply taking note of the increasing level of consolidation within urology, private equity's demand for investments within this clinical specialty will likely increase. The top five factors urology groups should consider when contemplating a private equity partnership include:

01. The importance of "monetizing" the value of historical physician shareholder ownership relative to forgoing non-clinical operational autonomy;

02. Local and regional market risks impacting the practice within the context of the changing reimbursement and regulatory programs, and increasing uncertainty in the post-COVID-19 health care industry environment;

03. The desire to increase the practice's operational performance and efficiency;

04. The need for working capital to invest and support practice infrastructure and growth (including the addition of more physicians, office locations and ancillary services); and

05. The overall cultural fit, track record and urology sector expertise of the potential private equity partner organization.

Before making a conclusion regarding whether private equity is right for your group, thoroughly explore the potential pros and cons based on the specific circumstances and characteristics of your practice. For urology groups with a stated goal of monetizing practice ownership, attaining the benefits of scale and growing the value of the enterprise, private equity will remain an attractive option in 2020 and beyond.

KEY POINTS

- **Despite COVID-19,** the urology sector remains an attractive area of investment for private equity because the demand for urological care is at an all-time high, yet the supply of urologists in the U.S. is relatively low.

- **Many industry experts** believe the immense financial and operational pressures facing independent physician groups as a result COVID-19 will catalyze increased levels of transaction activity in the second half of 2020, and beyond.

- **Private equity firms** usually seek to acquire a controlling interest in a urology group by "buying out" a majority ownership interest from the existing physician shareholders, who are guaranteed a percentage of personal productivity collections to the physician partners.

- **Private equity investment** in urology groups will be further supported by growth in the number of private equity firms seeking to invest capital within the clinical specialty.

- **At the highest level,** private equity firms bring physician shareholder liquidity, working capital and management expertise to partnerships with urology groups.

- **Cons to private equity** partnerships include loss of ownership and control of business aspects of practice and reduction in compensation to physician owners based on personal productivity.

- **Before a private equity** firm invests tens of millions of dollars to partner with a urology group, it will conduct comprehensive due diligence on the group, and will incur an average of $3-4 million on due diligence and other transaction expenses.

- **Urology groups exploring** potential private equity partnerships also need to conduct their own diligence on the private equity firms making partnership proposals (commonly referred to as "reverse diligence").

- **In a partnership transaction** with private equity, there are many contractual terms that are important to focus on in order to protect the interests of physicians both in the short- and long-term.

- **Prior to considering** a partnership with private equity, be sure to undertake a thorough review of the operational, financial, clinical, legal and regulatory aspects of your practice so you are aware of any potential areas of risk or liability.

ABOUT THE AUTHORS

Hector M. Torres, *Managing Director*
Health Care Investment Banking FocalPoint Partners, LLC

Hector M. Torres is a Managing Director and co-leader of the Health Care Investment Banking practice of FocalPoint Partners, LLC, a leading global investment banking and financial advisory services firm with offices in Los Angeles, Chicago, New York and Shanghai. With over 15 years of experience providing investment banking and financial advisory services to health care organizations nationwide, he has completed more than 25 M&A transactions with a cumulative value of more than $2.8 billion in the last six years alone. Most recently, Hector served as sell-side M&A adviser to Arizona Urology Specialists in its private equity partnership transaction with United Urology and Audax Group Private Equity. His clients include large physician practices and groups, national and multi-regional health systems, academic medical centers, health insurers, non-acute care providers, medical device companies and capital providers to health care entities.

Gary W. Herschman. *Member*
Health Care and Life Sciences Practice Epstein, Becker & Green, P.C.

Gary W. Herschman is a member of Epstein, Becker & Green, P.C.'s Health Care and Life Sciences practice, and serves on the firm's Board of Directors in addition to its National Health Care and Life Sciences Steering Committee. Gary is a health care attorney who focuses on mergers and acquisitions and other strategic transactions. This primarily includes advising physician groups (including urology groups and many other specialty practices) across the country on private equity partnerships, consolidations, merger and affiliations, as well as JVs, hospital-physician alignment, PSAs, Co-management, clinically integrated networks, ACOs, MSOs, IPAs, PHOs, and population health contracts. Gary also advises health care clients on regulatory compliance (federal and state), Stark, fraud and abuse, corporate compliance, HIPAA, government investigations, and civil and administrative health care litigation.

Aaron Newman, *Vice President*
Health Care Investment Banking FocalPoint Partners, LLC

Aaron Newman is a Vice President in the Health Care Investment Banking practice of FocalPoint Partners, LLC, a leading global investment banking and financial advisory firm with offices in Los Angeles, Chicago, New York and Shanghai. Aaron has more than a decade of experience in health care investment banking, debt capital markets and strategic advisory. Most recently, Aaron served as sell-side M&A adviser to Arizona Urology Specialists in its private equity partnership transaction with United Urology and Audax Group Private Equity. He specializes in the health care provider services sector, advising hospitals, health systems, physician practices and other provider entities on mergers, acquisitions and strategic advisory assignments.

CHAPTER 7

Electronic Health Records 2020 and Beyond

Robert Di Loreto, MD

The business of healthcare depends on exploiting medical providers. "Corporate medicine has milked all of the efficiency it can out of the system. With corporate mergers and streamlining, it has pushed the productivity numbers about as far as they can go. One resource that seems endless—and free—is the professional ethic of medical staff members. This ethic holds the entire system together. If doctors and nurses clocked out when their paid hours were finished, the effects on patients would be calamitous. Doctors and nurses know this, which is why they don't shirk. The system knows it too and takes advantage. By far the biggest culprit of the mushrooming workload is the electronic medical record, or EMR. It has burrowed its tentacles into every aspect of the health care system."[1]

Roughly 50% of total time spent per each patient encounter is taken up by completing the electronic chart. Other studies have shown that doctors spend 27% of their workday on direct clinical facetime with patients and 49% of their office day on EHR's and other desk work and to put it in even simpler perspectives, another analysis showed that "For every one hour spent with patients, doctors spend two hours in record keeping—which included afterhours time spent completing charts."[2,3,4] Similarly, administrator's ability to access quality data and analysis persists with documentation requirements for MACRA/MPS and APM programs. IT costs have not gone down and requirements for cybersecurity systems and HIPPA protection of IT systems is increasing. Most systems do not have fully integrated clinical protocol or pathway management tools that provide real-time management of disease states for practitioners as well as their patients that are mandated for care. Interoperability with shared patient data also remains an ongoing problem despite current CMS rules.

The HITECH act of 2009,[5] which budgeted over $60 billion to promote the adoption of health information technology and create a nationwide network of Electronic Health Records (EHR's). Most physicians recognize certain benefits including; remote access to the medical record, legible documentation, medication interaction checking, faster access to lab and imaging reports and (with some systems) a comprehensive time-line visualization of the patient's chart.

Key EHR complaints hinge upon:
- Poor workflow
- Too many clicks with slow response times
- System crashes
- Overload of physician-driven data entry
- Reduced face-to-face time with patients
- Overwhelming in-box load
- Prior Authorizations

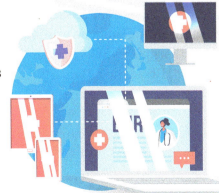

- Concurrent use of multiple hospital and private practice setting EHR's requiring different login/password settings—few of which interact with each other
- Afterhours time spent to complete records
- Lack of end-user feedback to vendor for improvements

Private practice Urologists generally have no control the selection process for hospital-based systems (which tend to be more hospital, primary care and corporate finance driven). Many physicians, unhappy with the EHR process, may not remember that certain areas (CCHPI, PE, ROS) have specific billing documentation rules courtesy of HCFA 1995/1997 E&M coding rules.[6] On a very high level, historic EHR coding is based on additive "bullet" points captured within a mandated number of required documentation areas. Other areas (Past Medical History, Past Family Social History, Past Surgical History, Medications, Allergies, reviewing documents/labs, referral letters, portal, patient access to note, etc.) are also required to be completed (or at least "touched") for maximum billing. CMS updates for 2021 may eliminate some of the original requirements but may create new EHR Coding issues.[7] Other rules (MACRA/MIPS)[8] as well as local insurance/healthcare demands can also mandate further documentation requirements with:

- Care-pathway/protocol adherence
- Patient Satisfaction Scores
- Coordination of Care
- Patient Engagement
- Patient Safety Measurements
- Public Health and clinical data registries reporting
- Ongoing PQRS/CQM – type reporting measures

EHR technology is advancing to automate some of the laborious input processes, but regardless the physician will always remain responsible for complete accurate documentation and appropriate billing codes.

This chapter will identify important areas in EHR and IT that large groups should be aware and have some basic knowledge of, particularly when considering a new EHR platform or upgrading an existing one. The following information will hopefully present some thoughts as well as suggestive measures for dealing with issues related to office based EHR's in the future.

Usability and Ongoing Issues

The lead statement from April 2019 in Fortune Magazine "Death by a Thousand Clicks"[9] below summarizes issues all medical practitioners are facing:

> "The U.S. government claimed that turning American medical charts into electronic records would make health care better, safer, and cheaper. Ten years and $36 billion later, the system in an unholy mess."

The basis of this article was, in summary, a patient in Vermont was seen by a local PCP circa 2012 for headaches different from previous migraines. The PCP suspected an aneurysm. Head CT was ordered through the clinics software system eClinicalWorks (eCW) but never transmitted. The patient died within two months. Upon investigation, eCW had "a dossier of troubling reports", Better Business Bureau complaints, and legal cases around the country. Forensic evaluation revealed multiple coding/performance issues, unbeknownst to physicians, that impacted patient care. The U.S. government sued eCW and was awarded a $155 million settlement that never went to a jury. Interesting kicker to entire case was "The U.S. government bankrolled the adoption of this software—and continues to pay for it." Or, as quoted in the article, "we should say: You do!"[9]

The beginning of this was the American Recovery and Reinvestment Act of February 2009,[10] signed by President Obama, which included a stimulus for electronic health records. The HITECH Act, of 2009[11] further moved more medical providers into EHR's using a stimulus package promoting adoption that rules that followed government "meaningful users" certification. Similarly, EHR vendors built systems to follow these rules—which primarily focused on billing documentation. Currently, 96% of hospitals and 85% of office-based physicians have "adopted" EHR's. Products remain clumsy, are not intuitive, don't talk to one another and force providers to spend more time entering data than taking care of patients. Numerous other medical legal cases were also investigated by Fortune were tied to software problems, user errors, corporate secrecy, gag clauses and hospital attempts withhold records. EHR safety projects, looking at usability and patient matching, have been shown in some systems to be accurate only 50% of time.[9] In April 2008, CMS renamed the EHR Incentive Program to "Promoting Interoperability" along with the associated initiatives of, "MyHealthEData" and "Patients over Paperwork", to promote patient data access.[12]

Physician Burnout

This is a major issue and felt to be a direct result of EHR Implementation. EHR training (or lack thereof) has been cited as a major factor in user satisfaction.[13] Studies have shown that "repetitive box ticking, and the endless searching on pull down menus create a cognitive burden that's wearing out todays physicians—driving increasing numbers into early retirement."[14] It has been shown that doctors spend 5.9 hours average time on EHR's (out of an 11.4 hour workday), compared to 5.1 hours spent with patients.[15] Merritt Hawkins, in 2018, found a staggering 78% of doctors suffered symptoms of burnout.[9] Increased in-box messages, particularly those EHR generated, have shown to be a factor in increased provider dissatisfaction and burnout.[16] Outdated regulatory requirements are also felt to be

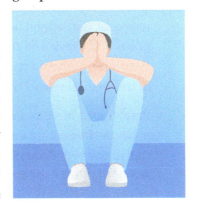

key to physician burnout. "A U.S. physician is a 'Data-entry' clerk, and typically needs to document diagnoses, orders, patient visit notes, and an increasing amount of low-value administrative data"[17] "The world we live in now, one where physician burnout gets worse every year and, by many estimates, is the new normal. That new normal is cyclical, and it goes something like this."[18]

- Increasing workload leads to burnout
- Physician burnout leads to poor patient outcomes and decreased profits
- Poor patient outcomes and decreased profits lead to increased workloads
- Increased physician workloads to to physician burnout
- Repeat ad nauseum

"What healthcare needs is innovation that subtracts steps from its weight. What is needed in the health tech world is something that reduces the menial tasks standing between physicians and the extremely meaningful work they do for patients."[18] Potential changes in CMS 2021 E&M coding rules MAY assist in this.[19]

EHR Documentation and New CPT Rules

The following is a very simple and strategic summary of current rules with explanation and strategy for implementation from the PYA group that all should consider.[22] The 2020 Medicare Physician Fee Schedule includes new documentation guidelines for office and outpatient-based evaluation and management (E/M) services effective January 1, 2019. The Final Rule also details a new payment methodology for E/M services effective January 1, 2021.

As part of its "Patients Over Paperwork" initiative,[23] the Centers for Medicare & Medicaid Services has sought input from physicians and other stakeholders on how to reduce the documentation burden associated with E/M services. With the new guidelines, CMS is simplifying documentation in two ways:

- When relevant information is already contained in the medical record, practitioners may choose to focus their documentation on what has changed since the last visit, or on pertinent items that have not changed, and need not re-record the defined list of required elements if there is evidence that the practitioner reviewed the previous information and updated it as needed. Practitioners should still review prior data, update as necessary, and indicate in the medical record that they have done so.

- Practitioners need not re-enter in the medical record information on the patient's chief complaint and history that has already been entered by ancillary staff or the beneficiary. The practitioner may simply indicate in the medical record that he or she reviewed and verified this information.

New and established office or outpatient visit codes 99202-99215 would eliminate history and examination as key components to select the E/M service level. Additional E/M documentation changes include the deletion of level one new outpatient visit code 99201, and revisions to codes for prolonged services with or without patient contact. History and exam are required, but not scored. The approved revisions to 99202-99215 require that a medically appropriate history and examination be performed: beyond this requirement, the history and exam do not effect coding. Instead, the E/M service level is chosen either by the level of medical decision making (MDM) performed, or by the total time spent performing the service on the day of the encounter.

Obviously new guidelines should require less documentation and would be easy to implement. However, the documentation structure in current electronic health records (EHRs) was developed based on 1995 and 1997 E/M guidelines.[24] Specifically, EHR templates are commonly designed to anticipate and populate the history and exam normal findings, as related to elements that are nearly always addressed. The physician then revises the findings to reflect any presenting abnormality. The provider's documented update and reference to prior history or exam must meet, in total, the history and exam elements required for the code level billed.

Some systems have moved away from date stamping every entry in the record as a visible documentation element on the legal record. As such, it may not be clear whether the physician cut and pasted the exam into the record from the prior visit or if he or she generated the documentation on that date of service. An additional statement may be needed to clarify this point.

CMS' new guidelines state that the provider can reference previous information and document an update from the last visit. There are at least two ways a provider can accomplish this:

- Use a free-form text field to reference relevant previous-visit documentation by date.

Example: "I have reviewed the history and exam documented in the previous visit note dated 1/5/2019, which are incorporated into today's note except for changes as documented below."

- Document the history and exam update in free-form text fields, unless documentation elements can be populated without normal findings automatically populating (e.g., review of systems or exam elements—constitutional, eyes, etc).

Under the new rule, a provider must reference a prior note that either:

- Was documented with the required elements for a given level of service.
- Further references a note containing required elements.
- Lists multiple visit dates which are relevant and account for the required elements.

For example, a provider could document an initial visit according to the 1995 or 1997 guidelines, and, then, the subsequent note could reference the history or exam previously documented and provide an update to meet a given level of service. EHR templates will need to allow for full documentation according to the 1995 or 1997 guidelines, as well as the ability to both reference the previous note and document an update.

CMS E/M Documentation Guidelines Implementation Checklist

As noted, there are numerous considerations that must go into determining whether the reduced documentation guidelines are a fit for your organization. The following checklist delineates a number of items to be considered, understanding that each requires additional analysis.

- Maintain 1995 or 1997 Documentation Guideline-based templates.
- Determine if CMS' new guidelines are a reasonable option for your providers.
- Create templates that allow for references with entry points for the date of the previous visit as well as updates.
- Determine if your EHR will allow providers to toggle between CMS' reduced documentation and other guidelines.
- Create policies and procedures representing your facility's interpretation of the guidelines.
- Train providers and perform periodic documentation reviews to monitor compliance.[22]

Interoperability

The ability of healthcare software systems "share" information, or Interoperability, is critical for patient care and remains an ongoing source of frustration for patients and providers.[25] Passage of the Health Information Technology for Economic and Clinical Health (HITECH) Act in 2009[11] and American Recovery and Reinvestment Act (ARRA) in 2009—both Acts forced healthcare providers to switch from paper to electronic health records.[26] The Medicare Access and CHIP Reauthorization Act (MACRA) of 2015 created a federal definition and metrics to measure national interoperability, specifically the electronic sending, receiving, finding, and integrating health information from outside sources AND using electronic information from outside sources in clinical decision making.[27] Sixty two percent of physicians surveyed have complained that the inability of technological platforms to connect with each other and share information is a major issue, both in 2016 and 2018.[29] Problems exist with Health Systems where different parts of the organization are on different EHR platforms, multiple other clinical systems and devices needing connection. Private practice physicians have similar local issues complicated by the need to interact with Health Systems simultaneously.

Government-controlled agencies have similar problems—where Medicare, Medicaid, VA and DOD records often do not communicate.[30, 31] On August 2, 2019 CMS published the Fiscal Year 2020 Medicare Hospital Inpatient Prospective Payment System (IPPS) Final Rule which included program requirements for Calendar Year 2020.[32] In this final rule, CMS continued its advancement of CEHRT utilization, focusing on burden reduction, and improving interoperability and patient access to health information. CMS is looking at penalizing and publishing nonparticipating software and Health Systems.[33] The Electronic Health Record Association has commented that "As written, the proposed rule would discourage innovation by imposing limitations on profit as well as compulsory licensing terms for new intellectual property, created through extensive investment in development." "Clearly this would have a chilling effect on innovation."[34] Time will only tell when this issue is resolved and we, the providers and our patients, will actually see open, shared patient records.

A relatively new technology, Fast Healthcare Interoperability Resources (FHIR) - pronounced FIRE—appears to have the ability to take information from disparate systems into Health Information Exchanges (HIE) and share with all participating software systems.[35] All of this is dependent on software vendors to have the ability to share information (which is mandated in the 2015 CERHT certification for EHR's.[36] "Information Blocking" between EHR systems as well as Health Care Systems remains an issue and is being looked at by CMS with potential penalties to software vendors or organizations.[37]

Choosing a System

Many urology groups have adjusted to the changes in healthcare and technology by upgrading their EHR two to three times over the past decade. Currently, LUGPA practices are using the following systems.

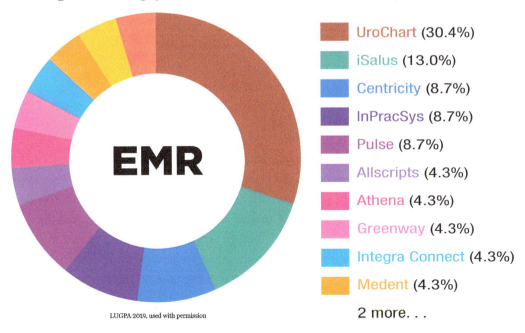

LUGPA 2019, used with permission

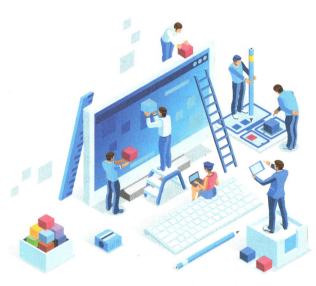

Outside EHR reviews can be of assistance but generally are primary care based and not Urology specific and often incorporate hospital-based systems in their reviews.[41,42] Past experiences, both positive and negative, should be transparently discussed with potential new vendors to determine if moving forward with a new product is a timely and reasonable choice. EHR company history, client volume, reputation, longevity, technology support, platform upgradability, colleague referral and product review are important components to consider in making a sound decision-making process. EHR demonstrations with a quick overview "on the fly" or in passing with limited patient information will often not translate to a large practice with thousands of historical charts and could be an opportunity for disaster. Multiple demonstrations and pilots may need to occur within a variety of pods or divisions for staff to provide collective input into the decision-making process. Final demonstrations need to be done in conjunction with a fully loaded program which should include real-time internet load testing, with simultaneous multiple users in different locations. Roles (physicians, medical assistants, check in/out staff, etc.) should be concurrently tested while IT support monitors system bandwidth requirements and system load comprehensively. The load of each additive user device on the access network can impact how the system performs and could require additional costly upgrades to current internet connections. Many vendors tout "any device, anywhere, anytime" use—without taking into consideration the impact of local Wi-Fi and internet connections, obvious increased bandwidth costs, the program or database capabilities the EHR is actually written on and, ultimately, the number of simultaneous users which can considerably slow down data transfer. Existing software; billing or lab systems, email, medical devices, etc. as well as staff browser use (including "Pandora®" type programs and video streaming) can additionally overload bandwidth circuits or even software resulting in poor performance.

The most distressing areas to busy physicians are the number of "clicks", flexibility of use, ease of data entry and screen to screen workflow which may be slow or at times redundant/nonsensical. This can create work and charting long after the office ends—particularly with future requirements. Current practice standards and workflows as well as customization opportunities also need to be considered in a comprehensive, strategic way. Many physicians do not realize that non-structured data entry (free form text, custom procedure or worksheets, generalized plan notes, PDFs, scanned imaging reports and information) can defeat the ability of the EHR product and practice to code appropriate billing levels and facilitate clinical decision making. This type of data, although often reviewed and/or utilized at the time of visit, typically has no bearing on the coding chosen as calculated by EHR products. This data often resides in large files and the ability to search and analyze, or share can be difficult unless proper additional software is employed. Given CMS's moves to Valued Based Medicine care, capturing this data has become very important and the EHR. System choice (upgrade or improvements) should consider Value Based Medicine factors including, but not limited to the ability to add as well as manage Clinical Guidelines and Pathways, manage Clinical Guideline and Pathway adherence with practitioners, track clinical outcome and costing data, report (hopefully on a near real-time basis) aberrations in care with the ability to factor in practice costing data to disease state management.

The ability of EHR programs to allow multiple users to access the system at the same time is critical to daily office operations. Physicians, nurses and staff need to be able to access the same chart simultaneously. That capability should be a standard function of any platform EHR. Use of support staff such as scribes or medical assistants (either on site or remote) accessing the same chart can lead to speedier documentation and can facilitate office throughput. Studies have shown that scribes allow an increased number of patients to be seen. Some medical providers and patients find this process uncomfortable as well as costly to the practice. Given the fact that some documentation may be structured (drill down answers in the EHR) as well as free text comments, issues may occur when physicians fail to review all data inputted that may be incorrect.[43][44][45]

Throughout the system decision process, attention needs to be paid to vendor support structure and access. Superuser's and/or key staff at busy office locations need to be trained at the practice level to handle routine or day-to-day issues—backed up by an in-house team of EHR/IT support staff with subsequent vendor support. Lack of real-time multi-level vendor support access or failure to provide (and correct) information regarding known bugs or technology defects to all users in a timely manner is critical. Vendors often provide stock answers such as "we have never seen this before" or "you are the only ones having this problem. These are untenable and should be supplanted with a solution-oriented feedback and a timely correction/ressolution process.

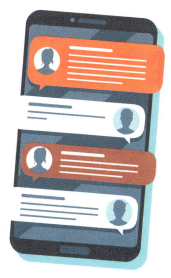

Formation of an ad-hoc user group (of multiple practices using the same program) that has regular internal dialogue as well as vendor input into changes and improvements into system should mandatory. This can be structured contractually with the vendor and/or easily implemented by having IT staff set up a "Google Groups" like messaging system/blog for real-time interaction amongst the participants (both internal and external to the practice) to share ideas, problems and solutions.[46] Key players from this group can act as intermediaries between the software users and vendor. The ideal situation would be regularly scheduled meetings, either face to face or web based, with a software company that was willing to "listen" to its users and move forward with appropriate suggestions to correct issues or improve functionality in a timely fashion.

Implementation strategy and training, once selection has been made, are critical to success. Having an internal team of a project manager(s), physician champions, nursing support staff, EHR analytics as well as in-house IT staff to analyze, as well as optimize, the software product and practice workflows is necessary. This same team, along with vendor trainers, should be used to roll out the training to all offices and staff. Additionally, the same team should institute periodic follow-up meetings with each office (both physicians and staff members). Many practices have used Agile project management sprint techniques in this process with great success.[47] Similarly EHR optimization with internal team participation and ongoing onsite "clinics" that include workflow improvement has shown can mitigate later issues. Analysis of administration burnout, EHR satisfaction, teamwork, and provider burnout was during the process. "After participating in sprint, 44% of clinicians indicated that the number of hours spent charting in the EHR had reduced. After sprint, more clinicians reported that the clinic team was working well together, providing excellent care, and that their use of the EHR had improved."[48] Of paramount importance is the ability of current or potentially new systems to meet current documentation rules.[49]

Data Analytics and Value Based Care

How documentation is done within an EHR has enormous impact in its usability from a data analytics standpoint. Data entered directly into specifically designed and mapped fields e.g. drop-down choices, prelabeled exam points or medication list selection would be considered discrete data and can fall short for more complex data capture needs. Free text notes, call logs, videos, Xray images or dictated and report summaries are examples of unstructured data.

Natural Language Processing (NLP) is a rapidly developing area of machine learning that can help to solve the unstructured data problem. NLP tools can identify key syntactic structures in free text and extract the meaning behind the narrative. The results can be used to generate new documents, like a clinical visit summary, or can be translated into codes for billing purposes. NLP is also used in speech recognition software to allow providers to dictate clinical notes that can be turned into text documents or mapped to standardized data elements for documentation and coding.[54] Optical character recognition (OCR) software can supplement the standardization process by turning static images, like PDFs or paper documents, into machine-readable text.[55] Eventually, the untapped wealth of information in images, audio, video, narrative text, environmental data, and other unstructured datasets, along with structured EHR data, will be able to feed AI programs that could provide critical insights into current and preventative patient care health management.

Security and Liability

In early 2019, two Michigan ENT providers were the first known physicians that closed their practice after a ransomware attack that encrypted their EHR and made it unusable. Rather than pay the ransom, they chose to retire and close their practice. Personal Health Information (PHI) hacking remains a huge issue for medical practices and health care institutions. 2017 studies from AMA and Accenture revealed that 87% of U.S. Physicians have experienced some form of a cybersecurity attack, with phishing cited by more than half (55%) of physicians who experienced an attack. In the first half of calendar 2018, there were 32 million patient records breached as compared to 15 million for the full 2018 year. 72% of these incidents were within the provider setting and caused by insider error, while roughly 10% were secondary to business associate issues. The bulk of these incidents were the result of hacking secondary to phishing and malware. "This data reinforces the need for health systems to build privacy programs that review 100% of accesses to patient data in order to prevent these breaches from occurring saving organization and patients post-breach costs"[61]

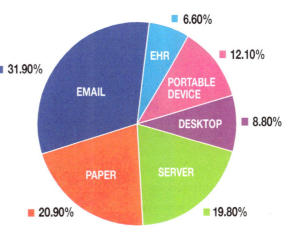

Record Breach Sources 2018

Multilevel internet security is needed in response to multinational hacking news reports.[62, 63] EHR (and respective embedded programs) will require security systems in place to meet existing CMS/HIPPA requirements and should be outlined in the original contract particularly since the Cloud software servers will be off-site.[64] In addition local networks and programs (email, browsers, internal program and external Health Information Exchange connections) need to be secured in order to meet these same standards. For the last several years, email has been the most likely cause of a healthcare cyber breach. These email incidents include phishing attacks, unauthorized email access, and misdirected emails.

EHR involvement had the least frequency of breaches of all practice sources in 2018, with Email being the largest.[65] Regular monitoring and updates are needed to be performed on both systems and local internet access restrictions for staff may need to be put in place to minimized risk. Policies, procedures and documentation requirements need to be in place as required by HIPPA.[67] Additionally, per CMS rules, "A covered entity must periodically review and update its documentation in response to environmental or organizational changes that affect the security of electronic protected health information."[68]

Staff training to open only recognized email messages and attachments is critical. Today, an additional "cyber-security" insurance policy is imperative. Many malpractice insurances have some cyber-attack coverage. Recommended separate cyber insurance policies should be (at a minimum):

- 1 million dollars for forensic/legal/recovery and downtime coverage
- 3 million is recommended for any patient liabilities, HHS penalties for failure to be up to date, and further legal costs that could potentially result in a class action lawsuit

As an aside, and related to PHI liability, is the issue of medical software companies accessing patient data—sometimes known to the practice, sometimes not. Many vendors, through their contractual process, "use" clinical information that is sold to research companies. The practice can only assume the data is de-identified (no PHI). If an EHR vendor inadvertently shares PHI info on a practice's patient, it is possible that the practice may end up as a party to a claim against the vendor. One must make sure all Business Associate's cover these issues and internal legal contractual review has occurred before signing contracts.

In addition, a practice may also be liable if the EHR software "fails" is some manner and mixes different patient information on different charts resulting in a malpractice action.[69] Sophisticated and updated firewalls that function real-time are required. Careful use of the internet and accepted sites should be monitored and regulated by the in-house IT team. It is recommended that as part of an internal IT team, there is a designated security officer. That individual would be responsible for monitoring abnormal activity on the network, unusual website activity and assuring that security measures are in accordance with CMS/HIPPA guidelines. In the event of a cyber-attack, the group should immediately contact FBI, local authorities, insurance carries, and initiate contact with the cyber policy providers.

There are some simple steps a practice can do to improve your security stance.[70]

➡ **Inventory assets:**
- Determine all software and hardware connected to your network as well as status of upgrades particularly related to security issues.

➡ **Secure Mobile Devices:**
- Many practices do have e-mail policies related to in-house e-mail but not specific to mobile devices which have more potential for loss.

- **Strengthen passwords:**
  - Often practices allow employees to share the same password for every login. Passwords should be 8 – 10 characters long and contain a mix of upper/lower-case letters, numbers and symbols.

- **Focus on staff education and training:**
  - Medical professionals and office staff benefit from regular training on good security and privacy practices. Train them to recognize malware and what to do if downloaded. Don't forward messages to everyone in practice.

- **Use encryption and get rid of outdated software:**
  - All devices and hardware should be encrypted. Often times outdated software, no longer supported by vendors, is still in use and no longer being updated.

- **Use a commercial grade firewall:**
  - Allowing entire internet traffic to be filtered for blacklisted attacks and, as well, allow network administrators to customize specific security protocols regarding web-browsing and e-mail communications.

- **Keep up with patching:**
  - Make sure ALL software, including medical devices, is updated on regular basis either monthly or on an automated basis.

- **Review contracts with IT service providers:**
  - Both internal IT support and their job responsibilities as well as managed service providers (MSP) and contractual responsibilities.

Thoughts moving forward and opportunities:

Outside Influences in Medicine: Newer mechanisms of data input beyond the "Dragon-like" systems may ease physicians' burden. The big 4 Tech Companies - Amazon, Google, Apple, et al.—are all entering the health care arena with spinoff businesses as well as products like "Transcribe Medical", "Alexa" which may significantly change EHR workflows. Their ability to leverage developmental abilities, financial, metadata analysis and Artificial Intelligence (AI)[71] may likely expedite data input and merge disparate healthcare databases as well as clinical decision making and research capabilities.[72,73,74] Additionally, collaborative relationships with other large businesses (e.g. Berkshire Hathaway) as well as their current employee and consumer base with their own EHR's will likely drive significant changes in both healthcare insurances, delivery and physician involvement.[75] Some reviews refute this and "suggest that Google and Apple stand to make a lot of money on health-related products and services. But none of their recent acquisitions or consumer plays will make a substantial impact where it matters most: On the quality and cost of U.S. healthcare." Reasons included the following:[76]

- Consumer Preferences Are Different Than Medical Needs
- No Major Tech Company Is Willing to Accept Medical Liability
- Tech Companies Will Face Major Data-Ownership Issues Ahead

Potential future relationships with business owners, insurance providers, third party administrators (TPA), large scale specialty based quality physician providers, and coordinated care managers using collaborative data with Clinical Guidelines may perhaps further move the needle towards better patient care, lower costs (to both patients and employers) and reduce the burden on providers.[77]

Clinical Cost Accounting: For years, this has been the holy grail for large hospital systems and has been one of the tools used to succeed.[78] There are limited opportunities for private practices. Consolidation of private practice groups, like LUGPA, should have the same ability to provide similar analysis. Data from practice EHR's, billing systems and general accounting, often which are in disparate systems, need to be accessible to a central data repository allowing clinical cost accounting with Adhoc reporting.[79] Information based on high level Relative Value Unit (RVU) data with averaged costs (general overhead, equipment, drug, staff, disposable, etc. costs) does not allow specific disease or guideline analysis, nor does it account for specific physician variability. Development of data outcome models based on specific ICD-10 and CPT analysis, coupled with clinical information and patient satisfaction scores would allow practices to view Clinical Costing, Outcome and Guideline adherence analysis on an almost real-time basis—critical for Value Based Medicine performance.[80]

Care Management: The Holy Grail moving forward today, is an intuitive single platform EHR that allows care management. Existing attempts generally are patchwork. Here's what typically happens in a typical care management workflow: a long-suffering

> - Causes a "Swiss Cheese Effect" (In an Excel-driven runaround, key information gets lost—especially information about a patient's risks and needs).
> - Impedes the ability to aggregate, analyze, and improve results.
> - Wastes valuable staff time.
> - Delays patient entry into the appropriate care management program.
> - Prevents staff from functioning at the top of their license.
> - Causes confusion (multiple emails and multiple staff reaching out to the patient—each representing a program-centric, not patient-centric, approach).
> - Prevents/delays the development of additional care management programs and patient populations."[91, 92, 93]

data analyst (or small team of analysts) consolidates multiple payer lists and targeted reports into one master spreadsheet, reconciles duplicates, performs Excel wizardry to reconcile formatting differences, matches the patient to an EMR or creates an EMR, and then emails patient list spreadsheets to care managers. After the patients are added (or declined) to the program, the data analyst must then manage the process of recording each patient's care management status back to the payer and capturing the activities needed to monitor and report on program performance resulting in the following;

In the Value Based Medicine world, this becomes an exercise in futility unless the EHR has the capabilities of incorporating Clinical Guidelines and Protocols with single platform documentation and interaction abilities between care providers, case managers as well as patients. Few, if any, EHR's have this capability at present. Ideally, the care coordinator would have the capability of interacting with multiple practices simultaneously as well as accessing insurance benefit data, TPA billing data, personal patient monitoring devices (ex, Blood Pressure, ECG, etc.) to be able to provide the best and most real-time longitudinal patient care.

Summary

EHR's are not going away. Changes in the healthcare world will probably alter the historic relationships between physicians, insurance companies and healthcare entities. Newer technologies and processes may ease the data entry burden, "assist" medical providers in complex decision making and potentially offer ongoing revenue streams. Hopefully the overall endpoint will be better patient care and a less stressful time for providers.

EHR 2020 and Beyond - Bibliography:

1. https://www.nytimes.com/2019/06/08/opinion/sunday/hospitals-doctors-nurses-burnout.html
2. https://www.healthcareitnews.com/news/ehrs-steal-primary-care-doctors-face-time-patients-study-finds
3. https://www.jwatch.org/fw111995/2016/09/06/half-physician-time-spent-ehrs-and-paperwork
4. https://www.healio.com/primary-care/practice-management/news/online/%7B063320c8-6954-45b8-89dc-3b293772d441%7D/physicians-spend-nearly-50-of-their-time-on-ehr-desk-work
5. http://www.hhs.gov/hipaa/for-professionals/special-topics/HITECH-act-enforcement-interim-final-rule/index.html
6. https://www.cms.gov/Outreoach-and-Education/Medicare-Learning-Network-MLN/MLNProducts/MLN-Publications-Items/CMS1243514.html
7. http://www.hhs.gov/hipaa/for-professionals/special-topics/HITECH-act-enforcement-interim-final-rule/index.html
8. http://www.hhs.gov/hipaa/for-professionals/special-topics/HITECH-act-enforcement-interim-final-rule/index.htm
9. https://khn.org/news/death-by-a-thousand-clicks/
10. https://en.wikipedia.org/wiki/American_Recovery_and_Reinvestment_Act_of_2009
11. https://www.asha.org/Practice/reimbursement/hipaa/HITECH-Act/
12. https://ehrintelligence.com/features/setting-the-stage-for-value-based-care-with-patient-data-access
13. https://ehrintelligence.com/news/ehr-training-cited-as-top-predictor-of-ehr-user-satisfaction
14. https://www.healthaffairs.org/doi/full/10.1377/hlthaff.2018.0699
15. https://journals.stfm.org/familymedicine/2018/february/young-2017-0121/
16. https://ehrintelligence.com/news/ehr-generated-inbox-messages-may-increase-physician-burnout
17. https://ehrintelligence.com/news/outdated-regulatory-requirements-key-physician-burnout-cause
18. https://www.idigitalhealth.com/news/health-tech-must-focus-on-subtracting-steps-from-physician-workflow
19. https://www.ama-assn.org/system/files/2019-03/february-2019-summary-panel-actions_0.pdf
20. https://www.advancedmd.com/learn/cms-releases-final-rule-2019-quality-payment-program/
21. https://www.cms.gov/Medicare/Medicare-Fee-for-Service-Payment/PhysicianFeeSched/index
22. https://www.pyapc.com/insights/implementing-cms-2019-e-m-documentation-guidelines/
23. https://www.cms.gov/newsroom/press-releases/trump-administration-puts-patients-over-paperwork-reducing-healthcare-administrative-costs
24. https://www.cms.gov/Medicare/Medicare-Fee-for-Service-Payment/PhysicianFeeSched/Evaluation-and-Management-Visits
25. https://www.beckershospitalreview.com/healthcare-information-technology/the-5-key-benefits-of-healthcare-interoperability.html
26. https://en.wikipedia.org/wiki/American_Recovery_and_Reinvestment_Act_of_2009
27. https://www.policymed.com/2016/02/understanding-medicare-access-and-chip-reauthorization-act-of-2015-macra-merit-based-incentive-payment-system-mips-and-a.html
28. https://www.formstack.com/blog/2019/legislative-history-healthcare-interoperability/
29. https://www2.deloitte.com/us/en/insights/industry/health-care/ehr-physicians-and-electronic-health-records-survey.html
30. https://www.politico.com/agenda/story/2017/03/vista-computer-history-va-conspiracy-000367
31. https://www.fedhealthit.com/2019/11/an-update-on-interoperability-with-dr-lauren-thompson/
32. https://www.cms.gov/newsroom/fact-sheets/fiscal-year-fy-2020-medicare-hospital-inpatient-prospective-payment-system-ipps-and-long-term-acute-0
33. https://patientengagementhit.com/news/cms-proposal-targets-information-blocking-patient-data-access
34. https://ehrintelligence.com/news/ehra-onc-interoperability-proposed-rule-discourages-innovation
35. http://hl7.org/fhir/https://healthitanalytics.com/features/fhir-is-blazing-a-path-to-patient-centered-data-driven-healthcare
36. https://www.cms.gov/Regulations-and-Guidance/Legislation/EHRIncentivePrograms/Certification
37. https://patientengagementhit.com/news/cms-proposal-targets-information-blocking-patient-data-access
38. https://ehrintelligence.com/features/choosing-an-electronic-health-record-cloud-vs.-on-premise-ehrs
39. https://www.selecthub.com/medical-software/ehr/cloud-based-ehr-systems/
40. https://ehrintelligence.com/news/ama-offers-guidance-for-ehr-vendor-selection-in-new-playbook
41. http://www.medscape.com/features/slideshow/public/ehr2016?src=wnl_edit_tpal&uac=113259SX
42. http://medicaleconomics.modernmedicine.com/medical-economics/news/ehr-report-card
43. https://www.physicianspractice.com/physician-productivity/medical-scribes-pros-and-cons
44. https://www.kevinmd.com/blog/2014/04/medical-scribes-threaten-patient-privacy.html
45. https://www.hcinnovationgroup.com/population-health-management/article/13029305/drilling-down-into-important-issues-around-the-use-of-medical-scribes
46. https://groups.google.com/forum/#!overview
47. https://en.wikipedia.org/wiki/Agile_software_development
48. https://ehrintelligence.com/news/ehr-optimization-sprints-may-help-to-boost-clinician-satisfaction

49. https://www.ama-assn.org/system/files/2019-03/february-2019-summary-panel-actions_0.pdf
50. https://en.wikipedia.org/wiki/Artificial_intelligence
51. http://sitn.hms.harvard.edu/flash/2019/artificial-intelligence-in-medicine-applications-implications-and-limitations/
52. https://healthitanalytics.com/features/health-information-governance-strategies-for-unstructured-data
53. https://healthitanalytics.com/features/explaining-the-basics-of-the-internet-of-things-for-healthcare
54. https://healthitanalytics.com/features/what-is-the-role-of-natural-language-processing-in-healthcare
55. https://en.wikipedia.org/wiki/Optical_character_recognition
56. https://www.urotoday.com/conference-highlights/asco-2018/asco-2018-prostate-cancer/104823-asco-2018-how-i-do-it-precision-medicine-for-prostate-cancer-in-the-real-world.html
57. https://www.urotoday.com/conference-highlights/asco-2018/asco-2018-prostate-cancer/104823-asco-2018-how-i-do-it-precision-medicine-for-prostate-cancer-in-the-real-world.html
58. https://www.ncbi.nlm.nih.gov/pmc/articles/PMC5433356/
59. https://www.medicaleconomics.com/med-ec-blog/success-precision-medicine-key-considerations
60. https://www.ncbi.nlm.nih.gov/books/NBK115574/
61. https://www.physicianspractice.com/technology/8-ways-thwart-hackers-and-improve-cybersecurity
62. http://www.computerworld.com/article/3088907/security/hacker-selling-655-000-patient-records-from-3-hacked-healthcare-organizations.html
63. http://www.newsmax.com/Health/Health-News/medical-identity-theft-id/2016/08/09/id/742866/
64. http://www.hhs.gov/hipaa/for-professionals/security/laws-regulations/
65. https://highside.io/blog/your-hipaa-compliant-email-messaging-apps-are-being-targeted-hacked
66. https://www.mddionline.com/device-cybersecurity-better-%E2%80%94-and-worse-very-connected-world-medical-devices
67. 45 C.F.R. § 164.316
68. 45 C.F.R. § 164.316(b)(2)(iii)
69. https://www.medscape.com/viewarticle/919804?src=wnl_tp10f_191219_mscpedit&uac=113259SX&impID=2189849
70. https://www.physicianspractice.com/technology/8-ways-thwart-hackers-and-improve-cybersecurity
71. https://en.wikipedia.org/wiki/Artificial_intelligence_in_healthcare
72. https://healthcareweekly.com/how-the-big-4-tech-companies-are-leading-healthcare-innovation/
73. https://healthitanalytics.com/news/ehr-metadata-could-enhance-clinical-decision-support-alerts
74. https://www.newsweek.com/amazon-health-care-jeff-bezos-telemedicine-1475154
75. https://healthcareweekly.com/how-the-big-4-tech-companies-are-leading-healthcare-innovation/
76. https://www.forbes.com/sites/robertpearl/2019/12/16/big-tech/
77. https://vxtrahealth.com/
78. https://www.healthcareitnews.com/news/how-merging-financial-and-clinical-data-saved-yale-new-haven-health-150-million
79. https://searchbusinessanalytics.techtarget.com/definition/ad-hoc-analysis
80. https://www.beckershospitalreview.com/finance/healthcare-cost-accounting-8-strategies-to-streamline-implementation-and-quickly-achieve-measurable-results.html
81. http://www.ama-assn.org/sites/ama-assn.org/files/corp/media-browser/public/arc/prior-auth-2017.pdf
82. https://www.healthcaredive.com/news/prior-authorization-moves-to-ehrs/528808/
83. https://www.urologytimes.com/article/prior-authorization-takes-its-toll-urologists
84. https://www.cchpca.org/sites/default/files/2018-11/FINAL%20PFS%20CY%202019%20COMBINED_0.pdf?utm_source=Telehealth+Enthusiasts&utm_campaign=bd7f7979d7-EMAIL_CAMPAIGN_2018_11_06_06_05&utm_medium=email&utm_term=0_ae00b0e89a-bd7f7979d7-353223937
85. https://www.cms.gov/Medicare/Medicare-Fee-for-Service-Payment/PhysicianFeeSched/index
86. https://www.cms.gov/Outreach-and-Education/Medicare-Learning-Network-MLN/MLNProducts/Downloads/TelehealthSrvcsfctsht.pdf https://blog.evisit.com/medicare-telemedicine-top-10-faqs
87. https://www.telehealthresourcecenter.org/big-changes-in-2019-for-medicare-telehealth-policy/
88. https://www.cms.gov/newsroom/press-releases/cms-finalizes-policies-bring-innovative-telehealth-benefit-medicare-advantage
89. https://www.cms.gov/newsroom/fact-sheets/contract-year-2020-medicare-advantage-and-part-d-flexibility-final-rule-cms-4185-f
90. https://www.cms.gov/newsroom/press-releases/cms-finalizes-policies-bring-innovative-telehealth-benefit-medicare-advantage
91. https://www.healthcatalyst.com/Six-Care-Management-Challenges-Healthcare-Must-Overcome https://broadviewuniversity.edu/2017/11/15/3-issues-affecting-health-care-management-today/
92. https://www.ahrq.gov/ncepcr/care/coordination/mgmt.html
93. https://www.optum.com/content/dam/optum/resources/whitePapers/Modern_Care_Management.pdf

KEY POINTS

- **Roughly 50% of total time spent per each patient encounter** is taken up by completing the electronic chart.

- **EHR technology is advancing to automate** some of the laborious input processes, but the physician will always remain responsible for complete accurate documentation and appro-priate billing codes.

- **New CPT rules** will affect the way in which documentation is recorded in the EHR.

- **The most distressing areas to busy physicians** are the number of "clicks", flexibility of use, ease of data entry, and screen to screen workflow with may be slow or at times redun-dant/nonsensical.

- **When contemplating a new EHR,** past experiences with EHR implementation should be dis-cussed with potential new vendors to determine if a new system is a timely and reasonable choice.

- **Throughout the system decision process,** attention needs to be paid to vendor support, structure and access.

- **Implementation strategy and training,** once selection has been made, are critical to suc-cess.

- **To minimize security risk,** regular monitoring and updates are needed to be performed on both systems and local internet access restrictions for staff.

- **Practices should regularly take steps** to improve their systems security.

- **Care management workflow** will continue to be an important part of EHR performance and implementation

Robert Di Loreto, MD

A board-certified adult and pediatric urologist, Dr. Di Loreto is President of Wayne-Macomb Consulting and a co-founder and past president of the Michigan Institute of Urology.

An innovator in health information technology, he developed a HCFA-compliant paper-based charting system that incorporated clinical protocols as well as internal audits 25 years ago. He serves as CMO for United Medical Systems (UMS) which provides mobile Urology medical services to hospitals, surgery centers and physicians' offices nationwide.

Dr. Di Loreto has extensive experience as a specialty-care physician and healthcare innovation. He consults for Urology medical malpractice reviews, medical practice management, clinical information technology, medical data analytics and electronic medical records companies. For more than 30 years, Dr. Di Loreto has served as a consultant and urology advisory panel member to the F.D.A.'s Center for Devices and Radiological Health.

Recently he served as CMIO for an EHR company and developed a new urology electronic medical record product based on Clinical Guidelines and Value Based Medicine with AI supported real-time clinical decision-making capabilities.

Additionally, he was also the founder and medical director for an organization that provides affordable advanced mobile medical services including cryo-surgical and laser treatments for prostate and kidney issues. He is former board chairman of Saint John Hospital and Medical Center, Detroit and on the board of Saint John Health System in MI. Dr. Di Loreto sits on the Board of Advisors for Vxtra Health and is its CMIO.

CHAPTER 8

Managing Human Resources in a Changing Health Care Environment

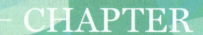

Laine Belmonte, MBA, PHR

The focus of health care organizations has swiftly changed toward an emphasis on patient engagement, patient satisfaction, and a positive office experience for the patient. To achieve this requires a change in how companies manage their human resources. With this shift, it is essential to recognize that staff and physicians who are more content with their employment experience are more likely to deliver better care, provide excellent customer service and increase productivity. How physicians and staff are managed and how they feel about their employment experience will ultimately determine patient outcomes, patient satisfaction, productivity, and overall company success.

The Role of Human Resources

Human Resources (HR) Management is a system of employing human talent effectively to accomplish the organization's goals. The role is vast and involves: recruiting, hiring, onboarding, training, performance management, business partnering, employee relations, compensation planning, benefits and leave administration and maintaining compliance with state and federal laws. Larger urology groups typically employ one or more people devoted to the HR role. Smaller groups may either assign the role to the practice administrator or outsource the HR functions.

An internal HR department can be a key contributor in shaping and supporting the company's culture. Human Resources should align with senior leadership to define the company's culture, then encourage employees and physicians to embrace it.

The Talent Landscape: Staff and Skill Shortages

Finding the right talent today is more challenging than ever as the demand for health care workers has increased, and supply has greatly diminished. According to the U.S. Bureau of Labor Statistics (BLS), employment opportunities for health care workers is projected to grow 14% by 2028, faster than the average for all occupations, adding 1.9 million new jobs. By 2028, Physician Assistant jobs are expected to grow 31%, nurse practitioner jobs by 26%, registered nurses by 12%, and physicians by 7%. This growth is being driven primarily by an aging population, specifically millions of baby boomers reaching retirement age, as well as an increase in chronic health conditions, including the need for urologic care.

Specifically, for urologists, although the number of practicing urologists has increased in recent years (1.1 percent from 2017 to 2018 according to the American Urologic Association survey, "The State of the Urology Workforce and Practice in the United States"), the population needing care is exceeding the resources available. In the same survey it was reported that the median age of practicing urologists is 56. With retirement on the horizon, a greater shortage of urologists is anticipated. To combat the shortage, practices are beginning to incorporate more Advanced Practice Providers into their practices as well as use telehealth as a means to manage their patient volume. As referenced in the above survey less than 12 percent of practicing urologists are using telehealth but it is expected to rise.

There are a number of mitigating factors precluding health care organizations from attaining required labor resources.

- Low unemployment rate in the U.S.- 3.5% as of February 2020.
- Inadequate capacity of medical residency and nursing school programs. American Association of Colleges of Nursing reported that more than 64,000 qualified applicants were turned away from nursing schools in 2016 due to insufficient faculty, preceptors, clinical sites and budgets. Additionally, there is lower federal funding of post medical school residency training, as reported in an article by Harvard Medical School.
- Competition for talent amongst health care organizations.
- Wage competition.
- Increased turnover.

The Society for Human Resource Management (SHRM) recently stated that 80% of HR professionals report difficulty filling professional health care positions, with their biggest challenges being a low number of applicants, competition, candidates with limited experience and local markets that don't supply enough qualified candidates. In general, it can easily take 2 to 4 months to hire clinical support staff.

As a result, health care companies can no longer rely on passive recruitment methods or traditional job placement ads to attract the right people. Instead, hiring managers and HR professionals must take a proactive approach to sourcing the right talent. The younger generation performs most of their job search using social media and their mobile devices. In order to capture this large talent pool, companies need to expand their social media presence and embrace recruiting methods that are mobile-friendly. This peer group is looking for companies whose web presence is fresh and appealing, reviews that are positive, interview experiences that are smooth and welcoming, and work environments that are innovative and fluid, that offer opportunities to learn and grow.

Another excellent resource for finding good talent is your existing employee population. Incentive programs such as Employee Referral Programs work well. These programs provide a modest cash reward to employees when their referred candidate is hired. Not only are employees an additional recruiting source, but good employees tend to refer good candidates. Doctors and management staff should also take responsibility for networking and helping the organization discover new talent, as they often are members of professional networks that attract the types of positions required by the practice.

Once a viable candidate is identified, it is essential to understand what that person is looking for in an employment experience, and to position the practice and job in a positive and desirable manner. It is important to be able to articulate how the practice is differentiated from similar work environments and what the practice can offer to that candidate to meet his or her expectations. Why would this person want to join your practice? What can your practice offer that the group down the road cannot? What is special about your organization?

Recruiting Urologists

Recruiting urologists also presents new challenges, as physician retirement is on the rise. The increased demand coupled with high physician turnover and a decreasing talent pool are forcing medical practices to retool their physician recruitment strategies.

Sourcing strategies for urologists vary and include placing advertisements on the company website as well as on professional websites such as the https://careercenter.auanet.org, https://careers.lugpa.org, and http://www.mdsearch.com; attracting physicians through social media avenues; engaging search firms; and networking through colleagues and educational institutions. It has also become a requisite for the practice leader to be involved in the recruitment process so he or she can articulate the practice's vision, long-term business strategy, and team culture at the physician level.

As part of any recruitment strategy, it is important to consider the demographic of the candidate and what he or she is looking for from a professional and personal perspective. Some physicians want to be involved in corporate decision making or cutting-edge technology; others prefer direct patient care with little to no involvement in practice operations or politics; and some desire both professional opportunities coupled with a solid work-life balance. A few particulars to be aware of during the recruitment process are:

- **Millennial urologists** tend to look for work-life balance and want transparency.

- **There has been an increase of female urologists** in the workforce (9.2% in 2018 vs. 8.8% in 2017 according to the AUA).

- **Female practicing urologists age 45 or older** are more likely to feel their work schedules do not leave them enough time for personal and family commitments, as suggested in an AUA survey.

- **Urologists, particularly those who are younger,** are migrating to urban areas, leaving rural areas with a scarcity of talent.

- **New urologists** are expecting to have a signed contract often before their last year of residency.

- **New urologists** are beginning to look for education loan repayment propositions as part of the offer package.

Ultimately, the recruitment strategy needs to align what physicians want with what the organization needs and can deliver. The recruitment process should include an explanation of the practice's business model and strategy, use of technology, role of partners, description of group dynamics, philosophy on patient care and satisfaction, day-to-day operations, and the perks and benefits offered as part of the package.

With a growing urologist shortage, the best defense is to begin recruiting at least 2 years in advance of the need and invest in a robust recruitment and retention strategy to ensure that new urologists who are brought on board are right for the practice and will stay for the long term.

Increased demand for health care workers and short supply leads to increased compensation. The compensation and benefits package offered is paramount to attracting and retaining the right talent. As competition is rising, wage offerings need to be competitive, if not aggressive. Benchmarking salaries and benefit programs against competitors is a necessity. Both compensation and benefits must be viable to compete for talent. When new recruits are considering a company for employment, they often evaluate many different facets of the offer, including the compensation, benefits, paid time off, organization culture, job description, expectations, who will be their manager, the physical space, work-life balance, etc. Therefore, the compensation and benefits package extended is a fundamental factor that remains essential, not only for the hiring process, but also for future retention of the physician.

It is important to determine the organization's compensation philosophy in terms of salaries relative to the market. Is compensation in the 90th percentile? Perhaps the 75th or 50th percentile is more feasible. The company's compensation strategy can vary for different positions. For instance, pay for mid-level employees may be in the 90th percentile because they are vital to the organization and are scarce in the local marketplace; licensed practical nurses may be paid in the 50th percentile if they are more plentiful and easier to attract. Whatever compensation strategy is chosen, it should be consistent across similar job groups, not only to avoid pay discrepancies that can lead to legal headaches, but more importantly, staff should feel they are paid fairly in comparison to the external market as well as compared to coworkers with a similar job scope and level within the organization.

As an organization gets larger, it is advisable to create a compensation structure to manage salaries. This entails placing groups of jobs and salary ranges into a hierarchy.

The salary range is the span between the minimum and maximum base salary an organization will pay for a specific job or group of jobs. The structure should take into consideration external market data coupled with internal salary data. This prevents having a large discrepancy between salaries for similar positions, which can negatively impact morale. An experienced Human Resources compensation specialist or compensation consultant can spearhead this type of project.

Benefits

The benefits offered by different organizations vary and may include:

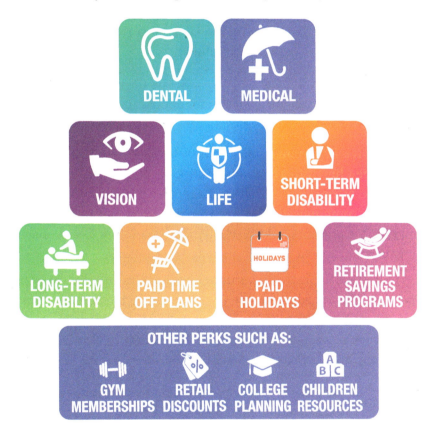

Different generations generally want different benefit offerings, an ongoing challenge for companies. There is a large generational shift taking place as Baby Boomers are remaining in the workplace longer, and Millennials have entered the workforce. According to the Bureau of Labor Statistics, 25.6% of Baby Boomers will continue to be in the workforce by 2022. Baby Boomers tend to value health care and retirement benefits, whereas Millennials are interested in career advancement and flexibility in their work schedules. The traditional "one size fits all" benefit offering will no longer satisfy this changing workforce. Instead, this shift requires organizations to be more creative in their delivery of benefit programs by offering benefit choices and giving employees more control over choosing the benefits that are important to them.

All Aboard!

Onboarding enables new employees to acquire the necessary knowledge, skills, and behaviors that lead them to become effective members of the organization. According to the Society of Human Resource Management (SHRM), half of all hourly workers leave new jobs in the first four months, and half of all senior executives leave within 18 months. These statistics are often due to poor onboarding practices—specifically, not having a clear understanding of the job or what is expected, not receiving the appropriate training, poor experiences with co-workers who are not helpful or friendly, or inadequate communication with the manager. Younger generations, in particular, are less tolerant of cumbersome or uninviting onboarding practices. Thus, the sooner new hires feel welcome and are familiar with the job and work environment, the quicker they will become satisfied, effective contributors.

Onboarding programs vary in length, complexity, and degree of formality, depending upon the organization. In general, a successful onboarding program should include these key elements:

- **Pre-boarding:** It is important for the company to make a positive first impression by providing the new hire with a clear job description, offer letter, benefit information, and explanation of the company culture. If there is a lag in start time, it is important to have periodic communication with the new hire. The manager, or in the case of a new urologist, the physician leader, should call the new hire to welcome him or her to the organization and answer any preliminary questions.

    It is also important to provide a warm welcome to a prospective physician on the first interview. The schedule for the first day should include meetings with key management staff and other physicians, as well as a lunch or dinner. During the second interview, it is essential to also invite the family to visit the office, attend a social function with other physician families, tour the area, etc.

- **Policies and Guidelines:** The new hire should receive education and information about company rules, regulations, and policies.

- **Job Description and Expectations:** It is important to provide a written job description and communicate performance expectations.

- **Workspace and Resources:** Workspace, equipment, and office supplies should be ready for the new recruit is first day on the job. In addition, it is helpful to provide necessary resources, such as an organizational chart; telephone and e-mail contact list; parking information; places to eat, etc.

- **Training:** The new hire should also receive any necessary computer, equipment, regulatory, or business training.

- **Company Culture:** Equally helpful is for a new staff member or physician to understand the organizational norms. He or she should be given a tour of the physical surroundings and in-person introductions to other employees, including a company leader. It is important for a new hire to feel connected to the new organization. It is also important to assign a "go-to" person or "mentor" for the first several weeks to create a support system for the new hire during the introductory phase of employment. This applies to new urologists too.

After the first month, the manager and/or HR should have a private conversation with the new hire to make sure he or she is acclimating to the job. A 30-Day New Employee Survey is a good way to gather this information. It's an opportunity to rectify any issues, gaps, or misconceptions, and is an excellent tool used to foster employee satisfaction and retention.

Onboarding of Physicians

Onboarding of physicians requires many of the steps above, with some notable distinctions. New physicians can get quickly discouraged by obstacles such as inadequate marketing that causes low patient volume, credentialing issues, poor management of patient scheduling that leads to low productivity, and disconnection from the culture or group dynamics. It is important for new physicians to understand the company's challenges, opportunities and priorities, as well as how they will contribute to its vision. The onboarding staff should also listen to the new physicians' concerns and ideas so they feel connected to a greater purpose early on. Additionally, it's important to help acclimate a new physician's family into the community.

Incorporating each of these elements into the onboarding strategy in a systematic way will maximize the success of the onboarding program and will serve as the foundation for integrating a new physician successfully into the organization.

Managing Employee Performance to Create a First-Rate Performing Team

Managing employee performance is an integral part of achieving desired organizational results. Performance management should be a continuous process of communication between a manager and employee throughout the year. Ideally, broad goals should be established at the leadership level, be broken down from department to department, and then be divided again to the employee level. This way everyone's performance goals are aligned with the goals of the organization, fostering greater opportunity for overall company success.

> **Some key areas to incorporate into a new physician onboarding strategy are:**
>
> - Timely attainment of credentialing and licenses.
> - Establishment of an orientation schedule that includes required employment paperwork, training, and introductions to key department managers and physicians.
> - Meeting with the CEO or physician leader who welcomes the physician and defines expectations for productivity and quality of patient care; discusses group dynamics and culture; and answers any questions.
> - Regular communication with the practice manager and/or HR regarding relocation questions, orientation, and practice operations specifics.
> - Training on electronic medical records and other practice systems and equipment.
> - Training on how to obtain needed clinical consults, tests, prescriptions, etc.
> - A pre-built patient schedule template with patients appropriately scheduled before the first day.
> - Assignment of a physician mentor from within the organization to foster integration into the culture and provide guidance to operational processes.
> - Discussion of the plan for marketing the new physician and establishing him or her in the community.

Providing employees with honest and constructive performance feedback is essential not only for the employee, but also to make sure the organization has a workforce that is productive and working efficiently. Providing consistent feedback to employees reinforces what they're doing well so they continue those behaviors and re-directs them when they are not doing things correctly.

The start of the year is an opportunity for the manager and employee to jointly set goals and determine specifically how those goals will be achieved. During this planning process, it is important to agree upon both the results and behaviors expected. The results to be achieved should be tied to the broader corporate goals, as well as encompass the employee's development goals.

Behaviors are equally important to assess because they represent how someone carries out the job and can affect the work culture. Regardless of how productive employees are, those who fail to cooperate or are difficult to work with can be disruptive and detrimental to the team dynamics. Thus, making sure employee behavior is consistent with the company's values and expectations is key.

Some organizations choose to formally evaluate staff performance one time per year and others may do it at regular intervals during the year. Whichever method is selected, that time can be used to assess the performance criteria and goals that were established at the beginning of the year and to document the outcomes in the form of written performance evaluation. The performance evaluation serves many purposes for the organization, including clarifying performance expectations; aligning performance and behaviors with the goals and values of the company; serving as a basis for administrative decisions (e.g., raises, bonuses, promotions); eliminating poor performers; and developing employee skills and capabilities. The performance management process is time-consuming and requires a great deal of effort from the managers. To reap the benefits associated with performance management, it is critical that the organization's leaders believe in and support it. Without that commitment, managers and employees will not see the value in putting forth the effort required to do justice to the process.

Gaining Insight about Employee Satisfaction

To gain insight about employee satisfaction, organizations can take several steps. Conducting exit interviews sheds light on why people leave. They are useful, however, it is often too late at that point to change the employee's mind about staying. A more proactive approach is conducting stay interviews, and/or surveying existing staff to gather information about what they like and dislike about working for the company. Stay interviews in particular, provide a platform for the employee to voice his or her concerns as well as articulate professional development goals. In turn, this gives the manager an opportunity to correct minor issues before they escalate and helps build a trusting relationship. Managers need to be mindful that stay interviews are not performance evaluations. Instead, they serve to provide the manager with genuine feedback about the organization and the person's employment experience. It's important for the manager to refrain from getting defensive or using stay interviews as an opportunity to highlight shortcomings. Managers should listen carefully, take notes, and discuss next steps; then share regular updates about progress toward the desired outcomes.

Employee satisfaction surveys provide another means of gathering an employee's perceptions and feelings about working for the organization. These surveys can be very effective to retain staff, increase productivity and improve morale. At the onset, it is essential to have the buy-in from the leaders of the organization before conducting an employee survey. Employees want to know that the leadership team will listen carefully to what they have to say, use the information to address concerns and identify improvement plans. In addition, these surveys are often best done anonymously as employees tend to provide more honest feedback.

The design of the survey is a key factor. Depending upon the organization's purpose for gathering employee satisfaction information (to improve morale, win an award, etc.), careful attention should be paid to the questions asked, the length of the survey and the ease by which the data can be reported and analyzed. According to SHRM, the survey should not take more than 20 to 30 minutes for an employee to complete. Otherwise, there is a risk of a low response rate. Using a numerical rating scale, such as 1 through 5, to rate responses is recommended. Open-ended questions can also be used, but they are harder to analyze due to the variety and volume of data that comes back.

Once the organization decides to launch an employee satisfaction survey, the managers should be informed and either HR or a business leader can introduce the survey to the staff either through email, a town hall, department meeting, or other communication mechanism consistent with the organization's culture. Upon completion, organizations will often form a cross-functional team to review the findings and devise action plans. Survey results and action plans can then be communicated back to the employees, bringing the process full-cycle. Tracking and analyzing this information, on perhaps an annual basis, will serve as a foundation to launch a successful retention strategy.

The Growing Concern of Turnover and Staff Retention

Turnover in health care today is on the rise, causing difficulty for organizations to retain good staff. According to an NSI study, hospital turnover was 19.1% in 2018 and projected to rise in 2019. This study also showed that more than 50% of new hires left within the first two years of employment. In 2018, MGMA reported single specialty practice turnover at 15.83% to 20% for clinical support staff and front office staff respectively. Why is turnover so important to understand? Turnover is expensive on many levels—the costs of turnover can be upward of 50% of the employee's annual salary. The costs vary depending upon the employee's role within the organization, his or her contribution, as well as how difficult it will be to replace the person. These costs include, but are not limited to, advertising, recruiting and interviewing, administrative time, onboarding and training, loss of productivity, impact on morale, burnout of existing staff and lost revenue while the position is unfilled. The impact of turnover also impacts productivity and overall company performance leading to further financial pressures, as well as inadequate patient and employee satisfaction levels.

Why is health care experiencing so much turnover? There are multiple factors influencing turnover today. One of the top reasons is burnout. Burnout happens when there's too much work to perform in a short amount of time, under stressful conditions and with less people. Patient volume is high, there are greater workloads and less staff. As staff leave, it's taking longer to replace them, causing staffing shortages, low morale and disengagement.

According to various sources, some of the main reasons people leave are:

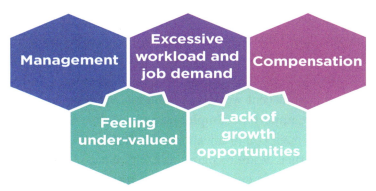

To address this growing problem, organizations must hold staff retention as a priority and place strategies in place to combat turnover. Each organization needs to assess its own staff and environment to identify why people are exiting. Some actions organizations can take to strengthen retention are:

- Evaluate hiring decisions and be sure the applicant's skills, goals and cultural fit are aligned with the organization.
- Provide a compensation and benefit package that is attractive.
- Help new employees become acclimated. Be sure they understand their role and have the tools, equipment and training to do their job. Help them to build relationships and understand how their role fits into the company's overall mission.
- Recognize achievements.
- Offer flexible scheduling if feasible.
- Ensure employees feel valued; allow employees to provide input; treat them with respect.
- Communicate company goals and current events.
- Provide opportunities for brief relaxation. Some companies have created relaxation rooms where employees can take a quiet break. Other companies have brought animals into the workplace as a form of therapy.
- Create a culture that is upbeat and encouraging.

To initiate a successful retention strategy, company management must understand why people stay with the company and what is important to the people the company is trying to retain. Individuals have their own assessment of the value vs. investment relationship—specifically, the value they are receiving from the job (professional satisfaction, compensation, benefits, personal relationships, etc.) compared to what they are investing (commitment, energy, time, sacrifices, etc.). When this is unbalanced and the perceived investment outweighs the value, the employee becomes dissatisfied and may look for a better value proposition elsewhere.

The impact of the manager must be considered. There is a long-standing saying that "people don't leave their jobs; they leave their managers." This statement continues to have validity and cannot be ignored. In a 2015 survey by Gallup, nearly 50% of employees left their jobs because of their manager. Of course, employees want good pay and benefits and decent working conditions, but what happens in between paychecks is often more important. Employees require clear and realistic expectations and goals; they want open communication with their manager, a reasonable workload and fair practices; they desire recognition from management and other employees; and they want to know that employees who are responsible and accountable are distinguished from those who are not.

EMPLOYEES STAY WHEN THEY ARE: PAID WELL, MENTORED, CHALLENGED, PROMOTED, INVOLVED, APPRECIATED, VALUED, ON A MISSION, EMPOWERED, TRUSTED

Additionally, top performers tend to need even more feedback, often in the form of greater challenges, expanded responsibilities, promotions, greater inclusion in leadership activities, and higher compensation. Breakdowns in these areas, which alter the value vs. investment relationship will cause employees to either become disengaged or resign.

Common Retention Strategies

Much can be learned from retention strategies that a wide range of organizations are finding successful. For example:

Compensation

- Conducting salary surveys and paying slightly above market rates
- Assigning a market adjustment to base salary
- Paying a differential for higher degrees, certifications, or hours worked outside the norm

Bonus and Recognition Programs

- Offering a retention bonus
- Providing bonuses for completion of special projects
- Offering sign-on bonuses to new recruits
- Implementing a recognition program such as employee of the month or peer-to-peer recognition

Career Development and Flexibility

- Providing career development opportunities or special training and education

- Offering flexible work schedules (e.g.: reduced work week, telecommuting, and flexible hours)
- Expanding paid time-off programs

Other Ways to Recognize Staff:
- A sincere "thank you" is free and is very effective
- Plan a special lunch or afternoon treat for an individual or department
- Note special achievements in a newsletter or company-wide email
- Send a recognition letter or certificate with balloons to the employee's office
- Provide additional time-off or comp time in exchange for going above-and-beyond
- Send a birthday or work anniversary card, and perhaps a gift to their home
- Invite them to a one-on-one lunch
- Arrange for a senior manager to stop by or call to say thank you

Especially in a tight labor market, it is increasingly important for organizations to be intuitive about what motivates their employees. One size does not fit all. It's important to have an array of awards, from monetary incentives and gifts to special experiences and non-monetary rewards. The employee value vs. investment relationship needs to be managed in a proactive way and must be considered when developing a retention strategy.

Retaining Physicians

As noted earlier, physician turnover and retirement have increased in recent years, placing greater emphasis on retention. The first one to three years of practice tends to be the most crucial time for physician turnover. According to a Physician Retention Survey released in 2013 by the American Medical Group Association (AMGA) and Cejka Search, physician turnover was 6.8%, up from 6.5% in 2011, and 5.9% in 2009. In addition, 36% of respondents expected that retirements would continue to increase, and roughly 74% of the groups surveyed expected turnover to stay around the same rate.

The study also found:

The average turnover rate for physicians in their second to third year of practice was 12.4%, with smaller groups reporting an average of 20.8%.

Nearly 85% of practices surveyed had an onboarding process for physicians.

Groups who assign a mentor during onboarding reported a lower overall turnover rate of 6% compared to the overall 6.8% turnover rate. Extended onboarding of physicians in the early years with a practice was connected to lower turnover during that time.

Turnover costs for physicians are far greater than for other positions. In fact, it is estimated that the loss of a full-time physician and the cost of recruiting a new one over a one-year time period are nearly 1.2 million.

Specifically, for urologists, a significant contributor of turnover, according to Dr. Raj Pruthi, professor and Chair of Urology at the University of North Carolina at Chapel Hill, is burnout. Surveys performed by the Mayo Clinic found that burnout in urologists was higher than average at 64%, compared to 54% for all physicians. There are numerous repercussions to physician burnout including depression, strained relationships at work and home, clinical errors and early retirement. Dr. Pruthi mentions in his article from the AUA's Daily News that the leading causes of dissatisfaction arise from more emphasis being placed on quantity verses quality of care and the high demands of the Electronic Health Records systems.

Having knowledge of the various drivers of turnover will help practices craft better retention strategies. Similar to conducting stay interviews for staff, it is essential to solicit the perceptions of the urologists before they get to an adverse stage in their employment. Physician Satisfaction Surveys are particularly effective. Based on the results, they will

Research suggests that there are three main reasons physicians leave a practice:

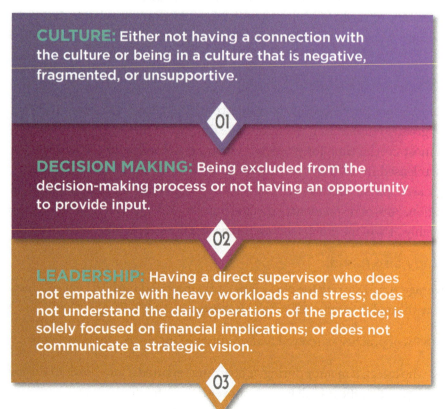

CULTURE: Either not having a connection with the culture or being in a culture that is negative, fragmented, or unsupportive.

01

DECISION MAKING: Being excluded from the decision-making process or not having an opportunity to provide input.

02

LEADERSHIP: Having a direct supervisor who does not empathize with heavy workloads and stress; does not understand the daily operations of the practice; is solely focused on financial implications; or does not communicate a strategic vision.

03

help the company uncover issues and identify actions that will increase satisfaction, and ultimately encourage retention.

Some common steps an organization can take to improve retention of urologists are:

- ✓ **Create a culture that is respectful,** where there is open communication and a collaborative style.
- ✓ **Communicate your company culture, core values, operating style and expectations** to urologist applicants. Be sure these are aligned when hiring.
- ✓ **Allow for autonomy and professional growth.**
- ✓ **Provide a reasonable balance** between work and personal life.
- ✓ **Beware of developing burnout situations,** and if they occur, investigate the reasons in order to identify solutions.

Senior Physicians Slow Down

In discussing recruitment and retention, it is prudent to acknowledge the sensitive topic of senior physician slowdown. Practices tend to view this as somewhat of a sore subject, and it certainly can be a complex one to approach. However, with the supply of physicians not anticipated to increase and the demand for physicians only becoming greater, retaining competent, senior physicians could be an advantage.

When senior physicians want to reduce their scope of practice, management must evaluate the practice needs verses the senior physicians' request as well as their partnership status, length of agreement, compensation, company benefits, and ownership assets. Since a slowdown entails a reduced scope of work and on-call responsibility, the senior physician's status would typically change. In private practices where senior physicians are often partners, they may lose their partnership status, accept a buyout payment, and become employees of the practice. A new employment agreement would then be created outlining the scope of responsibilities, company expectations, licensure requirements, paid time-off parameters, a revised compensation structure, and a description of company benefits. Generally, the new agreement would be renewed in one or two years. It is also advisable to encourage the senior physician to set a target date for retirement. This way both parties can benefit by planning accordingly for the future departure.

The Legal Environment

Many federal employment laws are based upon the number of employees in a company. As medical practices continue to join and form larger practice groups, they may be subject to an increasing number of federal and state employment laws. Management staff must be knowledgeable about these laws and ensure that work rules, policies, and practices are carefully designed and implemented per these regulations.

For example, it is unlawful in some states for companies to conduct blanket drug testing on all employees. In other states, it is a common hiring practice as substance abuse can negatively impact the company culture and productivity.

Here are additional federal employment laws that are especially important:

ADA (Americans with Disabilities Act): Applies to employers with 15 or more employees. It prohibits employers from discriminating against people with disabilities. Employers must also provide "reasonable accommodation" to individuals with disabilities.

ADEA (Age Discrimination in Employment Act): Applies to employers with 20 or more employees. Prohibits discrimination against employees based on their age, from age 40 or older.

COBRA (Consolidated Omnibus Budget Reconciliation Act): Applies to employers with 20 or more employees. It provides former employees, retirees, spouses, and children the right to continue their health coverage on a temporary basis, at group rates. Many states also have a "mini" COBRA law that applies to smaller employers.

FLSA (Fair Labor Standards Act): Applies to most employers.

It establishes minimum wage rates and rules regarding overtime pay for eligible employees.

FMLA (Family and Medical Leave Act): Applies to employers with 50 or more employees working each work day during 20 or more calendar weeks. Employees who qualify are allowed up to 12 work weeks of unpaid leave during a 12-month period for valid health-related reasons pertaining to either the employee or a family member.

Occupational Health and Safety Act (OSHA): Employers must comply with the safety and health standards and regulations established by OSHA. Employers also have a general obligation to provide employees with a workplace that is free from recognized hazards.

Title VII of the Civil Rights Act: Applies to employers with 15 or more employees. It prohibits employers from discriminating against employees and applicants based on race, color, religion, sex, or national origin.

Unlawful Discrimination and Harassment: It is unlawful to treat employees differently based on a protected classification such as race, color, national origin, gender, religion, disability, or age. Additionally, it is prohibited to engage in conduct that is considered sexual harassment or creating a hostile work environment.

Several of the laws outlined above require posting notices in the workplace that inform employees of their rights under the respective laws. Others, like FMLA, also require employers to state policies and provide forms to employees to comply with the law.

As companies grow, questions and issues surrounding employment increase, and it becomes necessary to handle these matters consistently and fairly. Accordingly, many companies benefit by drafting and maintaining an Employee Handbook that encompasses most, if not all, of the organization's policies and procedures. Employee Handbooks should always be reviewed by an attorney to ensure they are legally sound.

It is often the disgruntled employee who seeks legal avenues for dealing with a perceived, work-related offense. Whether there is a valid case or not, a court case can cost a great deal of time and money to defend. In general, there are some things an employer can do to avoid legal exposure:

- Know the employment laws and adhere to them.
- Treat employees equally, fairly, and respectfully.
- Be clear with staff about work-related expectations.
- Be straightforward and provide balanced feedback when addressing performance issues.
- Give employees a fair chance to improve if they are not meeting expectations.
- Document employee performance issues and progress over time. Focus on job-related matters and concerns (verses personal attributes and situations).
- Work with an attorney or other qualified professional to develop an employee handbook or to provide guidance on sensitive employee terminations.

Legal Representation

Some situations may call for assistance from an employment lawyer. For example, if an employee recently filed a complaint against the practice, and is now facing termination, it is wise to seek counsel prior to firing that person. It is also helpful to consult with a lawyer before making important decisions, such as discontinuing benefits or firing an employee who has had attendance issues due to a health-related reason.

What Can HR Do for the Medical Practice?

To successfully manage the future growth of a medical practice in this changing health care climate, emphasis must be placed on appropriate human resource planning. The ways in which the Human Resources Department can make an impact are by partnering with department leaders to manage the people-related issues and initiatives, implementing creative strategies to recruiting talent, hiring employees who are a good cultural fit for the organization, facilitating a successful onboarding process, developing ways to improve employee satisfaction and retention, creating pathways for professional growth and development, and encouraging a culture where employees feel valued.

Human Resources will also keep the organization in compliance with employment laws as well as assist the management team with appropriate handling of delicate employee-related issues. If there is no dedicated human resources function in the practice, it would be beneficial to consider incorporating one.

As an alternative to or an extension of an in-house HR department, a practice can utilize the services of a **Professional Employer Organization (PEO)**. A PEO provides an opportunity to outsource some or all of the human resources responsibilities, affording more time to focus on patient care. A business relationship with a PEO is one of co-employment whereby the PEO leases employees to the practice and thus shares many of the employment and legal responsibilities. In a PEO, the practice would report its employees' wages under the PEO's federal identification number, so employee liability would shift to the PEO. Some of the functions the PEO can provide are:

- Payroll & benefit administration, including unemployment and worker's compensation.
- Compliance with employment regulations.
- Maintaining employee files.
- Developing workplace policies.
- Training.
- Recruiting and hiring.

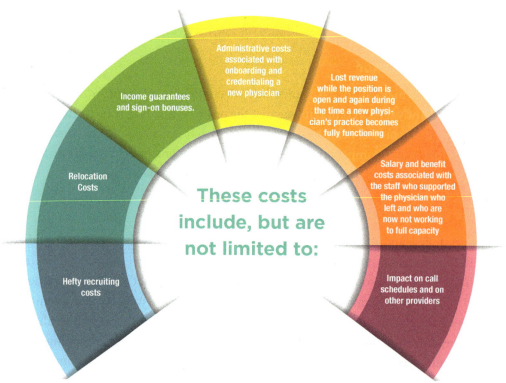

Some of the most common disadvantages of using a PEO are:

- Loss of control of basic employee processes.
- Loss of oversight of employee files.
- Less influence of the HR department.

PEO's are more commonly used in smaller practices. Before entering an arrangement with a PEO, the practice should evaluate the suitability of a PEO given its human resources/payroll needs and practice culture. Further, the practice should determine whether or not the particular PEO chosen can meet the practice's needs. Checking the PEO's references is strongly recommended.

Whether a practice chooses to employ an internal HR department or outsource some or all of its HR functions, a focus on human resources will benefit a practice given the various employment-related challenges facing health care organizations today.

KEY POINTS

- **The role of human resources involves** recruiting, hiring, onboarding, training, analyzing compensation and benefits, and maintaining compliance with state and federal laws.

- **The compensation and benefits package offered is paramount** to attracting and retaining the right talent for one's organization, and must be relative to the market.

- **Effective onboarding is important to retain physicians** who become effective members of the organization.

- **Managing employee performance** is an integral part of achieving desired organizational results.

- **To craft a successful retention strategy,** it is necessary to analyze turnover and why people leave the organization.

- **Managers need to be in touch with their employees** to gain insight into this relationship and how it affects performance and future employment.

- **When senior physicians want to reduce their scope of practice,** management must evaluate the practice needs verses the senior physicians' request as well as their partnership status, length of agreement, compensation, company benefits, and ownership assets.

- **Management staff must be knowledgeable** about federal and state laws and ensure that work rules, policies, and practices are carefully designed and implemented per these regulations.

ABOUT THE AUTHOR

Laine Belmonte, MBA, PHR

Laine Belmonte is the Director of Human Resources for Premier Medical Group, a multi-specialty medical practice. She has over 25 years of experience in Human Resource management, 6 years of which have been in health care. Ms. Belmonte's areas of focus include organizational development, talent management, employee relations, performance management, compensation and benefits.

CHAPTER 9

Diagnose and Manage Your Marketing Needs for Outcomes-Oriented Tactics

Jennifer L. Dally, MBA

Neil Baum, MD

Urology providers are trained to diagnose and treat urological conditions; however, few have ample training on how to market and promote their urological skills or practice. Yet today's discerning health care consumer requires the urologist to understand and deploy marketing initiatives to be competitive and maintain a healthy practice.

There are many approaches to leverage modern marketing practices. This chapter is designed to help you understand value drivers for today's consumer of health care and how you can prioritize and execute marketing initiatives to grow your practice and attract top talent.

Why Marketing is Essential

Practice marketing has changed dramatically in the last 20 years. The fact that you even have to be concerned about marketing your own practice is a new paradigm to many, so it's important to understand how today's health care consumer approaches their decision-making.

Many of today's popular brands are part of the reason health care consumers have become so discerning. Amazon, Nordstrom, Costco, Southwest Airlines, and Zappos have changed consumer's expectations of service, which has crossed over into all industries, including health care. Today's health care consumer expects:

- Quick access or speed of service
- To always be right
- Ability to review and learn as much as they want in advance
- Expert advice on demand
- Cost-efficiency

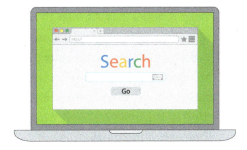

Let us consider the patient's journey before they arrive for a consultation. This overview of that journey maybe surprising:

01 They identify a potential health issue and consult "Dr. Google"

02 They then "socialize" their diagnosis by sharing it on their social networks to gather further information and recommendations from their "friends"

03 They review those recommendations by searching online for reviews, pouring through positive and negative comments

04 Once they select you, they do more online research to, essentially, earn their own medical specialty degree from the "University of Google"

05 Finally, they arrive at your practice for a consult...to validate their diagnosis or ask "any last questions"

06 Once they leave your office, they must validate your diagnosis and treatment plan by returning to their social network and "Dr. Google"

Sound familiar? Most providers today find their #1 competitor is "Dr. Google." Your role, in many patients' minds has evolved from their doctor to their health care coach.

Because the paradigm has shifted, so too are the ways in which physicians must communicate, educate, and interact with your patients. Much of that now needs to happen digitally before you even meet the patient. That mean traditional marketing methods aren't just as critical, but you need to consider all four primary marketing pillars: internal, traditional external, digital (including social media), and referral marketing.

Diagnosing Your Marketing Approach

Each urology practice has its own dynamic, from solo to group, rural to urban. Each practice also has varying types of competitive threats from hospitals, payors, or other specialties disrupting the marketplace. Regardless of those scenarios, there are fundamentals to diagnosing your practice's marketing needs to determine not only the best plan, but also to help prioritize time and budgets. The goal is to accomplish the benefits of marketing in the most efficient way, so time is maximized with patients while minimizing time executing marketing.

Consider approaching your marketing plan and execution much like you would diagnosing and treating a patient. Follow these five steps to achieve ideal outcomes for your practice:

01 **Understand your practice needs/goals:** This step not only helps clarify your priority areas for marketing, but also ensures everyone in your practice is "rowing the boat" in the same direction. First, align on your goals (or priority of goals) for your practice. Below are some sample goals:

- Grow your practice (either in patients or practitioners or both)
- Improve patient mix

- Reduce no-shows
- Reduce calls to office
- Improve patient engagement scores
- Improve patient compliance to treatment regime
- Improve office productivity (Yes, marketing tools can improve productivity while elevating patient satisfaction!)

02 **Know your target patient.** Outline your current patient demographic and decide if there is a niche you can most successfully serve. What patients do you seek to attract and what do you know about them? More specifically, what sources do your patients use to influence health care decisions?

03 **Assess your existing marketing assets and identify gaps.** Collect and review all your marketing materials, both physical copies and digital. How do your materials compare to competitors (it's easy to review competitor digital marketing efforts!). Are your materials current? Do they all consistently project the image of your practice?

04 **Create a plan with measurements of success.** Based on the above "diagnosis," create a prioritized list of marketing activities. The balance of this chapter will discuss the variety of marketing tools available to you. Remember it's not reasonable to execute everything mentioned in this chapter, rather use this "treatment plan" phase to focus on those most critical to the health of the practice.

05 **Monitor your effectiveness and adapt as you learn.** Just like treating a patient, you need to evaluate the effectiveness of your marketing and make changes to the regime. If something isn't working, it doesn't mean you should stop. Rather look at the evidence and determine if an adjustment is needed before abandoning the plan. Generally, that evidence gives you even greater insight into how you can make your marketing work harder for you.

While marketing efforts and spend should be aligned within the practice, it's important to designate one person to lead the effort. Experience shows when too many people drive efforts, you are less efficient in accomplishing goals. Using key performance indicators (KPIs) or establishing SMART (specific, measurable, achievable, relevant, time-based) goals can help you set expectations and allows the appointed person to drive without constantly seeking approval of smaller decisions by consensus.

Leveraging Modern Marketing Tactics to Achieve Outcomes

Marketing tactics for practices generally fall into one of four categories: internal, external, digital, and referral. These tactics all intersect and can work in concert when you plan your approach versus looking at them as stand-alone tactics. For example, the way your patients perceive their experience in the office (internal) may affect how they rate you online or refer you to their social network (digital & referral). Further, if you host an event or place an ad (external) you can drive people to your digital assets to learn more about the practice (digital).

A. INTERNAL MARKETING

Internal marketing can be considered low hanging fruit, which is readily available to every urologist. Further, the experience patients have in your office has a significant effect on their perception of care, their evaluation of you, as well as how they talk about you/your practice in the digital ecosphere (social media and ratings/review sites). Thus, working on internal marketing is not only an easier tactic to address—because you're likely already doing it without calling it marketing—but the most critical.

The primary audience for internal marketing is your staff, existing patients, and new patients interfacing with your practice:

- **Staff:** Believe it or not, your staff are the most powerful marketing tool you have! Before ever meeting with a physician in the practice, a patient interacts with at least one or more staff members, which shapes immediate impressions. Your staff members can be extremely influential if they are engaged, aware of your efforts, and their role in creating a superior customer experience. Consider, when you walk into a room and are greeted with warm welcome versus when you approach a desk and the person is distracted and doesn't address you immediately? How does that shape your perception? Generally, staff members interact with patients to a greater extent than physicians so whether it's their demeanor on the phone or customer service throughout the in-office experience, they significantly contribute to how a patient perceives the care received. Further, as your staff engage within their own community they are often seen as "expert sources" on practices. Prospective patients within their daily lives or social ecosphere will ask them about your practice. You want them to be both well-informed about your practice capabilities and enthusiastic about being on your team.

- **Prospective Patients:** From the time a prospective patient calls for an appointment, to their in-office and post-visit experience, prospective patients are evaluating each nuance to determine their confidence level in you as a practitioner. Are they stuck in a phone tree? Challenged to find a live staff member to talk to, or holding on the phone for extended wait times? Perhaps they're wondering why they haven't received a follow-up call. Each touchpoint has an impact. Put yourself in your new patient (or existing patient's) shoes and experience the journey. What would you expect and what improvements would you recommend?

- **Existing Patients:** This target audience can be a significant referral source! By informing and educating patients about your services and asking them to refer family and friends, they can extend the reach of your marketing efforts. For example, if you perform the no-scalpel, no needle vasectomy, and the patient has a good experience, it is easy to give the patient several packets of educational material to share with a few friends. You can expect one of every three patients will pass the material to friends or male siblings, resulting in new patients.

Internal marketing can be relatively inexpensive, but it is a slow process that requires constant effort to impress patients. Below is a list of tactics to consider:

- Avoid an extensive automated phone tree so every patient can easily speak to a human
- Use reminder text, phone or email, appointment reminders (but ask patients their communication preferences; it can by annoying to get all three when you have stated you prefer only text, for example)
- Refresh the waiting room décor or ensure that it is modern, clean, and has current and relevant reading material or videos
- Offer a phone/electronic device charging station in addition to water, coffee or tea
- Warmly greet each patient at each step of their in-office journey
- Reduce or consolidate paperwork; offer an option to complete it online prior to the appointment. Sixty percent of patients will choose a different provider if it means less paperwork
- Evaluate/monitor your speed of service. We are a culture of immediate gratification; 97% of patients are frustrated by wait times.[1] If a wait is unexpected, communicate the reason
- Provide patients with a tool to immediately assess satisfaction or ask them to rate you online (give them steps for where and how to rate your practice)
- Utilize medical portals to communicate follow-up, post-test results and allow patients to post questions without having to call
- Treat your patients with respect!

That last bullet shouldn't be taken lightly. *The Wall Street Journal* found health care consumers place more importance on a doctor's interpersonal skills than on clinical skills. Eighty-five percent of those polled said being treated with dignity and respect is an extremely important quality in a doctor, and 84% also said the same about good listening skills[2]. Further HCAHPS (Hospital Consumer Assessment of Health Care Providers and Systems) surveys found two factors linked to a decreased risk of readmission after discharge: doctors who thoroughly explained information to patients, and nurses with great listening skills[3].

B. EXTERNAL MARKETING

External marketing, simply stated, is any activity or event targeting prospective patients. Tactics in this pillar range from no- to low-cost to very costly. However, while some—such as advertising or direct mail—have a higher cost, they can be extremely efficient at driving patient volume without outlay of your/staff time.

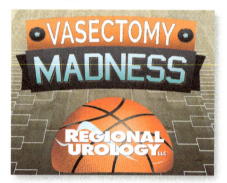
Billboard advertising during March Madness, Regional Urology Shreveport, LA

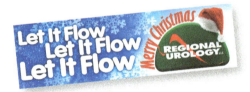

Many practices tend to shy away from advertising or direct mail due to the cost and fear of failure. But if you follow the steps stated in the beginning of this chapter regarding marketing planning—and understand that marketing spend is an investment in your practice—the return on investment can be significant. If your practice is interested in pursuing paid external marketing, it's highly recommended to find an agency or consultant who can help to strategically determine the best tools/spend to achieve your goals. While most wish to minimize consultant costs, a good partner will save you money in the long term.

The balance of this section is going to focus on no- to low-cost tactics designed to increase your visibility within your community, region, or even on a national level. While these don't require much outlay of expense, they do require time to plan, prepare and promote. Again, it's important to evaluate the merits of these tactics against your marketing plan, and continually evaluate their resulting impact on your practice goals.

Event Marketing

Event marketing strategies leave a lasting, focused impression of you/your practice on your target audience by grabbing their attention and providing them with an experience that resonates. In contrast to advertising, event marketing aspires to make quality individual impressions. The key to pulling off an effective event is to identify the target audience and create an experience that is valuable to them.

Seminars & Support Groups: Two examples of events your practice may wish to execute are seminars/talks or support groups. Both allow you to target audiences according to specific diseases, diagnoses, and treatments. Depending on your practice goals, you can even narrow the target audience to specific demographic groups, such as senior citizens or millennials. These, generally more intimate experiences, allow potential patients to get to know you and your practices' capabilities.

Selecting topics may seem daunting, but you have a terrific research tool in and out of your office every day! Are you seeing common trends, questions, or interests? Those are likely excellent and timely topics for seminars. In addition, the topics of wellness, nutrition, and cancer and disease prevention are universally appealing.

In terms of logistics, these events can take place at your local hospital, ambulatory treatment center, practices' reception area, or even the local library. Consider having a patient attend the meeting who has the diagnosis or who has received a treatment you are discussing. Patients who present can share their experiences, describe how the problem affected their quality of life, and how the treatment improved their life.

Sponsorships: Sponsoring community fundraisers or health advocacy programs are another way to elevate your practice awareness. These sponsorships can range from simply donating money in exchange for having your name included on promotional material, to a more-involved planning role to media interviews and speaking opportunities at the events. It's important the event(s) you select are aligned with your target audience. Activities like the ZERO Prostate Cancer Run/Walk or Bladder Cancer Advocacy Network (BCAN) fundraisers might be ideal depending on your practice capabilities.

Charity auctions are another sponsorship opportunity. You might consider offering your services as part of an auction for a school or local organization. For example, donate a no-scalpel, no-needle vasectomy to a local school's annual auction. You can be creative with how you title your donation, such as "School Tuition Getting You Down? A No-Scalpel No-Needle Vasectomy Is a Solution." A few men (or their wives) will probably call your office to make an appointment for the procedure. It's also likely your donated item will be the talk of the event!

Ethnic Marketing

Serving the health care needs of various ethnic populations presents a unique marketing opportunity to the culturally competent physician. Begin by identifying what ethnic community you would like to focus on. That may depend on the demographics of your area, your own ethnic background, and the languages spoken in your community. There are ethnic community websites and resources you can use to promote your practice to this discrete group.

Most ethnic groups have an effective word-of-mouth network. If you are accepted by a few members of the ethnic group, word will travel fast, and you can expect to become a lifelong provider of urologic care to their community. Another benefit to marketing to various ethnic communities is grateful patients often refer family members with urologic conditions from their native countries. If they know you can communicate with their relatives, they are likely to use you and your practice for their urologic care.

Authorship and Public Speaking

You are a subject matter expert in urology—and many of you specialize in treatments or procedures. As such, you have valuable knowledge to transfer to the general public. Writing articles/blogs or speaking are two ways to share your knowledge and areas of interest/expertise, while also promoting your practice.

Authorship: While it's not likely you will receive many referrals from an article authored for the *Journal of Urology*, writing articles/blog posts for local newspapers, magazines, and websites can drive patient volume. Writing articles for the lay media will increase your visibility, credibility, and ultimately, profitability.

You can create compelling and interesting articles about new procedures, treatments, a unique case with an excellent result, or the use of new technologies, such as the UroLift® to treat symptomatic BPH. An advantage of writing articles is the published article links can be posted to your website or social media accounts extending the shelf life (and improving your search engine ranking discussed in the Internet section).

Public Speaking: Few urologists are natural-born public speakers, but if you get started on the speaking circuit and acquire effective public speaking skills, you will be amazed at the increased demand for your speaking services and the commensurable increase in number of new patients. Through your speaking engagements, audiences have an opportunity to learn more about your medical topic and how it applies to their health. It also allows you to interact with potential new patients before and after the presentation.

Begin by contacting meeting planners at various church groups, service organizations, such as Rotary, Kiwanis, Lions Club, Knights of Columbus, and AARP, and patient advocacy organizations, such as the American Cancer

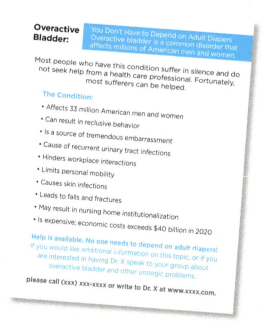

Figure 1: *Example of a Fact Sheet on Possible Meeting Topic.*

Society, American Diabetes Association, American Heart Association, and Us Too. Send the meeting planner a brief biography, which outlines your credentials. Consider attaching a fact sheet (**Figure 1**) and several articles, especially if you are the author on the topic.

In order to benefit further from the presentation, collect e-mail addresses of attendees and keep in touch with them by sending a newsletter (see **Figure 2**). You may also wish to send a fact sheet that includes highlights from your presentation with a call to action to schedule an appointment.

C. DIGITAL MARKETING

If you don't read anything else in this chapter, read this section! Digital marketing is one of the most influential tools available and you MUST secure your digital footprint. Your online reputation matters; you need to stay competitive by not only "being online" but ensuring information about you and your practice is updated and accurate.

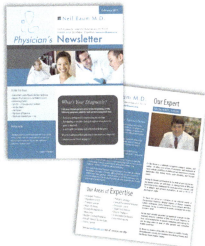

Figure 2: Newsletter sent to those who have been in the audience of a presentation

What is your digital footprint? At the core, it's the information about you and your practice that exists on the Internet. That online information is no longer just information you generate, such as websites, but also what others generate about you. While this subject is vast, this section highlights five core areas:

Website

Living in a digital world, a practice website is now a necessity . . . no matter the size of your practice. If you don't have a practice website, you are likely diminishing your new patient acquisition potential while also frustrating existing patients who wish to transact on your website. Your practice website can be used to accomplish many different marketing strategies, while also improving productivity.

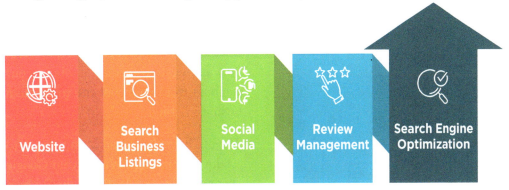

CHAPTER 9 | 147

Developing and maintaining a website doesn't need to cost a fortune, however, you need to have a plan. Most importantly, the website features and benefits should be reflective of your patient's desires. Health care websites no longer need to be endless pages of difficult to navigate information. Rather, they should validate who you are, be functional, and easy to navigate. Look at a few of your favorite brands and see how their websites are built. Key considerations include:

- Simple to navigate! (can't emphasize this point enough)

- Enable your patients to transact the way they want (pay bills, complete paperwork, schedule appointments, etc.)

- Keyword rich to help with search engine optimization (see below)

- Mobile friendly

It's critical your website be responsive. Responsive website layouts automatically adjust and adapt to any device or screen size. This is critical as more and more patients are using smartphones for all communication and transactions. Two-thirds of Americans own a smartphone, and 62% of smartphone owners have used it to look up information on a health condition[4].

Websites require care and feeding, which means periodically adding new content. Otherwise, your site won't be sticky, meaning viewers won't return. Further, updating content tells search engines, like Google or Bing, you are an active website; this improves your organic (non-paid) search rank.

Search Business Listings

The Yellow Pages are a mere memory since the intent of more than 87% of online searches is to search for the same info we used to find in that big yellow book—and more! Search business listings is an online entry that contains your business name, address, and phone number, along with other details. Many of these listings are generated by the directory, such as Google, Bing, or Yelp! They aggregate information about your business from your website to create a business listing.

If you haven't already, you need to claim your listings. Within your Google listing, for example, there should be a blue line that asks, "Suggest an edit-Manage this listing?" You then proceed through a series of activities to validate you have the right to manage the business profile. In this example, Google will send a postcard to the business address with a verification code. Once you receive the postcard, follow directions to enter the code. When you have the right to manage the listing, you can update inaccurate information and upload photos or other relevant data. At a minimum, you should include:

- Practice name (and associated physicians)
- Address
- Phone
- Website URL
- Hours
- Photos of your office from the exterior

Consider your search business listing as your digital office front! If a patient walked by and the lights are out and the landscaping is overgrown, would you walk in? Within the format of the listing, make it appealing. Pictures are worth a thousand words. In addition to the exterior of the building (for way finding), add a photo of the lobby, unique technology, an exam room, and the professional team.

As noted above, you likely have a business listing across multiple directories. Make sure you manage the key ones, including Google, Bing, and Yelp! Even some of the medical rating sites allow you to update your practice information. If you can't find a search business listing already established for your practice, create one. Simply type in the following phrase into your favorite search engine, "How do I create a business listing in Yelp!"

Social Media

The effectiveness and influence of social media is undeniable; it's no surprise urologists are embracing it as a major component of their digital marketing strategy. With leading social media sites, like Facebook, Twitter, LinkedIn and YouTube, it's never been easier to obtain or share content with your existing patients while increasing your visibility in the digital ecosphere. If your practice doesn't use social media and you are wondering if you really need a social media presence, the answer is YES!

Your patients expect to find you in the social ecosphere. According to Pew Research, nearly 80 percent of U.S. adults use at least one social media site, with the fastest growing segments being those aged 30-64. Interestingly, despite privacy concerns, people frequently share and ask health-related questions to help manage their health. Further, some studies indicate patients benefit from physician use of social media through increased access to care and enhanced perception of quality[5].

If you aren't a believer yet, consider these benefits to practices:

- Provides a vehicle for building relationships and a sense of community with existing patients

- Enables you to position your practice as a center of excellence

- Builds awareness of services and capabilities

- Provides an avenue for giving updates on practice news/events

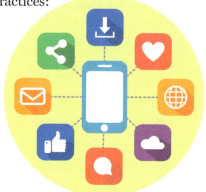

- Enables you to "listen and learn" about what's important to your patients

- Engages and helps develop relationships with thought leaders/influencers

- Highlights talent within your practice

- Gives your practice a "human face"

- Allows you to garner "market research"... you can ask followers questions to help inform changes in service

- Improves your search engine optimization (SEO)

Do you need to be on "all" social media platforms to have an impact? NO! Facebook and YouTube are the most widely-used social media platforms, and its user base is most broadly representative of the population of a whole. A smaller percentage of Americans use Twitter, Instagram and LinkedIn. You need to select the social media platform(s) that works best for you and your patients. Start by asking them where they would expect to find you or wish to engage with you.

Getting started with social media doesn't need to be overwhelming. Once again, make a plan!

- Define your objective
- Understand your audience: where are they and where do they expect to find you?
- Define your "tone" (e.g., are you serious, funny, ivory tower, guy/gal next door?)
- Establish your publishing themes (e.g., what topics you will address in your posts?)
- Establish and commit to a regular posting schedule

When it comes to content, there are two types: original and curated. Original content is anything you generate, such as text or blogs, photos, videos, or infographics. Curated content is gathering existing available information on a topic and sharing it because it adds value to your target audience. Leveraging curated content is a great way to regularly post, while also bringing your followers value with relevant, timely information. When you post curated content, add a brief comment on why you believe this content is relevant to your audience. (See section in this chapter titled, "Making a YouTube Video: There's A Steven Spielberg Inside All of Us")

Once you have social media sites, alert your patients and ask them to "like" or "follow you." You can also add links embedded in social media icons to your website to direct people to your social pages. Build your presence by liking and following influencers in your community and related groups. Don't be afraid to engage with followers. When you respond, ensure you are both professional and familiar; patients want to feel like they have a personal connection.

Lastly, develop a social media policy for your practice. Define who can post to the site and set clear guidelines to ensure you remain HIPAA compliant. Be clear about the "nevers:"

- Never ID a patient; address patients as a collective group
- Never engage patients on personal health questions; have them call the office
- Never diagnose!

Connecting with existing and prospective patients on social media can be enjoyable! You can explore patterns and trends shaping how your patients perceive their health and well-being.

Review Management

Research shows 91% of people regularly read online reviews; 84% trust online reviews as much as a personal recommendation. And, according to Inc Magazine, they make decisions quickly! Sixty eight percent form an opinion after reading between one and six online reviews. So, if you haven't embraced online reviews, the time is now! Your "webutation" is at stake.

What patients have to say about you, both positive and negative, can be easily posted on a variety of review sites. For good or bad, this posting remains indefinitely and can impact your practice both positively or negatively! According to Harvard Business School, a one-star increase in ratings can increase revenues by 9% of most businesses.

As we noted in the beginning of this chapter, a patient's medical journey includes evaluating online reviews. Patients will check your reviews, whether they were referred by the most prestigious physician in the community or their best friend. Potential patients want to get a feel for the urologist before scheduling an appointment; they want to read first-hand from other patients what they liked and didn't like about you and your practice.

Take these steps to be aware of and manage your online reputation:

1. Google yourself! Regularly monitor and see what patients are saying. Remember, any feedback, even in the form of a negative review, is a gift. Gaining knowledge about what patients say about you and your practice is incredibly insightful.

2. Act on negative reviews. Depending on the forum, you may be able to post a response. On most ratings websites, responses are posted for all to see, so do not include details that would breech patient confidentiality. Consider your tone when responding. While we all feel defensive when seeing a negative remark, it doesn't send a positive message to viewers if you take a defensive position. Rather, patients expect to see negative reviews, but are often looking for how you handle the feedback. Unless it's a clear case of incorrect facts, simply thank them for their feedback. Again, remember feedback is a gift! If patients have a consistent complaint, there is likely opportunity for improvement. (Note: if the review is clearly not about you or your practice, you can contact the review website and ask for it to be removed. They won't remove negative reviews, but some, with evidence, will remove inaccurate information.)

3. Tip your online reputation balance in your favor. There's nothing unethical about making patients aware of the opportunity to post an online review of your practice. Proactively ask for their review and provide them with instructions for posting reviews to Google, Yahoo, Yelp! and Bing. You can marshal support from established patients—and help their waiting time go faster—by queuing up a computer in the reception area, or handing them a laptop or tablet with access to consumer ratings websites. **Figure 4** is an example of an in-office kiosk that enables quick patient feedback.

Just like other aspects of digital marketing, there are companies that specialize in review management if you'd feel more comfortable. Just ensure you select a partner that specializes in health care reputation management as our profession has unique needs. A partner should be able to track and report online reviews, as well as aggregate and funnel those incoming reviews to third-party sites that publish.

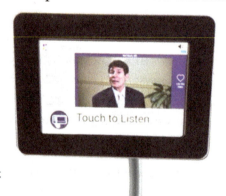

Figure 4: *Kiosks located in each exam room.*

Search Engine Optimization (SEO)

In order to acquire new patients, search engine optimization (SEO) has become a necessary tool in the digital marketing landscape. SEO is the practice of getting a website to rank highly in the search engine results page. In other words, it determines where your practice lands in the list of choices served up following a search. When a potential patient searches for "urology physician near me" into a search engine, you want your name to show up on the first page of search results.

Effectively managing your SEO is a bit of art and science. Because there are extensive SEO practices, it's a worthwhile investment to have your website partner, or an SEO consultant, help you optimize for search. Below are a few tips to help improve your chance for search engines to find you and your practice. Ranking factors are always evolving, but those that have a significant impact on SEO ranking include:

- A secure and accessible website
- Mobile friendliness
- Page loading speed
- Social signals (having social media accounts linked to your site)
- Regularly adding new content to your page (blog postings or social media posts, for example)
- Optimized content (effective use of keywords)

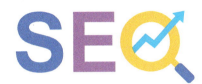

Keywords are the words or phrases in your web content that make it possible for people to find your site via search engines. Search engines take the words or phrases and connects the searcher with results; consider Google a matchmaker. Its job is to figure out, based on the keywords or phrases, the best match for marriage. You need to be in the dating pool (first page search results) to have a chance at getting to the altar.

A list of keywords for urology practices is included at the end of the chapter. If you are interested in exploring more specific terms for your market, Google has a tool, AdWords, it not only tells you how many people are searching a particular keyword every month; but also provides related keywords. Another way to define keywords is ask your patients what words/phrases they used while searching for various urologic topics or to find your practice.

To leverage keywords in your digital marketing tools, you'll want to incorporate them into website copy, blogs, social media posts, etc. A caveat: keyword density should be no more than approximately 3% to 5% of the article or Google will penalize you for "keyword stuffing" by lowering your ranking.

D. REFERRAL MARKETING

The last of the marketing pillars, referral marketing, is one of the most overlooked yet most powerful. Consider the last time someone you trusted spoke highly (or negatively) of a product or service. When you needed a similar product or service, did you recall their passionate feelings (positive or negative)? While online/digital reviews are impactful, there is nothing more powerful than word of mouth. There are three primary direct referral sources:

1 **Referring Physicians/Professional Peers:** While most professional referrals come from primary care, don't forget to identify and monitor other potential sources. Those could include: nurses, urgent care clinics, emergency departments, pharmacists, case managers, dentists, dieticians, podiatrists, or chiropractors to name of few. When a patient comes to your practice from a referring physician, it's especially critical both for the referring physician relationship, as well as the continuity of care, that you make additional effort. Below are some tips to consider if you aren't already deploying:

- Give the patient top priority in seeing them promptly
- Thank the referral source with a note or call
- Follow up with clinical findings and progress reports
- Make sure the patient is happy with care
- Make yourself readily available for consults with referring physicians
- Send patients back with a personal thank you note

Also, with referring physicians, it's also important to understand how much influence the office staff in a primary care practice has in the referral. Some physicians have a list of preferred physicians, but it's the office that makes the initial call. Make sure you are recognizing those staff members and find a way to consistently remind them of your appreciation!

2 **Current/Past Patients:** There is no better source of referral than a happy and healthy patient (or family member). They are a talking billboard for you. The two most critical steps in activating these referral sources is first to ask them to refer you! It's an easy transition in a conversation when they are thanking you for their health to graciously ask if they have family or friends who would benefit from your expertise to recommend you now...or in the future. (Remember, nearly 90% of people will act on making a recommendation if asked!) Second, when you are asking them to be a referral source, ensure they are armed with information to pass along. You can also remind them of your website and of course, social media sites!

3. **Community Resources:** Don't forget those community resources that can influence referrals. Both men and women have very unique relationships with their stylist or barber and will discuss uncomfortable issues and personal problems such as ED or incontinence. Another resource where people share intimate knowledge is their attorney. It's a good idea to network with these resources in your community and ensure they know about your capabilities or know where to direct prospective patients for information about your practice.

As you execute on referral marketing tactics, it's especially important to track the source of new patients. Information should include contact information, referral volume, and payer (i.e., the insurance coverage of patients). Most current practice management systems enable you to document this information. If your tool(s) do not, consider searching for a simple customer relationship management (CRM) software that can help you track, store and recall information.

Once you have a referral tracking tool, you can create a set of simple numerical or alpha codes to indicate the referral source. When you have a new patient, enter the appropriate code into your practice management system. After several months of gathering this data about referral sources, you will begin to see trends or patterns. You may uncover new sources you were not aware of as well as find referral sources to develop further. Also, if a referral source has stopped making referrals to your practice, you should proactively reach out to identify if there is a problem that you can address or fix.

Conclusion

Physicians must navigate an ever-evolving health care world; this is especially true when it comes to attracting and retaining patients. Those who plan and invest—time and resources—thrive. Others will fall behind. While marketing can be overwhelming, it is manageable. When viewed through the lens of a patient diagnosis and treatment model, the marketing activities right for you and your practice become clear.

With a well-developed marketing plan, your practice can most effectively utilize a variety of tools in the mix, including internal, external, digital, and referral marketing. As you develop your plan, execute your actions, and measure your results, remember:

- Marketing is an ongoing process. Your approach will adapt to changes in goals, patients' needs, and the health care industry. You will learn through the journey.

- Marketing is an investment—of both time and resources. While you want to track your results and measure effectiveness, it's also important to remember you won't achieve outcomes if you don't put anything into the process.

Finally, always put the patient at the center of your marketing efforts. Improving their experience, outcomes and health will ultimately make your practice healthy.

BLOGGING AND YouTube VIDEOS

Blogging for Beginners

Urologists who plan to develop a social media presence can consider blogging. Blogging is free and can be accomplished reasonably quickly. The process allows you to communicate with your existing patients, and also attracts new patients to your practice. The only expense is your time. A user-friendly blog site is **wordpress.com**. **Wordpress.com** has a tutorial, which can provide you with a few steps to create a blog site, enter content, and publish your material.[6]

Blogging is defined as website maintained with regular entries (posts), which invites comments by viewers. This is the uniqueness of blogging as it allows feedback from those who visit your blog site. A blog site becomes interactive and creates a dialog between your existing patients and potential new patients—that's difficult to do on a website.

There is a 3-step formula:

1. Develop a hook or an enticement in the title to capture the attention of viewers,[7]

2. feature a relevant message to identify with your viewer,

3. include a call to action where the viewer can connect to your website or your practice to find solutions to their medical problems.

You need to make your blog interesting and worth taking the time to read. Start by beginning your blog with a startling analogy, simile, statistic, or metaphor. For example, if you are writing about prostate cancer you might begin with the statistic that nearly 40,000 men die each year of prostate cancer, which is twice the capacity of an NFL sports stadium. That comment usually grabs the attention of the reader.

After developing a blog, you will want to check your traffic using the blog sites analytics. This gives you information on the number of viewers that you have, how long they are spending on your blog, and

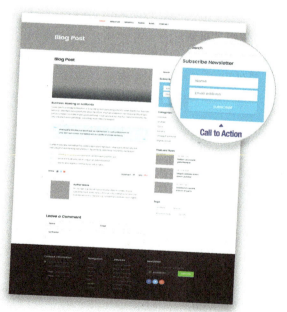

Figure 3: *An effective call to action*

and how many are connecting to your website. This is valuable information you can use to tweak your blogs and identify what works and what to abandon.

Finally, you need to provide a call to action. This means motivating your readers to visit your website, call to your practice, and become a patient. The easiest method is to offer something free on your website in exchange for the viewers e-mail address. (**Figure 3**) is an example of an effective call to action.) Now you add the potential new patient to your e-mail list and send them newsletters from your practice.

MAKING A ▶ YouTube VIDEO:

There's A Steven Spielberg Inside All of Us

YouTube has become the most popular video-sharing platform on the Internet. Urologists have the ability to create their own fame with short Web "TV shows" broadcast on YouTube. Furthermore, YouTube has become the second most popular search engine,[8] and, for that reason, it is vitally important for urologists to have an online YouTube presence.

To broadcast yourself, you need a video camera, an iPad, or even iPhone can be used to capture excellent quality videos. If you aren't comfortable being onscreen, think about creating a video using free recording software voicing over a PowerPoint presentation.

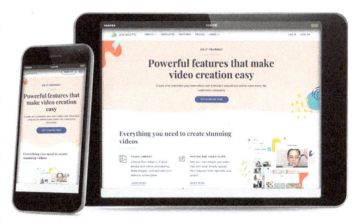

You can also use still photos to create an online montage using Animoto (**www.Animoto.com**).

Once the video is created, it can be used in multiple ways. It can be uploaded to YouTube and other video sites; added to blog posts; embedded on on embedded on your website; loaded onto the office EMR and used to educate patients while in the exam room. Google and other search engines are attracted to video. Therefore, create a title that contains the keywords to optimize how your video is found and indexed by search engines.

After you have recorded your video, it's simple process to start uploading it to YouTube. All you need is a Google ID or Gmail account. If you don't have an account, you can create one at no cost on **www.youtube.com**.

A Partial List of Urologic Keywords

urologist, urology, kidney doctor, urine doctor, kidney, kidney disease, kidney cancer, kidney stones, prostate, prostate cancer, treatment prostate cancer, surgery for prostate cancer, robotic surgery, robot, laparoscopy, radiation for prostate cancer, X-ray therapy, brachytherapy, high intensity ultrasound for prostate cancer, HIFU, chemotherapy for prostate cancer, metastatic prostate cancer, Stage 4 prostate cancer, prostate infection, blood in the urine, urinary tract infection, cystitis, bladder infection, unable to urinate, urinary retention, urinary incontinence, leaking urine, loss of urine, diapers, incontinence, pelvic organ prolapse, prolapse, POP, dropped bladder, cystocoele, rectocoele, uterine prolapse, bladder lift, bladder repair, mesh, mesh repair, bladder cancer, male infertility, low sperm count, pregnancy, testicle cancer, testis cancer, scrotal pain, painful urination, vasectomy, male sterilization, contraception, erectile dysfunction, ED, impotence, poor erection, penis, hard on, STD, sexually transmitted disease, VD, gonorrhea, syphilis, discharge, discharge from penis, clap, interstitial cystitis, IC, bladder pain, female sexual dysfunction, FSD, pain with intercourse, painful intercourse, lack of sexual desire, decreased sexual desire, lack of orgasm, anorgasmia, absence of orgasm, vaginal dryness, vaginal atrophy, atrophic vaginitis, infertility, male infertility, problem with pregnancy, no sperm, semen analysis

1. Health Information Services, LLS. "Addressing Patient Wait-Time Woes." 2014
2. Weinacher, A, MD. "Press Ganey again? Strategies for improving the patient experience." https://stanfordhealthcare.org/
3. Patient Experience Journal. "The relationships between HCAHPS communication and discharge satisfaction items and hospital readmissions." http://pxjournal.org/cgi/viewcontent.cgi?article=1022&context=journal. 2014
4. Smith A. US Smartphone Use in 2015. Pew Research Center. http://www.pewinternet.org/2015/04/01/us-smartphone-use-in-2015. Published April 1, 2015. Accessed July 29, 2015
5. Ventola, C. Lee. "Social Media and Health Care Professionals: Benefits, Risks and Best Practices." P&T. July 2014.
6. https://learn.wordpress.com/get-started/
7. Baum N, Titles are terrific-creating titles that attract attention. J Med Pract Manage 2014 Nov-Dec;30(3):166-7
8. YouTube-The second largest search engine. Social Media Today, August 2013, http://socialmediatoday.com/socialbarrel/1650226/second-largest-search-engine-infographic

Non-cited Resources:

Baum N., Henkel G. Marketing Your Clinical Practice-Ethically, Effectively and Economically (4th Edition). Jones and Bartlett, 2014.

Jackson R. The changing game of practice marketing. Podiatry management. 35(6);65-68.

KEY POINTS

- **Most providers today find their #1 competitor is "Dr. Google."**

- **To achieve ideal outcomes,** create a marketing plan by understanding your practice's needs and goals; knowing your target patient; assessing existing marketing assets and identify gaps; measuring success and adapting as you learn.

- **Designate one person to lead the marketing efforts**—too many people involved prove to be less efficient.

- **The primary audience for internal marketing is your staff,** existing patients, and new patients, making the customer experience, easy check-ins and décor prime opportunities to boost referrals.

- **If your practice pursues paid external marketing,** it's highly recommended to find an agency or consultant to help strategically determine the best tools and spend to achieve your goals.

- **Event marketing strategies** leave a lasting, focused impression of your practice on your target audience by grabbing their attention and providing them with an experience that resonates.

- **Most ethnic groups have an effective word-of-mouth network.** Serving the health care needs of various ethnic populations presents a unique marketing opportunity to the culturally competent physician.

- **If you get started on the speaking circuit** and acquire effective public speaking skills, you will be amazed at the increased demand for your speaking services and the commensurable increase in number of new patients.

- **Digital marketing** is one of the most influential tools available and you MUST secure your digital footprint. This includes utilizing your website, search business listings, social media, review management, and search engine optimization.

- **Google yourself,** manage your online reputation and respond to negative reviews.

- **Utilize key words** in this chapter to rank higher on search engines and incorporate them into website copy, blogs, social media posts, etc.

- **Never forget the power of word of mouth** and show appreciation to your referring physicians and health care professionals, patients and community organizations.

Jennifer L. Dally, MBA

Jennifer is the Founder and Chief Attunement Officer of Attune Marketing Group. Jen has more than 25 years of health care marketing experience. Her tenure working for integrated delivery systems, health care/pharmaceutical advertising agencies and a fortune 500 health care consumer packaged goods company provides her with a unique perspective on how to help practices and health care organizations achieve their marketing goals within the constantly changing health care environment. In addition to coaching, she is a frequent speaker, guest lecturer and contributing author within the health care industry.

Attune Marketing Group coaches physicians on how to improve their practice outcomes through marketing and strategy and offers a collaboratory of experts within a variety of marketing disciplines to efficiently execute.

Neil Baum, MD

Dr. Neil Baum is a Professor of Clinical Urology at Tulane Medical School. He is the author of seven books on practice management and medical marketing. His first book, Marketing Your Medical Practice–Ethically, Effectively, and Economically, has sold over 175,000 copies and has been translated into Spanish. His latest book, The Three Stages of a Medical Career was published in March 2017 by Greenbranch Publishing.

CHAPTER 10

Credentialing & Privileging

Mia Frausto, BSB, CPCS

Few processes in a medical practice have a greater impact on the provision of care or on reimbursement than credentialing. Credentialing is the process of applying to health care entities, such as hospitals or ambulatory surgery centers, for access to their services and to insurance carriers for inclusion in their provider panels. In addition to credentialing a provider with a hospital or ambulatory surgery center (also referred to as a "facility"), Privileging must also occur to secure membership on the Medical Staff or Allied Staff at a facility. Credentialing establishes the qualifications of licensed medical professionals and validates their training and experience to provide a specific array of health care services.

Credentialing is a multifaceted process that is best initiated as soon as the decision is made for a health care provider to join a practice. The main purpose of credentialing is to verify a provider's qualifications. Credentialing variations range from the perspective of a group practice, a facility, or an insurance carrier. Although the work is similar, state rules and regulations influence the requirements for each organization. For information on your state rules and regulation, you can contact your local state agency. You can also contact the U.S. Health and Human Services (HHS) at **www.hhs.gov** to be directed to your state agency. If your entity is accredited, you can refer to your accrediting standards provided by the accrediting agency. Some of the accrediting agencies are The Joint Commission (TJC) and the Ambulatory Association for Ambulatory Health Care (AAAHC).

Many steps in credentialing are time-sensitive and interdependent. In other words, some credentialing steps may not be taken until others have been satisfied. For example, professional liability coverage cannot be secured until a state medical license is active. The state medical license is dependent on the medical board securing original source documents from training programs, hospitals, surgery centers, etc. Consequently, completing each step to meet the requirements is essential. Since individual state requirements for licensure vary, it is important that you are familiar with requirements at the state and national level for licensure/certification, as well as being familiar with the unique requirements of each insurance carrier. Credentialing is its own distinct process and should not be confused with the insurance carrier contract participation process.

Privileging and Credentialing are not one-in-the same. For appointment to the Medical Staff or Allied Health Staff at a facility, credentialing is the first step and then Privileging, based on the verifications achieved. All information obtained for credentialing and privileging is presented to the Organized Medical Staff for review. A provider wanting to perform specific activities at a facility must be appointed to the facility for the desired privileges being requested. The privileges are requested on a Delineation of Privileges (DOP) form, and the provider must have completed some training in the requested privileges. The training must be verified through the method of primary source or secondary source. The method accepted is identified in the organization's policies and procedures and/or bylaws. Licensed practitioners who can practice independently can be granted clinical privileges.

Selecting the Credentialing Coordinator

The Credentialing Coordinator may also be referred to as Credentialing Specialist, Credentialer, or Medical Staff Professional (MSP).

Processes do not occur on their own. Consequently, selecting the right person to lead your credentialing efforts is crucial. The Credentialing Coordinator must be detail oriented, organized and capable of managing multiple deadlines. Effective communication skills are essential since a tremendous amount of information will flow verbally, through email, fax, and in some situations hard copy documents are still required. As insurance carriers and facilities require provider recredentialing on staggering time schedules, tracking pertinent dates, deadlines and consequences are vital to the success of this area.

In most practices, new providers cannot begin employment without being credentialed by a large majority of the most frequently occurring insurers. By laying out these guidelines and expectations up front, it creates realistic expectations for both the new provider and office staff assisting in the process. One misstep can be costly to the practice and to the new provider.

Similarly, insurance carrier recredentialing occurs typically on three-year cycles while facilities (hospital and ambulatory surgery centers) recredentialling typically occurs on two-year cycles. Essentially, the Insurance carrier or facility can choose to credential prior to the recrendentialing cycle ending so they can avoid overlooking the recredentialing due date(s). Although insurance carriers and facilities typically send out reminders to the provider or provider office, it is important for the Credentialing Coordinator or designee to track recredentialing cycles, so they do not run the risk of missing a recredentialing cycle. You should not depend solely on a reminder from the carrier or facility.

When the Credentialing Coordinator is knowledgeable in all scopes of credentialing, the practice is at a great advantage. Knowing what is needed for the practice in conjunction with what to expect from outside sources helps the Credentialing Coordinator know how to deal with the various outcomes that can occur. Some practices may not have an experienced Credentialer or Medical Staff Professional (MSP) and may need to use other staff to manage this responsibility. In either case it is beneficial for that person to have the tools and resources necessary to keep them up to date on any credentialing trends or changes.

On the national level, there is the National Association of Medical Staff Services (NAMSS) located online at **www.namss.org**. They can provide information on joining to enhance the education for the MSP and offer educational conferences that are held annually in different states. They can also address inquiries about the state or local chapters, if available in your state. Additionally, there are books that can be purchased through NAMSS and other sites, such as HCPro, are located online at **hcmarketplace.com**.

Key Professional Relationships

Maintaining key contacts in each insurance company may prove helpful as front-line personnel change or as processes are modified—often without formal notice to the provider or the provider's practice. As more carriers eliminate local provider representatives and consolidate processes at the national level, resolving time delays or determining what is needed to move an application forward may seem impossible if key contacts are not maintained. As documents are received from various insurance carriers, always enter names, phone/fax numbers, titles, and addresses into your business contact list. When the need arises, you may not have the luxury of waiting on e-mail responses or returned phone calls.

It is also helpful to develop a professional relationship with the Insurance Commissioner or Department of Insurance in any state in which you do business. This should be done well in advance of any "ask" you may ever have or conceive to have of them. Having these contacts and relationships built over the years will serve you well in several areas. A single phone call from the State Insurance Commissioner's office can jumpstart a stalled process or make a topic that was previously an insurmountable issue for the carrier seemingly disappear instantly. These departments carry a tremendous amount of influence on the carriers. They also can provide useful information on state laws and guidelines.

Understanding the laws regarding health insurance, contracting, and provider participation in the states in which you maintain a presence is essential. For example, some states require a carrier to retroactively set the effective date of a qualified new provider as the date of application upon request. If you are not familiar with the laws in your state, you may miss out on opportunities. When sending in the application packet, a cover letter should be enclosed detailing the state law and requesting retroactive date treatment. Without this additional letter, the carrier is under no obligation to make the effective date retroactive—potentially causing a significant financial loss to the practice.

Some states also recognize provisional credentialing, as detailed in the National Committee for Quality Assurance (NCQA) standards. Most insurance carriers seek NCQA accreditation and may permit provisional credentialing when a provider requests it. Provisional credentialing typically requires the provider to have:

- A Current valid State License to practice
- Current completed and signed State application with attestation
- Current professional liability (malpractice)

Complying with the laws set by your state and accrediting body, if applicable, is mandatory. Learn more at **www.hhs.gov**.

The Responsibilities of the Practice

The practice should start onboarding a provider by securing all documents available from the provider, including, but not limited to, copies of the provider's driver license or passport, current curriculum vitae, passport-size photo (when available), explanations of any previous malpractice claims, state medical licenses, DEA certificates, and provider numbers already secured. The new provider checklist, **Figure 1** is designed to assist the Provider in understanding the why, what, when, and how of the credentialing onboarding process. **Figure 2** is designed to track the receipt of the required documents and information identified on **Figure 1**.

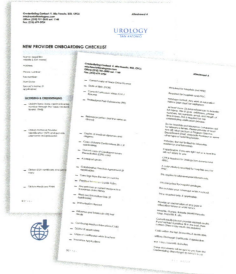

Figure 1: New Provider Onboarding Checklist

Most applications can be filed online or through the Council for Affordable Quality Health Care (CAQH) at **www.caqh.org**—the credentialing coordinator or designee should take advantage of this method when given the choice. In some cases, insurance carriers only give the provider the option of using CAQH, thus CAQH must be kept current and is required to be attested to every 120 days so the company accessing the provider information has accurate data.

▶ STATE MEDICAL LICENSE

Often, physicians who are coming out of residency will not have a Medical License in your state unless they happened to have attended Medical School or Residency in the state. Some states require residents to have a medical license while they are enrolled in the programs. The earlier you can start, the better off you will be as some states are more difficult to obtain a license in than others. The practice should ensure it clearly understands the requirements for state medical licensure since most of the credentialing process is dependent on this document. Even if a physician has not trained in your state and has not completed his Urology residency, many states allow the physician to secure a medical license after one year of post medical school training. For example, if the provider attended a medical residency in Ohio, but has not yet completed the residency program, he

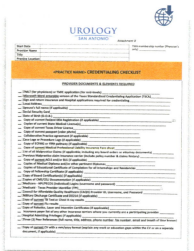

Figure 2: Credentialing Checklist

may be able to secure a Texas medical license after only one year of post-medical school training. This provides an opportunity to move the application process up by several months.

Some states have an extensive test that must be passed while others merely depend on the fact that the provider successfully graduated from medical school. Knowing state rules is important, as realistic timelines should be established at this point with the provider. Some states require that the provider make a personal appearance to sit for an interview, which presents a time issue in order to arrange time off from residency or fellowship training while the state board can accommodate the interview, arrange travel, etc. The earlier the process of acquiring a license, the greater the likelihood of avoiding licensing delays.

Know the idiosyncrasies of your state license laws. For example, some states issue medical licenses secondary to the first state license that a provider may possess. This means the provider cannot give up the first license in the future because the new license is tied to it.

Some states require specific attendance in a class to educate the provider on state specific medical law, expectations, and the role of the medical board in the state. While this should not be a significant issue, it does often present logistical issues to the out-of-state provider who has limited time to travel, prior to arriving permanently in the state to fulfill this requirement.

▶ FEDERAL DEA LICENSE

Concurrently with the state medical licensure process, the provider's Federal DEA license should be verified. If he or she does not hold a DEA license, work with the applicant to apply for one online. Due to the opioid crisis, the DEA has enforced additional requirements when registering or renewing a DEA. The DEA's registration address must match the practice address on the provider's state medical license. While this requirement may seem insignificant, it can be challenging to larger practices with multiple suites within one building. The DEA requires the exact suite number match that of the provider, even if delivery does not occur in that suite number. Under no circumstances should a provider be allowed to have his/her home address on a DEA certificate.

▶ STATE NARCOTIC LICENSE

The practitioner is responsible for ensuring that the prescription conforms to all requirements of the law and regulations, both federal and state. Typically, a state narcotics license is dependent on the possession of both an active medical license (from the same state) and an active Federal DEA License. This license will take 30 to 60 days from application submittal to receiving the license in most states. You will not be able to apply for this license until the prior two items have been completed. Logistically, this extends the time horizon required to bring a provider on board and positively reinforces the theme of beginning the entire process as early as possible. Not all states require this license, so it is important for you to find out what your state requires.

▶ PROFESSIONAL LIABILITY COVERAGE

In general, malpractice coverage has prerequisite requirements of an active medical license (from the same state), an active Federal DEA license and an active state narcotics license, if applicable. This application will need to have an effective date in advance of the provider arriving as the next steps typically require an active malpractice policy, not one that has an effective date sometime in the future. The malpractice carrier needs to review the applicant's claim history (if any exists) and will want to know what type of surgical exposure the applicant will be potentially performing. It may be best to have one of your existing providers work with the applicant to select the surgical procedures he/she may be performing since a misstep here could further delay facility privileges.

▶ MEDICARE

You can apply to Medicare for credentialing once the provider has an active state medical license; an active Federal DEA license; an active state narcotics license, if applicable; and an active professional liability (malpractice) policy. Use the on-line application, through the Provider Enrollment Chain and Ownership System, to avoid significant processing delays. Find out which region you are in based on your state, so you know which contractor manages enrollments. (i.e., Novitas manages Part B applications for Medicare in Texas). To help avoid delays, put the provider's anticipated start date on the Medicare application. Medicare will credential a provider only 60 days prior to the actual start date. It is important to start this process first because many commercial insurance carriers require Medicare approval before they will credential a provider.

▶ HOSPITAL PRIVILEGES

Typically, hospital privilege applications require an active state medical license; an active federal DEA License; an active state narcotics license, if applicable; and an active professional liability (malpractice) policy. It is best to have an existing provider assist the new provider in choosing which privileges to request since many health systems require training, experience, and case logs before approving privileges for some procedures. Asking for everything rarely reflects the reality of the new provider's needs and opens the door to hospital privilege delays. Credentialing committees or medical executive committees, at the hospitals may not meet frequently, so it is best to understand the requirements for approval of temporary privileges. Temporary privileges are not automatically granted. When requested, they require approval separate from the normal hospital privilege process. While waiting for temporary approval, or if not granted initial approval, a provider can request to observe an active provider at the facility.

▶ AMBULATORY SURGERY CENTER (ASC) APPOINTMENTS

If the provider will be utilizing an ASC to perform surgery, submit the application concurrently with the hospital application. ASC approval processes often parallel hospital processes so know the timeline for approval and plan accordingly. If your practice has ownership in an ASC, it is important that your Credentialing Coordinator or designee keeps the provider credentialing files for the practice separate from the credentialing file that is managed for the ASC. For example, when the malpractice insurance is updated for a provider and the information is put in the provider's credentialing file for the practice, there should be a separate file that is maintained for the ASC. The practitioner credentialing and privileging checklist, The activity calendar, **Figure 3** is used to assist in tracking all the documents and information required for the ASC. There are many variables that can affect processing timeframes. The ASC and hospital processing times are similar, which is between 60-90 days. Processing timeframes are affected by the size of the ASC or hospital, and staff size.

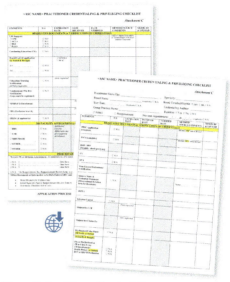

Figure 3: *Practitioner Credentialing & Privileging Checklist*

All surgery centers and hospitals have committees to assist in the decision making. The Medical Executive Committee (MEC) is just one of those committees. This committee makes recommendations relating to, but not limited to, quality of care, appointments, reappointments,

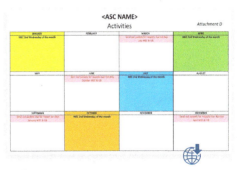

Figure 4: *Activity Calendar*

clinical conduct, clinical competency and clinical privileges. Keeping track of when these meetings occur is crucial, so the Credentialing Coordinator or designee has all necessary documents required and completed before the MEC meeting date. An activity calendar is helpful so you can view a snapshot of each month that the MEC is held. The activity calendar, **Figure 4**, which can be used for other activities, such as but not limited to, Governing Body, Quality Improvement Committees, and Quality of Care.

▶ COMMERCIAL INSURANCE CREDENTIALING

Many carriers utilize a standardized state application through CAQH that helps reduce the application time. It is critical to maintain a list of insurance carriers accepted by the practice keep it updated. Many regional, smaller and mid-size carriers are aggregating their payer networks in plans, such as PHCS-Multiplan, which allows for a single application to gain access to hundreds of carriers. The key to all these applications is to make certain that when submitted, an application is completed in its entirety. An insurance carrier can and will return an application if any part is missing or incomplete. Retaining electronic copies of the applications, along with a timeline of contacts, is essential.

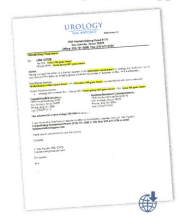

Figure 5: *Sample letter*

Sending paper correspondence via trackable delivery methods and retaining the delivery confirmation is highly recommended. A carrier stating, they have lost an application packet or never received it will not be an unusual occurrence. Proving correspondence transmission and knowing with whom and when you spoke with an insurance carrier representative is crucial. As previously mentioned, knowledge of your state laws is essential in this area, as you may need to specifically request special assistance or conditions by referencing certain state laws or guidelines. Again, this is an area that most Insurance Commissioners offices are more than willing to help you with and can provide you as much information and education as you need to facilitate a smooth process.

These applications can take anywhere from a couple of weeks to process to three to six months before a provider is fully credentialed. Even after the provider is credentialed, the next step is for the insurance carrier to add the newly credentialed provider to the existing group contract and data enter the provider's demographics in its claims payment system. If the provider does not require credentialing and only needs to be added to the group contract, a Link letter will be required. **Figure 5** shows a sample letter. This tool should be on your letterhead and requires specific information to link the provider to an existing group's Tax Identification Number (TIN). Often, a well-placed phone call to your Insurance Carrier Provider Representative will help expedite the process. Periodic status follow-up is recommended through the approval process. Utilize a Status

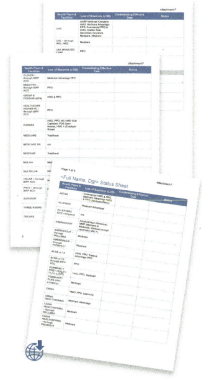

Figure 6: *Status Sheet*

Sheet, similiar to **Figure 6**, to assist in tracking the submission, follow-up, and completion of applications submitted to payers and facilities.

Some insurance carriers do not have a provider representative assigned to a specific practice so you will need to contact the Insurance Carrier's Provider Relations department to ensure the entire process is completed timely. It is wise to follow up with provider relations or provider enrollment, at a minimum, every 30 days, to ensure nothing falls through the cracks. Additionally, it is important to keep your provider roster accurate and current. Terming or inactivating a provider with the contracted Insurance Carrier, network or facility after the provider leaves the practice is necessary to ensure the entity has accurate and complete demographic information on file for your practice. Understand that each entity's termination process differs to ensure you submit as requested. Submit a request in writing (**Figure 7**) to terminate a provider who will be leaving or has left the practice. Terminations vary by health plan or network, so this tool is helpful when they ask for a termination notice on letterhead. Use a checklist, similar to **Figure 8**, to assist in tracking the termination request's submission and receipt.

It is important to keep the demographic information current and accurate with any health plan or network in which you participate. Federal and state regulations require quarterly validation of directory information and updates to provider demographics to ensure their provider directories are up to date. This safeguards members, so they can locate the provider for whom they are searching. It also warrants prompt payment and filing of claims. To locate more information about your state's rules and regulations on this this matter visit **www.hhs.gov**. Use something similar to **Figure 9** when you are asked to provide an update on letterhead. Other times you may be given a tool that is specific to the health plan or network to request demographic updates.

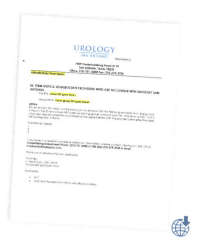

Figure 7: *Term Notice Letter*

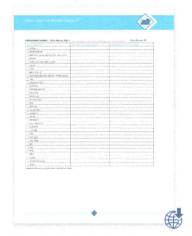

Figure 8: *Termination/Inactive Process Checklist*

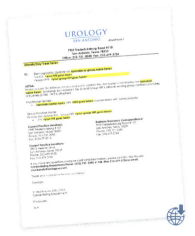

Figure 9: *Provider Demographic Update Letter*

When Enough is Not Enough

There may be occasions when a carrier refuses to credential a provider in its network. In most instances, these situations occur due to network sufficiency or are related to a specific issue with the provider's work history, which may not have been disclosed during provider negotiations or contracting.

Network sufficiency refers to an insurance carrier's contention that enough urologists are already under contract, and the market needs no additional urology specialists to meet its beneficiaries' needs. Depending on your group's market position, you can leverage its participation by insisting that Network sufficiency refers to an insurance carrier's contention that enough urologists are already under contract, and the market needs no additional urology specialists to meet its beneficiaries' needs. Depending on your group's market position, you can leverage its participation by insisting that all urologists in the group provide call coverage. Having even one non-contracted provider will result in unintended out-of-network charges to the patient. An option for groups with market dominance is to notify the carrier that the group may exit the agreement if the additional provider is locked out of the network. Contacting your state's Department of Insurance also may provide leverage, especially if there is an "Any Willing Provider" statute in place. Any Willing Provider laws basically state that a provider must be allowed to participate if he or she is willing to accept established terms, accept allowable fees, and will otherwise meet minimum credentialing requirements. For government payers, a similar approach may be taken by contacting your CMS (Centers for Medicare and Medicaid Services) regional office at **www.cms.gov/Medicare/Coding/ICD10/CMS-Regional-Offices.**

Thoroughly vetting incoming providers is imperative. You do not want to leverage your group's participation in a plan only to discover that your incoming provider has had licensing or clinical care issues in a prior position. Every state's medical board has a process in place which permits file review by the public. If there is any doubt about a candidate's credentialing viability, it is better to identify those issues prior to contracting.

To protect the medical group, you also may wish to consult legal counsel to incorporate these items into your employment agreements:

1) That incoming providers may not start work until credentialing has been substantially completed for all major government and commercial payors in your market, and

2) Incoming providers may not start work until privileges are in place with all facilities in which the physician or advanced practice provider will render care.

Incorporate into your recruitment process a specific discussion about pending litigation, prior issues with credentialing or privileging, or other significant legal matters, which might limit the provider's ability to provide care.

Should a candidate misrepresent past clinical activities, criminal issues, or fitness for employment, the group has a variety of legal remedies. No remedy is better than prevention, so incorporating specific provisions, which permit without cause termination of an employment agreement—even before employment begins—is an important step in protecting your group's reputation and financial integrity. Employment agreements should address credentialing, and your legal counsel should advise on how to clearly delineate the circumstances, which may trigger separation.

Typically, a provider has no issues being credentialed; however, the length of time to complete the process with the insurance carriers may vary greatly. Many carriers require Medicare and/or Medicaid provider numbers to be in place prior to approving participation. With increased automation, the process has accelerated. Nonetheless, the group should foster internal discussions to determine which carriers must be credentialed prior to a provider's start date. For example, a recently graduated urology resident who is learning clinic flow may be able to start with only Medicare credentialing complete. Thus, as the patient base builds, so does the provider's competency with the practice's workflows. In other instances, there may be specific key carriers that a group must serve, and that must be complete prior to the provider's start of employment. Remember, a partially credentialed provider should not be scheduled to take call until the provider can see most, if not all, insured patients.

Some carriers permit retroactive billing, making the effective date coincide with the submission date of a fully completed, accurate carrier application. Check with individual carriers about their retroactive billing policies. Please remember that if a provider ultimately is denied access to the carrier's network, the patient may not be billed for those services unless an advanced beneficiary notice (ABN) has been secured. An ABN outlines that a specific service may not be covered by the insurance carrier and the patient may be responsible for payment. Securing ABNs on all patients is prohibited by many carrier contracts and represents a less-than-optimal approach to conducting business in a fair, ethical manner. Know and follow each carrier's policy on credentialing.

There is never an instance in which a partially credentialed provider should bill using another provider's number. Services should be billed only by the individual providing the service.

Automated Solutions

Cost-effective, efficient credentialing software exists, and practices are encouraged to fully utilize available resources to track due dates, storekey documents, and complete standardized or customized forms. The cost often is minimal; the productivity afforded by many

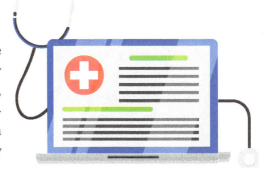

of these products easily justifies the monthly per-provider cost. Automating your credentialing also helps eliminate the possibility of missing renewal dates for any required licenses or certificates, and any other expirables you need to track. It is important to research a few different software companies to find out which one works best for your credentialing and/or privileging needs.

The Best Solution is to be Prepared

There are many opportunities for delays, misunderstandings, and even logistical issues. Complex processes result in misplaced documents, missed deadlines, and unintended delays. Even seemingly simple logistical issues can become larger problems as schedules become tighter and options become fewer as the process nears completion.

From the perspective of the provider that is transitioning from one practice to another, the process remains essentially the same in that each step must still be covered. Unless the new provider is currently practicing in the same state, it is unlikely that any appreciable time savings will be realized. In fact, some steps, such as the malpractice process, may take longer as there will be more data for the underwriter to review in this case.

Once you have the provider setup and confirmations begin to arrive from insurance carriers, it is time to begin bringing other components of the practice into the picture. These involve the practice's practice management (billing/collection) system, insurance claims clearinghouse, electronic medical record (EMR), and accounting systems.

Many of these licenses and facilities require annual or biennial renewal. Knowing when to prepare recredentialing documents is essential. Do not depend solely on notices you may receive. Remember that some carriers send important notices directly to the provider, which means you must be attentive to timelines and essential documents.

In summary, start as early as possible to give your practice time to deal with issues that will arise. Utilize employees who are detail oriented and highly responsible to ensure that a smooth, controlled, and streamlined process is accomplished. Set realistic expectations for both the practice and incoming provider. Realize that steps will not always go perfectly, and that assistance will be required to help facilitate the credentialing process.

Staying Current with Trends and Changes

Credentialing and privileging requirements can change at any time, so it is important to stay ahead of any changes by attending credentialing seminars, webinars and accessing other relatable resources that provide information on the latest credentialing trends and requirements. Know your rules and regulations within your state. If you must meet standards through an accrediting body, know their standards too. Sometimes, the requirements are the same and other times they are different. It is important to be knowledgeable of any requirements that affect your practice or facility.

CREDENTIALING CHECKLIST

Physician Name _____

	Agency	Date Requested	Date Received	Notes
State Medical License				
DEA License				
State Narcotics License				
Malpractice Coverage				
Medicare				
Medicaid *(if applicable)*				
Hospital Privileges				
ASC Privileges				
Commercial Insurance				
Commercial Insurance				
Commercial Insurance				
Commercial Insurance				

KEY POINTS

- **Credentialing is the process** of applying to health care entities, such as hospitals or ambulatory surgery centers, for access to their services and to insurance carriers for inclusion in their provider panels.

- **For appointment to the Medical Staff** or Allied Health Staff at a facility, credentialing is the first step and then Privileging, based on the verifications achieved.

- **The Credentialing Coordinator** must be detail oriented, organized and capable of managing multiple deadlines.

- **Maintaining key contacts in each insurance company** may prove helpful as front-line personnel change or as processes are modified—often without formal notice to the provider or the provider's practice

- **It also is helpful to develop a professional relationship** with the Insurance Commissioner or Department of Insurance in any state in which you do business.

- **Understanding the laws regarding health insurance,** contracting, and provider participation in the states in which you maintain a presence is essential.

- **Start onboarding a provider** by securing all documents available from the provider, including copies of the provider's driver license or passport, current curriculum vitae, passport-size photo, explanations of any previous malpractice claims, state medical licenses, DEA certificates, provider numbers already secured, etc.

- **Know and follow each carrier's policy on credentialing.**

- **Credentialing and Privileging requirements can change at any time.** Stay ahead of any changes by attending credentialing seminars, webinars and accessing other relatable resources.

Mia Frausto, BSB, CPCS

With seventeen years experience as a credentialing specialist for hospitals, ambulatory surgery centers, health plans, and private physician practices, Mia Frausto holds a Bachelor of Science in Business Administration and is a Certified Provider Credentialing Specialist (CPCS). She also is a member of the South Texas Association of Medical Staff Professionals (STAMSP). Knowledgeable in the TJC, NCQA, and AAAHC accreditation standards, Ms. Frausto specializes in project management and quality assurance as they relate to facility privileges and medical practice credentialing.

CHAPTER 11
Negotiating Third-Party Payments: A Never-Ending Challenge

Jerri Wilson-Durbin

"How many of you actually read and understand the payer contracts you sign?" This question was posed by a health care attorney to physicians and administrators at a seminar focused on managed care contracting. I estimated fewer than half of the room raised a hand.

With declining reimbursement and financial security at risk, how can such a critical issue be ignored or lack the required attention? Many practices fail to prepare or implement steps for the management of payer contracts. There is no guide, roadmap, or instruction manual for this function, as each market, practice, and payer are different. It is human nature to avoid difficult issues and negotiating with an insurance company is the great unknown and the dark abyss combined. The collection of data necessary to properly negotiate is time consuming and overwhelming. Getting the payers to the table for negotiations and a mutual agreement on the terms of a contract can take months, years, or even disappear into the bureaucratic black hole. The payers benefit from the advantage of comparable provider data, which practices cannot legally have. All of this and more results in the feeling that the odds are stacked against the medical practice. Although this all sounds so negative, you can achieve positive results by understanding your challenges, and strategically setting goals with reasonable expectations. So, what can be done to successfully negotiate contracts for urology?

Preparation, Patience, Data, Data, and More Data

Implement steps and processes to facilitate negotiations that will provide results in third-party negotiations:

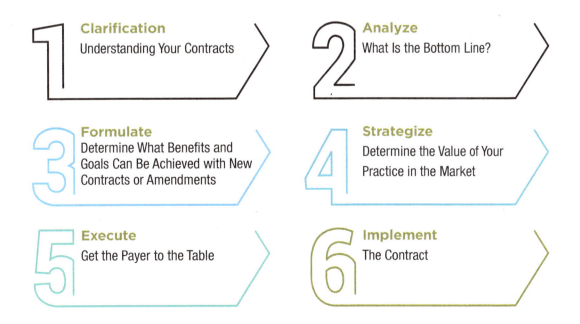

STEP 1: Clarification – Understand Your Contracts

Understanding the terms of each contract is extremely important. Viewing the data in a comparison format can ensure a clear vision that is not a perception, but factual and informative.

Create an in-depth analysis and comparison of each payer. Once created, a spreadsheet will identify payer contracts in need of attention and determine obstacles and opportunities. Include the following list of important details for each contract:

- List major payers, identifying products such as PPO, HMO, Medicare Advantage Plans, etc.
- Terms of the contract, deadlines and terminations, or auto renewal
- Percentage of the practice's business
- Type of contract
- Reimbursement rate
- Lines of service: lab, pathology, imaging, radiation, etc.
- Other pertinent information: denial rate, denial by service, request for records, etc.

With regular updates, this information is an excellent benchmarking tool for your administrative team. Monitor progress with monthly meetings including key staff members apprised of all aspects of dealing with the payer. For example, administration may have an entirely different view of expectations than the billing manager. Create a payer specific shared calendar, which includes meetings, goals, contract terms, renegotiation, and any other pertinent dates. It's important to remind members of your management team that contractual rate sharing is not allowed between medical practices under antitrust laws, which prohibit practices from sharing reimbursement rates.

Study the Payer Mix; the percentage of your market is PPOs, HMOs, or Advantage Plans. This information is useful when preparing proformas and budgets. It will also allow you to watch both growth and changes in your market, specifically in aging geographical areas.

A list of obstacles and roadblocks that the practice experiences will identify which payers are labor intensive. A dive by payer can reveal which payers are presenting a higher overhead resulting from difficult precertification policies, overly cumbersome processes, or a high percentage of denials.

Terms

FFS

Payer 1 Contract Comparison			
Evergreen	Not Covering Cost/Refer to Outside Lab		
Market 32.77%	HMO 18.55%	PPO 8.42%	MCR Adv 5.80%
Hospital E&M	XX% of 2018	XX% of 2018	XX% of 2018
Surgical	XX% of 2018	XX% of 2018	XX% of 2018
Office	XX% of 2018	XX% of 2018	XX% of 2018
Office E&M	XX% of 2018	XX% of 2018	XX% of 2018
DME	XX% of 2018	XX% of 2018	XX% of 2018
Drugs/Injectables	XX% of 2018	XX% of 2018	XX% of 2018
Urodynamics	XX% of 2018	XX% of 2018	XX% of 2018
Biofeedback	XX% of 2018	XX% of 2018	XX% of 2018
X-Ray	XX% of 2018	XX% of 2018	XX% of 2018
Ultrasound	XX% of 2018	XX% of 2018	XX% of 2018
Radiation	XX% of 2018	XX% of 2018	XX% of 2018
Lab	XX% of 2018	XX% of 2018	XX% of 2018
Cytology	XX% of 2018	XX% of 2018	XX% of 2018
Pathology	XX% of 2018	XX% of 2018	XX% of 2018

01 High volume of records request after the claim is paid

02 High volume of records request due to modifier 25 after the claim is paid

03 Extremely long hold times for representatives

04 Incomplete explanations when requesting refunds

05 Receiving demographic denials/COB updates that payer has not updated

06 Receiving denials for no coverage; actual issue is patient needs to update COB

07 Payer advising patient the claim was denied due to coding, when service is not covered, for example, ED

08 Not enough information provided on the EOB for denied claims

Numbers used in the tables are for illustrative purposes only, unless a source is stated.

Add additional data for a more in-depth review by analyzing volumes and reimbursement by CPT code. Is the practice being reimbursed properly? Practice management software programs assist with the testing of the contracts to ensure accurate reimbursement rates. List the results of reimbursement errors and bundle testing. Review each line of service (E & M, Hospital, Ultrasound, Imaging, Radiation, etc.) by CPT code and volume. Review reimbursement for higher volume codes, versus reimbursement for lower volume codes.

Many contracts offer a different rate for visits compared to lab, imaging, etc.

Take note of the "year of Medicare reimbursement" used for the contract percentage. Even a small increase can have a positive result. E & M Codes increased in 2019. (CMS national payment)

CPT Code	2019 InfoDive Avg. National Visits/Urologist	2018 MCR National Reimbur Rate	2019 MCR National Reimbur Rate	2019 Increase	% Increase
99213	1,396	$74.16	$75.32	$1,619.07	1.56%
99214	1,263	$109.44	$110.28	$1,061.15	0.77%
Potential Increase in Revenue				$ 2,680.22	
Potential Increase in Revenue for a Group of 20 Urologists				$ 53,604.31	
Potential Increase in Revenue for a Group of 40 Urologists				$107,208.62	

[1] InfoDive® Reports: Eval & Mgmt Codes and Average Medicare Reimbursements, IntrinsiQ Specialty Solutions, Inc.

STEP 2: Analyze – What Is the Bottom Line?

Understanding the details of practice reimbursement is vital. Equally important is the other side of the equation, the expense side: What is the cost to the practice to perform each service?

Determine the Breaking Point, or Bottom Line, for Each Service

Do reimbursement rates cover costs, and what is your profit? How much of a margin do you need to ensure the physicians receive a fair compensation? When should you walk away from a service line or contract?

Each line of service must be calculated independently, with the knowledge from both the revenue and expense side. Office visits and procedures, pathology, lab, urodynamics, medications, imaging, radiation, etc., will all require independent analysis.

First, the revenue side of the equation:

What is the revenue for work performed in the office? (Excluding all lab, imaging, etc., as all ancillaries will be calculated separately)

E & M Reimbursement Data	
E & M CPT Code Volume for 10 Urologist *InfoDive Average Per Urologist for 2019 was 3,585*	35,850
E & M Collection for 10 Urologist *InfoDive Average Per Urologist for 2019 was $369,281, Utilizing National Avg. Reimbursement Rates*	$3,690,810
Avg. Collections Per Visit E & M Codes **Each Physician Average will be different due to Level of Coding, Payer Mix, and Volume (New vs. Established)** Avg. Reimbursement New Patients Avg. Reimbursement Established Patients Avg. Reimbursement Consult Patients *InfoDive Average Collection Per Urologist for 2019, Utilizing National Avg. Reimbursement Rates*	
Numbers used in the tables are for illustrative purposes only, unless a source is stated.	

[1] InfoDive® Reports: Eval & Mgmt Codes and Average Medicare Reimbursements, IntrinsiQ Specialty Solutions, Inc.

Next, the expense side of the equation:

A detailed chart of accounts and proper cost centers allows the practice to calculate and analyze the overhead cost of each line of service. However, when calculating the expense side of the equation, it becomes labor intensive to calculate only the E & M expense, as there are also added visits to consider, such as visits without an associated E & M code.

This table provides a simple concept of viewing the average cost per visit. A deeper look will be required, with considerations that include levels of coding, removing surgery scheduling expenses, etc.

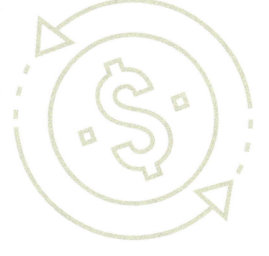

When reviewing expenses, another factor to consider is the volume a payer brings to each line of service. For example, by adding a high-volume payer for a lab test, even one that reimburses at a low rate, may accomplish benefits for the service line as a whole, by reducing the expense per test.

Remember to make allocations to all the lines of service for central types of expenses like administration, IT, billing, and call centers.

Average Expense Per Visit	
Other Visits without an E & M Code (Vasectomy, Biopsy, Cystoscopy, Etc.)	1,250
Total Visits with and without E & M Codes (35,850 + 1,250)	37,100
Total Office Collections	$4,800,000
Includes all Office Collection but excluded all Ancillaries such as Medications, Imaging, Labs, Radiation, Etc.	
Avg. Collections Per Visit	$129.38
Total Office Expenses (No Physical Compensation or Benefits) **using 60% overhead**	$2,880,000
No Ancillaries such as Medications, Imaging, Labs, Radiation, Etc.	
Average Cost Per Visit	$77.63
Average Net Profit Per Visit	$51.75
Estimated Compensation to Physicians:	
Net Office (Total Office Collections minus Total Office Expenses	$1,920,000
Net Hospital	$1,000,000
Net All Ancillaries and Other Revenue	$5,020,000
Average Compensation Per Physician (Based on 10 Physicians)	$502,000
Numbers used in the tables are for illustrative purposes only, unless a source is stated.	

Example of Lab Testing

MCR Reimb $18.00

PAYER A ONLY

Revenue	Reimb	Volume	Revenue	
Payer A	$22.50	5,000	$112,500.00	125% of MCR
		5,000	$112,500.00	
Expenses		**Volume**	**Expenses**	**Avg. Per Test**
Rent		5,000	$2,000.00	$0.40
Staff		5,000	$5,000.00	$1.00
Supplies		5,000	$80,000.00	$16.00
Admin, Billing			$10,000.00	$2.00
			$97,000.00	
Net Lab			**$15,500.00**	

PAYER A & B COMBINED

Revenue	Reimb	Volume	Revenue	
Payer A	$22.50	5,000	$112,500.00	125% of MCR
Payer B	$16.20	20,000	$324,000.00	90% of MCR
		25,000	$436,500.00	
Expenses		**Volume**	**Expenses**	**Avg. Per Test**
Rent		25,000	$2,000.00	$0.08
Staff		25,000	$9,000.00	$0.36
Supplies		25,000	$375,000.00	$15.00
Admin, Billing			$10,000.00	$0.40
			$396,000.00	
Net Lab			**$40,500.00**	

Numbers used in the tables are for illustrative purposes only, unless a source is stated.

STEP 3: Formulate – Determine What Benefits and Goals Can Be Achieved with a New Contract or Amendment

What are the reasons for new negotiations? After completing the calculations of reimbursement versus cost, does the evaluation identify financial goals or benefits? The reason for a new or amended contract may not be about reimbursement rates. Increasing fee-for-service reimbursement rates is tough, and sometimes an impossible feat, so what are other options or benefits? What are other options to consider or products that are being offered in your market?

▶ Benefits of a Group vs. Individual Contract

As health care continues to see the merger of smaller medical groups into large and even larger groups for the benefit of ancillaries and economies of scale, a "group contract" makes more sense. The burdensome task of placing a new physician on contracts is greatly reduced. Once the practice is covered under one contract, the process is streamlined, with no wait time for the physician to be placed on the plan and no "out of network" issues.

▶ Incentive Programs

Many payers offer incentive programs to direct lines of services of preferred partners or facilities. Incentive programs can provide bonuses to the practice for compliance of these referrals, but typically the bonuses are small and short lived. Look at this as an opportunity that can open the door for communications for other topics.

▶ Addition of New Services

Urology practices continue to create new lines of service, such as physical therapies, urogynecology, and chemotherapy. A review of all CPT codes will ensure these lines of service are included in your contract.

▶ Improvement of Processes

MGMA reported in its October 2019 Annual Regulatory Burden Report, "There is no shortage of opportunities to reduce regulatory burdens on physician practices." Participants reported the overall regulatory burden on the medical practice had increased 86% over the past 12 months (2019). Reach out to the payer for discussions regarding improvement of processes, such as prior authorization requirements, the appeals process for denials, audits, and number of records for medical necessity. Make recommendations for efficiencies and potential cost-saving solutions for both the payer and the practice.

▶ Fee for Service (FFS) Contracts

Even though margins grow smaller and smaller, medical practices have spent hours strategizing to justify an increase in reimbursement. When recently polling 12 medical groups, 11 reported no increases in FFS contracts in the last five years; however, two were able to develop strategies and were successful in reversing cuts in their rates. One large group was able to negotiate a rate increase on office services, by offering their ASC as an option, resulting in a lower overall spend for the payer.

A Health Care Finance article from October 2018, by Jeff Lagasse, Associate Editor, states the percentage of health care payments tied to value-based care reached 34% in 2017, but this still leaves the majority of reimbursement tied to FFS. Some areas of the country are slow to adopt other types of plans. Recently, when requesting a meeting with our largest payer in the market for discussions on value-based and incentive plans, our organization received the response, "Performance-based contracts are not being offered at this time." Even though the transformation from FFS to value-based care will take time, if you have not started to generate data, get started now. Be prepared to align incentives for both the providers and payer.

▶ Value-Based Care and Sharing Savings Contracts

Value-Based Quality Care, Accountable Care Organizations (ACOs), Merit-Based Incentive Payment (MIPs), Alternative Payment Models (APMs), and Episodes of Care all share the same basic goals: to maintain or improve the quality of patient care and to deliver care more efficiently to reduce expenditures; this all requires a partnership between the payer and provider. The complex balance between providing value, while promoting quality patient care is measured in different models and programs.

ACO organizations continue to make a big push to recruit PCPs into their organizations, accomplishing cost-reduction goals by steering patients to selected groups of high-quality, low-cost facilities and providers. Urology groups must participate with these ACOs to receive referrals from these PCPs. Now, many of these ACOs are offering insurance products of their own.

Pay for Performance or Shared Savings contracts track financial reductions of ED visits, readmissions, length of stay, and infection rates—all positive steps resulting in savings and potential financial rewards to the urology practice. If you are not tracking these types of measures, get started. This is an excellent opportunity to prove your value and ability to manage costs. Identifying these opportunities will interest payers, bringing them to the table. With a shared savings to the payer and a potential bonus reward to providers, both sides win.

Health Day news reports, "Of the 10 most common outpatient conditions treated in the U.S. emergency departments, urinary tract infections and kidney stones can be the most expensive, according to a new report." (Preidt 2013).

Median Price for Kidney Stone ED Cost	**$ 3,437**
New Patient Level IV Office Visit (Medicare Rate)	**$ 168**

▶ Bundled Payments or Episode of Care

A CMS Innovation Center Episode Payment Models January 2020 article states, "Episode payment models incentivize participants to look across settings at the beneficiary's treatment needs to improve coordination, reduce expenditures, and maintain or improve quality by thoughtfully determining optimal treatment processes and opportunities to deliver care more efficiently." (2020). Since 2013, seven models have been tested. The process began with the testing of specific procedures or hospitalizations in order to offer a set price for the scope of services required. In 2018, CMS announced a bundled payment model, Bundled Payments for Care Improvement (BPCI), which provides a single payment to participants who take on the financial risk for a urinary tract infection episode. Many medical groups offer this type of bundle or episode of care to payers and self-insured employers. This model is used often for services, such as orthopedics and colonoscopies.

▶ Risk Contract

A risk contract requires a significant commitment from both the payer and the practice. Both parties acquire the financial risk when collaborating on reimbursement. Many administrative hours are required for the enormous commitment of research, implementation of technology, tracking utilization, clinical outcomes, administration and measuring the performance of the plan. This type of contract fosters a commitment to proper utilization while monitoring quality of care.

STEP 4: Strategize – Determine the Value of Your Practice in the Market

What do you bring to the table? What part of the market do you represent? What sets you apart in the market? What are the practice's strengths and weaknesses? Payers view urology as another line on the budget, a "cost center" to manage. The payers are focused on reducing expenses or, at a minimum, maintaining a neutral budget. So, what added benefits or qualities are offered to make the practice appealing to the payers? View the data as if sitting on the payer's side of the table.

Take into consideration the size of your group. What is the ability of the payer to provide medical coverage for urology in your geographical area without your practice? Does a large percentage of the market share represent power? Size has made a difference in reimbursement for the mega-medical groups and is a strategy often used. Although when I interviewed a few medical groups that dominate or have significant numbers in their market, none were successful in negotiating significant increases in reimbursement. But at minimum, the practice size should provide leverage to get the payers to the table for negotiations. But what are other negotiating attributes?

Measurable qualities and features, such as quality, utilization, cost, and patient satisfaction are essential factors to tie to the success of the practice, so benchmark these measurable events to learn from and improve upon them.

Measure **quality** and outcomes such as infection rates, return to the OR, and length of stay.

Benchmark the **utilization** of CT, MRI, ultrasound, cystoscopy, and lithotripsy.

Calculate and evaluate the **cost** of referrals and services ordered by the practice. Since all services performed and "ordered" are associated or tied to each physician, gain an understanding and comparison of pricing in your market. Do you know which facilities provide low or reasonable rates for imaging?

Make pricing comparisons and understand the "going" rate of urology services. Internet websites, such as Health Care Blue Book are resources for comparisons on pricing of medical services. These sites attract the interest of patients and employers with high deductible plans.

What do your **Patient Satisfaction Surveys** reveal? Take patient feedback seriously. Yes, many times these surveys are no more than a platform for unhappy patients to vent or retaliate. Nevertheless, these public sources are viewed by patients and payers. Many ACOs mandate the medical groups to promote these surveys. Act on the feedback as quickly as possible:

- Utilize services that report negative posts immediately by email to the practice.
- If possible, reach out to the patient, listen, make apologies, and take corrective action.
- Inform and address concerns with staff.
- Inform physicians in a timely manner when there is a negative review post regarding patient care.
- Track and advertise the positive postings, which is an excellent marketing tool.

This is an easy way to promote the practice during negotiations. Highlight what the practice does well and improve on the rest.

STEP 5: Execute – Getting the Payer to the Table

Bring your game and be prepared to share your knowledge with a clear strategy. Now it all boils down to collaboration between the payer and practice.

In 2018, urology represented only 1.54% of the total Medicare Part B expenditures; therefore, urology is not always at the top of the list of priorities or the focus for payers, so just getting them to the table can be a challenge. Be focused and prepared; introductory meeting requests are often met with hesitation and delays, with no interest, and as a burden. The first request should be a written communication that supports the mutually beneficial reasons for the meeting, along with a few supporting factors to pique interest.

Once the required tasks are completed and objectively reviewed, the value of the practice determined, what else will motivate the payer for negations? Research the metrics and measurements of their programs. What accomplishments is the payer looking to achieve in the market? Communicate with other practice administrators. What strategies have worked for them? Use all your resources to gain an understanding of what the payer is looking for, including the payer's website, insurance brokers, and health care attorneys.

Being persistent is a key factor for keeping your practice on their radar:

- Request the first meeting in person, face-to-face.
- Build a good relationship with your representative.
- Place reminders on the calendar to send friendly emails to the representative, keeping the process moving forward.

- Look for opportunities to make connections with the right people within the payer organization. Does anyone within the practice (physicians, administration, and the practice's attorney) have a connection, serve on a common board, or know "someone" that knows "someone" within the payer's organization?

- Attend meetings and functions where introductions of the payer's representative might be made.

Be prepared for initial communication with the payer:

- Place all topics for discussions in written form to ensure all are covered in a clear and precise manner.

- Invite the payer to your facility to show off the professional environment.

- Emphasize the group's commitment to be "good citizens," willingness to comply with facility requirements, and participate in incentive programs that benefit both parties.

- What sets the practice apart from others in the market?

- Begin discussions with the easy wins and commit to long-term improvements

    • Reductions in ED, utilization of low-cost designated facilities, etc.

    • What improvements are easily measured and manageable?

Be proactive:

- Keep the top incentive of both parties in mind.

- Ask for everything you want up front, with an understanding that you will not achieve all.

- Provide solutions, not obstacles.

- Avoid conversations that give ultimatums; there will be no winners.

- Be prepared to counter offer.

- Know your breaking point and be prepared to make difficult decisions. It is critical to know when to walk away from the table.

Keep your data current and up to date. By the time negotiations are completed, some data may have changed. You may be required to reinvent the strategic plan along the way, but you have the data to support the decisions to be made.

STEP 5: Implement – The Contract

The basic terms are agreed upon, but now for the contract itself. Be tolerant, and do not get discouraged; be prepared for this process to take some time. Expect negotiating strategies, such as delays, last-minute changes, and unacceptable contract language. But continue to work toward transparency to build an efficient and effective partnership.

▶ New vs. Amendments

When possible, push for an amendment instead of a new contract as contracts are becoming lengthier and increasingly more complex. A new contract can easily take several months for the payer's legal team to produce. As new contracts become lengthier and more complex, attention to each detail of the contract is necessary. Any and all amendments should be mutually agreed upon and signed by both parties.

Each aspect of the contract is as important as the next. Is the best option a multiyear contract? If the contract has a term date, require a lengthy window of time to negotiate before the contract expires. Also, some contracts allow rate inflators, which provide an increase with long-term contracts. If the contract is evergreen, require the opportunity for renegotiations or amendments every year or two.

Common language in payer contracts typically reads that the payer can amend the contract at any time without practice approval. Or only allow the provider 30 days to object in writing before it automatically goes into effect. A 90-day notice should be a minimum timeline but should not be allowed at all.

Practices must require a mandatory notice of any changes to the contract, requiring two forms of notification, such as an email and a certified letter; a posting on their website is not sufficient notification.

Confirm the ability to utilize a third party if required in arbitration.

Prior to signing a contract, request the administrative policies, guides, and manuals to review.

Required Terms:

- Number of days to submit a claim after the service date
- Credentialing/network requirements
- Scope of services/unlisted services or codes
- Reimbursement policies/rates/fee schedules
- Fee changes/notifications
- Prior authorizations
- Claim submission deadlines

- Claim denial dispute procedures
- Timely payment of claims
- Term and auto renewals
- Notice of periods for renegotiation and termination
- Statute of limitations on claims, claims resolution, appeals processing and timing

Understand your state's rules and regulations. Some states require the payer to notify providers of changes to the contract, but others do not.

Invest the time, be vigilant and committed. All of this and more is required to achieve successful changes.

> **When negotiations fail, when do you walk away from the table?**
>
> After attempts to correct discovered inefficiencies, yet negotiations have failed, it is time to make a final determination of whether to terminate the contract. The next steps are difficult as there are many unknown factors to attempt to measure. Once a contract no longer meets the practices' cost of doing business, the decision is an easy one, correct? No, the decision to terminate a payer contract does not only require analyzing the financial data, but also includes a comprehensive study of the following factors:
>
> - What percentage of the market does the payer represent?
> - What is the anticipated payer growth; what will the market look like in 5 to 10 years?
> - What are the anticipated products the payer is expected to introduce?
>
> Reach out to your resources again, practice administrators, hospital administration, insurance brokers, and the payers themselves for anticipated future market and growth information.
>
> **Will the decision for termination have an impact on referrals?**
>
> Does the practice have a large number of referring physicians on the plan? Will PCPs be more apt to refer patients to a urology practice that can handle all their patients, rather than dealing with the task of tracking which patients can be directed to which urologist? Large numbers of PCPs participate in ACOs and clinically integrated networks, which mandate the direction of the PCPs referrals.
>
> - The decision should be considered long term and final.

If there were a shift in the market, will the board of directors and physicians continue to support this termination? Once a contract is terminated, and the payer has replaced urology services with another provider, a decision to renegotiate can be difficult and the result could be even lower rates than previously offered. Even after several years, be aware that once the relationship is terminated, it can be very difficult to recreate a positive outcome for the practice.

But the bottom line is, even with all these considerations and uncertainty, a contract which reimburses below cost is unsustainable.

▶ The Process of Termination

Abide by the company's by-laws for direction and approval of such a decision. This is a big decision so many discussions will have taken place, and most likely a vote by a board of directors or governing body will be required. The practice's physicians should be informed throughout the decision-making process, keeping all informed of the relevant factors.

Prepare a notification letter of termination to the payer.

- Address the letter to the designated contact listed in the contract.

- Include the effective date of the termination. The contract will state the amount of notice required.

- Review and abide by all terms for termination required in the contract.

- Provide the reason for termination and be clear if with or without cause. If termination was the result of a breach, state the breach and list the history and attempts made for correction. Include all pertinent information to support the decision.

- Provide the practice's relevant names, addresses, email addresses, and phone numbers for future communications.

- Make the delivery by certified letter or a type of delivery with proof of delivery and signature.

- Follow up to ensure your practice has been removed from the payor website and list of physicians.

Produce a scripted and informative announcement for the physicians and staff.

- Physicians and staff members will require instructions to communicate with patients. Some patients could decide to continue with the urologist with out-of-network terms.

- Inform the patients by written communication and patient portals, with a minimum of 90 days' notice.

Provide referring physicians notification with the reason for termination.

The final negotiations in many circumstances are settled at the last minute. As you work though the necessary steps, stay focused on the facts. You have clarification of the current contracts, the breaking point for each urology service line, a clear vision on the contractual changes desired, and the unique qualities of the practice in the market. You have made the determinations required to make the hard decisions.

When feeling the odds are stacked against a successful negotiation, stay focused throughout the process on the achievements being made. You have taken the necessary steps, you know urology, you know the practice, and you possess the factual data to make the right decisions. Do not underestimate the power of this knowledge, but whatever the outcome you are equipped with all the facts to make the final decision with Preparation, Patience, Data, Data, and More Data.

Lagasse, Jeff. "Health Care Payments Tied to Value-Based Care on the Rise, Now at 34 Percent." Health Care Finance News, 24 Oct. 2018, www.healthcarefinancenews.com/news/healthcare-payments-tied-value-based-care-rise-now-34-percent.

"MGMA Regulatory Burden Report." MGMA Regulatory Burden Report, Oct. 2019, www.mgma.com/getattachment/a6acc774-b5ce-44b1-b98c-d6dcc824db60/MGMA-Annual-Regulatory-Burden-Report-Final.pdf.aspx?lang=en-US&ext=.pdf.

"CMS Innovation Center Episode Payment Models." CMS Innovation Center Episode Payment Models, Centers for Medicare and Medicaid Services, Jan. 2020, innovation.cms.gov/Files/reports/episode-payment-models-wp.pdf.

"Medicare Part B Physician/Supplier National Data - CY2018 Q1, Expenditures and Services by Specialty." Centers for Medicare and Medicaid Services, 2018, www.cms.gov/Research-Statistics-Data-and-Systems/Statistics-Trends-and-Reports/MedicareFeeforSvcPartsAB/Downloads/Specialty2018.pdf.

Preidt, Robert. "Costs of ER Visits Vary in U.S., Study Finds." Consumer HealthDay, 27 Feb. 2013, consumer.healthday.com/general-health-information-16/emergencies-and-first-aid-news-227/costs-of-er-visits-vary-in-u-s-study-finds-673861.html.

KEY POINTS

- **Successfully negotiate contracts for urology** by implementing steps and processes to facilitate negotiations for in third-party negotiations.

- **Understand your contracts** by creating a spreadsheet to compare payors.

- **Analyze the bottom line** by calculating each line of service independently, with the knowledge from both the revenue and expense side.

- **Formulate** by determining which benefits and goals can be achieved with new contracts or amendments.

- **Value-Based Quality Care, Accountable Care Organizations (ACOs), Merit-Based Incentive Payment (MIPs), Alternative Payment Models (APMs), and Episodes of Care** all share the same basic goals: to maintain or improve the quality of patient care and to deliver care more efficiently to reduce expenditures.

- **ACO organizations** continue to make a big push to recruit PCPs into their organizations, accomplishing cost-reduction goals by steering patients to selected groups of high-quality, low-cost facilities and providers.

- **Pay for Performance or Shared Savings contracts** track financial reductions of ED visits, readmissions, length of stay, and infection rates—all positive steps resulting in savings and potential financial rewards to the urology practice.

- **Strategize** to determine your practice's value in the market. Benchmark measurable qualities and features, such as quality, utilization, cost, and patient satisfaction to tie to the success of the practice.

- **Get the payer to the table** with a written request that supports the mutually beneficial reasons for the meeting, along with supporting factors to pique interest.

- **Implement a contract** and continue to work toward transparency to build an efficient and effective partnership.

Jerri Wilson-Durbin

Jerri currently is the CEO of Urology Clinics of North Texas. In her two decades in this position, she has taken the physician's vision of a multi-location practice covering the Dallas and mid cities of the DFW metroplex, and watched it become a reality. This was accomplished working in tandem with her board of physicians and developing a team approach to management. UCNT, originally a 7-physician practice, has grown through mergers and strategic initiatives to 45 physicians, 18 locations, with a complementary array of ancillary services.

Immediately prior to being the CEO, Jerri was the CFO of UCNT and previously held progressive administrative, management and financial leadership positions in private medical practice management as well as a decade of financial management in hospital and post-acute care services.

CHAPTER 16

Service Line Agreements with Hospitals

Alan J. Beason, MS, FACMPE

The relationship between hospitals and their medical staff is a delicate balance. The hospital seeks provider alignment with its goals through support of its programs and initiatives. Providers desire practice autonomy and a way to boost their income.

Initially, hospitals rewarded physicians' allegiance through payment for call coverage and hospitalist services. Using employment contracts and professional services agreements, hospital executives leveraged the employer-employee relationship to influence physician behavior. The hospital's goal was to bring efficiencies into their operations that would lead to reduced costs and increased profits. In the fee-for-service era, this was enough.

As payment mechanisms evolve from volume to value-based, success depends upon a new paradigm. It is not enough to use protocols that address efficiency and expense reductions. Strategies must also improve measurable quality performance against defined metrics and demonstrate better patient outcomes. Driven by the hospital's desire to thrive under the new payment paradigms, there is a growing prevalence of hospital Service Line Agreements (SLAs).

Hospital service line agreements are also known as Clinical Co-management Agreements (CCMAs). For simplicity, the term service line agreement will be used in this narrative.

Background

The intent of an SLA is to promote activities that align provider interests with the hospital through improving patient outcomes, reducing costs and increasing value for the care rendered (Gamble, 2011). Provider engagement may range from supporting clinical enhancements to involvement in the management of the service line program.

The terms of an SLA are often incorporated into an employment contract or professional service agreement with the provider. Alternatively, the SLA may be part of a separate contract between the hospital and an independent provider or autonomous practice.

The SLA may allow practitioners to preserve a degree of autonomy while aligning with the hospital's goals. SLAs may be a viable alternative for hospitals considering practice acquisition and provider employment. SLAs may allow the hospital to avoid extensive capital outlays to purchase assets as well as employ the providers and staff of the acquired practice.

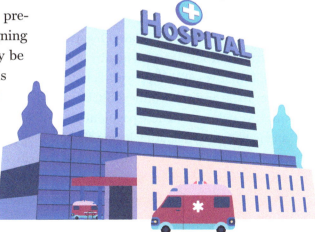

The use of an SLA may allow providers and hospitals to counter the resurgence of private equity acquisitions of practices (A.D. Winkler, personal communication, November 3, 2019). Although a service line agreement cannot match the potential returns of such a stock investment strategy; it does offer a conservative paradigm that allows the provider to benefit from increased income without sacrificing practice ownership and autonomy.

Cardiology and orthopedics were early adopters of service line agreements. Even urology, which tends to focus upon outpatient care, may find benefit in SLAs. Inpatient urology services, such as robotic procedures; collaboration on quality reporting and performance improvement initiatives; reduction in infection rates and operating room turnover times; and acute episodic care, are candidates for SLAs. Each of these activities benefits the hospital by increasing its scope of services and the efficiency by which they are delivered.

Even hospitalists may enter into a co-management agreement with a hospital. The SLA with hospitalists typically defines roles and responsibilities among the providers delivering inpatient care. It also addresses "provider engagement throughout the patient care episode, with focus around handoffs and signoffs during the episode" (Vora, 2017, p. 3).

Adaptable to Evolving Payment Mechanisms

Service line agreements are adaptable to the changing health care environment. In the fee-for-service era, SLAs sought to achieve cost savings through improved efficiencies. Simple changes in practice patterns often resulted in significant savings. Examples such as early morning rounds and enhanced discharge planning reduce average length of stay. Value-based payment models reward providers for meeting quality thresholds by closing care gaps and improving the overall outcome of care for the patient.

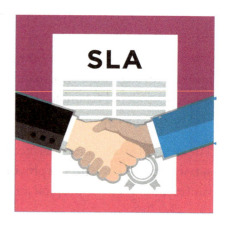

Likewise, Accountable Care Organizations (ACOs) and Medicare Shared Savings Programs (MSSPs) reward quality initiatives and cost savings. Under Bundled Payment Care Initiatives (BPCI), payers set a price for all services tied to a condition or procedure. To be profitable under BPCIs, providers must collaborate to purge expenses and improve outcomes. These payment parameters make SLAs desirable for both providers and facilities participating in bundled payment care initiatives. Expense reduction at all points of care by the provider, including outpatient, inpatient, and post-acute care, along with improved quality metrics and patient outcomes are key to success under a fixed payment system. For these reasons, payers embrace SLAs as a desirable enhancement to the health care system.

> Along the continuum of alignment, Service Line Agreements offer the independent practice an opportunity o develop a hospital-based program that meets the clinical needs of its patients and to demonstrate commitment to a health system without forfeiting practice control. SLAs also allow the hospital to identify those non-negotiables in the clinical arena and to assess the physicians' level of engagement in terms of quality and cost measures.

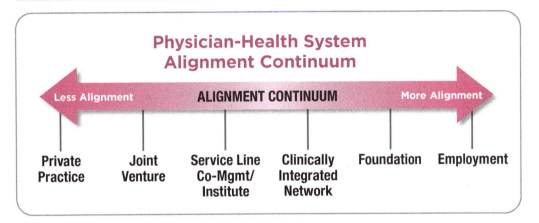

▶ Advantages and Disadvantages

Service Line Agreements offer distinct benefits as well as potential drawbacks. Hospitals use SLAs as the framework to align providers with the goals of the institution. Those objectives may be enhanced patient outcomes, improved quality reporting, increased efficiencies and increased profits. As the environment changes, the contractual terms of the SLA need to evolve. The revisions may be as simple as including an addendum that specifies new metrics and the effective time interval.

The main drawback of SLAs is the investment of time and resources required by the facility and providers. The service line must ensure compliance with ever-changing rules and regulations. Participants must remain actively engaged and committed to changing patterns of behavior in the pursuit of excellence.

▶ Culture Change

A successful service line embraces a culture change for all parties. Achieving operational efficiencies and cost savings require new behaviors such as adopting new practice patterns and care protocols. An already demanding practice may make provider commitment to the service line difficult. In a similar manner, the hospital must commit key leadership and financial support to make the service line successful. Providers and institutions must adopt a collaborative and collegial mindset. This facilitates open communication and data sharing. All parties must commit to being change agents and active participants to make the service line successful.

Types of Service Line Agreements

There are four broad types of SLAs (Greeter, Harrison, & Ropski, 2016). The common theme among the various SLAs is that the arrangement promotes closer alignment and synergy between the providers and the hospital.

The first general type of SLA is the traditional service line agreement. There is no new corporate entity required. This format involves only one provider group serving the hospital under a contractual agreement. Typically, individual physician participation toward the base fee and performance for incentive payment is tracked with the resulting overall payment for the contributions by all providers issued to the practice. It is then up to the practice to allocate the revenue from participation in the service line among the providers.

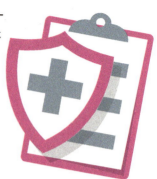

The second model involves the creation of a new entity for the service line. This allows individual physicians within a group to opt in or opt out. It also allows participation by providers from multiple groups. The new entity contracts with the hospital to manage the service line. In turn, the hospital pays a management fee to the newly created entity, which then compensates the participating providers for their services.

The third general format for an SLA involves the creation of a joint venture management company by the hospital and providers. The joint venture management company then contracts to manage the hospital's service line. This option involves complex legal issues. The Stark Laws, Anti Kick Back Laws, and False Claims Act are of concern under this model. Due to the complexity and heightened legal risk, this option is the least common strategy. The emergence of Accountable Care Organizations (ACOs) and Medicare Shared Savings Programs prompted potential rulemaking exemptions to the Stark Law and associated safe harbors. If enacted, these revisions may have a positive impact for this SLA model.

The fourth SLA model is a joint service line oversight arrangement. Under this model, the hospital and providers create a joint oversight committee. This joint oversight committee, which is part of the hospital's overall organizational structure, manages the service line. It has the authority to address clinical, operational and administrative issues specific to the service line. Multiple practices and providers can participate under this model. Separate SLAs or employment contracts address provider roles, responsibilities and compensation arrangements.

Financial Arrangements

The financial arrangements for service line agreements have two components. The first component is a base or fixed fee. "The fixed fee is typically determined by an hourly rate required to perform specific duties, such as medical directorship duties, attending meetings, on-call coverage, etc." (Dunn, 2012).

It focuses upon payment for services rendered to the service line and not rewarding provider accomplishments. This compensation is set in advance for a specific time interval, such as a year. The base or fixed fee is typically set at an hourly rate for services rendered. There is usually a cap on the base or fixed fee for which a provider is eligible.

Incentive payments, which may be considered the "variable payment" or "variable fee" are the second component of service line compensation. The incentive payments promote behavior changes to meet performance standards and metrics.

The variable fee includes any incentive payments for meeting quality or other benchmarks. Here, incentives should only be paid if quality benchmarks are either improved or are at a truly high-performing level. In other words, hospitals and ambulatory surgery centers must be careful not to reward stagnant or low-quality levels of quality or outcomes performance. Doing so could put them at risk for compliance issues. (Dunn, 2012). The base fee may be paid monthly or quarterly. The incentive payment may be paid annually.

The use of Work Relative Value Units (wRVUs) is increasingly common as the basis for compensation in hospital SLAs since they consider physician productivity. A simple calculation that considers the wRVU conversion factor at the median (total compensation/median wRVU = $$ conversion factor) can be applied to that specific physician's normal hourly production level (how many wRVUs does the physician or similar physicians produce in 2,080 hours of work?) If the physician produces an average of 3.50 wRVUs per hour, one could multiply 3.50 * a calculated conversion factor of (for example) $54.56 to determine an hourly rate for the SLA work of $190.96. Since physician agreements should be assumed to be subject to Stark Laws, care should be taken in deciding on the compensation component to ensure it considers cost, income, and/or market rates. The ease with which these items may be considered varies since some service areas may have limited market data available; some may have a higher cost basis (it costs more to practice medicine in an urban area than it does in a rural area); and payer mix may depress market rates below fair market value for the services being performed under the SLA.

Non-Compete Covenants

To be effective, the providers serving a service line must have access to proprietary data. The service line agreement will invariably address the confidentiality of this data and competitive information to which the provider has access. In addition, the SLA will likely include a non-compete covenant.

According to Jennifer Breuer and John D'Andrea on behalf of The Advisory Board's Health Care Law Roundtable's Law Review,

> While it may not be advisable to restrict where physicians may perform clinical services in a co-management arrangement, it is essential to consider whether to impose a non-competition covenant more closely tailored to the management relationship and the services to be performed under a co-management agreement. Appropriate covenants would include a prohibition on ownership of a competing hospital or technical service line and a prohibition on providing similar management, administrative, medical director or similar services for a competing hospital (Breuer & D'Andrea, 2011).

The language regarding non-compete covenants found in employment agreements may serve as a reference in creating the non-compete provisions in a service line agreement. For example, it may have geographic restrictions such as defined zip codes or counties where the provider may not practice during the effective term of the SLA or for a set interval after the conclusion of the agreement. In large metropolitan areas where competing health systems coexist, careful consideration should be given to the provisions of the non-compete agreement and its effective duration. Differing provisions should be included depending upon whether the provider or the hospital terminates the agreement. For example, if the hospital terminates the agreement, the non-compete provisions may be less restrictive or waived altogether.

Regulatory Considerations

There are several federal laws governing fraud and abuse that impact financial relationships between hospitals and providers. Violators run the risk of criminal penalties, civil fines, exclusion from the Federal health care programs, or loss of the medical license from the respective state medical board (Office of Inspector General, A Roadmap for New Physicians – Fraud & Abuse Laws).

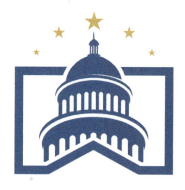

The Stark Law (Physician Self-Referral Law) prevents providers from referring patients for designated health services to organizations in which the provider or members of the provider's immediate family have a financial relationship or ownership interest, typically exceeding five percent. The Stark Law exemption allows providers to refer to such facilities when the compensation arrangements do not vary upon patient volume or the number of referrals to the facility. The compensation must be consistent with fair market values and be commercially reasonable (MGMA, Physician Self-Referral (Stark) Law).

Federal Anti-Kickback Law states:

> anyone who knowingly and willfully receives or pays anything of value to influence the referral of federal health care program business, including Medicare and Medicaid, can be held accountable for a felony.

(Office of Inspector General, Fact Sheet – Federal Anti-kickback Law and Regulatory Safe Harbors, 1999, November).

Several safe harbors allow certain business practices to proceed.

The Civil Monetary Penalties Act prohibits a hospital from paying a physician to restrict services to a Medicare or Medicaid patient. Penalties for violation of the Civil Monetary Penalties Act include steep fines plus exclusion from the Medicare and Medicaid programs (Office of Inspector General, Special Advisory Bulletin—Gainsharing Arrangements and CMPs for Hospital Payments to Physicians to Reduce or Limit Services to Beneficiaries, 1999, July).

These federal laws focus upon federal programs such as Medicare and Medicaid. Individual states may have comparable laws that impact patients insured through commercial plans. For further discussion of Stark and related laws, see Chapter 1.

Not-for-profit institutions must comply with IRS rules that prohibit inurement. Failure to do so could jeopardize the institution's not-for-profit status. The resulting obligation to pay certain taxes can have a devastating impact upon the financial health of the institution. An accountant or legal professional familiar with such arrangements should review the agreement (IRS, Exemption Requirements – 501(c)(3) Organizations).

A professional familiar with the laws and issues should review the contracts. The agreement should define the bonus thresholds in advance of the compensation interval. The compensation should reward progressive improvement in the defined metrics. Rewards for stability in the metrics is justifiable in certain instances. However, the typical strategy is to increase the threshold over time to promote continuous improvement. A fair market valuation is prudent before finalizing the agreement. A periodic review ensures that the SLA remains compliant as the regulatory environment and market conditions change. The fair market analysis should include a review of similar arrangements in the region in which the providers operate. However, the analysis should also look at arrangements outside of the market. The fair market analysis outside of the market provides protection in case the local competitors made a mistake in interpreting the governing regulations and inappropriately structured the SLA or its compensation arrangements.

Finally, the service line should keep detailed records. In addition to minutes of meetings, these records should include documentation of provider time spent working to support the service line. This may be through attendance at meetings and related activities. These records justify the payment of the base or fixed fee for direct provider services for the service line. Also, the records should prove that achievement of performance thresholds justified incentive payments to providers. The service line should keep these records for an interval sufficient to defend an audit or investigation. Usually keeping such records for ten years is enough unless an investigation is underway.

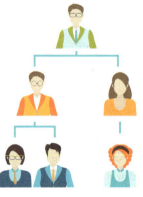

Organizational Structure

Careful consideration should go into designing the structure of the service line. There should be provider representation from each practice involved in the service line. It may also be desirable to include administrative representatives of the practices. The structure should include hospital departments that affect the service line's operations and efficiency. All representatives should be strong advocates for the service line. They should be recognized leaders with the practice or hospital. It is important that they are empowered to lead change.

An organizational chart clearly depicts participants with their responsibilities and lines of accountability. It will show committees and their composition. The administrator-physician dyad model works well when selecting leadership for the various committees. This allows for input from clinical and administrative perspectives. In a simple service line arrangement, the structure may only consist of an oversight committee. The organization of more complex service lines may consist of a steering committee overseeing the activities of several subcommittees that manage specific aspects of the program.

Documentation of the governance structure defines responsibilities and relationships in the chain of command. It will establish oversight responsibilities and authority to empower change. It provides accountability for the committee participants and aligns the activities of the various committees with the overall mission of the service line.

Successful service lines have written business plans. The business plan includes the budget by which the service line will operate and serves as the benchmark to measure financial success. Some of the initiatives cited in the business plan may include expanding relationships and cooperation with other practices or hospital departments. Goals may be the review and update of existing protocols to improve efficiencies and outcomes or participation in a bundled payment care initiative.

Including the hospital's Compliance Department in the service line structure is wise. The Compliance Department should offer more than traditional coding audits. It should stay current on issues involving collaborative activities by hospitals and its providers.

The environment in which the service line operates is dynamic, so updates are often necessary in the format and operations of the service line.

In the November 16, 2011, issue of Becker's Hospital Review newsletter dealing with Integration and Physician Issues, Rebecca Bales and Robert Minkin noted,

> Hospitals with a healthy compliance culture seemed more successful with co-management arrangements. When hospital management was fluent in language that described Stark and IRS excess benefit concerns, there was better acceptance of the constraints on compensation, and the exceptions for incentives were more clearly communicated. Hospitals with good compliance were also better at defining roles and responsibilities, which ultimately reduced conflict in their arrangements (Bales & Minkin, 2011).

Operational Considerations

A successful service line will attack the status quo. The existing processes need to be thoroughly scrutinized. New protocols can bring significant time and cost savings. Replacing "tried and true" methods for new ways of doing business will be the single most challenging aspect of managing the service line. It requires change agents dedicated to implementing new ways of thinking and addressing the service line's operations.

The service line should periodically analyze all aspects of care from intake to post-discharge services to identify opportunities for improvement. For example, reducing operating room turnover time to increase surgery volume is a typical project for a surgical service line. Other departments of the facility that impact the service line hold similar opportunities for improvement. Increased patient volume, reduced waiting times, improved patient satisfaction, and enhanced service for the provider are among the benefits of process improvement reviews.

In the value-based era, providers are accountable for post-acute care costs. Ineffective post-op protocols and discharge planning, or the lack thereof, may hinder the efficiency of the total patient care experience, detract from patient outcomes, or negatively impact total costs. Careful review and improvement in post-discharge care and the choice of post-acute care provider is particularly important in programs that are at risk for the total costs of care. Medicare Shared Savings Programs and Bundled Payment Care Initiatives are two examples of programs that hold providers accountable for these aspects of care.

Supply chain factors can influence costs and efficiency. Seeking the best price structure from a vendor requires a degree of compromise. Sometimes, a product may be less expensive from a different source. Losing that item from a vendor contract could undermine a favorable overall discount based upon volume or exclusivity. Service aspects, such as timely delivery and support, can be equally important. Physician preference should be a consideration, but not the only determinate. Often, selection of products requires physicians to change their behavior. Adapting to a product that may not be their first choice or using an item that comes from a different vendor than the one with whom they have had a long-standing relationship, are behavior changes that can have a significant impact upon costs.

Human resource costs are typically the largest single expense for health care providers. Controlling these costs is a way to improve the service line's profits. Using excessive or inappropriate staffing can drive personnel costs. Using personnel to the upper limit of their license makes the best use of human resources supporting the service line. Identifying opportunities for improvement and implementing the change is challenging. This is especially true when dealing with personnel.

Continuous Process Improvement

Much of a service line's work involves process improvement. Therefore, participants can expect to be involved in Lean Six Sigma as well as Failure Mode Effect Analysis activities. The Lean and Six Sigma methodologies are accepted strategies for identifying waste and purging it from a process (American Society for Quality, What is Six Sigma?). An emerging strategy being embraced by health care organizations to discover, quantify and avert potential failures is Failure Mode Effect Analysis or FMEA (American Society for Quality, Failure Mode and Effects Analysis. Given that purging waste and eliminating potential failure points in the continuum of care are goals of any health care provider, these methodologies will likely be a key focus of a service line's activities.

Metrics

According to management guru Peter Drucker, "If you can't measure it, you can't improve it" (Lavinsky, D. The Two Most Important Quotes in Business). This principle is prevalent in successful service lines. It involves establishing a base line and benchmarking progress against it. Data will identify outliers. Sharing data will trigger the competitive nature of providers to excel and outperform their peers. It is for this reason that data analytics and open sharing of data is critical to successful service lines.

According to Scott Slagis, MD, of the Tuscon Orthopaedic Institute and medical director for the orthopedic SLA, and his administrative counterpart, Mr. Stuart Katz, director of the hospital's orthopedic surgery department and the SLA administrative manager:

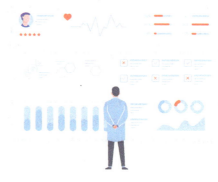

> ... one of the biggest challenges in creating an SLA is agreeing on metrics by which to measure the physicians' and hospital's success. The hospital and physician group have to agree on not only what to measure, but also how to measure it, what the goal is, who is responsible for achieving the goal and who is responsible for measuring.
> (Becker's Hospital Review, 2012)

For years, payers, especially Medicare, have been placing greater emphasis upon quality metrics. Payment is contingent upon meeting or exceeding pre-established performance benchmarks. These performance goals are often scalable over time as payers seek greater values through quantifiable improvement.

Thriving service lines collaborate with payers to measure performance and identify performance improvement opportunities. A successful service line monitors performance and identifies providers that need help to meet or exceed performance thresholds.

Given health care's rapid pace of change, there needs to be flexibility built into the metrics and benchmark values that affect incentive compensation. The metrics that dictate incentive payments should change as need dictates and not revised only at contract renewal.

Starting a Service Line

For a facility that wishes to establish a service line or a provider seeking to join an existing venture, the challenges are many. There are many similarities in the process to create a service line or join an existing one. Understanding operational, financial, and regulatory issues is an important first step. Having clear expectations regarding the time commitment and performance improvement activities tied to participation in a service line is vital.

When a service line does not already exist, enlisting a skilled negotiator to bring the parties together is helpful. This individual's roles are to identify issues, guide discussions, and help the parties reach consensus.

All parties should have clarity on the structure, goals and activities of the proposed service line. The parties need to understand that cultures and past relationships may be a barrier. Time and unified efforts can overcome these obstacles. A new culture of trust, transparency, and collegiality should set the tone going forward. Realistic goals and expectations are vital as is a commitment to succeed. Alignment and empowerment focus activities in pursuit of goals to which the parties agree.

Consensus on the key issues brings clarity to who should be the participants and representatives. The governance and organizational structure define the responsibilities, and accountability for the organization. The objectives of the service line often reveal the traits sought in the service line manager. Skills should include the ability to build consensus, serve as a change agent, and focus activities upon the goals of the service line.

These issues are among the key topics providers and hospital executives should consider when creating a service line. As conversations among the parties gain traction, the vision for the service line will come into focus. Goals and objectives will become clear. The identification of projects will lead to the assignment of teams. In a short period of time, the service line will be operating as a viable entity.

Joining a Service Line

Many of the same steps to develop a service line apply for a practice or individual providers considering joining an existing service line. Since the venture is already in place, the prime concern for the providers or practice considering joining a service line is the due diligence process.

It is important to understand the structure of the service line. A clear understanding of the governance provisions, organizational structure, participants and activities is vital.

The contractual terms and financial conditions merit special attention. What are the base compensation and incentive payments? What are the expectations for time and service to earn the base compensation? What is the cap on base fee payments and incentive compensation? What are the metrics and criteria to earn incentive compensation? Does the contract pass fair market review? What is the duration of the contact? What are the conditions for termination? These questions are among the important issues to explore during the due diligence process.

There may be an opportunity to negotiate these terms. Legal and financial experts should review the arrangement and offer their advice.

Complementary Alignment and Integration Strategy

Service line agreements offer several advantages to the respective parties. They provide a legal framework for facilities and providers to collaborate. Service line agreements promote a cohesive culture that embraces change. They encourage provider alignment without practice acquisition plus the employment of providers and staff. Service line activities provide experience with strategies necessary to flourish under value-based care.

Financial success for facilities and providers is contingent upon cooperation and collaboration. Experience under a service line agreement may be the beginning of a practice integration strategy.

Flexibility for Evolving Models of Care

As value replaces volume to become the payment mechanism of choice, new care models and provider arrangements are emerging. These ventures allow providers and facilities to succeed in evolving reimbursement models and benefit from participation in Accountable Care Organizations (ACOs) and Clinically Integrated Networks (CINs). The goals and advantages of service lines mirror those of an ACO or CIN. Incentives encourage facilities and providers to increase quality and outcomes while reducing costs. They share the common traits of being data intensive, culture driven and modeled upon adopting new models of care. They force participants to view care on a holistic level and seek improvement at every step in the process.

Conclusion

Facilities and providers find that SLAs promote a collaborative relationship to improve outcomes and reduce costs. These arrangements offer several advantages to the participants that embrace these strategies.

An SLA establishes the legal structure for facilities and providers to share the financial benefits of their collaboration. It offers base compensation to facilities and providers for work that supports the service line. Facilities and providers receive incentive payments for achieving defined performance measures and improving patient outcomes.

These financial rewards bring providers into closer alignment with the facility's goals. It also makes the facility more receptive to supporting the providers through the changes required to succeed.

The financial rewards through an SLA meets the provider's desire for increased compensation. The facility benefits from improved reimbursement under new payment models.

An SLA allows providers to maintain a degree of independence and autonomy. The SLA offers a strategy for the practice to remain independent while the group collaborates with the hospital to add its services under the hospital's spectrum of care. The facility gains the providers' support without a sizeable capital expenditure to buy the practice and employ the providers and staff.

SLAs can be structured and operated to comply with regulatory issues such as the Stark Law, Anti-Kickback Laws and Civil Monetary Penalty Laws. It is important to engage accounting and legal professionals in any contractual considerations.

Participation in an SLA is a good precursor to participation in emerging care and payment models. There is tremendous synergy in operating under a service line agreement with participation in Accountable Care Organizations and Clinically Integrated

Networks. Efforts to improve quality and reduce costs are common among these care paradigms; therefore, the experience gained under an SLA is transferable to these other models.

Participants in service line agreements benefit from data analytics. The preponderance of data becoming available to health care providers leads to identifying opportunities for improvement such as population health and care management strategies. The support of a service line structure helps the participating providers benefit from the data and embrace emerging care management strategies.

A favorable experience with a service line agreement may encourage expansion of the relationship of the practice or provider with the facility. It may lead to acquisition of the practice and provider employment. These arrangements complement the terms and conditions of the service line agreement.

Service Line Agreements are a proven alignment strategy for providers and facilities. The SLA provides a legal framework for closer alignment to increase quality and patient outcomes while reducing costs. As value-based care becomes the reimbursement model of choice, these agreements become an increasingly important strategy to be successful in the ever-changing health care system.

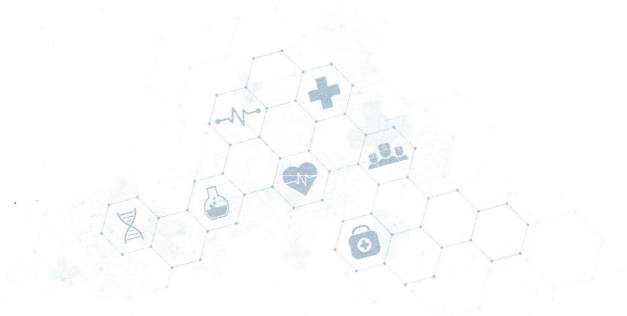

American Society for Quality. (n.d.). Failure Mode and Effects Analysis (FMEA). Retrieved December 4, 2019, from https://asq.org/quality-resources/fmea

American Society for Quality. (n.d.). What is Six Sigma? Retrieved December 5, 2019, from https://asq.org/quality-resources/six-sigma

Bales, R. & Minkin, R. (2011, November 16). Top 10 Lessons Learned from "Mature" Co-management Arrangements. Retrieved October 6, 2019, from https://www.beckershospitalreview.com/hospital-physician-relationships/top-10-lessons-learned-from-qmatureq-co-management-arrangements.html

Becker's Hospital Review. (2012, March 20). SLAted for Success: Creating Service Line Agreements to Drive Hospital Quality. Retrieved October 6, 2019, from https://www.beckershospitalreview.com/hospital-key-specialties/slated-for-success-creating-service-line-agreements-to-drive-hospital-quality.html l

Breuer, J. & D'Andrea, J. (2011, November 10). The Law Review: Structuring co-management agreements. Retrieved on October 28, 2019, from https://www.advisory.com/daily-briefing/2011/11/10/law-review-considerations-in-structuring-co-management

Dunn, L. (2012, June 15). What Can Be Paid for Co-Management Arrangements? Retrieved October 29, 2019, from https://www.beckershospitalreview.com/hospital-physician-relationships/what-can-be-paid-for-co-management-arrangements.html

Gamble, M. (2011, November 28). Co-Management Agreements 101: Basic Principles to Know. Retrieved October 6, 2019, from https://www.beckershospitalreview.com/hospital-transactions-and-valuation/co-management-agreements-101-basic-principles-to-know.html

Goldfischer, Evan R & Carpenter, David (2017, June). Hospital Service Line Agreements – A Changing Paradigm. LUGPA Integrated Urology Practice Forum - Philadelphia.

Greeter, A, Harrison, T., & Ropski, L. (2016, November). Physician Empowerment in the Hospital: An Overview of Clinical Co-Management Agreements White Paper. Retrieved October 25, 2016 from https://docplayer.net/42490240-Physician-empowerment-in-the-hospital.html

IRS. (n.d.). Exemption Requirements – 501(c)(3) Organizations. Retrieved December 5, 2019, from https://www.irs.gov/charities-non-profits/charitable-organizations/exemption-requirements-501c3-organizations

Lavinsky, D. (n.d.). The Two Most Important Quotes in Business. Retrieved December 5, 2019, from https://www.growthink.com/content/two-most-important-quotes-business

MGMA. (n.d.). Physician Self-Referral (Stark) Law. Retrieved December 5, 2019, from https://www.mgma.com/advocacy/issues/federal-compliance/physician-self-referral-stark-law

Office of Inspector General. (n.d.). A Roadmap for New Physicians -Fraud & Abuse Laws. Retrieved December 5, 2019, from https://oig.hhs.gov/compliance/physician-education/01laws.asp

Office of Inspector General. (1999, November). Fact Sheet – Federal Anti-kickback Law and Regulatory Safe Harbors. Retrieved December 5, 2019, from https://oig.hhs.gov/fraud/docs/safeharborregulations/safefs.htm

Office of Inspector General. (1999, July). Special Advisory Bulletin – Gainsharing Arrangements and CMPs for Hospital Payments to Physicians to Reduce or Limit Services to Beneficiaries. Retrieved December 5, 2019, from https://oig.hhs.gov/fraud/docs/alertsandbulletins/gainsh.htm

Vora et al. (2017). The Evolution of Co-Management in Hospital Medicine. Retrieved October 6, 2019, from https://www.hospitalmedicine.org/globalassets/practice-management/practice-management-pdf/pm-17-0019-co-management-white-paper-m1.pdf

KEY POINTS

- **Driven by the hospital's desire** to thrive under the new value-based payment paradigms, there is a growing prevalence of hospital Service Line Agreements (SLAs).

- **Under Bundled Payment Care Initiatives,** payers set a price for all services tied to a condition or procedure, requiring provider collaboration to improve outcomes and purge expenses to be profitable.

- **The main drawback** of SLAs is the investment of time and resources required by the facility and providers to ensure compliance with ever-changing rules and regulations.

- **There are** four broad types of SLAs:

  - a traditional service line agreement, which does not require a new corporate entity.

  - second model involves the creation of a new entity for the service line.

  - the third general format for an SLA involves the creation of a joint venture management company by the hospital and provider.

  - the fourth SLA model in which the hospital and providers create a joint service line oversight committee.

- **The financial arrangements** for service line agreements have two components: a base or fixed fee, or incentive payments, also referred to as the "variable payment" or "variable fee.

- **Regulatory considerations include** The Stark Law (Physician Self-Referral Law)the Federal Anti-Kickback law, and Civil Monetary Penalties Act that prohibits a hospital from paying a physician to restrict services to a Medicare or Medicaid patient.

- **Many of the same steps** to develop a service line apply to a practice or individual providers considering joining an existing service line.

- **SLAs provide** a legal framework for facilities and providers to collaborate and promote a cohesive culture that embraces change.

Alan J. Beason, MS, FACMPE

Alan J. Beason, MS, FACMPE, is a senior health care consultant based in Shreveport, Louisiana. He has extensive senior-level experience in medical group practice management, hospital administration and professional association governance. During his tenure with a large health system, he supported physician practices and network administration through service on the physician network's Clinically Integrated Network Steering Committee, development of new care models and affiliation strategies, plus contributions to provider quality reporting and improvement activities. He has experience in provider recruitment and contracting, as well as compensation arrangements. He served as the CEO/Administrator for regional cardiology practice and collaborated in its integration into a large health system.

His commitment to enhancing the prestige of the medical group practice profession is demonstrated through his service as a Past Chair of the American College of Medical Practice Executives and the Inaugural Chair of the Certification Commission of the Medical Group Management Association. He was designated a Distinguished Leader of the Medical Group Management Association, served as a past board member, and was its representative as the only non-physician member of the National Physician Advisory for the United Health Group.

CHAPTER

Urology Coding

Mark N. Painter
M. Ray Painter, MD

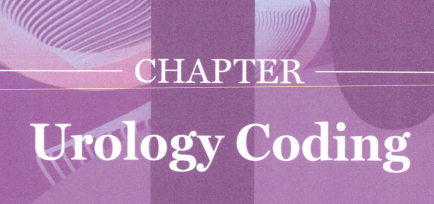

Urologists, APPs, billing staff and practice managers should all have a fundamental understanding of both procedure and diagnosis coding, as these skills have a direct effect on third party payment for the services your practice provides. The fundamentals of coding are an important part of the education that the practice should be routinely providing to assure that the group is up-to-date in understanding the coding systems and the important compliance issues that surround the use of the code sets.

Equally important is training on the appropriate medical record documentation of services. Without these essential skills for providers, billers and practice managers, the practice may well be unknowingly providing uncompensated services.

The documentation, coding, and reporting of services follow the 80/20 rule. Eighty percent of procedures are regularly provided—these procedures represent the majority of `coding situations that you will encounter. The remaining 20% requires more work, knowledge, and understanding to correctly code.

In this chapter, we will provide "tips" on high dollar and high-frequency topics. **The tips will increase the accuracy of payments, decrease the risk of takebacks, and save you time.** "Pitfalls" for most major topics are also presented. **Pitfalls alert you to common mistakes and how to avoid them.** Improving your documentation, coding, and reporting result in more accurate health care data, payments, and fewer take backs.

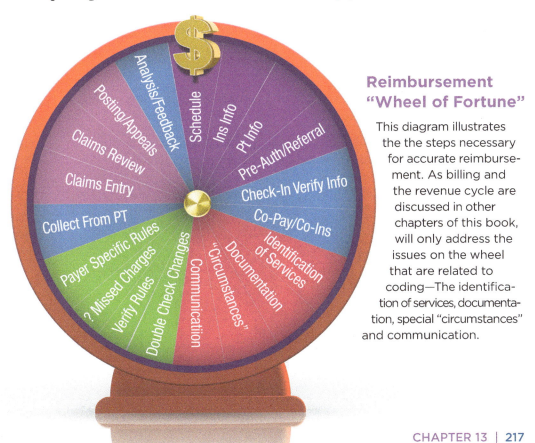

Reimbursement "Wheel of Fortune"

This diagram illustrates the the steps necessary for accurate reimbursement. As billing and the revenue cycle are discussed in other chapters of this book, will only address the issues on the wheel that are related to coding—The identification of services, documentation, special "circumstances" and communication.

OVERVIEW

The System

The coding system is complex, but not complicated. You can usually understand each issue if you drill down to its lowest denominator. Urology coding consists of both structural and functional components.

The Structure of the Coding System

- **HCPCS (Health Care Common Procedural Coding System) has two levels**
  - **Current Procedural Terminology (CPT®) developed and published by the American Medical Association.**
    - Including coding vignettes developed by the AMA to further define the procedure description to assist in use of the codes and development of Relative Values assigned to the codes, and;
  - **HCPCS Level II** codes developed and published by the Centers for Medicare and Medicaid Services (CMS).

- **International Classification of Diseases,** 10th Revision, Clinical Modification (ICD-10-CM) is:
  - **A modification of ICD-10** is updated annually by the National Center for Health Statistics (NCHS) with permission from the World Health Organization (WHO).
  - **ICD-10** is copyrighted by the WHO, which owns and publishes the classification.

- **Payment Rules:**
  - **CMS** publishes the most complete set of documentation, coding, and reporting rules.
  - **Private payers** develop their own rules, usually a modification of the CMS rules. Many of these rules are not published.

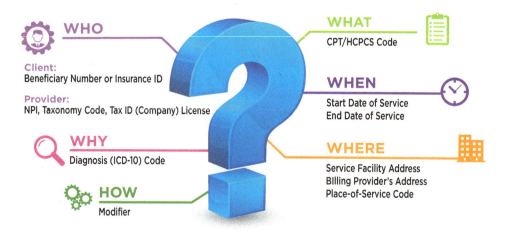

The Functions Needed to Code

Functions required to report a service:

- Identification of the service provided and the reason for providing the service.
- Documentation of that service and the reason for the service being provided
- Identify and document any special circumstances encountered.
- Communication of that service to the appropriate members of the team:
    - Select the most accurate procedure or service code.
    - Select the most accurate diagnosis codes.
    - Report the service using the appropriate reporting rules for that entity/payer.

⚠ PITFALLS

- **Knowing the rules without having a full understanding of their application leads to inaccurate reporting.**

    Years ago, we hired a very bright Coding "expert." She was very conscientious and could quote the rules verbatim. Unfortunately, when presented with a new coding scenario she often made mistakes. She did not understand how to apply the rules.

- **Trusting without verification.**

> **WC Fields once said: "Trust everyone but cut the cards."**
> Cut the cards in all aspects of your practice. Reevaluate the knowledge and effectiveness of your team. The status quo may not be good enough. There could be a better way.

💡 TIPS

- **Study** each issue until you fully understand the concept.

    For example: Knowing the definition of the -25 modifiers is important. **Understanding** the concept of when to use and when not to use the modifier is essential.

- **Keep an open mind** when reading the suggested tips. Do not dismiss them because they are different from the way you do things now.

Identification, Documentation, and Communication

Identification, documentation and communication are key to successful urology coding. Appropriate use of modifiers, detailed documentation, and accurate communication lead to accurate reporting. Mastering these three steps will result in higher collections and fewer take backs.

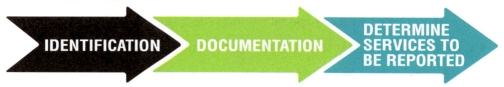

Identification

The physician/APP is the one who knows what services were performed and the reason each service was provided. Capturing that information at the time of the encounter is the most accurate way to identify all services.

The recommended process:

1. **Identify** all services.
2. **Select** the most accurate CPT® code.
3. **Document** the reason each service was provided. Select the appropriate ICD-10 code.

The Physician/APP must work with the team (yes, it takes a team) to develop a system that provides the most efficient process.

We recommend that each team focus on high-volume services first.

NOTE: 20-30 service codes and 40-50 ICD-10 codes typically identify 80-85% of all services provided by a Urologist.

⚠ PITFALLS

- **Urologist/APP** not selecting appropriate CPT/HCPCS and/or ICD-10 code for communication to billing staff:
  - **Incorrect use of templates** in the electronic medical record (EMR).
  - **Incorrect use of search tools** or outdated shortcut list.

💡 TIPS

- **Educate clinic and support staff** on the correct use of templates.
- **Educate clinic on the proper use** of the shortlist.
  (see discussion under communications).
- **Educate clinic on the correct** use of the search tool.

NOTE: While coding can be accomplished using printed code books, computer applications that assist in the selection of codes may be more efficient. Examples throughout the chapter will reference the **AUAcodingtoday.com** program for illustration.

> **Example:** You perform a ureteroscopy procedure. The EMR suggested **code 52353**
>
> 1. **Enter *5235*** (If a wider range of codes are needed, enter list digits. E.g., #52* or #523*
>
> 2. Click **"Go"**
>
> 3. All the codes in that range will appear
>
> 4. Based on the procedure performed, select the most accurate code from the list of alternatives presented.

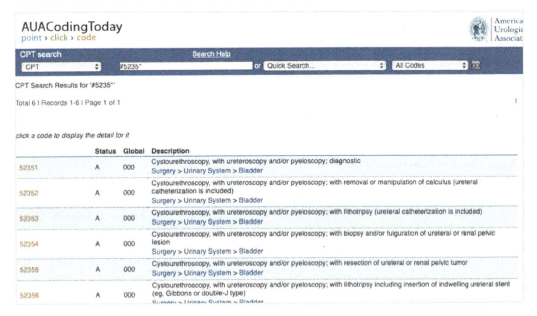

*Disclosure: **AUACodingToday.com** is provided to the American Urological Association for its members by Physician Reimbursement Systems, Inc. in which the authors have financial interest.

⚠ PITFALLS

- **EMR** does not list all the services provided.

💡 TIPS

- **Urologist and staff** work together to reevaluate and update the codes yearly.
- **Update/revision** of the shortlist available in most EHR systems.
- **Remove older codes** and codes with missing digits or other errors.

CHAPTER 13 | 221

Documentation

Documentation tells your story. Documentation communicates the service provided and the reason for that service. The old adage applies, "if you didn't document it, you didn't do it." In short, if there is no documentation to support the service it will not be paid.

The urologist or APP should document, in detail, all services and the reason for each service.

⚠ PITFALLS

- **Incomplete** documentation of a service.
- **Documentation** does not explain that a service is an exception to the global payment rules.
- **Failure** to document all services.
- **Missing or delayed** documentation.

💡 TIPS

- **Educate** the clinical staff on the documentation necessary to justify a modifier.
- **Demonstrate** the revenue lost due to missing information.

Identify Circumstances

Report all services that are not a part of the global payment. Do not report services that are a part of the global payment. Add the appropriate modifier to any procedure or service provided in the global that is not a part of the global payment and is subject to denial for that payer.

⚠ PITFALLS

- **Billing for follow-up appointments** prior to billing surgical services.
- **Reporting of services** included in other service(s) provided.
- **Lack of documentation** for all services/circumstances provided.

💡 TIPS

- **Timely submission** of documentation and coding is essential. This should take place within 48 hours after performance of the procedure/service.
- **Documentation** must support modifier use.
- **Do not report** a secondary procedure performed to facilitate the primary procedure.

- **Report** the secondary procedure performed for another reason. If bundled, add the appropriate modifier.
- **Physician/APP** must understand the modifiers and global payments to provide complete documentation.

Communication

The goal of the entire "Urological Coding Game" is to report all services and submit clean claims (claims without errors or omissions) for each encounter. Timely and accurate communication between the clinical staff and the billing department is a vital step in this process. Clean claims will save the practice time and money and increase income. Investment in training and developing processes is worth the effort and time.

⚠ PITFALLS

- Documentation for a service is not included in the medical record.
- Missing or incorrect modifiers on billable secondary service on day of primary procedure.
- Missing or incorrect modifiers to report billable services provided during a global period.
- Delayed physician dictation causing global period denials.
- Delayed/missed/incorrect claims submission due to inconsistent processes.

💡 TIPS

- Develop a shortlist for each place of service.
    - Start with 50 most commonly provided procedures and diagnosis codes.
    - Urologist/APP and billing staff review list for accuracy.
    - Finalize the shortlist.
  - Make shortlist available to the provider for each patient (paper or electronic).
  - Educate physician/APP on required documentation for each service.
  - Determine the appropriate way for the provider to convey reason for procedure with short list.
  - Mark the services/reasons for each patient.
  - Communicate to coding and billing staff.
- Educate the billing and/or coding staff on the clinical reasons for use of modifiers.

- Develop and maintain payer-specific guidelines for modifier use by circumstance.
- Educate the billing and/or coding staff on the clinical reasons for use of modifiers.
- Educate billing and/or coding staff for modifier definitions and appropriate usage.
- Demonstrate lost revenue to physician/APP through the show of timely filing losses.
- Develop penalty for late dictation submission.
- Develop practice wide processes for communication.
- Allow for cross-training of personnel.
- Developed accurate and consistent double checks and compliance programs.

The Global Concept and Modifiers

Appropriate use of modifiers is vital to correct urological coding. One must understand the underlying "global concept" to master modifier use.

The Global Concept

> **According to CMS rules,**
> Payment for the primary procedure includes payment for pre-operative services, all components of surgery, and postoperative care.

Remember, only the primary procedure is paid. Secondary procedures and other services provided during the global period are not paid unless accompanied by the appropriate modifier. Modifiers communicate the reason that service is an exception to the global rules. ***The service must meet the definition of the modifier.***

The concept of the global is described in the CPT® coding manual. Each surgical service includes:

- Local anesthesia.
- Pre-operative visits after the encounter in which the decision for surgery is made.
- Immediate and typical post-operative care.

Medicare and other payers have expanded the definition of "included services" and have prescribed a specific number of days for four global period definitions. It is important to know which services tare not included in the global period.

Medicare Chapter 12 40.1.B. Services Not Included in the Global Surgical Package:

- The initial consultation or evaluation to determine the need for surgery for a major surgical procedure.
- Services of other physicians, not in the same practice.
- Visits unrelated to the diagnosis for which the surgical procedure is performed, unless the visits occur due to complications of the surgery.
- Treatment for the underlying condition.
- Diagnostic tests and procedures.
- Surgical procedures during the postoperative period which are not re-operations or treatment for complications.
- Treatment for postoperative complications, which requires a return trip to the operating room (OR), a dedicated procedural room, or endoscopy suite.
- If a less extensive procedure fails, and a more extensive procedure is required.

Example: Global days

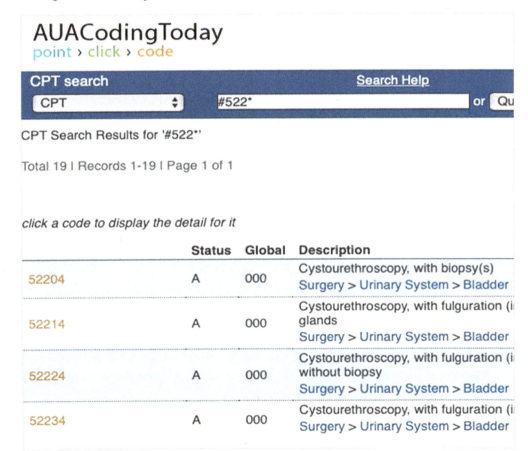

⚠ PITFALLS

- Failure to report unrelated services during the global period.
- Lack of documentation to support reason service should be reported separately.
- Failure to report service provided after the global period.

💡 TIPS

- The physician/APP and/or coder should identify the services that are exceptions to the rule. Documentation should include the reason for providing that service. These two steps are vital to accurate urological coding.
- Global rules do not apply to "XXX" Global procedures. Note: Although global rules do not apply to "XXX" procedures same-day services some payers may require modifiers.
- There are many services that are not a part of the global payment. Report these services in addition to the primary procedure. No modifier required.

Examples:
- Pathology and radiological services.
- Some procedures such as 51798-ultrasound PVR; 51741-Uroflow.

Code			Description
51798	A	XXX	Measurement of post-voiding residual urine and/or bladder capacity by ultrasound, non-imaging Surgery > Urinary System > Bladder
51800	A	090	Cystoplasty or cystourethroplasty, plastic operation on bladder and/or vesical neck (anterior Y-plasty, vesical fundus resection), an procedure, with or without wedge resection of posterior vesical neck Surgery > Urinary System > Bladder
51820	A	090	Cystourethroplasty with unilateral or bilateral ureteroneocystostomy Surgery > Urinary System > Bladder

- Education should include appropriate documentation required to justify modifier use. Provide physician/APP with a global period list for commonly performed procedures. List of the global periods can be found on the CMS.gov website as 85-95% of payers follow Medicare global periods. **AUAcodingtoday.com** and other coding tools also list global periods.

Global Period Examples

Global Days	CPT Code	Procedure/Service
XXX (Global rules do not apply)		
	51798	Measurement of post-voiding residual urine and/or bladder capacity by ultrasound, non-imaging
	74160	Computed tomography, abdomen; with contrast material(s)
	76705	Ultrasound, abdominal, Limited
	84153	Prostate specific antigen (PSA); total
0 Days (Day of procedure only)	52000	Cystoscopy
	52240	Cystourethroscopy, with fulguration and/or resection of; LARGE bladder tumor(s)
	52356	Cystourethroscopy, with ureteroscopy and/or pyeloscopy; with lithotripsy including insertion of indwelling ureteral stent
10 Day (Day of procedure + 10 days postop)	53265	Excision or fulguration; urethral caruncle
	54160	Circumcision, surgical excision other than clamp, device, or dorsal slit; neonate (28 days of age or less)
	54160	Circumcision, surgical excision other than clamp, device, or dorsal slit; neonate (28 days of age or less)
	55100	Drainage of scrotal wall abscess
90 Days (Day before, day of, + 90 days postop)		
	52601	Transurethral electrosurgical resection of prostate, including control of postoperative bleeding, complete (vasectomy, meatotomy, cystourethroscopy, urethral calibration and/or dilation, and internal urethrotomy are included)
	55250	Vasectomy
	55840	Prostatectomy, retropubic radical, with or without nerve sparing;

Modifiers

Modifiers inform all interested parties that the service is an exception to the global rules. As stated in the old country-western song, "You've got to know when to hold them, and know when to fold them. It is as important to know when not to use a modifier, as it is to know when to use a modifier.

Modifiers for Bundled Procedures

If the procedure was not a component of the primary procedure or performed to facilitate the primary procedure, the procedure should be reported with the appropriate modifier. *The reason for performing the procedure must meet the definition of the attached modifier.*

Payers define included services as "bundled." Bundled services are conceptually based on clinical work overlap. Not all bundled procedure rules make sense clinically.

CMS has developed a bundling rule set called the National Correct Coding Initiative (NCCI). CMS is responsible for the development and maintenance of NCCI, which is maintained by a contractor and updated quarterly. Private payers develop or purchase their own bundling edits, usually a modification of NCCI. The NCCI and other bundling edits determine payments and denials for services reported for the same date of service.

The appropriate modifier must be attached to the secondary procedure to allow payment.

⚠ PITFALLS

- Failure to check bundling edits.

- Overuse of modifiers: Some conscientious coders, obviously not understanding the rules, apply incorrect or unneeded modifiers to secondary procedures.

- Underuse: Misinterpreting the rules and failure to add a modifier when one is justified.

💡 TIPS

- Multiple procedures performed on the same day should be checked to see if they are "bundled" by the payer rules. (The edits were developed for all procedures performed at the "same encounter." However, the computer cannot identify an "encounter," therefore, the bundling edits apply to all same "calendar day" services provided)

The Medicare bundling edits (NCCI), are most easily checked using an electronic software.

For Example:

① **Enter** up to **20 codes** in the **"Bundling Matrix"** of **AUACodingToday.com**.

② **Click "Analyze Codes."**   ③ **View** analysis.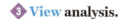

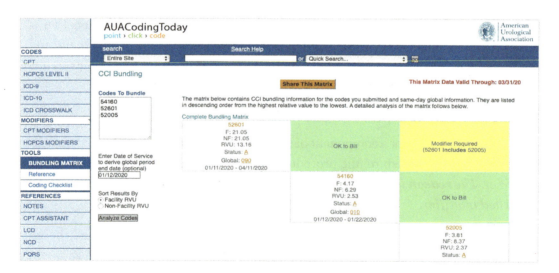

52601 is the primary procedure. The analysis shows that 54160 is not bundled and should be reported without a modifier. 52005 can be billed with the appropriate modifier if it was performed for reasons unrelated to the procedure 52601.

*Most private payer edits can be checked on their website.

- Develop a keen understanding of the global payment concept.

- Do not report a procedure/service performed as a component of the primary procedure. (Procedures that are included in a global payment).

- Apply the correct modifier only if supported by documentation. Develop a profound understanding of the global concept and appropriate modifier use.

- Be diligent in assessing each service to determine if a modifier should be added and which modifier is appropriate.

- Attach the modifier to all services that meet their criteria as an exception to the global payment.

- Report all services that are not a component of the primary procedure or performed to facilitate the primary procedure. If a code is listed as unbundling never allowed, the service will be denied regardless of modifier. If documentation supports a modifier, it may be reported and appealed. Payment, even on appeal, with accurate documentation is not guaranteed.

Modifiers-59

Modifier 59 is the modifier of choice for most bundled procedures (see the X modifiers for Medicare).

CPT definition: Distinct Procedural Service not ordinarily encountered or performed on the same day by the same individual.

Documentation must support:
- different session,
- different site or organ system,
- separate lesion, or
- different procedure or surgery,
- separate incision/excision,
- separate injury (or area).

⚠ PITFALLS

- Adding –59 to any procedure that is bundled, regardless of the reason the service was performed.

💡 TIPS

- Use only for private payers. (Use "X(EPSU)" modifiers for Medicare).
- If you cannot determine the private payers bundling edits, apply the Medicare bundling rules. However, if the secondary procedure, meets the definition of the -59 modifier, bill the procedure with the –59 modifier even if NCCI edits state "unbundling never allowed."

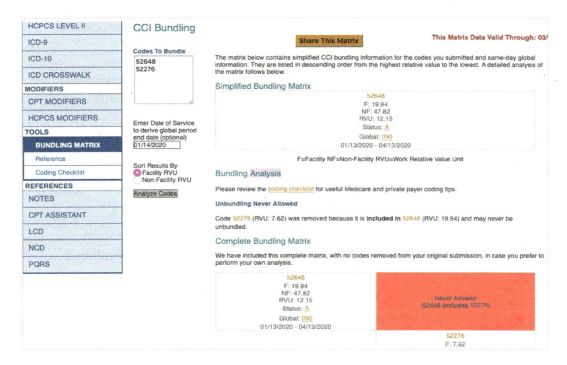

For Examples: using AUACodingToday:

SCENARIO 1.

Patient had a pre-existing urethral stricture and the internal urethrotomy was performed to treat the stricture and Laser vaporization of prostate performed.

SCENARIO 2.

VIU was performed to facilitate the performance of Laser vaporization of prostate.

1. **Enter** codes into bundling matrix.
2. **Scroll** down to bundling analysis.
3. **Results** show that 52276 is bundled into 52648 and cannot be unbundled.

SCENARIO 1.

Coding: Patient had a pre-existing urethral stricture and the internal urethrotomy was performed to treat the stricture.

>   **Medicare** – Report 52648 only.
>   **Private** – Report 52648 and 52276-59.

SCENARIO 2.

Coding: VIU was performed to facilitate the primary procedure.

>   **Report** only 52648.
>   **Do not report** 52276 to Medicare or private.

X(EPSU) Modifiers

The **X modifiers** were developed by Medicare to replace the −59 modifier to provide more detailed data as to why the modifier was justified.

-XE

Separate Encounter:
a service that is distinct because it occurred during a separate encounter.

> **TIPS**
> - Does not require a separate site of service.
> - Documentation should clearly indicate two separate encounters on the same calendar date.

-XP

Separate Practitioner –
a service that is distinct because it was performed by a different practitioner.

> **TIPS**
> - Can be used for the same encounter or different encounters.
> - Use only if the two practitioners are in the same specialty and practice.
> - Documentation must include medical necessity of both visits.
> - Do not use if a procedure code exists that includes all services provided by both practitioners.

-XS

Separate Structure –
a service that is distinct because it was performed on a separate organ/structure.

> **TIPS**
> - Kidney (cortex + renal pelvis), ureter, bladder, urethra, prostate, etc. are all separate organs/structures.

-XU

Unusual Non-Overlapping Service –
the use of a service that is distinct because it does not overlap usual components of the main service.

> **TIPS**
> - Same practitioner, same encounter, same organ or structure, and the service is not a component of the primary procedure.

- Do not use to report services to accomplish the same goal (such as laparoscopy converted to an open procedure).

Modifier –50

Bilateral Procedure:

Unless otherwise identified in the listings, bilateral procedures that are performed at the same session, should be identified by adding modifier 50 to the appropriate code.

💡 TIPS

- Cannot be used with services identified as bilateral.
- Cannot be used with services that cannot be performed bilaterally due to anatomy.

💡 TIPS

- Apply –50 to a procedure performed bilaterally. List only once.

Global Modifiers for Procedures

Modifiers to be added to a procedure, during the global period of a previous procedure, to convey the reason it should be reported separately.

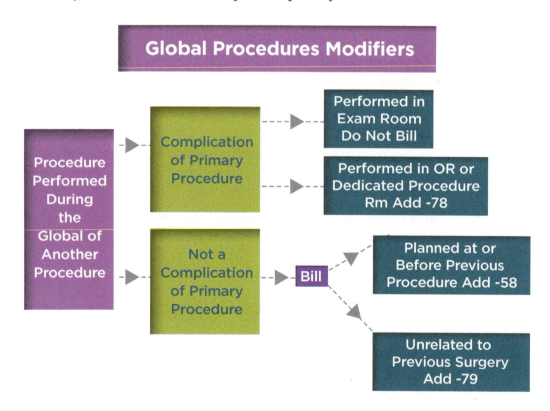

Modifier −58

Staged or related procedure or service by the same physician during the postoperative period:

USES

- Planned or anticipated (staged);
- More extensive than the original procedure; or
- For therapy following a surgical procedure.

PITFALLS

- Failure to document plans for a future procedure at the time of the original procedure.

TIPS

- Document planned procedure/service and the reason for procedure/service in the operative note of the original procedure or in the medical record prior to initial procedure/service.

Modifier −78

Unplanned return to the operating/procedure room for a related procedure – "complication."

TIPS

- Can be applied to a procedure performed for a complication during the global period in a dedicated endoscopy suite or procedure room in the office.
- Do not use for procedures performed in a routine exam room, in the office, ER, or hospital room.

Modifier −79

Unrelated procedure or service

TIPS

- Do not use for a complication of the previous surgery.
- A new unrelated diagnosis is required.

Global Modifiers for E & M Services

Modifiers to be added to an E & M service, during the global period of a procedure, to communicate the reason it should be reported separately

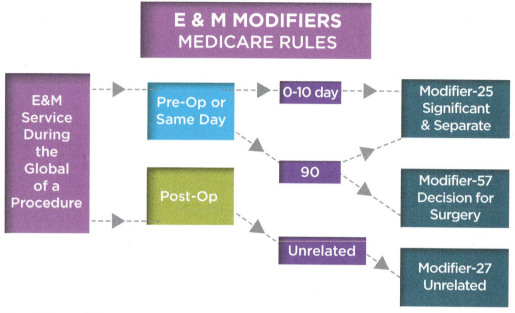

Modifier –57

Decision for surgery: An evaluation and management service that resulted in the initial decision to perform the surgery.

TIPS

- Use only for an E & M Service provided the day before or the day of a 90-day global procedure for Medicare.
- Try applying to an E & M Service provided the same day as a zero or 10-day global procedure for a patient with private pay insurance if the payer denied the claim using modifier-25.

Modifier –25

Significant, separately identifiable evaluation and management service by the same physician on the same day of the procedure or other service:

PITFALLS

- **Overuse:** Applying the modified to services that do not fit the definition.
- **Underuse:** Failure to add the modifier to services that comply with the definition.
- Lack of supporting documentation.

TIPS

- Add modifier -25 to any E & M Service, provided on the same day as a procedure if this service meets these two criteria. **The documentation must justify both "separately identifiable" and "significant."**

  - **Criteria #1. Separately identifiable**
    - Discussing/treating the primary disease process, following the procedure.
- Discussing/treating a disease different from the disease for which the procedure was performed.

  - **Criteria #2. Significant**
    - The service was medically necessary and required "significant" additional time and effort. (Significant has not been specifically defined. We recommend that documentation should convey to the "auditor" that this service required medical decision making effort (see E/M below)).
- A separate diagnosis is not required. Use the appropriate diagnoses for both the E & M service and the procedure.

Modifier -24

Unrelated E & M service by the same physician during a postoperative period.

PITFALLS

- Overuse: Applying the modified to services that are a part of the postoperative care or in addressing a complication that is included in the global payment, according to the rules.
- Underuse: Failure to add the modifier to services that should be reported.

TIPS

- In providing this service, check the global of any previously performed procedure.
- Add modifier -24 to any E & M Service provided during the postoperative global days of a procedure if this service is "unrelated" to the procedure.
- Do not add modifier -24 to any routine postoperative care service or a complication of a previously performed procedure, if the date of this service is within the global period of the procedure for Medicare.
- Some private payers do not bundle complications into postoperative care, and therefore the services should be reported separately using the -24 modifier.

Other Modifiers

Modifier -22

When the work required to provide a service is substantially greater than typically required, it. Documentation must support:

- Substantial additional work.
- Clinical reason for the additional work (i.e., increased in intensity, time, technical difficulty of the procedure, severity of the patient condition, physical and mental effort required).

TIPS

- Document the relative extra time it took to perform the procedure (i.e., 50%, 2X, etc. of the normal time for that procedure).
- Document the reason it took extra time and effort.

Evaluation and Management Services

Evaluation and Management services (E & M) are the most commonly provided and billed services for most urologists and APPs. The CPT coding manual list E & M codes by place of service and type of encounter. Each section defines services by the amount of work provided and documented.

The American Medical Association has announced significant changes to the documentation requirements or E & M services provided in the office setting beginning January 1, 2021.

We will break this section into two parts, "Office and other outpatient settings" and "Other categories of service." Report services provided in the office setting before January 1, 2021 under current guidelines similar to those listed in the "Other categories of service" section.

Selecting the correct E & M service code:

STEP 1 **Determine the place of service** (Office, Hospital, etc.)
STEP 2 **Determine the category** (new patient/Establish patient
STEP 3 **Determine the correct level** (components or time)

TIPS

- A new patient is one that has not had any service provided by a Physician/APP in the same group and the same specialty within the last three years.
- Facility-based initial visits
    - The initial encounter of that admission by a physician/APP of a specific specialty and group,

- Even if the patient is an established patient for that group,
- Even if the patient has been seen during a different hospitalization.
  - Some private payers still pay for consults for the initial visit of a referred patient.

Base the selection of the appropriate code on either components or time. First, we discuss office and other outpatient-based services.

Office and Other Outpatient Setting

Background

The January 1, 2021 changes will replace a system first introduced in 1992. The 1992 system was further clarified by The Centers for Medicare and Medicaid Services (CMS) in 1995 and again in 1997. Most payers and physician groups adopted the new guidelines. Several attempts to make changes failed. In 2018, CMS proposed a significant revision of the payment structure. The physician community objected strongly.

The American Medical Association, the steward of the CPT® system, proposed a rework of the coding system for the most highly utilized section of these codes. CMS accepted the proposed changes to be implemented on January 1, 2021.

Summary of Changes for 2021

Documentation for new and established patients will require a medically appropriate History and Physical Examination. The physician or the staff can collect the information. The physician /APP must review the information. The extent of the History and Physical examination is not counted in the selection of the appropriate code in this category. The selection of the appropriate service level provided and documented by the physician or APP is to be based on the elements of Medical Decision Making or Time.

Time

For coding purposes: Total time for office or other outpatient services is the time spent by the physician and/or other qualified health care professional on the date of the encounter. Services must pertain to patient care throughout the date of service.

Total time does not include staff time. Count only the time of the physician or other qualified health care professionals. New codes will include time ranges for each code and a new code for extended time. The new code will replace the current extended time codes.

Medical Decision Making

Medical Decision Making (MDM) consists of 3 elements:
- The Number and Complexity of Problem(s),
- Amount and/or Complexity of Data, and
- The Risk from the complications, morbidity and or mortality of Management Decisions made during the visit.

The system recognizes 4 levels of MDM corresponding to the levels of service available:

- 99202- 99205
- 99212-99215

Code 99201 has been deleted since MDM does not apply to code 99211.

MDM requires that 2 of the 3 elements meet or exceed the level for the defined level of service. The AMA released a table as a guide to appropriate MDM levels the table can be found at: https://bit.ly/amadocument.

Tips and Pitfalls:

As the system is new:

- We encourage each group to study the rules as published, continue to document medically appropriate services provided, and,
- Get extra training available from qualified sources.

Other Categories of Service

Time based E & M coding

Office and Other Outpatient visits (2020) and for Home Health, Home Visits, etc. (2020 and 2021)

- Total time includes overall time spent face to face with the patient
- Document substance and amount of time spent in discussion
- Documentation must reflect that over 50% of the time was spent counseling or coordinating care

Tips. Time listed in the CPT description and included on the PRS pocket card are averages, not threshold times.

Inpatient setting, (2020 and 2021)

- Count total floor time:
  - The overall time spent with the patient and or family
  - The time spent dealing with other health care professionals.
  - Chart review and documentation
  - Care provision
- The items discussed must be included in the document
- Documentation must reflect that over 50% of the time was spent counseling or coordinating care
- Again, the times listed are averages

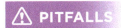
PITFALLS

1. **Failure** to document the exact time spent.

    Tips. Document exact time spent, not approximate or a range

2. **Misinterpreting** time listed for each code as minimum time instead of an average time.

    Tips. Select code closest to the actual time spent.

Code Selection Based on Components or Elements of Service.

Initial visit codes require that all three elements listed below must meet or exceed the level of service reported. For subsequent or established patients only two of three components must meet or exceed the level of service selected. Below is a brief introduction to the three components.

History consists of three elements:

- History of Present Illness (HPI),
- Review of Systems (ROS), and
- Past Medical, Family, and Social History (PFSH).

HPI – A chronological description of the development of the present illness from the first sign and/or symptom to the present.

- Includes a description of the sub-elements:
    - Location,
    - Quality,
    - Severity,
    - Timing,
    - Context,
    - Modifying factors, and
    - Associated signs and symptoms significantly, related to the presenting problem(s).

ROS is an inventory of body systems and is:

- Obtained through a series of questions
- Identifying signs and/or symptoms, which the patient may be experiencing or has experienced
- Ensuring each system addressed must be specifically documented

PFSH – Contains three sub-elements:

- Past Medical history
- Family history
- Social history

Physical Examination: The PE may be supported by either the 1995 or 1997 Medicare Documentation Guidelines. The 1995 guidelines count systems examined and the number of comments per system. The 1997 guidelines developed for specialty practice are more detailed.

Medical Decision Making (MDM): MDM includes three sub-elements: Number of Problems or Diagnosis, Amount of Data, and the Amount of Risk. The following table provides a summary of the documentation requirements.

ELEMENT: TABLE OF RISK

Level of Risk	Presenting Problem(s)	Diagnostic Procedure(s) Ordered	Management Options Selected
Minimal	• One self-limited or minor problem (eg, cold, insect bite, venipuncture, tinea corporis	• Lab tests w/venipuncture • Chest x-rays • EKG/EEG • Urinalysis • Ultrasound (eg, echocardiography) • KOH Prep	• Rest • Elastic Bandages • Superficial dressings
Low	• Two or more self-limited or minor problems • One stable chronic illness (eg, well controlled hypertension, non-insulin dependent diabetes, cataract, BPH) • Acute uncomplicated illness or injury (eg, cystitis, allergic rhinitis, simple sprain)	• Physiologic tests not under stress (eg, pulmonary function tests) • Non-cardiovascular imaging studies with contrast (eg, barium enema) • Superficial needle biopsies • Clinical laboratory tests requiring arterial puncture • Skin biopsies	• Over-the-counter drugs • Minor surgery with no identified risk factors • Physical therapy • Occupational therapy • IV fluids without additives
Moderate	• One or more chronic illnesses with mild exacerbation, progression, or side effects of treatment • Two or more stable chronic illnesses • Undiagnosed new problem with uncertain prognosis (eg, lump in breast) • Acute illness with systemic symptoms (eg, pyelonephritis, pneumonitis, colitis) • Acute complicated injury (eg, head injury with brief loss of consciousness)	• Physiologic tests under stress (eg, cardiac stress test, fetal contraction stress test) • Diagnostic endoscopies with no identified risk factors • Deep needle or incision biopsy • Cardiovascular imaging studies with contrast and no identified risk factors (eg, arteriogram, cardiac catheterization) • Obtain fluid from body cavity (eg, lumbar puncture, thoracentesis, culdocentesis	• Minor surgery with identified risk factors • Elective major surgery (open, percutaneous or endoscopic) • Prescription drug management • Therapeutic nuclear medicine • IV fluids with additives • Closed treatment of fracture or dislocation manipulation
High	• One or more chronic illnesses with severe exacerbation, progression, or side effects of treatment • Acute or chronic illnesses or injuries that pose a threat to life of bodily function (eg, multiple trauma, acute MI, pulmonary embolus, severe respiratory distress, progressive severe rheumatoid arthritis, psychiatric illness with potential threat to self or others, peritonitis, acute renal failure) • An abrupt change in neurologic status (eg, seizure, TIA, awareness, sensory loss	• Cardiovascular imaging studies with contrast with identified risk factors • Cardiac electrophsiological tests • Diagnostic endoscopies with identified risk factors • Discography	• Elective major surgery (open, percutaneous or endoscopic) with identified risk factors) • Emergency major surgery (open, percutaneous or endoscopic) • Parenteral controlled substances • Drug therapy requiring monitoring for toxicity • Decision not to resuscitate or to de-escalate care because of poor prognosis

Selecting the Correct Level

As noted above, the selection of the appropriate code may be based on either components or time. The below figures provide a graphic representation of the requirements for each code in the outpatient setting.

⚠ PITFALLS

- Lack of recorded Hx or PE to support MDM documented.
- MDM not documented to include all considerations.

💡 TIPS

- The physician must review the History
- In the inpatient setting,
  - Note review of history included in the medical record.
  - Update changes as needed.
  - The patient encounter is down coded due to lack of medically appropriate PE.
- Document all systems examined/observed during the visit.
- Medical decision making should be the primary determining factor for approprivate code selection.
- For subsequent/established patients, since only two of three elements are needed, perform only medically necessary physical exam.

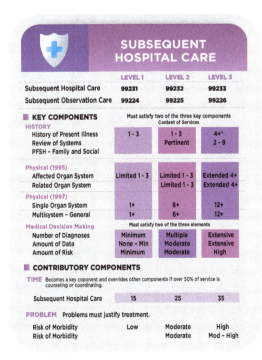

KEY POINTS

- **The documentation, coding, and reporting of services** follow the 80/20 rule—80% of what you do is repetitive so learn it well. 20% requires more work, knowledge, and understanding—this applies to accurate coding to obtain payment.

- **Knowing the rules** without having a full understanding of their application leads to inaccurate reporting.

- **Study each issue** until you fully understand the concept.

- **Identification, documentation and communication** are key to successful urological coding.

- **Appropriate use of modifiers** is vital to correct urological coding. One must understand the "global concept" to master modifier use.

- **If the procedure** was not a component of the primary procedure or performed to facilitate the primary procedure, the procedure should be reported with the appropriate modifier. The reason for performing the procedure must meet the definition of the attached modifier.

- **Evaluation and Management services (E & M)** are the most commonly provided and billed services for most physicians and APPs.

Mark N. Painter

Mark N. Painter is a managing Partner of PRS Consulting, LLC, the CEO of PRS Urology Service Corporation and the Vice President of Coding, Reimbursement Information for Physician Reimbursement Systems, Inc. (PRS) and CEO of Relative Value Studies, Inc. Since co-founding PRS in 1989, Mr. Painter has served as the primary coding resource for the PRS products currently produced and marketed in conjunction with 9 National Specialty Organizations including Hotlines, Coding Manuals and quick reference tools, the Internet based application **codingtoday.com** and seminars. He serves as an expert to legal counsel, bio device companies, medical directors, and pharmaceutical companies.

M. Ray Painter, MD

M. Ray Painter, MD, a board-certified urologist, has devoted the last 30 years to assisting physicians and their practices with documentation, coding, and billing. Dr. Painter is Co-Founder and President of PRS network and Physician Reimbursement Systems, Inc. (PRS). He is founder and CEO of the PRS Educational Foundation. He served as a member of and then a consultant to the American Urological Association's Coding and reimbursement committee for 23 years. Most recently as developed and teaches a virtual course to teach urologist what they need to know about the coding and billing system and the Advanced Coding and Billing for coders and billers.

Dr. Painter authored for a number of years and then co-authored with Mark Painter, an informative monthly article for Urology Times for 20+ years and has written many articles on documentation, coding, billing, and collections for the likes of The Journal of Urology, AACU News, the ACS Bulletin, etc. He lectures nationwide on topics related to coding and reimbursement, Practice Management, contract medicine, and the future of the health care system.

CHAPTER

Billing and Revenue Cycle Management

Twila J. Puritty, MBA

Medical billing is complex. The variety of ancillary services provided in many urology practices adds another level of intricacy to an already complex process. Over the past decade, there has been a continuous stream of new procedures, new drugs, and ever-evolving changes to the treatment protocols of many urologic conditions and cancers. The complexity in urology billing requires specialized expertise, continuous monitoring of key indicators, and a dedication to ongoing education.

This chapter will break down revenue cycle management into key process areas that follow the lifecycle of a billed service. The key areas include authorizations and referrals, time of service collections, accurate coding, contractual reimbursement, insurance billing, patient billing, revenue cycle analysis, refunds to patients and insurance companies, and bad debt collections.

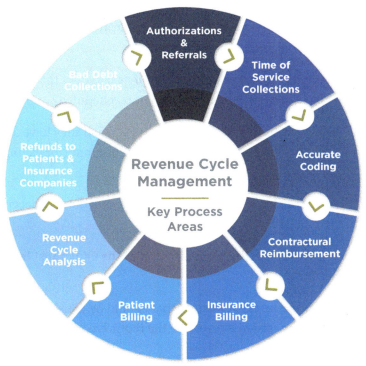

For many reasons beyond the scope of this chapter, urology practices nationwide are responding to the reality that insurance carriers are shifting more of the cost of medical care to patients through increased deductibles, higher coinsurance percentages, higher copayments, and other shared payment arrangements. Financially successful groups have responded to this shift by supporting robust Time-of Service (TOS) collections initiatives.

The first step in developing an effective TOS collections program is for key leaders to agree on a TOS collections philosophy. The philosophy of a financially successful urology practice supports processes and protocols that appropriately require patients to pay their out-of-pocket (OOP) amount at the time the patient receives services in the practice.

It can't be overstated that buy-in from leadership is vital to a successful TOS program. Gaining consensus on the topics and questions below will set the practice on the path for success. Answers to the following questions will assist leadership in defining their philosophy and commitment to appropriate TOS collections:

- Is there a commitment to allocate resources to the project?
- Does leadership understand that all departments within the practice will have some responsibility for the success of the project?
- What happens if the patient is unable or unwilling to pay the amount due?
- Will patients be expected to pay past due amounts before they are seen?
- If a patient has an account written off as bad debt that balance must be paid before the appointment is scheduled?
- Will patients be dismissed from the practice if they have a large bad debt balance? If so, is there a dollar amount (for example, $5,000) that will trigger the dismissal?
- What are the terms of budget payment plans that are acceptable to the group?
- Who can override the requirement that the OOP must be paid before being seen?
- What are the broad guidelines that should be considered when making the decision to override the requirement?
- Are there disease states or other conditions that will not be subject to the TOS collection protocols?
- Does the group want to establish OOP collections guidelines for elective or other non-urgent surgeries?

After developing the policies and procedures, the leaders must be willing to enforce those that support the TOS collection protocols. A provider who routinely overrides the TOS policy is openly communicating to colleagues and staff that TOS policies are optional and do not need to be followed. To maintain the integrity of the TOS policies, key leaders in the group need to promptly address these overrides with the offending provider.

Time-of-Service Collections

With few exceptions, a scheduled office visit or procedure triggers the revenue cycle process. Assuming accurate health insurance information is obtained at the time of scheduling, the first step is to determine if there will be an OOP amount due from the patient. Answering some basic questions will guide the staff on next steps in the process.

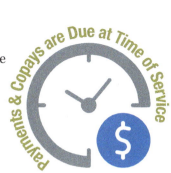

- Does this visit need a referral?
- Is an authorization required for the visit or the service?
- Is the scheduled visit or service covered by the patient's insurance?
- Has the patient's deductible been met?
- Will there be a co-insurance amount due?
- Does this service require a co-payment?
- If the patient has a secondary insurance policy, does the policy require a co-payment or deductible?
- Does the patient have an outstanding balance?
- Does the patient have an account that has been written off to bad debt?

Depending on a group's practice management (PM) system, calculating a patient's OOP amount may be a fully or partially automated process. In the absence of PM system functionality, the process will be more time consuming but still worthwhile. Through contact with the insurance companies, either electronically or via phone, the OOP estimators will gather deductible, co-insurance, and co-payment amounts from both primary and secondary insurance payors. Staff who calculate the OOP estimates should work a week ahead on each clinic and ancillary schedule.

Once the amount is calculated, the billing estimator calls to inform the patient of the amount that will be due when they arrive for the appointment. Some OOP amounts can be quite large. Notifying patients a week in advance is a courtesy. The intent of the call is to give patients an opportunity ask questions about the amount that may be due, eliminate any unpleasant surprises during check-in, and provide an opportunity for patients to learn about budget plan options, if needed. To aid in effective communication with the patient, consider developing a script to help estimators effectively communicate the practice's collection policies and respond to patient concerns or objections.

A practice may decide that phone calls are not necessary if the amount is less than a pre-determined amount (for example, $25.00).

After talking with the patient or leaving a voicemail, information regarding the amount due needs to be documented in the PM system where the reception staff can easily find it. Additionally, the estimator should enter relevant information from the call with the patient or document that a voice message was left for the patient. This sharing of information between the estimator and front desk staff increases the success of collecting because the reception staff can rebut patients' claims that they were not informed payment was due at the time of service.

Some groups may opt for an automated service to notify patients of OOP amounts. The drawback to an automated service is the lack of two-way communication. Patients cannot ask questions or learn more about payment options. The reception staff may not know if the call was received or even went to the correct phone number.

On the day of the appointment, during the check-in process patients are informed of the amount due. If a patient is unable to pay the amount due but wants to keep the appointment, consider offering a budget plan, which requires that payments be charged to a credit card or debit card that the practice keeps on file. To accomplish this, a practice needs a secure and compliant program for storing the card information and a protocol for charging the payments to the cards. Patients who do not have a credit or debit card can be encouraged to apply for health care financing through credit services, such as CareCredit®. These health care financing services offer short-term financing options with no interest. If the patient refuses to pay the amount due or commit to a budget plan secured by a credit or debit card, the receptionist should graciously offer to reschedule the appointment for another day. When faced with rescheduling the appointment, many patients pull out their checkbooks or credit cards.

Appointments added to the schedule since it was worked by the estimator should not be neglected in the pre-collection process. Ideally, a staff member should be assigned to review the upcoming daily schedule and work up the accounts as described previously. There should be an attempt to reach the patient in advance of the appointment.

Some practice management systems have kiosks or other electronic devices for patient check-in. Through the kiosk, the patient is notified of the amount due and pays with a credit or debit card.

Time-of-service collections do not end once the patient has left the front desk. A practice should also develop processes for collecting out-of-pocket amounts for procedures, labs, and imaging that are added on and performed during a patient's appointment. To accomplish this, patients need to be informed that the add-on service may require an additional payment. The estimating staff needs to be notified so they can determine if additional payment is needed. When patients are notified of the amount due, they have the option to proceed with the service and pay the amount due when they check-out, or schedule the service for another day.

In addition to bringing more revenue into the practice, effective time of service collections save money by reducing the number of statements sent to patients and the number of accounts requiring more intense collection efforts.

▶ Accurate Coding

Before money enters the urology practice's revenue cycle, the physician services need to be coded for billing purposes. Accurate coding is essential to maximizing appropriate reimbursement and minimizing days in accounts receivable. This requires competent, well trained coders. The American Urological Association has many coding resources for coders who may struggle with urology coding. It may be helpful to encourage coders to join a medical coding association. Some associations have chapters throughout the country that provide continuing education and networking opportunities, including the American Academy of Professional Coders (**www.aapc.com**) and American Health Information Management Association (**www.ahima.org**).

▶ Improved Chart Documentation

Coders should only code what is documented in a patient chart. At times, coders may struggle to find documentation in the patient chart to support the services provided. A practice can bridge these gaps in documentation by encouraging good communication between the coding staff and providers. This could be in the form of one-on-one conversations between a provider and coder, coding tip emails from the coding department to one or all providers, or coding presentations to providers.

Compensation models may impact how a provider will respond to suggestions for improved documentation. In some cases, it may be necessary for physician leadership to drive provider behavior related to appropriate documentation.

▶ Coding Audits

Validating good coding practices can be accomplished with internal and/or external coding audits. An internal coding audit can be accomplished by assigning a senior coder an audit schedule, or rotating the internal audit between all coders. While the preferred frequency of coding audits is quarterly, performing semi-annual or annual audits is better than skipping internal audits entirely.

In an internal audit, charts are randomly selected in each of the following categories: New Patient Office Visits, Established Patient Office Visits, and Consult Office visits. Within each of the categories, up to 15 charts are reviewed, five charts each for Level 3, 4, and 5 office visits. To verify the correct level of service and accurate diagnosis, the coder should review the office notes, medical history forms, lab, pathology, and imaging reports.

External coding audits are another option. They can be costly but are more likely than an internal audit to uncover institutionalized processes or issues that need improvement.

Billing

After services are appropriately coded, the charges are ready to submit for payment. With few exceptions, urology billing is comprised of two components: billing to insurance companies and/or billing patients.

A basic, yet critical step in billing is to assure all services performed are captured for billing. Most practice management systems have reports to identify scheduled services that were not billed. For the reporting mechanism to work, all services and procedures must be scheduled. If it is possible that a drug, injection, procedure, or other service could be done without being scheduled, the group should develop other audit mechanisms to ensure that every charge is captured for billing.

Insurance Billing

Most medical insurance claims are filed electronically. However, there are still scenarios where the only choice is to submit a paper claim form. Practices should strive to submit insurance claims, whether on paper or electronically, on a daily basis. The benefits of electronically filing include: savings on postage, paper, and administrative time.

Electronic claims can be filed directly to a payor or through a claims clearinghouse. Direct filing of claims means the claims go directly from the PM system to the insurance carrier. Claims clearinghouses are companies that electronically receive all electronic claims from a practice and then send them to the various insurance companies. Using a claims clearinghouse is preferred over filing claims directly. A good clearinghouse service will scrub claims; meaning they check all claims for errors, which are withheld from filing. A claim error log is then returned to the practice to correct errors. In many cases, not all, the PM system dictates the clearinghouse a practice uses, which allows the practice to benefit from the vendor's support with any clearinghouse issues.

Using a clearinghouse that scrubs claims does not mean claims will not be denied. Reviewing denied claims must be a priority in a billing department. The person doing the review should be looking for recurring issues and new trends in denials. Thorough claims denial review will reveal areas for improvement within the billing department. Some denials will highlight areas of additional training needed for coders or staff members. Reviewing denied claims can also catch errors made by payors. Insurance company consolidation has resulted in many unnecessary denials and payment errors. These errors occur more frequently during the transition from one payment platform to another. For example, claims start being denied as "out of network" or payments are denied or inappropriately bundled with another payment. Reviewing denied claims improves the chances of catching the errors and reporting them to the payor.

There are other options for working denied claims. There are denial management software programs that can be integrated with an EHR or PM systems. These systems can extract denial information from the PM system and then group the data for more efficient resolutions. Another option for managing denials is to contract with an outside vendor that provides denial management services.

Patient Billing

Most patients want their physicians to receive payment for the services provided. If the patient's out-of-pocket costs are not collected at the time of service, the practice will incur the expense of sending patient statements. Patient statements may be processed within the practice or electronically sent to a service that will print and mail them for a fee. Some practice management systems can email statements to patients. Each practice should research their options and select the most cost effective and efficient process.

To save money and reduce patient confusion, many practices do not send statements to patients until AFTER the insurance company has paid the claim. Each practice decides how frequently a patient will receive a statement and the number of statements a patient will receive before the account is considered past due. Unfortunately, it is still common for practices to send a statement every 30 days until either the account is paid or the account is moved on to the next phase of the collection process. Instead of 30-day intervals between statements, consider experimenting with a 10- or 15-day interval for quicker collection.

Not all patient statements will be successfully delivered. This applies to both statements mailed or emailed. Return mail should be diligently worked. Ideally, addresses should be updated immediately to prevent additional statements going to the wrong bad address. Most practice management systems allow an account to be placed on hold, meaning no more statements go out, until a good address is obtained. If accounts are placed on hold, it is imperative to regularly review the "hold from billing" report. Some medical practices have discovered that tens of thousands of dollars were uncollectable because accounts were placed on hold and then forgotten about.

Patient Billing – The Collection Phase

After sending a pre-determined number of statements, the account may move to a pre-collection phase. In this phase, the patient may be sent a collection letter or called by an in-office collector. The intent of the pre-collection phase is to inform the patient that the account will be sent to an outside collection service if it remains unpaid. If an account remains unpaid after pre-collection efforts, the balance will be written off as bad debt and sent to an outside collection service.

Outside collection services vary in effort, methods, costs, and services provided. A practice should thoroughly research outside collection agencies. Below is a partial list of things to consider when selecting or changing collection agencies.

- What is their fee?

- Will they offer a lower fee if accounts are turned earlier in the aging process (for example, when the accounts are 60 days old versus 120 days old)?

- How are the accounts worked? Do they only send letters, or do they also make calls?

- If they make calls, where is the call center local, in a different region of the country, or outsourced overseas?

- Do they understand that their collection efforts are a reflection of your medical practice? Will they perform pre-collection services that don't generate a fee?

- If a payment on a collection account crosses in the transfer to their office, will they waive their fee?

- Can accounts be recalled from the agency if the group wants to end the collection efforts?

- Does the agency accept the accounts electronically or are paper documents required?

- How easy is it to report payments on bad debt accounts that are sent to the practice?

- Is their collection report easy to reconcile to the PM system?

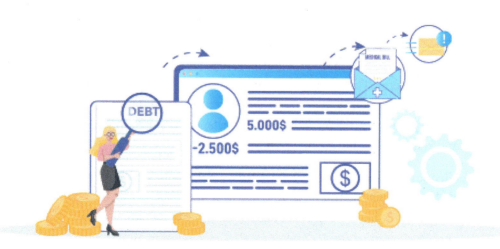

Though it takes time, someone in upper management should regularly review accounts written off to bad debt. If it is not possible to review every account, the manager should review the accounts on some regular interval to identify emerging patterns. Identifying the patterns can lead to opportunities for improvement.

Through reviewing bad debt accounts, a practice discovered that more clinical lab services were being applied to patient deductibles. In response, the practice started working up lab services for TOS collections. In another instance, the manager noticed that many services and procedures added during patient appointments were being written off as bad debt. The practice's response was to implement TOS collection procedures for services added during the patients' appointments. In another example, the manager noticed that a large volume of surgery charges were being written off as bad debt. The group's solution was to require OOP amounts to be paid before an elective surgery could be scheduled.

Payment Posting

There are many options for processing payments from insurance companies or patients. Payments collected at the time of service will be posted by the practice. Payments from insurance companies may come in the form of a paper check with a paper remittance advice, or be electronically deposited in the group's bank account, which is then electronically posted to patient accounts. How a group receives payments from insurance companies is dictated by its practice management system and the insurance company paying the claim. When options are available, opt for electronic deposit and electronic posting of payment.

For payments due from patients, it is important to provide options for patients to make their payment. Many patients like to make their payments on-line. If this is accomplished through the group's website, make sure the payment icon is easy to locate on the website's landing page. Other patients may prefer to mail their checks, or call the office to make a credit card payment.

Health care lockbox services are another option for receiving payments. These services range from very basic to quite complex and expensive. The basic services provide mail boxes for accepting electronic and paper mail. The hardcopy documents are copied or scanned and then delivered to the practice electronically or via a courier. In addition to accepting all payments and automatically depositing them into the group's bank account, the more sophisticated lockbox services create customized interfaces to electronically post payments directly into the PM system.

After all payments are posted either electronically or manually, the system should flag payments that are less than the amount the payor is contractually obligated to pay. The variances should be researched and acted upon.

All businesses should have effective internal controls to identify suspicious transactions, errors, and other inconsistencies. Since large sums of money flow through urology offices, segregation of duties should be enforced. For example, staff members who take payments or open mail should not post payments or prepare the bank deposits. A practice should conduct a review of segregation of duties and internal controls every 2-5 years. The review can be done internally by upper management or outsourced to an accounting or law firm.

The Key Performance Indicator Report

The Key Performance Indicator Report is a good way to capture the critical elements of the revenue cycle. Practices and PM systems have different names for this report. The basic components of the report are:

- Total charges for the month.
- Total payments for the month.
- Total write-offs/adjustments for the month.
- Total Accounts Receivable (AR).
- Days in AR—The calculation for monthly days in AR will differ from an annual calculation. Tracking monthly is preferred.
- Daily charges based on work days in the month.
- Daily payments, based on work days in the month.

Enhancements to the basic data include:

- Physicians vacation days in the month.
- Physician work days in the month.
- Charges per Physician Work Day.
- Payments per Physician Work Day.

The Charges and Payments per physician work day calculations show large differences in monthly charges and payments that occur during months there are a lot of vacations. Theoretically, charges and payments per physician work day should remain relatively stable even if physicians come and go from the practice.

The same format can be used to capture the key performance indicators by provider, location, procedure, drug or type of visit.

DESCRIPTION	January-17	February-17	March-17	2017 Mo Avg	2016 Mo Avg	2015 Mo Avg
CHARGES	$ 3,020,160	$ 3,304,205	$ 4,171,399	$ 3,498,588	$ 3,423,754	3,507,212
PAYMENTS	$ 1,539,244	$ 1,435,502	$ 1,796,472	$ 1,813,981	$ 1,950,998	$ 1,591,956
WRITEOFFS	$ 1,908,233	$ 1,853,852	$ 2,098,809	$ 2,228,340	$ 2,305,057	$ 2,061,694
REFUNDS	$ 20,475	$ 23,922	$ 54,236	$ 37,451	$ 24,901	$ 19,216
COLLECT %	42.05%	43.54%	44.37%	43.18%	45.22%	43.45%
TOTAL AR	$ 3,534,186	$ 3,603,466	$ 3,933,821	$ 3,700,659	$ 4,015,200	$ 3,308,302
DAYS IN AR	31.10	31.52	25.59	30.41	32.05	29.12
Daily Charges	$ 166,550	$ 168,964	$ 181,365	$ 171,679	$ 177,673	$ 154,679
Daily Payments	$ 75,825	$ 73,405	$ 78,107	$ 74,674	$ 81,004	$ 60,476
Work Days Per Mo	21.0	20.0	23.0	21.33		
Phys Work Days	183.0	152.5	175.5	170.33		
Phys Vac Days	4.0	25.5	30.5	20.00		
Chgs Phys Work Day	$ 19,452	$ 22,014	$ 23,768	$ 21,745		
Pmt Phys Workday	$ 9,036	$ 9,564	$ 10,236	$ 9,612		

Accounts Receivable Aging Reports

Accounts receivable aging data is a terrific tool for measuring the overall financial health of the practice. Closely monitoring the number of days in outstanding receivables due from payors and patients will identify collection issues early so internal processes can be adjusted if needed. Very small changes in a billing department, such as a new employee, can start a cascade of events that can quickly reduce cash flow. The methods of monitoring AR will be dictated by the practice's PM system and the creativity of the practice administrator or billing manager.

Month-to-month comparison of the aged accounts receivable is an easy way to spot and stop a negative trend. Below is a helpful format of the report:

DATE	Total	0-30	%	31-60	%	61-90	%	91-120	%	91-121+	%
June-19	3,922,721	2,894,968	73.80	411,885	10.50	243,208	6.20	94,145	2.40	278,513	7.10
July-19	3,444,654	2,552,488	74.10	406,469	11.80	124,007	3.60	89,561	2.60	272,127	7.90
Aug.-19	3,896,426	2,891,148	74.20	444,192	11.40	171,442	4.40	66,239	1.70	323,403	8.30
Sept.-19	4,002,186	2,865,565	71.60	588,321	14.70	152,083	3.80	112,061	2.80	284,155	7.10
Oct.-19	4,248,124	3,173,348	74.70	475,789	11.20	135,939	3.20	144,436	3.40	318,609	7.50
Nov.-19	4,015,168	2,806,602	69.90	630,381	15.70	212,803	5.30	62,227	1.50	305,152	7.60
6 Mo. Avg	3,921,547	2,864,020	73.05	492,840	12.55	173,247	4.42	94,445	2.40	296,993	7.58

Patient Responsibility					
	Oct	Nov	Dec	2019 Mo Avg	2018 Mo Avg
0-30	$27,156.49	$27,420.40	$34,606.67	$29,727.85	$28,863.61
31-60	$49,339.27	$35,998.12	$60,911.15	$42,668.70	$53,711.09
61-90	$54,901.22	$56,811.60	$50,001.15	$53,904.66	$49,009.04
91-120	$20,114.01	$31,468.51	$30,182.44	$27,254.99	$30,050.10
121+	$128,907.54	$130,068.58	$133,430.56	$130,802.23	$121,222.68
Total	$280,418.53	$281,767.21	$309,131.97	$284,358.42	

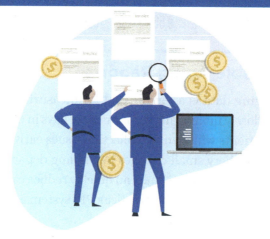

Insurance Responsibility					
	Oct	**Nov**	**Dec**	**2019 Mo Avg**	**2018 Mo Avg**
0-30	$3,064,422.01	$2,331,290.58	$3,091,894.98	$2,829,202.52	$2,902,004.86
31-60	$402,286.75	$555,455.05	$550,688.09	$502,809.96	$536,321.23
61-90	$93,105.02	$128,711.11	$228,124.58	$149,980.24	$200,338.56
91-120	$71,007.58	$42,302.22	$140,875.12	$84,728.31	$112,401.52
121+	$169,062.60	$150,021.27	$138,830.88	$152,638.25	$255,460.00
Total	$3,799,883.96	$3,207,780.23	$4,150,413.65	$3,719,359.28	

Other Revenue Cycle Management Reports

▶ *Time of Service Collections*

Generally, people pay attention to what is measured. Weekly sharing of this data with the managers' responsible for TOS collections and surgery pre-payments will likely result in increased collections. Reporting collections per clinic, rather than limiting it to the collective total, provides better comparative and accuracy of data at each facility.

The sample report below includes Elective Surgery pre-payments. This data does not need to be reported with TOS collections, but it should be tracked somewhere. The results should be shared with staff responsible for pre-collecting OOP amounts for elective surgeries.

Accounts sent for outside collection efforts – Track the following data per month:

- Total dollars sent to the agency per month
- Number of accounts sent to the agency per month
- Average balance per account sent to the agency.
- Amount collected by the agency per month

Main Office	East Office	West Office	Weekly Total	Daily Average	# Clinics Main	# Clinics East	# Clinics West	Average Collect per Clinic Main	Average Collect per Clinic East	Average Collect per Clinic West	Surgery Prepay	Total Collections
$21,822.17	$3,674.07	$4,298.34	$29,794.58	$5,958.92	20	6	6	$1,320.05	$606.06	$566.27	$6,155.70	$37,553.98
$23,902.55	$10,001.58	$4,699.45	$38,603.58	$7,720.72	24	5	9	$1,012.66	$1,188.62	$1,106.24	$3,278.48	$45,021.22
$22,609.09	$6,297.62	$3,518.09	$32,424.80	$6,484.96	22	7	7	$1,078.77	$519.14	$924.50	$2,871.92	$37,691.29
$23,104.99	$9,402.21	$3,722.61	$36,229.81	$7,245.96	24	4	9	$993.07	$852.48	$1,461.64	$3,309.80	$33,661.53
$20,141.14	$5,521.00	$5,820.04	$31,482.18	$6,296.44	19	6	7	$1,062.58	$851.17	$822.86	$1,044.93	$30,901.62
$111,579.94	$34,896.48	$22,058.53	$168,534.95		109	28	38				$16,660.83	$184,829.64

Outside Collections	Oct	Nov	Dec	Totals	Mo. Avg
Amount sent to Agency	$26,822.00	$22,109.00	$30,552.00	$79,483.00	$26,494.33
Amount Coll by Agency	$8,697.00	$9,411.00	$5,102.00	$23,210.00	$7,736.67
# of Accts sent to Agency	78	72	110	260	86.66%
Collection %	32.42%	37.20%	16.70%	86.32%	28.77%
Avg Coll per Acct	$111.50	$130.71	$46.38	$288.59	$96.20
Avg Amt Turned Per Acct	$278.10	$322.28	$283.90	$294.76	$294.76

(Implementing Robust TOS collection efforts will drastically improve these statistics).

▶ Collections by Charge Category

Most practice management systems allow for grouping of similar CPT® codes in charge categories. For example, all CT scans are grouped in a category, E&M Codes are grouped, etc. Charge Category reporting allows analysis at the charge category level and helps narrow down where reimbursement issues may be occurring. If Charge Category reporting is not available, the data can be recorded in a spreadsheet for analysis. A Charge Category report should include the following;

- Charges and payments per month, per category
- The number of services per category
- Average collection per service in the category
- Average collection percentage per category

Charges Zero Paid

There are legitimate reasons that a charge would be fully written off. It could be that the charge is bundled with another service or was performed during a global surgical period. After weeding out legitimate reasons a review may find charges written off inappropriately.

Charges Paid In Full

If a payor is paying the full charge it could be that the group's charge is less than the payors allowed amount for the service. This could be a signal to increase the price of the service.

Est PT Office Visits	January	February	March	Current Yr Mo Avg	Collection % Avg Pmt per	Prior Yr 1 Mo Avg	Collection % Avg Pmt per	Prior Yr 2 Mo Avg	Collection % Avg per 2017
Charge Count	1,958	1,907	2,044	1,970	60.22%	2062	70.14%	1958	58.17%
Charges	$184,675.00	$195,007.00	$233,324.00	$204,335.33		$191,903.33		$222,558.34	
Payments	$141,988.06	$141,204.41	$140,887.81	$140,360.09	$69.80	$140,101.00	$67.67	$130,625.02	$66.63
INPATIENT HOSP CARE									
Charge Count	58	36	41	45	56.58%	52	51.49%	54	48.42%
Charges	$10,004.00	$7,882.00	$7,762.00	$8,549.33		$8,552.92		$9,011.75	
Payments	$7,401.27	$3,701.82	$3,901.66	$5,001.58	$107.81	$4,812.26	$85.20	$4,368.42	$80.03
X-ray									
Charge Count	198	177	185	187	22.11%	211	21.65%	199	27.01%
Charges	$37,978.00	$32,079.50	$33,146.00	$34,401.17		$39,888.22		$28,222.65	
Payments	$7,707.78	$8,364.41	$6,750.71	$7,607.63	$42.76	$8,697.06	$40.97	$7,336.34	$38.37

Other areas recommended for detailed review are collections for drugs, DME, and procedures with other expensive consumables. UroLift and Rezum would be included in that category.

For buy and bill drugs, a report should be produced to check that all drugs are billed with the correct number of units and that the reimbursement exceeds the cost of the drug. Even the most conscientious staff can make mistakes when entering the number of units for a drug injection. (This detailed review is not necessary if the practice management system automatically enters the correct number of units for each injection.) Costly mistakes WILL be made when the units are manually entered.

If the PM system can't produce a report that groups like drugs together for quick review, of units and total payments, it is worth the effort to confirm that the payments for Xofigo®, Provenge®, and other very expensive drugs cover the cost of the drugs.

This can be done electronically IF the practice management system allows the cost of the drug to be entered into the system. If not, tracking can be accomplished with a simple spreadsheet. For one urology group, this tracking mechanism was instrumental in identifying a Xofigo® infusion that had been posted with 1 unit. The infusion would not have been found on an AR report because the practice was paid for 1 unit with the balance of the charge being written off.

Reviewing data on drugs and other expensive consumable items helps identify reimbursement issues that might go unnoticed. Some examples of issues that may be discovered are:

- A group's charge for the drug has not kept up with the increasing cost and reimbursement of the drug.
- A payor's allowed amount is below the cost of the drug.
- Patient OOP amounts are not being collected.

The revenue cycle manager or other designated person should thoroughly review AR and Key Performance Indicator (KPI) reports then dig into and find answers to any unexplainable discrepancies.

If robust reporting on the critical aspects of billing data is not available in the PM system, a urology practice might benefit from a subscription to InfoDive. Through a partnership with Amerisource Bergen, LUGPA members can access InfoDive for a reduced fee.

Costs of Revenue Cycle Management

In addition to continuous monitoring of all aspects of the revenue cycle processes, a practice should also monitor how much the billing department is costing the practice. The simple calculation is the ratio of billing department expenses to total collections. The calculation can be performed, monthly, quarterly, or annually. The expense items should include, staff salaries and benefits, workers compensation insurance, travel and training, IT, books (coding books are expensive) and publications, statement processing, office supplies, consulting fees, outsourced collection fees, software and software maintenance, hardware and hardware maintenance, credit card processing fees, and capital expenditures. The ratio of expenses to collections should be monitored over time. If the ratio is too high perhaps an outside billing service should be considered.

Another measure of the financial efficiency of the billing department is the ratio of total billing department expenses to total number of claims filed in a defined period of time. If the costs per filed claim continue to climb, the efficiency of the department may be eroding.

Revisiting Time of Service Collections

A practice can realize dramatic positive results by embracing appropriate TOS collections. The following statistics are real data from a group that began a regimented TOS program in early 2014.

In 2013 providers in the practice saw 16,669 patients. In that year 903 accounts totaling $502,615.00 were sent to collections. The average balance on the accounts turned to outside collections was $556.61. In 2018 providers in the practice saw 21,810 distinct patients. 903 accounts totaling $285,995.00 were turned to outside collections. The average balance on the turned accounts was $316.72.

In that five-year period, the group added providers and doubled their annual charges and annual collections. The billing department grew from 8 to 11 employees. Even though 25% more patients were seen in 2018 compared to 2013, and the total charges and payment doubled, the same number of accounts were sent for outside collections. The total dollars sent to the outside collection agency dropped by 43%. The average balance on the turned accounts dropped by 43%.

In an era of increasing expenses and lower reimbursement, home runs are hard to find. Implementing an appropriate Time-of-Service Collections initiative can be that elusive home run for your practice. Being financially proactive in your collections process will guarantee that your practice will be a winning team!

KEY POINTS

- **Buy-in from leadership** is vital to a successful Time of Service collection program.

- **Obtain health insurance information** at the time of scheduling to determine the out-of-pocket amount due and notify the patient in advance.

- **Offer patients a budget plan,** billed to a debit/credit card or credit services if they cannot pay.

- **Accurate coding is essential** to maximizing appropriate reimbursement and minimizing days in accounts receivable.

- **Reviewing denied claims** must be a priority in a billing department. (Denial management software programs can be integrated with an EHR or PM systems).

- **After sending a pre-determined number of statements,** the account may move to a pre-collection phase, and if unpaid, to an outside collection agency.

- **All businesses should have effective internal controls** to identify suspicious transactions, errors, and other inconsistencies. Since large sums of money flow through urology offices, segregation of duties should be enforced.

- **Refunding overpayments** to insurance companies or patients is an important step in revenue cycle management.

- **The Key Performance Indicator Report** is a good way to capture the critical elements of the revenue cycle.

- **Accounts receivable aging data** is a terrific tool for measuring the overall financial health of the practice.

- **Reporting Time of Service collections per clinic,** rather than limiting it to the collective total, provides better comparative and accuracy of data at each facility.

Twila J. Puritty, MBA

Twila Puritty serves as Practice Administrator of Wichita Urology Group, in Wichita, KS. With more than 25 years of experience in practice management, Ms. Puritty has developed expertise in facilitating growth initiatives and maximizing shareholder value. Since joining Wichita Urology in 2013, she began and completed the ground-up construction of a 10,000 sq. ft. radiation oncology center, successfully implemented in-office dispensing, added nine new outreach clinics and began an infusion program.

CHAPTER 15

Maximizing Productivity: APPs and Scribes in the Urology Practice

Diane Bonsall, MSN, APRN, ACNS-BC
Evelina Kaminski, MSN, APRN, AGCNS-BC
Gordon Lang, MSN, APRN, FNP-C
Amanda Licea, MPAS, PA-C
Marcia O'Brien, MSN, APRN, FNP-C

Maximizing Resources in the Urology Practice

As medicine continues its trend toward value-based payments, shortages of urologists and an expanding universe of patients who need urologic care, the maximization of resources is an essential element in today's urology practice. Efficiency is key to helping address clinician burnout, enhancing the group's ability to improve patient flow and maximizing reimbursement for services provided.

As independent urology groups continue their evolution of practice, Advanced Practice Providers (APPs) and scribes can play an important role in maximizing resources to enable the group to remain competitive in today's health care market.

Who are Advanced Practice Providers?

Advanced practice providers are medical professionals with advanced education that allow them to assess, diagnose, and treat patients, similarly to physicians. The two types of APPs are advanced practice registered nurses (APRNs) and physician assistants (PAs). APPs are frequently referred to as "mid-level providers," however, this title is neither a legal nor academic term. "Mid-level" is misleading and can imply that the provider provides middle level of care. It is preferable that APPs are referred to by their professional title, APRN or PA.

This chapter discusses how to incorporate APPs into a large urology group where physicians are seeking assistance caring for a growing patient population. If physicians or managers are seeking an APP to join their practice, they will need to advocate for APPs and educate their colleagues and patients about the value APPs bring to the practice.

Advanced Practice Registered Nurses

APRNs are registered nurses (RN), with a master's degree or higher, within one of the four advanced practice nursing roles. The four roles are: nurse practitioners (NP), certified nurse anesthetist (CRNA), certified nurse mid-wives (CNM), and clinical nurse specialists (CNS). NPs serve as primary and specialty care providers, "who are responsible and accountable for health promotion, disease prevention, health education, and counseling as well as the diagnosis and management of acute and chronic diseases" (National Council of State Board of Nursing, 2019). Nurse anesthetists work primarily in hospitals and surgery centers, and provide care and advice related to the delivery of anesthesia (National Council of State Board of Nursing, 2019). Nurse midwives "provide a full range of primary health care services to women throughout the lifespan, including gynecologic care, family planning services, preconception care, prenatal and postpartum care, childbirth, and care of the newborn" (National Council of State Board of Nursing, 2019). Clinical nurse specialists are versatile providers whose roles range from direct patient care, to research coordination, to administration. According to the National Board of Clinical Nurse Specialists (2019), clinical nurse specialists are clinicians whose specialty may be defined by population (e.g. pediatrics, geriatrics, women's health), setting (e.g. critical care), disease or medical subspecialty (e.g. diabetes, oncology), type of care (e.g. psychiatric or rehabilitation), and type of problem (e.g. pain, wound care).

APRN education programs are at the masters or doctorate level, and in most circumstances, applicants must first be trained and licensed as an RN with several years of work experience before being eligible to apply for an APRN program. Once trained and licensed, APRNs must maintain and renew their state license every two years as well as their national credentialing every five years. Credentialing is maintained through either the American Association of Nurse Practitioners (ANPP) or the American Nurses Credentialing Center (ANCC), and licensing is maintained through the specific state board of nursing in which the APRN practices. Practice hour requirements and continuing education (CE) requirements vary by state, making it important for practices and APRNs to be aware of their specific state requirements. ANPP and ANCC also have different CE requirements, but both require a specific number of practice hours, CE hours in the field of practice, and pharmacology CE hours.

Physician Assistants

The American Academy of Physician Assistants (2019) states,

> Physician Assistants (PA) receive a generalist medical education that makes the profession uniquely flexible and able to adapt to the evolving needs of the US health care system based on a curriculum used in medical schools.

All aspiring PAs must obtain a bachelor's degree. While a particular field of undergraduate study is not required, successful applicants often possess bachelor's degrees in physiology, chemistry, mathematics, or biology. In order to obtain the physician assistant-certification designation, the PA must graduate from a master's degree program accredited by ARC-PA (Accreditation Review Commission on Education for the Physician Assistant) and pass the Physician Assistant National Certifying Exam (PANCE). Upon certification, PAs maintain licensure through the state medical board in which they practice.

PAs must also work to maintain their certification. The National Commission on Certification of Physician Assistants uses a 10-year certification cycle divided into periods. During every two-year period, professionals must earn at least 100 continuing education credits. At the end of each 10-year cycle, PAs must pass a recertification exam, the Physician Assistant National Recertifying Exam (PANRE).

What are the differences between APRNs and PAs?

Although the job duties, practice settings, and scope of practice are similar for PAs and APRNs, differences do exist. In a growing number of states, APRNs can practice and prescribe without any kind of collaborative agreement with a physician, whereas PAs always need to have a collaborative agreement with a physician (**NurseJournal.org**, 2019). APRNs and PAs training also differs. PAs adhere to a disease-centered model while APRNs follow a patient-centered model and can be explained as follows:

The nursing model looks holistically at patients and their outcomes, giving attention to a patient's mental and emotional needs as much as their physical ailments. The medical model places a greater emphasis on disease pathology, approaching patient care by looking primarily at the anatomy and physiology systems that comprise the human body (**NurseJournal.org**, 2019).

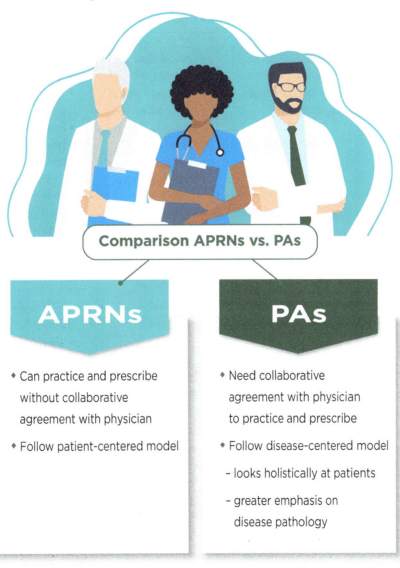

Comparison APRNs vs. PAs

APRNs
- Can practice and prescribe without collaborative agreement with physician
- Follow patient-centered model

PAs
- Need collaborative agreement with physician to practice and prescribe
- Follow disease-centered model
  - looks holistically at patients
  - greater emphasis on disease pathology

Prescriptive Authority

Prescriptive authority privileges vary from state to state for APPs. Generally, APPs can prescribe most medications, including controlled substances schedules III-V. The ability of APPs to prescribe schedule II substances varies by state and practice location.

HOW DRUGS ARE CLASSIFIED IN THE US

	DESCRIPTION	EXAMPLES
SCHEDULE 1	Drugs with no currently accepted medical use and a high potential for abuse. They are the most dangerous drugs of all the drug schedules with potentially sever psychological or physical dependence.	• Heroin • Lysergic acid diethyiamide (LSD) • Marijuana (Cannibis) • Methylenedioxymethamphetamine (Ecstasy) • Methaqualone • Peyote
SCHEDULE 2	Drugs with a high potential for abuse, with use potentially leading to severe psychological or physical dependence. These drugs are also considered dangerous.	• Combination products with less than 15mg of hydrocodone per dosage unit (Vicodin®) • Cocaine • Methamphetamine • Hydromorphone (Dilaudid) • Meperidine (Demoral) • Oxycodone (OxyContin) • Fentanyl • Dexedrine • Adderall • Ritalin
SCHEDULE 3	Drugs with a moderate to low potential for physical and psychological dependence. Schedule 3 drugs abuse potential is less than Schedule 1 & 2 drugs, but more than Schedule 4.	• Products containing less than 90mg of codeine per dosage unit (Tylelnol® and codeine) • Ketamine • Anabolic steroids • Testosterone
SCHEDULE 4	Drugs with low potential for abuse and low risk of dependence.	• Xanax® • Soma® • Darvon® • Darvocet® • Valium® • Ativan® • Talwin® • Ambien® • Tramadol®
SCHEDULE 5	Drugs with lower potential for abuse than Schedule 4 and consist of preparations containing limited quantities of certain narcotics. Schedule 5 drugs are generally used for antidiarrheal, antitussive, and analgesic purposes	• Cough preparations with less than 200mg of codeine per 100ml (Robitussin AC) • Lomotil® • Motofen® • Lyrica® • Paropectolin®

Scope of Practice

The scope of practice of APRNs is dictated by the State Board of Nursing, and PAs by the State Medical Board. Therefore, the scope of practice varies from state to state. APRN scope of practice falls into three categories: full practice (13 states plus Washington, D.C.), full or reduced practice (11 states), and reduced or restricted practice (26 states). APRN practice authority is constantly evolving and frequently debated, therefore it falls upon the APRN and the practice/facility to remain current with state specific rules and regulations. PAs are required to be licensed by the state board of medicine in which they practice and, as with APRNs, their scope of practice and supervision requirements vary by state. APP scope of practice is a widely debated topic:

> Existing state-based laws and regulations limit the effective and efficient use of the health workforce by creating mismatches between professional competence and legal scope-of-practice laws and by perpetuating a lack of uniformity in these laws and regulations across states. State laws limit needed overlap in scopes of practice among professions that often share some tasks and responsibilities, and the process for changing the laws is slow and adversarial. *(Dower, Moore, & Langelier, 2013).*

It is important to be able to differentiate between professional and legal scope of practice. It is not uncommon for an APP's legal scope of practice, dictated by the state, to be more limiting than the APP's actual training or professional scope of practice:

> "Professional scope of practice, often referred to as professional competence, is a profession's description of the services that its members are trained and competent to perform. Legal scope of practice refers to state laws and regulations that define the services that may and may not be provided by members of each profession. *(Dower et al., 2013).*

National and state professional associations maintain guides that assist their members in keeping abreast of licensing, credentialing, and scope of practice requirements.

Roles and Responsibilities

Across the United States, urology APPs can be found in outpatient clinics, surgery centers, assisted living/rehabilitation facilities, and inpatient hospital settings. Specific duties vary according to the provider's education and training as well as the collaborative agreement with the supervising physician. As APPs gains experience in their role as a urology specialist, they can continue to expand the breadth of patients and diagnoses they provide care for.

Most urology APPs practice in outpatient clinics. APPs see common new and established urology diagnoses, not limited to but including urinary tract infections, benign prostatic hyperplasia, elevated prostate specific antigen, prostate cancer, pelvic pain, overactive bladder, kidney stones, hematuria, incontinence, hormone replacement therapy, sexual dysfunction, vasectomy consults, and common post-operative visits. The APP performs physical exams, evaluates imaging and laboratory results, identifies differential diagnoses, and formulates a plan of care. While urologists are frequently in the operating room, an APP typically works exclusively in the outpatient clinic, ensuring that patients can always be seen in a timely manner.

APPs play a valuable role in on-call/after-hours duties. While an MD must always be available for surgical cases, the APP can ease the MD's burden by acting as the first-call resource. APPs can triage after-hours patient calls, which mainly consist of medication questions, post-operative concerns, and symptom management. These are problems that the APP routinely deals with in the clinic setting. However, it is important that the APP have a physician easily accessible for advice or guidance.

Utilization of APPs in after-hours care in a hospital setting is dictated by an APP's experience and training. Given a potential need for surgical intervention, often the on-call physician handles contact from hospital-based providers. However, the physician should be able to delegate specific tasks to the APP, such as difficult catheter insertion, urethral dilation, and catheter irrigation. The ability of the APP to safely and effectively perform these skills should be evaluated on a case-by-case basis between the APP, the supervising physician, and the facility. Delegating routine post-operative and inpatient rounds to APPs leaves the MD the time to focus on more acute and critically ill patients. APPs can coordinate peri-operative visits, coordination of care, and discharge planning in the inpatient setting.

State laws and practice acts vary regarding the amount of training and necessity of formal certification required of the APP to assist in the operating room. Utilization of APPs in the operating room setting requires hospital credentialing but, in most circumstances, this is easily attained. Compared to APRNs, PAs are more often trained to assist in the operating room. In addition to their APRN license, APRNs are required to hold a Registered Nurse First Assistant (RNFA) certification through The National

Commission for the Certification of Surgical Assistants (NCCSA). However, urologists often work with other well-trained surgical assistants in the operating room, which allows the APPs to see patients in the outpatient and/or inpatient setting.

Procedures

The use of APPs for some urologic procedures is becoming more common in busy urology practices. As urologists spend more time with complex patients and operating, appropriately trained APPs can perform procedures in the clinic setting. One study found that from 1994-2012, Medicare claims by APPs for cystoscopy increased by over 7,000%, prostate biopsy increased by 4,000%, and renal ultrasound increased by 24,000% (Langston et al., 2017a). These numbers draw attention to the increased role APPs play in urology groups and highlight the need for urology practices to utilize APPs for procedures. The specific procedures performed by APPs, are dictated by practice and facility policy, but more importantly by the supervising physician. Commonly performed procedures are cystoscopies, prostate biopsies, prostate ultrasounds, urodynamics, complex urinary catheter insertions, hormone pellet insertions, and renal ultrasounds.

The ability of an APP to perform a cystoscopy remains a controversial subject. Nurse-led cystoscopy clinics in the United Kingdom and Australia are common but remain a heavily physician performed procedure in the US. When discussing the APP's ability to perform cystoscopy, the two main focuses are the technical and diagnostic aspects of the procedure. For example, cystoscopy for ureteral stent removal can be quickly and easily performed by a well-trained APP. However, cystoscopy for a urinary tract symptom or hematuria evaluation is more complicated to implement in practice. The British Association of Urologic Surgeons (2007) has developed a cystoscopy training program that has been adopted by the Society of Urologic Nurses and Associates (SUNA). These guidelines recommend observation of a minimum of 10 physician performed cystoscopies followed by a minimum of 50 APP performed cystoscopies supervised by the physician. Following certification, the APPs are routinely audited in person or via video recordings. It is widely agreed that US based APPs should not routinely perform unsupervised cystoscopies for bladder cancer surveillance or hematuria evaluation (Urology Times, 2013). This is dealt with on a case-by-case basis, and a solution for this controversy may be for the APP to perform the procedure while the physician monitors (either in person, or via remote monitoring). This allows the APP to take the time to evaluate proper patients for cystoscopy, explain procedural risks and expectations, and perform cystoscopy. Meanwhile, the physician only needs to be available during the evaluation of the urinary tract.

Prostate biopsies are another procedure that has been heavily performed by physicians, but in the right scenario can be effectively performed by an APP. Like cystoscopy, most outcome data on APPs performing prostate biopsies have come from the United Kingdom. This data has found that an APP can safely and effectively perform a prostate biopsy with similar quality to that of a physician (Turner & Pati, 2010). The Emory University Department of Urology has developed an APP prostate biopsy training program, and now most of the prostate biopsies at the institution are performed by APPs (Urology Times, 2013). This training program requires supervision of 50 APP performed prostate biopsies by a physician followed by periodic evaluation of the APP. Muta Issa, MD, from Emory University, states that, "Prostate biopsy and cystoscopy are repetitive and mechanical, making them relatively straightforward to learn and be proficient at. They are performed in high volumes and therefore tend to take up a good portion of the urologist's time and effort." (Urology Times, 2013).

Research

Practices that engage in clinical research will also find benefit in including their APPs as assistant or co-investigators. "Nurses in clinical research may practice in centers with numerous resources devoted to research and have a more defined scope of practice; at centers with fewer resources, however, nurses may function more as generalists, assuming activities ranging from direct patient care to administrative responsibilities." (Castro et al., 2011). The major responsibilities for any nurse involved in clinical research is ensuring research participant safety, study integrity, and ongoing maintenance of the informed consent process, all within the context of effective and appropriate clinical care. As the national and international clinical research enterprise expands, investigators, health policy makers, regulators, and sponsors of clinical research must understand the pivotal role of nurses (Castro et al., 2011).

Collaboration with Physicians

Physician-APP collaboration is, "a process in which a nurse practitioner works with one or more physicians to deliver health care services within the scope of the practitioner's expertise, with medical direction and appropriate supervision as provided for in jointly developed guidelines or other mechanisms as provided by the law of the state in which the services are performed." (United States Code of Federal Regulation, 2019). Effective and positive physician-APP collaboration should be based on open communication, mutual trust and respect, and recognition of the value of the skillset that each party brings to the relationship. Collaborative practice, while very interdependent, allows for a great degree of autonomy and self-governance. (Hamric, Hanson, Tracy, & O'Grady, 2014).

Supported by research on the benefits of collaboration. APPs enhance the delivery of comprehensive care for patients leading to improved quality of care and increased patient satisfaction. Optimal use of APPs allows the physician to focus on complex patients. It increases physician appointment availability to accommodate new patient visits and decreases wait times for patients. A collaborative practice of APPs with physicians leads to best practice value-based care. (Cairo et al., 2017). There are many factors that influence the physician-APP relationship. Practice size, patient volume, patient demographics, and types of procedures performed are a few aspects that need to be considered when deciding on the best collaborative physician-APP model. State laws governing APP supervision also play an important role.

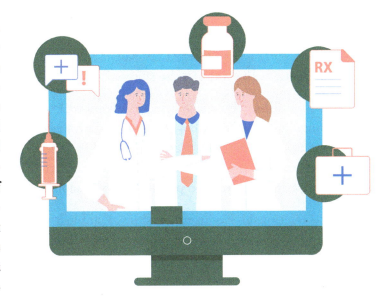

There are two main categories of physician-APP relationships. The first is a one-to-one approach. Urologists hire one APP specifically to work with them on an individual basis. The APP is tasked with caring for this physician's patient population and works and reports directly to that physician. The second model is a shared model where one APP works with several urologists and assumes duties and care for their patients.

As expected, there are advantages and disadvantages to both models. Working with multiple MDs increases an APP's productivity; and bigger patient population between multiple MDs allows APP's schedules to be filled quickly. Also, the APP becomes experienced with a variety of urologic conditions, procedures, and interventions. Although a standard of care is preferred, there is often practice variation amongst physicians. This exposure can be both challenging and beneficial for the APP. Working with multiple physicians requires the APP to be organized, flexible, communicative, and accessible. Conversely, in a one-to-one model, the communication and organizational aspect of practice is more straightforward. It is easier to find time to discuss patient cases and details of treatment plans. It is also easier to resolve conflicts and misunderstandings since only two parties are involved. In a well-functioning one-to-one model, the APP is in tune with their supervising physicians' treatment plans, which improves efficiency of that APPs practice. There is, however, potentially less diversity in patient population and fewer opportunities for the APP to become familiar with a wide variety of disease states and procedures.

How to Recruit an Advanced Practice Provider

A practice looking to increase patient satisfaction and practice revenue will find the right candidates with some of these suggestions:

01. Use a recruiter who specializes in Advanced Practice staffing. These recruiters have experience with successful sourcing, screening, and placement of APPs. They are well informed on state laws regarding scope of practice, prescriptive authority, and physician supervision rules.

02. Build relationships with universities. Establish a preceptorship and mentorship program where experienced APPs precept students and soon-to-be graduates. This provides an opportunity for physicians and other team members to become familiar with the student and decide whether they are a good fit for the practice. It is also a valuable opportunity for students to learn about the field and decide if it is a good match for them.

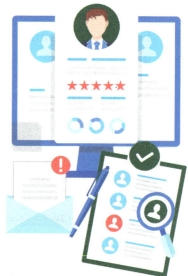

03. Build relationships with medical facilities. This provides opportunities for APPs looking for different clinical settings and work schedules. It is also a great way to recruit registered nurses looking to transition to an advanced practice role.

04. Build relationships with the community. Attend health fares and community events, such as fundraisers. Remember that advanced practice providers often have family members who use health care services or are patients themselves. Being involved in the community is a powerful and effective way to introduce people to your company and your company's mission and values.

There are some important differences between hiring a physician and an advanced practice provider. When looking for a new position, a vast majority of physicians rely on word of mouth and professional connections. APPs are less likely to use their professional networks and use more conventional methods such as job boards. APRNs and PAs use job boards such as, CareerBuilder and Indeed, in addition to specific nursing and PA job boards. APRNs and PAs are active on sites like LinkedIn while physicians are more likely to use physician-specific sites, such as Doximity and Sermo. It is important to understand that the recruitment cycle and time to hire is also very different for physicians and APPs. Physicians typically complete their training over the summer. APRNs and PAs finish their training in the fall or spring. APPs are less likely to sign annual and bi-annual contracts, which make them more available throughout the year. Additionally, the average time to hire a physician is 180 days compared to less than ninety days for APPs (Ascendo Resources, 2019).

Onboarding and Training

All newly hired APPs, regardless of previous urology experience, need time to become accustomed to new electronic medical record systems, clinic workflow, and collaborating physicians' patient population and practice preferences. Realistically, this onboarding period can last between four weeks and three months. During this time, it is recommended to slowly increase patient load and allow for proper physician support while seeing patients. It is also important to acknowledge the difference between new graduate APPs and APPs with previous work experience (urology or otherwise). New graduate APPs are still becoming comfortable in their new role as a provider, as well as the urology specialty, and will likely require more mentoring and support from other APP or physician counterparts.

For APPs with prior urology experience, onboarding can typically be accelerated, but it is important to assess their prior patient population, understanding of current treatment guidelines, and prescribing tendencies. Training and onboarding need to be tailored specifically based on their background. For example, if an APP is coming from a predominantly female urology background but will be seeing more male patients in their new role, training needs to be specified to fit their new role.

APPs with no prior urology experience need to be on-boarded slowly, receive more support resources, and be evaluated for understanding and competency along the way. Shadowing their collaborating physician(s) or other APPs is a valuable tool for APPs new to urology. Shadowing exclusively can last between two to four weeks, allowing the APP to understand the patient population and Electronic Medical Record (EMR). Following this, APPs can begin seeing patients in collaboration with a physician, like a medical student or resident. Allow the APP to perform the history and physical examination and formulate a plan to present to their collaborating physician. Throughout this time, the APPs schedule can be filled with future appointments.

Resources for newly hired APPs can range from APP mentors, to online modules, to textbooks. The American Urological Association (AUA) provides an online curriculum for its members called the AUA University, in which specific training modules can be selected for the APP to complete. Well known by urologists, The Pocket Guide to Urology by Jeff Wieder, is a valuable resource for APPs as well as numerous other textbooks.

Retaining the Ideal Candidate

According to a 2011 Compensation and Employment Survey, the top five reasons APPs change jobs are salary, advancement opportunity, hours/shifts, location preference, and desire for more responsibility (**AdvancedPractice.com**, 2012). According to a survey conducted by PracticeMatch (2016), 43% of participants are unwilling to relocate any distance for a new job, and only 20% say they are willing to relocate. In order to develop a competitive offer and retain the APP, consider the following:

- Develop a comprehensive, clinical training plan for the new APP regardless of years of experience, and training with the EMR, billing, documentation, and company structure.

- Provide a path for professional development with specific goals and objectives. Offer quarterly incentive pay or a performance-based end-of-year bonus.

- Create a support system for newly hired APPs, whether it is the supervising physician or an experienced APP.

- Issue competitive continuing education (CE) and conference allowance with paid-time-off. These educational hours will be used towards APP recertification.

- Offer a flexible schedule whenever possible.

- Offer a competitive salary, which depends on a multitude of factors:
  - Geographic region and cost of living
  - Years of experience
  - Education level
  - Certifications
  - Additional training or specialized skills

According to Jeff Morris, a surgeon, coach, speaker, and physician executive leader, "Hiring an APP should be taken as seriously as bringing a physician into your practice. A solid recruitment and selection process, including behavioral-based interviewing, will ensure the APP you hire is a good fit for your practice, the other team members, and the patient population that you serve" (Morris, 2016).

Financial Advantages of Employing Advanced Practice Providers

The American Board of Urology predicts a 20% decrease in full-time practicing urologists by the year 2035, while predicting a 43% increase in APPs working within the urology specialty. Simultaneously, individuals over the age of 65 are the fastest growing demographic in the United States (McKibben, Kirby, Langston, Raynor, & Pruthi, 2016) thus, increasing the demand for quality medical services. There is a rising need for urology practices to incorporate and retain well-trained APPs into their practice.

The efficient hiring and retention of APPs requires careful balancing of several considerations, including optimizing remuneration, incentives, and billing practices. The

Center for Health Care and Leadership Management conducted a 2018 survey titled "PA and NP Workplace Experiences Survey," which delineated the most important considerations for APPs when accepting an offer from a medical practice. Ninety-one percent of respondents noted their top concern was the salary and benefits package (Roberson, 2019). A 2015 PA Salary Survey showed half of all practices offer PAs a base salary coupled with a production bonus. In addition, a 2018 Advanced Practice Registered Nurse Survey showed 34% of NPs were offered a base salary with a production bonus (Stokowski, McBride, & Berry, 2018). Incentivizing APPs based on production is beneficial not only in generating additional revenue for the practice, but also in tracking APPs individual financial contribution to the practice. APPs collect more in pay when offered a production bonus, which can then increase the employee's job satisfaction, and therefore, decrease a practice's turnover rate. Recent data reveals medical practices with a "higher non-physician provider (NPP) to physician ratio (0.41 NPPs per physician or more) report greater expenses; they also report earning more in revenue after operating costs than practices with fewer NPPs (0.20 or fewer NPPs per physician), regardless of specialty" (Medical Group Management Association, 2018).

An advantage of hiring an APP versus adding an additional physician to the practice extends beyond monetary considerations. The use of an APP can be tailored to an individual physician's needs: a surgery-heavy urologist can task an APP with pre-operative and post-operative clinic visits along with rounding on patients post-operatively in the hospital. This maximizes the surgeon's time in the operating room. Urologists preferring to focus on in-office procedures and more complex patients can direct their APP to concentrate on new patient visits with less complicated presentations and post-procedural evaluations. The way a practice intends on employing an APP should be made explicit during the interview process. Additionally, APPs are performing more in-office procedures, with over 81% performing procedures independently and over half of APPs performing moderately complex procedures (Langston et al., 2017b).

Billing Considerations

If a practice intends to use "incident-to" reimbursement, several considerations must be made." Incident-to" billing allows for a practice to collect 100% of the Medicare Physician Fee Schedule (MPFS) for a given service, however strict standards must be adhered to (Wallace & Polacheck, 2017). Wallace & Polacheck (2017) state that the Office of Inspector General (OIG) specifies the following policies regarding "incident-to" billing.

- Services and supplies must be:
  - Furnished in a non-institutional setting to non-institutional patients.
  - An integral, though incidental, part of the physician's services during diagnosis or treatment of an injury or illness.

- Commonly furnished without charge or included in the physician's bill.

- Of a type that are commonly furnished in a physician's office or clinic.

- Furnished under the physician's direct supervision.

- Furnished by the physician, practitioner with an "incident to" benefit, or auxiliary personnel.

* Services and supplies must be furnished in accordance with applicable state law.

* Auxiliary personnel or a supervising physician may be an employee or an independent contractor.

* Claims for drugs payable administered by a physician as defined in section 1861(r) of the Social Security Act to refill an implanted item of durable medical equipment (DME) may only be paid under Part B to the physician as a drug "incident to" a physician's service under section 1861(s)(2)(A).

Because physicians must be present when their APP provides services, some medical practices are questioning the continued use of 'incident-to" billing. The OIG began auditing medical practices in 2012, levying fines for noncompliance ranging from $10,957 to $21,916 per false claim (Wallace & Polacheck, 2017). Since auditing began, negligent practices have been fined, in some cases, more than $1 million (Wallace & Polacheck, 2017). Additionally, up to five years of incarceration is considered for knowingly submitting false claims.

Billing under the National Provider Identifier (NPI) of APPs reimburses at 85% of the MPFS. Practices billing through each individual provider's NPI will have clear information on the individual contribution of each provider under their umbrella. "Incident-to" billing can mask the contribution of an APP within a practice because services rendered are billed exclusively through the physician's NPI. A practice can utilize "incident-to" billing if it implements clear policies, explicitly documents compliance with "incident-to" requirements within patient charts, and continuously monitors emerging regulatory developments as outlined by the Center for Medicare and Medicaid Services (CMS) and OIG.

Scribes

Regardless of the practice setting, providers face an increased burden of documentation and reporting. The growing regulation and payer requirements places practices at risk for revenue loss. Coupled with this are the increasing requirements for EMR implementation and these EMRs' increased complexity. When time spent dedicated to computer work increases, the amount of time spent with patients suffers. Incorporating scribes is a way to address the evolving requirement for documentation while preserving quality patient interaction. ScribeAmerica, a national scribe agency, defines a scribe as a physician collaborator who fulfills the primary secretarial and non-clinical functions of the busy physician or mid-level provider. Scribes specialize in medical data entry into a paper or electronic medical record system and in instituting efficient workflow process, thus increasing the medical provider's capacity to provide direct patient care" (2019).

Many medical staffing agencies offer scribes for hire and scribe-centered agencies can be found nationwide. The educational and experience background of scribes can vary widely. The individuals working as scribes are often students in a pre-med or allied health major who are looking to gain medical experience while they complete their degrees. It is important to know the qualifications of the individual you are contracting, as there are no accepted minimum qualifications for scribes.

When thinking about incorporating scribes into the urology group, consider the following points.

01 Engage group members in the decision to use scribes. Assess the level of clerical burden and EHR frustration to inform the decision making.

02 Consider a pilot program using a subset of clinicians. Track productivity, time savings, chart quality and clinician satisfaction.

03 Consider the return on investment (ROI) is adequate for the use of scribes. Naturally, there is a financial ROI resulting from increased productivity, but also consider the non-financial ROI of burnout reduction and clinician engagement and fulfillment.

04 If you hire scribes, make sure to treat them as essential team members. They should receive proper training and support.

When hiring a scribe, several qualifications are important to consider. These include previous experience in urology; excellent spelling, computer, and keyboarding skills; and an understanding of medical terminology. A skills assessment to evaluate typing speed and accuracy, and a medical vocabulary test is also worth consideration. When hiring a scribe from an agency, be sure to request evidence of these types of evaluations.

PayScale (2019) reports the 2019 median hourly rate for scribes nationwide at $12.30/hour. Pay varies by location, experience, and complexity of the assignment. Cost to the practice will likely be higher as most scribes are employed through an agency and not as a direct hire. Agency placements can allow for better coverage of clinic needs by utilizing several scribes per assignment to ensure adequate staffing in the event of a scribe needing to cancel a shift due to illness or vacation.

Many groups that use scribes report increased productivity that allows for an increase in patient visits as well as an increase in RVUs. Real time data entry is improved, that translates into fewer notes to be entered at the end of the day, resulting in better work-life balance for clinicians. Many also report that their interactions with patients are improved by using a scribe.

Challenges exist, of course, to using scribes. One of the first questions often asked is about cost. How does the group pay for the scribe? Should an individual provider be responsible for the cost or should the group pay for the service? Further challenges include the education, training and quality assurance processes, the buy-in for the use of scribes by the group and the manner in which scribes are allocated.

When thinking about incorporating scribes into the urology group, consider the following points:

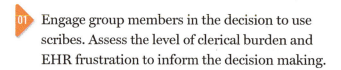

How Medical Scribes Help Physicians

- Increased productivity allowing for increased patient visits and RVUs
- Improved real time data entry means fewer notes to be entered
- Allows for better work/life balance for physicians
- Improved patient interaction

01 Engage group members in the decision to use scribes. Assess the level of clerical burden and EHR frustration to inform the decision making.

02 Consider a pilot program using a subset of clinicians. Track productivity, time savings, chart quality and clinician satisfaction.

03 Consider if the return on investment (ROI) is adequate for the use of scribes. Naturally, there is a financial ROI resulting from increased productivity, but also consider the non-financial ROI of burnout reduction and clinician engagement and fulfillment.

04 If you hire scribes, make sure to treat them as essential team members. They should receive proper training and support.

Conclusions

A key metric for contemporary urology groups is to increase patient volume and improve efficiency. The reduction of administrative burden on clinicians is one way to enhance these areas. By adding APPs and scribes to the practice, APPs can expand capacity; take same day appointments; be the leader of clinical service lines, such as prostate cancer clinics; and engage in the group's research program. The addition of scribes in the practice also can enhance productivity, reduce EHR fatigue for the clinician and improve the overall patient experience.

REFERENCES

AdvancedPractice.com. (2012). Recruiting advanced practice providers (APP's) for hospital and clinic-based practices. Retrieved from http://www.maprainc.org/wp-content/uploads/2013/10/2012_MAPRA_Recruiting-advanced-Practice-Providers.pdf

American Academy of Physician Assistants (AAPA). (2019). *PA Education-Preparation for Excellence* [PDF version]. Retrieved from https://www.aapa.org/wp-content/uploads/2016/12/Issue_Brief_PA_Education.pdf

Ascendo Resources. (2019). 6 Differences Between Recruiting Physicians & Advanced Practice Providers. Retrieved from https://ascendo.com/6-differences-between-recruiting-physicians-advanced-practice-providers/

The British Association of Urologic Surgeons. (2007). *Flexible Cystoscopy Training and Assessment Guideline* (2nd ed.). Retrieved from https://www.baus.org.uk/_userfiles/pages/files/Publications/BAUN%20BAUS%20Flexible%20Cystoscopy%20Guidelines%20-%20November%202017.pdf

Cairo, J., Muzi, M. A., Ficke, D., Ford-Pierce, S., Goetzke, K., Stumvoll, D., Sanchez, F. A. (2017). Practice Model for Advanced Practice Providers in Oncology. *American Society of Clinical Oncology Educational Book*, 37, 40-43. Retrieved from https://ascopubs.org/doi/full/10.1200/EDBK_175577?url_ver=Z39.88-2003&rfr_id=ori%3Arid%3Acrossref.org&rfr_dat=cr_pub%3Dpubmed

Castro, K., Bevans, M., Miller-Davis, C., Cusack, G., Loscalzo, F., Matlock, A. M., ... Hastings, C. (2011). Validating the Clinical Research Nursing Domain of Practice. *Oncology Nursing Forum*, 38(2). doi: 10.1188/11.onf.e72-e80

Dower, C., Moore, J., & Langelier, M. (2013). It Is Time to Restructure Health Professions Scope-Of-Practice Regulations to Remove Barriers to Care. *Health Affairs*, 32(11), 1971–1976. doi: 10.1377/hlthaff.2013.0537

Hamric, A. B., Hanson, C. M., Tracy, M. F., & O'Grady, E. T. (2014). *Advanced Practice Nursing: An Integrative Approach* (5th ed.). Philadelphia, PA: Saunders.

Langston, J. P., Duszak, R, Jr., Orcutt, V. L., Schultz, H., Hornberger, B., Jenkins, L. C., Nielson, M. E. (2017a). The Expanding Role of Advanced Practice Providers in Urologic Procedural Care. *Urology*, 106, 70-75.

Langston, J. P., Orcutt, V. L., Smith, A. B., Schultz, H., Hornberger, B., Deal, A. B., Pruthi, R. S. (2017b). Advanced Practice Providers in U.S. Urology: A National Survey of Demographics and Clinical Roles. *Urology Practice*, 4(5), pp. 418-424.

McKibben, M., Kirby, W. E., Langston, J., Raynor, M. C., & Pruthi, R. S. (2016). Projecting the Urology Workforce Over the Next 20 Years. *Urology*, 98, pp. 21-26.

Medical Group Management Association (MGMA). (2018). *New MGMA Data Shows Medical Practices Utilizing More Non-Physician Providers are More Profitable, Productive* [Press release]. Retrieved from https://www.mgma.com/news-insights/press/new-mgma-data-shows-medical-practices-utilizing-mo

Morris, J. (2016). Optimizing the Value of Advanced Practice Providers. Retrieved from https://www.studergroup.com/resources/articles-and-industry-updates/insights/august-2016/optimizing-the-value-of-advanced-practice-provider

National Board of Clinical Nurse Specialists. (NBCNS). (2019). What is a CNS? Retrieved from https://nacns.org/about-us/what-is-a-cns/

National Council of State Board of Nursing. (NCSBN). (2019). APRNs in the US. Retrieved from https://www.ncsbn.org/aprn.htm

NurseJournal.org. (2019). Nurse Practitioner Vs. Physician Assistant. Retrieved from http://nursejournal.org/nurse-practitioner/np-vs-physician-assistants/

PayScale. (2019). Average Medical Scribe Hourly Pay. Retrieved from https://www.payscale.com/research/US/Job=Medical_Scribe/Hourly_Rate

PracticeMatch. (2016). One-Third of Advanced Practice Clinicians on the Move—New Survey from PracticeMatch Reveals Job Preferences, Goals of NPs and PAs. Retrieved from https://www.practicematch.com/employers/recruitment-articles/one-third-of-advanced-practice-clinicians-on-the-move.cfm

Roberson, J. (2019, October 4). Survey Uncovers Ways Employers Can Enhance the PA Workplace: Formal Orientation, Onboarding, Leadership Structure, and Productivity Reporting Important to PA Workforce. Retrieved from https://www.chlm.org/survey-uncovers-ways-employers-can-enhance-the-pa-workplace/

ScribeAmerica. (2019). FAQ. Retrieved from https://www.scribeamerica.com/faq/

Stokowski, L. A., McBride, M., & Berry, E. (2018, November 28). Medscape APRN Compensation Report, 2018. Retrieved from https://www.medscape.com/slideshow/2018-aprn-compensation-report-6010997

Turner, B. & Pati, J. (2010). Nurse Practitioner Led Prostate Biopsy: An Audit to Determine Effectiveness and Safety for Patients. *International Journal of Urological Nursing*, 4(2), 87-92.

United States Code of Federal Regulation. (2019). 42 CFR 410.75 - Nurse practitioners' services. Retrieved from https://www.govregs.com/regulations/expand/title42_chapterIV_part410_subpartB_section410.75#title42_chapterIV_part410_subpartB_section410.75

Urology Times. (2013). Non-physician providers: Allied or disparate? Retrieved from https://www.urologytimes.com/modern-medicine-feature-articles/non-physician-providers-allied-or-disparate

Wallace, M. & Polacheck, J. (2017, July 19). *"Incident to" Billing in Health Care: Navigating Complex Requirements and Ensuring Compliance* [PDF version]. Retrieved: http://media.straffordpub.com/products/incident-to-billing-in-health-care-navigating-complex-requirements-and-ensuring-compliance-2017-07-19/presentation.pdf

KEY POINTS

- **The American Board of Urology** predicts a 20% decrease in full-time practicing urologists by the year 2035, while predicting a 43% increase in Advanced Practice Providers (APPs).

- **The use of APPs for some urologic procedures** is becoming more common in busy urology practices.

- **APPs are medical providers with advanced education** that allows them to assess, diagnose, and treat patients, similarly to physicians. The two types are advanced practice registered nurses (APRNs) and physician assistants (PAs). PAs adhere to a disease-centered model while APRNs follow a patient-centered model.

- **Across the United States, urology APPs can be found** in outpatient clinics, surgery centers, assisted living/rehabilitation facilities, and inpatient hospital settings.

- **In a growing number of states, APRNs** can practice and prescribe without any kind of collaborative agreement with a physician, whereas PAs always need to have a collaborative agreement with a physician.

- **A solid recruitment and selection process,** including behavioral-based interviewing, will ensure the APP you hire is a good fit for your practice.

- **Delegating routine post-operative and inpatient rounds to APPs** leaves the MD the time to focus on more acute and critically ill patients.

- **As APPs gain experience in their role as a urology specialist,** they continue to expand the breadth of patients and diagnoses for which they provide care.

- **Effective and positive physician-APP collaboration** should be based on open communication, mutual trust and respect, and recognition of the value of the skillset that each party brings to the relationship.

- **Adding scribes to the practice** can increase efficiency and reduce clinical EHR burden.

Diane Bonsall, MSN, APRN, ACNS-BC

Diane Bonsall completed her undergraduate degree at the University of Pennsylvania in Philadelphia. She then spent several years in the pharmaceutical industry providing clinical monitoring and regulatory compliance support to investigators and study sponsors. After returning to school she received her Master of Science in Nursing from the University of Texas at Austin. Currently, she holds her Advanced Practice Registered Nurse license as a board certified Clinical Nurse Specialist (CNS) with prescriptive authority. Since 2014 she has been in practice with Urology Austin.

Evelina Kaminski, MSN, APRN, AGCNS-BC

Evelina Kaminski completed her Master of Science in Nursing from the School of Nursing at University of Texas at Austin in 2017. In 2017, she also received her Advanced Practice Registered Nurse certification from the Texas Board of Nursing and her Clinical Nurse Specialist certification from the American Nurses Credentialing Center. She also holds an Advanced Oncology Clinical Nurse Specialist certification. She currently practices at Urology Austin at their Radiation Oncology clinic, which specializes in treatment of prostate cancer.

Gordon Lang, MSN, APRN, FNP-C

Gordon Lang is a Nurse Practitioner in Austin, TX and has specialized in urology since 2015. He received a bachelors degree in nursing from Indiana University and a masters degree from Georgetown University. His areas of interest are prostate cancer and men's health.

Amanda Licea, MPAS, PA-C

Amanda Licea is a Board Certified Physician Assistant (PA-C), who received her Master of Science in Physician Assistant Studies in 2012 from Texas Tech University Health Sciences Center. She is nationally certified by the National Commission on Certification of Physician Assistants. Amanda currently works with Dr. Peter Ruff, who has a special interest in minimally invasive robotic surgery for the treatment of prostate, fine kidney and bladder cancers and as well as urologic malformations. Prostate cancer management and post-prostatectomy recovery are Amanda's primary focus.

Marcia O'Brien, MSN, APRN, FNP-C

Marcia O'Brien is a Board Certified Family Nurse Practitioner, who received a Master's in Science in Nursing at University of Texas at Tyler in 2016. She collaborates with Dr Brett Baker, Dr Jeff Kocurek, Dr Michael McClelland, and Dr Herb Singh at Urology Austin in the inpatient and outpatient setting. Her areas of interest are prevention and treatment of urinary tract infections, interstitial cystitis, overactive bladder, neurogenic bladder, and chronic pelvic pain syndrome in male and female patients.

CHAPTER 16

Medical Imaging

Benjamin Lowentritt, MD, FACS

Medical imaging has been a core part of urology practices for decades. The use of imaging techniques in commonly performed outpatient urological procedures, such as ultrasound for prostate biopsy, and fluoroscopy for cystoscopy and extracorporeal shock wave lithotripsy (ESWL) has led to further adoption of these technologies in the office setting. As urology practice has evolved, additional applications have emerged requiring more advanced imaging options, such as magnetic resonance imaging (MRI) in the diagnosis and treatment of prostate cancer, dual-energy X-ray absorptiometry (DEXA) scans in the monitoring and management of patients treated for advanced prostate cancer, and computed tomography (CT) for the evaluation and management of kidney stones.

Since the early 2000s, urology groups have felt the pinch of declining reimbursements. As a result, many groups looked to expand their services, and some incorporated diagnostic imaging services as part of this effort. While in the past this may have been to capture revenues that were previously sent to other facilities, the shift to value-based payments creates an opportunity to focus on quality and cost control by keeping imaging services in-house.

The amount and types of imaging services frequently used in the evaluation and management of urologic disease has increased as it has throughout medicine. Previously, practices may have incorporated an ability to do intravenous pyelography (IVP) and/or ultrasound, however, most imaging used now is with more advanced techniques, such as a CT scan, MRI, positron emission tomography (PET), and other nuclear medicine services. Furthermore, these services are not only diagnostic in nature, as the advancements in less-invasive treatments frequently are accomplished using image-guided techniques. Increased use of biopsy for kidney lesions and metastatic lesions from prostate cancer and the potential for localized chemoablation of lesions in the genitourinary organs will likely drive care that was previously only offered within an interventional radiology suite into the urology practice or affiliated facilities.

A urology group's financial commitment to launch an imaging line of service, maintain equipment, and manage ambulatory supply chain services can be daunting. Some imaging centers and ancillary center builds have risen into millions of dollars in overhead and buildout. In addition, the legal implications and ramifications of multi-specialty or urology group facilities must be carefully considered to stay clear of laws prohibiting self-referral. Reports from various third-party payors and others have also suggested that insurers previously questioned the high costs of imaging services and have worked to restrict coverage of them in certain markets.

With changes in health care, including the passage of the Affordable Care Act, and the Medicare Access and CHIP (Children's Health Insurance Program) Reauthorization Act of 2015 (MACRA), incorporating imaging into the services of a practice not only has the potential to add revenue, it has the potential to meet goals of health care reform.

WHY CONSIDER IMAGING SERVICE?

Although the development of new payment models has not significantly impacted urology to date, implementation of these payment models is growing in other fields. Incoming payment models impact Medicare Part B services (not Part A Hospitals, Home Health, Part C Medicare HMOs, or Part D Drugs) and are focused on quality and cost measurement, reporting, and payment adjustments. MACRA's goal has been to facilitate the Department of Health and Human Services' (HHS) desire to achieve better patient quality and value.

As the newer payment models and quality initiatives are implemented, physicians see the possibilities of imaging centers and ancillary services. These include quality control bundled and alternative payment options, and the opportunity to be positioned as more affordable care, especially when compared to similar services as offered by hospitals and hospital systems.

Many urology groups have found that startup costs for an imaging center can be significant, with the price of the equipment and facility build out alone moving into high-expense categories. Groups may hire paid consultants to help create business plans, proformas, and certification strategies in order to structure the ownership and make certification of their imaging centers easier and more manageable.

Urologists may choose to share the financial risks of opening an imaging center with another entity such as a hospital, an imaging center, or a multi-specialty group. Many groups have weighed various options of strategic partnerships due to costs, scheduling, and other considerations.

Three-way joint ventures, involving a hospital, multi-specialty group, or other physician groups, are now surfacing with transactions underway. Although in the past, hospitals and groups have seen each other as competitors, they now view each other as complementary entities and sometimes allies. There have been new models of joint ventures recently involving medical practices that share the same office building. Many groups come together to build an ambulatory surgery center or imaging facilities in their shared space as a cohesive revenue stream.

Under this conjoined model, no single group practice must be financially at risk for the equipment, scheduling, coding, or billing. Instead, they are only financially at risk for their anticipated piece of the capacity of the diagnostic imaging center in their respective specialty or area. A potential downside of partnering with a hospital or hospital system is that most of these arrangements establish payment rates at the hospital level. While this can be advantageous in a fee-for-service model, it limits the value added in a total-cost-of-care (TCOC) model.

For all the various models, a critical component to success is ensuring there will be enough patient volume and an appropriate payor and scheduling mix to warrant making such significant capital and personnel investments.

Imaging center financial risk can be lofty regardless of the model. Many groups have tied their financial success to the success of their imaging center and have created shared revenue streams. Shared revenue streams can be useful as groups move toward joint ventures and can incent the appropriate behaviors for facility growth. As a part of a shared imaging or ancillary service venture, physicians in a group might have to give personal guarantees on loans used to finance the project, meaning their personal wealth would be jeopardized if the center or facility fails.

Medical imaging covers a broad cross-section of diagnostic procedures. MRIs, CT scans, PET scans, mammography exams, ultrasounds, radiology, and bone density screenings are just some of the diagnostic services offered by leading, independent medical groups and imaging clinics.

Potential legal concerns for physician development of imaging centers is important as physicians should be aware of the federal Stark law, which prohibits physicians from referring Medicare and Medicaid patients to entities in which they have a financial interest. Although the current Stark ruling includes an in-office ancillary services exception that allows referring physicians to open imaging centers under certain conditions, urology groups should be mindful of how they set up their group dynamics and coordinate scheduling, billing, and care. The in-office exception is only available for group practices, so physicians who cannot meet that criterion could run afoul of Stark. Current efforts for Stark reform focus on the changing dynamic of payment models, acknowledging that controlling the costs and scope of ancillary services, like imaging, are hindered when physicians or groups are not allowed to manage those services themselves.

Other laws, including the federal anti-kickback statute and state certificate-of-need laws, also should be weighed by physicians who are planning a diagnostic imaging center. With a well-structured business plan and the proper legal advice, urology group centers can easily launch in a legally sound way. Many groups have worked in conjunction with bodies or associations to reach appropriate certification standards rather than running the risk of being outside of certification and/or legal bounds.

As mentioned, the capital required to start a diagnostic imaging center can be substantial. A small operation could cost anywhere between $500,000 to $1 million to build and equip while a large one could cost $5 million to $8 million. Depending on the urology groups' goals and desires, there may be a unique opportunity to keep costs down while continuing to drive revenue forward. Certifications and other fees (consulting, overhead, construction costs) should be worked into the overall proforma for the facility plan and should be reviewed as a part of a consistent timeline for launch.

IMAGING MODALITY OPPORTUNITIES IN UROLOGY

As with all aspects of urologic medicine, the options and indications for imaging, as well as the complexity, continue to expand. Use of advanced imaging can be included in the evaluation and management of many benign and malignant genitourinary conditions, and this may present opportunity for incorporation into an integrated urology practice. Examples of imaging modalities that are commonly used in urologic practice include:

▶ ***Plain Film/Fluoroscopy:*** X-ray imaging is commonly used in different stages of kidney stone care for treatment planning prior to ESWL, verification of stent placement, and monitoring of treatment results. Fluoroscopy, either through integrated cystoscopy tables or C-arm, has a wide variety of use within urology. It is integral to the performance of endoscopic procedures such as ureteroscopy, but also can be used to verify instillations of medications into the upper tract. Fluoroscopy capabilities also can be used to augment functional studies of the bladder and allow video urodynamics for better analysis of complex pelvic floor and voiding dysfunction. With the widespread availability of digital imaging, fluoroscopy can often be used to obtain plain films. Because these modalities require radiation, appropriate safety and monitoring protocols need to be established, as mandated by state agencies. Typically, this will require radiation badges, standard operating procedures, and possibly a formal radiation safety officer.

▶ ***Ultrasound:*** Ultrasound imaging has become integral to urologic care, to the point that it can be seen as an extension of good GU workup in many cases. Hematuria workups, monitoring of small renal masses, evaluation and monitoring of voiding dysfunction, and evaluation of kidney stones and flank pain are some of the most common diagnoses seen in a typical urology practice. Furthermore, the use of trans-rectal ultrasound for prostate biopsy and workup of BPH has made this technology essential for a high volume of urologic procedures. Ultrasound services can be executed in many different ways, including physicians performing scans themselves, full integration of ultrasound technicians to work alongside the physician or separate machines for use in the office setting and procedure areas/ASC.

▶ **CT Scan:** CT imaging is often a critical piece in evaluation of a number of urologic conditions, including GU malignancies, kidney stone disease, and hematuria workup in higher risk patients. This modality adds the additional option of including contrast enhancement, which can help in diagnostic yield for certain conditions. While non-contrast scans can be very helpful in the assessment of urolithiasis, most other indications within urology benefit from the addition of intravenous contrast. The use of contrast requires a physician to be on-site and immediately available due to the possibility of an allergic response. In addition, while most urologists feel comfortable evaluating components of the GU system, it is advisable to have radiologist overreads for most CT scans as there may be findings outside the typical focus of urology. The technology for CT scans has continued to evolve, but most GU indications can be evaluated with a 16-slice scanner (as opposed to more expensive 64 slice or higher scanners). As with plain imaging and fluoroscopy, this modality uses radiation and requires appropriate safety and monitoring protocols.

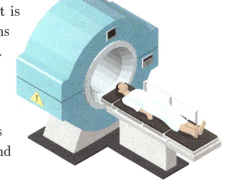

▶ **MRI:** The use of MRI has rapidly expanded in urology due to increased utility in evaluating patients for prostate cancer. The use of multi-parametric MRI has become a key component to the workup of many patients with a history of an elevated PSA and for many men choosing active surveillance for prostate cancer. It also has uses for staging of GU malignancies as well as for evaluation of complex renal cysts, pelvic floor abnormalities, and pain evaluations. While there is the potential for significant improvement in quality control and specialization by establishing MRI services within a urology practice, there is also a significant expense and a need for radiology overreads.

▶ **MRI/US Fusion:** While not specifically an imaging modality, the increased use of MRI in evaluating patients before a prostate biopsy has been accompanied by the development of technology to allow MRI findings to be incorporated into an ultrasound-guided biopsy. These MRI/US fusion technologies have seen rapid adoption within urologic practice. How to structure provision of these services requires an understanding of the potential costs and benefits of the procedure. The only additional billable service in this workflow is additional mapping and segmentation of the radiology images to incorporate targets and prepare the information for integration with the biopsy platform. The biopsy itself is billed just as with any ultrasound-guided biopsy. There is also often additional software required for either or both the radiology and urology facility to facilitate this process. Many third parties provide case or daily rates to rent the necessary equipment, or a group could purchase their own. Regardless of the mechanism, these procedures often require organization to optimize use of the equipment and to develop a core group of urologists comfortable with the techniques.

Considerations for how to incorporate this service may include the volume of patients needing this approach, the potential increase in treatments if cancers are found in earlier stages, and the potential to lose patients to other practices if the service is not provided.

▶ **PET Scan:** Positron Emission Tomography (PET) is typically paired with CT scan to evaluate for evidence of metastatic cancer. Specific radioactive tracers are injected into the patient that concentrate in areas of metastases. While not traditionally a very frequently used modality in the evaluation of GU malignancies, there have been a series of advances and promising developments that utilize this technology. Traditional FDG-PET scans can be used for evaluation of certain bladder and testicular cancer patients, and the NaFl PET scan appears to deliver information superior to bone scan for identification of metastatic disease, but this is not currently widely available commercially. The renewed interest within urologic oncology surrounds the use of PET imaging technology with newer tracers, including fluciclovine F-18 (Axumin®), and PSMA (prostate-specific membrane antigen) ligands. These have shown ability to identify sites of metastatic prostate cancer at lower PSAs than traditional imaging, providing more accurate staging but also the possibility of improved success for salvage therapies. Increasing options and indications will likely increase the number of these procedures being done, and developments including tracers for renal cell carcinoma, pairing with MRI, and fusion may expand the use in urology further in the coming years.

IN-OFFICE IMAGING VS. A TRUE IMAGING CENTER:

There is a difference between in-office imaging and an imaging center. In-office imaging defines the integration of imaging into an existing urology group as defined by the in-office exception under Stark.

In-office imaging defines the integration of imaging into an existing urology group as defined by the in-office exception under Stark. Imaging modalities that fall underneath this consideration include the following services:

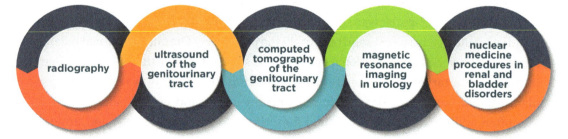

An imaging center on the other hand is a free-standing medical facility that provides medical imaging for routine and diagnostic imaging. The types of imaging that may be done in an imaging center may include x-ray, ultrasound, MRI, CT scan, nuclear imaging, PET scan, and other imaging services.

Though hospitals may also have their own imaging facilities, many medical imaging centers are in a free-standing building and are independent of hospital facilities. Satellite hospitals, or smaller scale acute care facilities, may also be equipped with a medical imaging department or imaging facility. Typically, only hospitals and acute care facilities are equipped with the ability to perform all types of imaging. A smaller medical imaging center will typically specialize in a specific type of imaging or in specific diagnostic care.

For practices that choose to bring imaging in-house, an additional concern needs to be addressed regarding formal diagnostic reads by a radiologist. Some modalities, such as plain-film or ultrasound, may be focused enough on a specific location to allow a well-trained urologist to make a full diagnostic read. However, more advanced imaging, such as CT, MRI, and PET scans may allow a urologist to do a focused analysis for a specific GU pathology, but the images should be evaluated for further pathology in other organ systems. Many radiology groups provide off-site "overreads" for this situation. When setting up this kind of arrangement, typically the radiologist will bill for the professional services, while the urology group would receive technical fees. With enough volume, a urology group could seek a part or full-time employment arrangement with a radiologist or group.

Choosing one or more radiologists to work with in this model provides an opportunity to develop and partner with radiologists focused on GU imaging. Effort should be made to partner with a specific individual or small subset of trusted radiologist(s) as opposed to a general pool so as to decrease variability. Especially with advanced imaging modalities like MRI and PET, a collaborative arrangement can ensure reliability of the reads and elevate care for the patient.

CHECK CONTRACTS, COMPETITION

Urologists should research potential contracts with payers before starting any kind of imaging center or diagnostic ancillary service facility. Payers scrutinize these types of facilities because they are concerned about the potential for abuse by referring physicians. Urologists can get ahead of any potential problems by vetting their respective geographic payor contracts prior to beginning any serious conversations about construction costs or build.

Imaging center politics could also create tension with a physician group's relationship with a local hospital by creating competition between the two. Urology groups would be wise to vet any potential issues with their hospital and/or imaging center colleagues prior to embarking on any imaging or diagnostic ancillary endeavor.

The following are considerations urology groups should take in determining their geographic market assessment while laying the foundation of a diagnostic imaging business plan.

UROLOGY GROUP DIAGNOSTIC IMAGING MARKET ASSESSMENT:

1 Is there an imaging market opportunity?

2 How do we know this opportunity exists?

3 What must be done to capture the opportunity in our respective geography or group?

- Identify diagnostic imaging service area and expertise
- Demographic analysis
- Competitive analysis
- Modality use rate analysis
- Conduct physician and physician office staff interviews
- Conduct employee interviews
- Financial opportunity analysis
- Identify the lowest physician utilization of imaging services due to lacking technology and inefficiencies in operations
- Increase market share via marketing and improved operational processes
- Determine if there is an opportunity to create a multi-modality free standing facility outside of the hospital

The following is a summary of some action items a urology groups should put into place as a part of their proforma and market research planning:

▶ Utilization

- Improve operational processes
- Increase equipment availability
- Upgrade equipment
- Introduce new diagnostic/treatment options
- Improve customer service

PREPARING AND APPLYING FOR ACCREDITATION:

When building or acquiring diagnostic imaging equipment or a center, The Joint Commission (TJC) is designated by the Centers for Medicare and Medicaid Services (CMS) as an approved accreditor for modalities including CT, MRI, PET, and Nuclear Medicine Services.

As a urology group, the technical component (TC) of advanced diagnostic imaging services requires that you become accredited to receive Medicare Part B Payments under the physician fee schedule.

Providers of MRI, CT, PET, and nuclear medicine imaging services are required to follow standards from TJC's Comprehensive Accreditation manual for Ambulatory Health Care (CAMAC), which includes the following attributes: Qualifications of medical personnel and medical directors, quality assurance, and quality control programs to ensure the safety, reliability, clarity, and accuracy of diagnostic imaging.

As a diagnostic imaging center or urology group with imaging services, the following information and documentation should be a part of the accreditation process:

- Performance/Quality Improvement Data
- Infection Prevention & Control surveillance data
- Infection Control - Plan
- Analysis of a high-risk process
- Environment of Care data, including Statement of Conditions (SOC), if applicable
- Access to computer for surveyor 'sign-off,' regarding current Environment of Care and any Plans for Improvement, if applicable
- Environment of Care management plans and annual evaluations
- Environment of Care team meeting minutes
- Organization chart
- Map of the organization, if available
- List of all sites eligible for survey
- List of locations where services are provided, including anesthetizing locations
- Reports or lists of patient appointment schedules
- List of contracted services
- Name and extension of key contacts who can assist surveyors in planning tracer selection

MARKET SHARE

- Increase imaging marketing efforts
- Develop a marketing plan and new marketing materials for secondary service area referring physicians
- Investigate pre-certification services through diagnostic imaging associations and governing bodies

One of the most difficult decisions for a new urology group imaging center is the selection of equipment. Traditionally, most purchasers of equipment will utilize past relationships with vendors, and therefore, physicians may not understand the details of all contractual expectations. Purchasers also may not comprehend all the options that are available by modality. The equipment criteria selection process for this project utilizes a team approach of including radiology technologists, managers, directors, administrators, and consultant expertise.

Equipment vendor presentation meetings should be scheduled and site visits to similar facilities should be planned based on initial presentations. For the site visits, it may be useful for urology group leaders to create specific criteria in a scoring grid for what made the most sense to satisfy partnership, technology, service, and cost.

A strategic timeline for the imaging center facility should be quantified in order to solidify the overall opportunity, cost considerations, and overall start-to-build timeframe. Weekly and monthly tasks should be broken down into specific steps, so errors and challenges can be kept to a minimum.

Group leadership should identify respective leaders and a project management team to be tasked with specific roles and responsibilities as the diagnostic imaging center unfolds. Project managers should calendar their decision-making meetings and be in continued communication as their respective project delivery unfolds. The more succinct and specific timelines and consistent messaging a group can create, the better the overall outcome and process for staying on task for both short-and long-term successes.

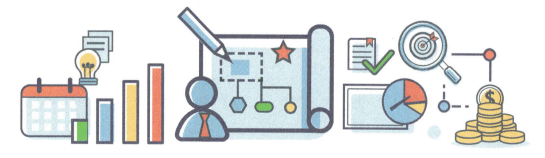

SAMPLE UROLOGY GROUP IMAGING CENTER TIMELINE AND SCHEDULE:

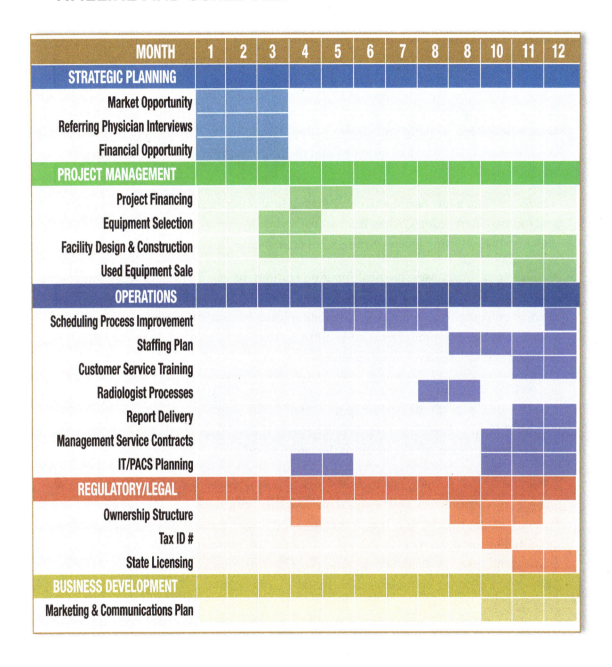

Selecting the Design and Project Management Team

When selecting an architect, designer, and contractor, a urology diagnostic imaging center should look for professionals who have worked on prior imaging projects. Different modalities have unique needs, such as magnetic and radiation shielding, cryogenics, plumbing, cooling, electrical, lighting, and insulation requirements that are vastly different from other medical installations.

A urology group should never accept a boilerplate, or standard contract from the contractor, architect, or designer. A specific line item to include in all contracts is that a bid is considered final when accepted and that any change orders will be at the cost of the bid recipient.

There are quite a few barriers to entry for medical imaging startups, including capital and industry connections. When it comes to capital requirements, urology groups should consider the following when working to open a diagnostic imaging center.

▶ *Investors.* Diagnostic medical imaging equipment can be pricey. Single imaging devices routinely can cost in excess of $1 million. To secure adequate startup capital, startup entrepreneurs often need the help of strategic investors who are knowledge about medical entrepreneurism and willing to financially participate in the launch of a urology group's medical imaging endeavor.

▶ *Leasing.* Medical equipment leasing can substantially lower the upfront cost of launching a for-profit medical imaging center. In the long run, you will pay more than you would in purchase financing. But the upside is that leasing makes it easier to turnover your equipment and upgrade to the latest models.

▶ *Partnerships.* In many instances, urologists or urology groups can form partnerships in order to distribute risk and financial burden. Urology groups should carefully proceed by researching partnership business structures before making any commitments to potential business partners or to their own respective group members. It is essential to understand how the structure of these partnerships may impact the ability to show value in the evolving world of health care payment reform.

CONCLUSIONS

Like many creative efforts undertaken by integrated specialty groups, the idea of starting an imaging center can seem daunting and risky. However, as payment models change, even Stark restrictions are being reconsidered and likely to be reformed. The ability to perform state-of-the-art, specialty-specific advanced imaging will likely be an essential component for the groups trying to achieve both overall cost-control and quality care management.

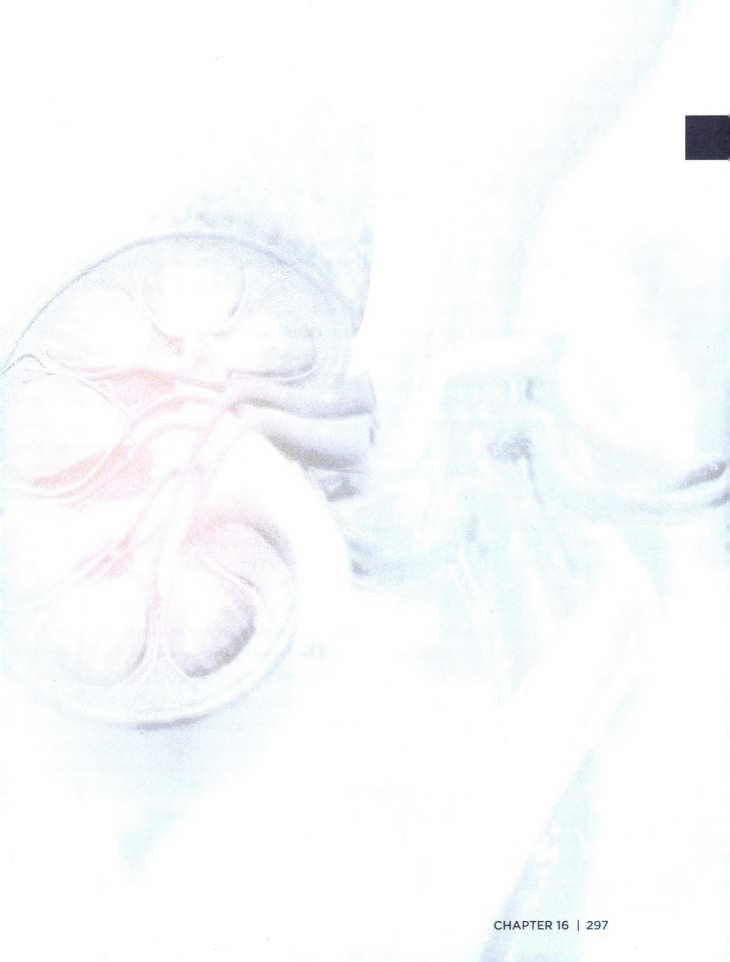

KEY POINTS

- **The shift to value-based payments** creates an opportunity to focus on quality and cost control by keeping imaging services in-house.

- **Incorporating imaging into the services of a practice** not only has the potential to add revenue, it has the potential to meet goals of health care reform.

- **Some imaging centers and ancillary center builds** have risen into millions of dollars in overhead and buildout.

- **Urologists may choose to share the financial risks of opening an imaging center** with another entity such as a hospital, an imaging center, or a multi-specialty group.

- **Group leadership should identify respective leaders and a project management team** to be tasked with specific roles and responsibilities as the diagnostic imaging center unfolds.

- **When selecting an architect, designer, and contractor,** a urology diagnostic imaging center should look for professionals who have worked on prior imaging projects.

- **Medical equipment leasing** can substantially lower the upfront cost of launching a for-profit medical imaging center.

- **Physicians should be aware of the federal Stark law,** which prohibits physicians from referring Medicare and Medicaid patients to entities in which they have a financial interest.

- **For many modalities, arrangements will need to be made for formal read to be performed by radiologists**

- **Providers of MRI, CT, PET, and Nuclear Medicine Imaging Services** are required to follow standards from The Joint Commission's Comprehensive Accreditation manual for Ambulatory Health Care.

- **Certifications and other fees** (consulting, overhead, construction costs) should be worked into the overall proforma for the facility plan and should be reviewed as a part of a consistent timeline for launch.

ABOUT THE AUTHOR

Benjamin Lowentritt, MD, FACS

Benjamin Lowentritt, MD, is the Medical Director of the Prostate Program at Chesapeake Urology Associates. In this role, he has led the development of programs for patient education, advanced prostate cancer management, bone health, MRI/US fusion, and active surveillance. He is also the Director of Robotics and Advanced Laparoscopy. He is a graduate of Harvard College and Baylor College of Medicine, completed his Urology Residency at the University of Maryland and a fellowship in Robotics, Laparoscopy and Endourology at Tulane University.

CHAPTER

Establishing a Urology-Specific Laboratory

Nicholas A. Maruniak, MD
Candy M. H. Willets, MT (AAB)
E. Scot Davis, BA, MPA, MBA, CMPE
Adam J. Cole, MD
Stephanie Evans, BS, MT

Orchestrating the setup of a laboratory can be a challenge. Using a guide developed by the Clinical Laboratory Standards Institute (CLSI), as a reference can help. The *Quality Management System: A Model for Laboratory Services* guideline provides a plan and systematic approach to organizing start up, maintaining quality, and continued improvement of laboratory processes and services.

12 Quality System Essentials to Establish a Successful Laboratory

A Quality Management System (QMS) uses twelve quality system essentials (QSE) that outline the framework necessary for establishing a successful laboratory:

1. Organization
2. Personnel Equipment
3. Documents and Records
4. Information Management
5. Personnel
6. Equipment
7. Purchasing and Inventory
8. Process Management
9. Event Management
10. Assessments
11. Client Services
12. Process Improvement

This chapter describes each aspect of a Quality Management System necessary to establish a successful lab. It explains how to execute each step by implementing scalable tasks either through manual or automated methods that are dependent on the size of the practice's laboratory—and are geared specifically to an individual urology group.

Key Questions to Consider

Before setting up, expanding, or improving a lab, the practice should develop an ad hoc committee or assign a key physician to work with the administrative team/lab director to address the following questions:

- What is the margin of income the practice earns from its lab services?

- Does the practice routinely look at additional tests that could be brought in-office to increase the margin?

- Has the practice reviewed its existing payer contracts to potentially negotiate higher lab rates?

- Does the practice have the latest equipment to maximize the number and variety of tests that can be performed?

- Is the clinical staff adequately trained on the latest equipment and procedures to ensure the highest output of the lab?

- Does the practice have a lab manager who understands Clinical Laboratory Improvement Amendments (CLIA) regulations and maintains good policies and procedures to avoid any licensing entanglements?

- Has the practice engaged in any discussions with a third-party lab service to determine the feasibility/profitability of outsourcing its lab?

- If so, are the providers agreeable to giving up control of its lab samples to a third-party?

- Does your state allow for client billing arrangements for commercial insurance?

- If so, has your practice reviewed these regulations with legal counsel to determine your practice is compliant with insurance contracts?

Establishing a Quality Assurance Program

The starting point for organizing and detailing all processes in the laboratory and the beginning of establishing a Quality Assurance Program is to purchase a three-inch, three-ring binder with 12 indexes corresponding to the 12 quality system essentials. Each section must include the policies, procedures, and forms that specifically relate to the practice. Most references for these sections are taken from regulations and guidelines set forth in the CLIA 1988 laws and regulations, specific state governing agencies, and chosen accrediting agencies. This binder will serve as a compass in all decisions and tasks necessary for operation.

BASIC COMPONENTS

▶ Organization

Designing an organizational chart for members involved in the laboratory is critical to the lab's support and success. This organization section should be written in parallel with the personnel section. The organizational chart will identify key players within the organization and define roles and responsibilities for the team needed to staff the laboratory.

▶ Personnel

Hiring qualified, licensed personnel with experience is the optimal choice. However, under the CLIA guidelines and specific state requirements, staffing a physician-operated laboratory may not require licensed personnel. These decisions could depend upon the level of complexity of the test menu. Job descriptions specify the work processes and tasks authorized for persons with a specific job title. It is required that employees who make professional judgments regarding diagnostic testing or interpretations possess

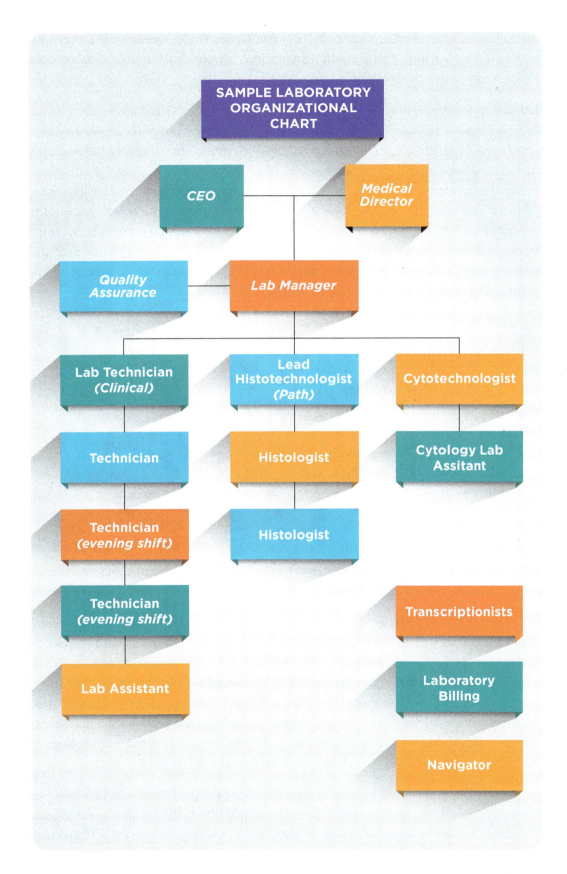

the theoretical and practical educational background and work experience, in accordance with federal, state, and local accrediting agencies. Any physical requirements, such as, lifting heavy reagents, should also be noted.

Laboratory positions may require that staff can pass a color-blind assessment. If the practice houses both a clinical and pathology laboratory, the pathologist may also serve as medical director, technical consultant, and clinical consultant. Other positions within the laboratory include phlebotomists, laboratory assistants, grossing technicians, medical laboratory technicians, medical laboratory technologists, histotechnicians, histotechnologists, cytotechnologists, laboratory manager, and possibly a quality assurance consultant. Initial training and six-month and annual competencies must be documented for each position in the lab. In the case of laboratory technicians and technologists, it is useful to have a training/competency form for each piece of equipment or instrumentation staff will be using.

▶ Facilities and Safety

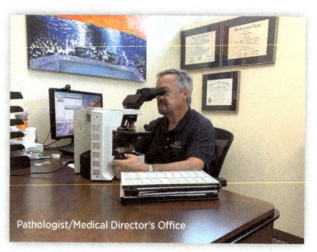
Pathologist/Medical Director's Office

When planning and designing the floor plan, it is important to understand the use of Lean design principles for routing the flow of specimens through processes to eliminate wasted steps and time. Creating flow charts and spaghetti diagrams aid in visualizing the path a specimen takes from accessioning to archival. One must take into consideration the amount of space needed for instrumentation, work benches, flame resistant cabinets, reagent and specimen storage, waste closets, and the ergonomic accommodation of personnel.

Consideration should be given to the placement of the microbiology and histology departments, as well as the chemical and biohazardous waste areas with respect to patient care areas. These departments are odorous. The space needed to accommodate a full-service clinical and anatomic pathology laboratory depends on instrumentation, specimen volume, and number of employees. Off-site climate-controlled storage may be necessary for 10 years of archived blocks and slides if these cannot be housed on location. If the lab is limited to clinical and pathology services without microbiology, it may be able to operate only five days a week on a single shift.

The safety manual should have a written Exposure Control Plan that includes the Occupational Safety and Health Administration (OSHA) Blood-borne Pathogens Standard. A material safety datasheet (MSDS) and/or a safety data sheet (SDS) manual containing information on all reagents used in the practice is a requirement. Other safety policies and procedures include, but are not limited to: a Disaster Plan, Tuberculosis Exposure Plan, Ergonomics and Noise Assessment Plan, and Bioterrorism Plan. All staff should have annual documented safety training.

▶ Employee Safety and Health

It is recommended that all laboratory employees undergo a pre-employment drug screening and baseline testing for Hepatitis B and HIV. Employees should have copies of their current immunizations on file. If the employee cannot show proof of Hepatitis B vaccination, it is the responsibility of the employer to provide the vaccination free of charge. If the employee recalls having the vaccination series, a positive titer is sufficient.

In the event of a post-exposure or accidental needle stick, documentation must be thorough and coordinated through a Workers' Compensation approved provider. Post-exposure testing should be performed on the employee and the source patient if available. Optional post-exposure prophylaxis should be offered to the employee. If it is not offered onsite, it is necessary to partner with a local facility that offers the treatment. It is important to have these policies, procedures, and contacts in place prior to an occurrence since the window for treatment is within 72 hours.

▶ Hazardous and Non-Hazardous Waste

There are multiple types of waste in the laboratory that need to be sorted and discarded accordingly: The most obvious is ***routine trash*** that can be removed by standard means.

Secured waste is required for discarding documentation containing patient information. Services are available to properly shred and discard any protected health information in compliance with federal and state regulations.

Depending on the amount of testing performed, there will be a fair amount of ***biohazardous waste*** that requires an annual biohazardous waste permit, special red bags, boxes, sharps containers, and a scheduled waste removal service. Most companies charge by the pound for incinerating biohazardous waste and by the number of scheduled pickups. If the lab performs a high volume of microbiology testing, the amount of biohazardous waste generated while plating sensitivities by manual methods will be greater than if the lab were to perform microbiology by automated methods.

Chemical waste is a large byproduct of the pathology laboratory. Fifty-five-gallon drums are needed for the safe disposal of chemicals used during the fixation, processing, and staining processes. Adequate space or a specific "waste" closet or room is necessary to house full drums, boxes, and bags awaiting removal. These are to be kept in a sanitary and safe fashion away from the eyes of patients and other clinic guests.

DOCUMENTS AND RECORDS

▶ Quality Management System

The Quality Management System (QMS), compiled in the binder and easily accessible on the practice's internal website, is the set of documents and records for the laboratory. It defines the standardization of document formats for policies, procedures, and forms and describes the process for the creation, approval, archival, and destruction of documents and specimens.

> **For example:**
> - Paper requisitions are to be kept for two years and then securely shredded
> - Quality control records are kept for two years
> - Tissue blocks and microscopic slides are retained for 10 years
> - Records retained electronically are stored indefinitely.

This information should be readily available in the QMS and verified against accrediting agency regulations on a regular basis. Hardcopy versions of policies and procedures should be stored in binders, with a master copy on a thumb or external hard drive. An electronic document control system is an excellent solution for inspection readiness, compliance education, and meeting continuing education requirements. It ensures that staff members have immediate access to current procedures and forms to perform their work; that revisions of the procedures and forms are automatically tracked when changes are made for compliance and archival purposes; that annual employee sign off is documented on procedures for competency documentation; that date/time stamps are provided for the required final approval by the medical director before a procedure or form can be put into use.

▶ Procedure Manuals

Procedure manuals are paramount in standardizing processes. Technical procedures should follow the CLSI guidelines for correct procedure format. This format is easy to follow, with clearly identifiable sections and headings to locate information quickly.

Each department should have its own manual detailing step-by-step directions listing each reagent, calibrator, quality control material, and other supplies used in a testing process. The manual should include other valuable information related to testing, including, but not limited to: specimen collection and required volume, rejection criteria, stability, interfering substances, acceptable ranges, critical values, and any additional pertinent information.

▶ Calibrations and Quality Control Binders

Calibration and quality control schedules are dictated by the volumes, equipment and shifts in the laboratory. Chemistry analyzers generally need Quality Control (QC) performed every eight hours if the lab operates three eight-hour shifts. Most analytes require weekly or monthly calibration. Electrolytes are calibrated every eight-hour shift and require the running of QC every shift.

For special low volume immunochemistry tests, like Estradiol, it is more cost effective to batch weekly or monthly as opposed to running every shift for one or two specimens.

Most Laboratory Information Systems (LIS) maintain quality control information for the clinical laboratory; however, in addition to LIS, it is recommended to also retain hardcopy verification of these system checks.

The easiest way to maintain calibration and quality control information is to use a binder system. For each instrument in the clinical lab, it is best to use four three-inch, three-ring binders to separate the year quarterly and then by monthly dividers. All instrumentation calibrations and QC printouts should be filed in reverse of chronological order by month.

Other monthly records that need to be maintained are temperature logs for freezers, refrigerators, and ambient temperature and humidity charts, incubator temperatures, quarterly and monthly maintenance logs, specimen rejection logs, specimen referral logs, reagent logs, corrective action logs, and communication logs, to name a few.

The pathology equipment calibration and QC logs can be housed in one large binder separated by dividers for each piece of equipment. When the inspection window nears, laboratory staff will have all documentation organized and ready for review.

INFORMATION MANAGEMENT

▶ Laboratory Information Systems and Electronic Health Record Integration

When considering a Laboratory Information System (LIS) to support the laboratory infrastructure, one must bear in mind that a singular platform that can support clinical, microbiology, pathology, and molecular pathology is the optimum choice. It is important to inquire about the level of support that is provided when purchasing software. It is also helpful to know the cost of interfacing with each workstation, label printer, electronic health record (EHR), and reference laboratory, and the annual maintenance costs involved. To interface individual laboratory platforms, various EHRs, and reference laboratories can be a challenging and time-consuming endeavor that requires a skilled and experienced information technology team. A deliberate initial investment could avoid a lot of back end work.

The practice's EHR will also dictate whether lab staff can receive orders electronically in the LI.S. With the advent of meaningful use, all laboratory orders and results should flow electronically. Some practices are still manually hand ordering tests from paper requisitions; however, a bi-directional interface between the LIS and EHR will reduce data entry time and clerical errors.

The laboratory should be able to accommodate both ways of ordering tests. Hardware and software validation should be performed and documented after installation. It is extremely important to have not just one, but several backup drives, with frequently scheduled backup times to prevent any data loss. This cannot be stressed enough. It would also be beneficial to have all equipment on adequate backup power supplies to prepare for power outages. A battery backup should have the capacity for a 45-minute run time to complete any batch, so work is not lost.

Procedures need to be put in place to add new users and limit access and functions. It is not recommended to use a single log-in credential for an entire group of people: e.g., clinical lab. Every user should be individual, identifiable, and traceable. Compliance with the Health Insurance Portability and Accountability Act is mandatory in the laboratory, and each user should maintain patient privacy and confidentiality and have a signed agreement of compliance filed.

Procedures should be in place for requests for patient information, cancer reporting, and requests for patient material. There also needs to be annual documentation proving that formulas, whether produced in the instruments' software or via the LIS, are calculating results correctly. LIS downtime procedures and manual reporting forms will also be of benefit in the case of planned software upgrades or unscheduled emergencies or service outages.

▶ Practice Management and Billing Software

There are many choices when it comes to practice management and billing software suites. These can be installed separately or built together. It is helpful to investigate each solution thoroughly for its user friendliness; ease of patient check-in; scanning capabilities for identifications and insurance cards; insurance plan libraries; appointment setting and cancellation functions; qualified diagnosis codes to Current Procedural Terminology® code matching; ease of generating reports; inputting multiple fee schedules; submitting claims; and processing refunds.

▶ Meeting Medicare Requirements for Pathology

To be considered a group practice and bill for pathology and clinical laboratory services, the group must bill for those services under a single tax ID number. The pathologist must be contracted to be a member of the group for at least a one-year term. The pathologist must be licensed to practice medicine in each state where patient specimens are taken.

The following applies only to billing pathology services for Medicare patients. To bill globally for the professional component of the pathologist's services (reading of the slides), the pathologist must perform his or her readings in the location where the clinicians see patients, unless 75% of the pathologist's services are dedicated to the group practice. This becomes important if the pathologist is NOT a full-time employee of the group, and the group has satellite offices. If the pathologist provides more than 75% of his or her services to the group, the group can bill globally, regardless of where the patient specimens were collected.

If the pathologist is an independent contractor and works for multiple groups and doesn't provide 75% or more of his or her services to the group, only the offices where the pathologist reads slides onsite can bill Medicare globally for patients seen by clinicians who provide the full range of their services in that office. If the group has multiple satellite offices, patient specimens collected in those locations can be processed in the central pathology lab and read by the pathologist in the central lab; however, the group can only bill for the technical component. The pathologist must bill for his or her professional component separately. In this case, the group can act as the billing agent for the pathologist and charge him or her a fair market value billing fee.

▶ Process Management

Process Management is initiated by documenting the processes in the laboratory's path of workflow. Opportunities for improvement can be identified by developing process flowcharts and analyzing every step of specimen testing, from receipt to result. Through understanding and controlling the processes, management becomes more effective in meeting the requirements and more efficient in the use of human and other costly resources. Standardizing procedures and processes are important to the seamless operation of the laboratory and needs to be examined on a continuous basis.

▶ Event Management (Incident Reports)

The purpose of event management is to identify any occurrence that is nonconforming to the routine pattern of business and medicine and to recognize systematic problems to gain management's commitment to removing the cause. These include all occasions of verbal or written customer complaints, nonconforming quality control or reagents, product recalls, mistakes or problems in work operations, Information Technology (IT) breaks, and/or issues with report delivery.

Internal Quality Training forms are used when a documented error needs to be brought to the attention of the offender or management and does not necessarily result in a progressive discipline counseling form. These are used to quantify repetitive errors within some system, process, or personnel.

IT Systems Failure Reports quantify and identify failures within the network, ranging from practice management software, the laboratory information systems, and multitude of EHRs that may be connected to the IT infrastructure. These could be any breaks in hardware, software, or middleware connections that are not syncing properly.

Any work-related injuries, near misses, or medical device related deaths need to be documented in the laboratory's event management system and must be reported to the appropriate agency—for example, the Food and Drug Administration—in accordance with the facility's policies.

Common events in the pathology department are situations where "missing" tissue is documented as a QA incident. For example, a 12-core prostate biopsy kit may have been received in the laboratory with only 10 cores in vials. The two omitted cores are considered missing, documented, and a courtesy call is placed to the provider for confirmation. More often than not, the specimen was not taken at biopsy.

Checklists for missing specimens at embedding, microtomy, and missing block and slide documentation are necessary to trace specimens at each phase of processing within the department if a misplacement is discovered.

PURCHASING AND INVENTORY

When shopping for equipment, it is wise to compare at least three brands, makes, and/or models. It is necessary to consider the footprint of the equipment, the square footage of laboratory space available, and whether the unit is a countertop or floor model.

> **Other concerns to address:**
> - Will the equipment use distilled water in cube form or require an installed water unit?
> - What are the electrical and LIS interface wiring requirements and ventilation, temperature, and humidity needs?
> - Will the equipment fit through the exterior and interior doorways for installation?

Other necessary purchases include reagents, calibrators, quality control materials, and any other consumable materials necessary to perform the job functions. It is always helpful to compare prices with several vendors and to have a secondary vendor in the case of shortages or back orders. Vendor pricing contracts should be reviewed on a yearly basis as vendors will raise the cost of supplies without notification.

Minimum levels must be created for all consumables to ensure that an adequate supply is always available. Reagent expirations need to be closely monitored, and stock must be continuously rotated to the front to eliminate waste. Availability of dependable and reliable test kits and supplies is essential to the seamless operation of the laboratory.

A document or binder should detail which vendors have been selected to provide reagents and supplies; how they are distributed, managed, and reordered; associated costs; and contract renewals, if applicable.

Opting for an electronic ordering system for materials management, in lieu of a traditional inventory checklist and a label gun to mark receivables, could be ideal when there are multiple locations to stock. There is an advantage to standardizing items purchased at higher volumes for negotiating pricing with suppliers. With high-tech ordering systems, the use of handheld barcode scanners can reduce time counting inventory and checking in items.

▶ Equipment

Equipment decisions for the laboratory are dictated by the test menu offered and by considering the current or anticipated volumes. Cost effectiveness of running tests in-office versus sending them out to a reference laboratory is a major consideration.

A cradle-to-grave process for the acquisition of equipment must be developed. Master binders for clinical laboratory and pathology laboratory equipment can be created to track the history from request to decommission. Each piece of equipment has its own section with an equipment record that lists its name, manufacturer's name, model number, serial number, inventory tag ID number, purchase price, service agreement details, date of receipt, date of entry into service, decommission date, final disposition, and a section for additional comments.

Any service or repair, maintenance, and calibration records that need to be maintained for the life of the instrument should be kept in this section.

▶ Histology

In a low-volume pathology laboratory, it is customary to accession cases into a ledger book and handwrite biopsy cassettes and slides. As the volume grows, other solutions like preprinted labels or cassette and slide printers that will save time and increase patient safety are available.

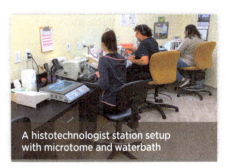
A histotechnologist station setup with microtome and waterbath

A stationary area under a fume hood is required when grossing specimens. Annual air quality tests should be performed and documented to determine the potential for employee exposure to formaldehyde, xylene, ethanol, and other hazardous reagents.

Grossing techs must have at least the equivalent of a two-year science degree to qualify for performing this task. It is prudent to hire a grossing tech/lab assistant to gross as opposed to paying histotechnologists to perform this duty when their time is most valuable processing and sectioning tissue.

Tissue processing can take place in a variety of rapid tissue processors offering standardized and customizable processing protocols. Instrumentation is available for processing smaller batches from 72 to 600 blocks a run. Some instrumentation can be programmed to process overnight and will not need manual reagent changes. A single embedding station is sufficient for smaller volumes; however, a secondary embedding station will serve as back up, additional support, and can reduce the delay between embedding and sectioning. A reserve paraffin wax melter is handy when refilling the embedding station(s) and eliminates the wait time for wax chips to melt.

A broader view of two additional histotechnologists stations, the slide and cassette printers, autostainer (under a hood), and two microwave tissue processors.

Automated Stainers and cover slipping equipment.

Histotechnologists' work areas will require a minimum of 40" x 24" of counter-top space to arrange a microtome, water bath, block rack, and ample drawer space for various tools and accessories, such as, brushes, extra blades, and slides. A single-drying oven shared between the histology and cytology departments will suffice if there is not room or capital available to purchase two.

Manual stain lines and cover slipping by hand are acceptable with lower volumes; however, with increasing caseloads, automated stain lines and cover slipping equipment would improve turnaround times and standardize staining processes for both histology and cytology specimens. The same applies when performing special stains and Immunohistochemistry (IHC) stains.

▶ Urine Cytology/Fluorescence in Situ Hybridization

The cytotechnologist should have a workspace that could double as a cyto-prep area with ample workspace to process specimens. Required equipment includes:

- One to two centrifuges for spinning the 60ml conical tubes
- A manual stain line under a hood
- A dark room to house a fluorecent microscope with camera attachment for scanning Urine Cytology/ Fluorescence in Situ Hybridization (FISH) slides
- A bright field microscope for scanning cytology slides, and a computer workstation
- A - 20° C freezer for reagent probe and slide storage stability near the workstation

The cytology methodology can be accomplished by the manual filter method or cytospin automated thin prep method. FISH can be performed utilizing Abbott's (UroVysion) or the Cellay method. Automated FISH readers, such as Abbott's BioView platform, allow for walk away scanning and imaging solutions for volumes of up to 200 slides.

▶ Hematology

In the hematology department, options include a small "single mode" instrument that performs a three-part differential as opposed to a five-part differential. This will save on reagent costs for a low volume test. Accreditation requires determining what criteria should reflex to a manual differential. The medical director or pathologist chooses if these will be performed in-office or sent out to a reference laboratory. For smaller options, staining can be done by hand; higher volumes may require automated solutions.

▶ General Chemistry

The general chemistry instrumentation should boast a test menu specific to a urology practice. At a minimum, it should include:

- Blood Urea Nitrogen/Creatinine (BUN/CREA)
- Basic Metabolic Panel (BMP)
- Complete Metabolic Panel (CMP)
- Hepatic Panels
- Magnesium, Phosphorus, Uric Acid, and urine chemistry assays

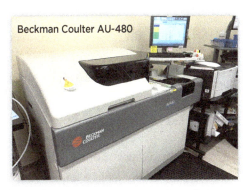

Beckman Coulter AU-480

If affiliated with an ambulatory surgery center and Prothrombin Time/Partial Thromboplastin Time (PT/PTT) is not offered as a pre-op, it can be helpful to add them to the test menu to determine if these can be performed within 48 hours of collection. Most coagulation assays are performed onsite using a point-of-care (POC) handheld instrument for Clinical Laboratory Improvement Amendments (CLIA) waived testing.

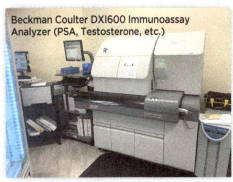

Beckman Coulter DXI600 Immunoassay Analyzer (PSA, Testosterone, etc.)

▶ Immunochemistry

An adequate immunochemistry analyzer should handle the bulk of serum testing and include the Prostate-specific antigen (PSA), fPSA, and %fPSA,

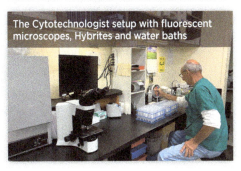

The Cytotechnologist setup with fluorescent microscopes, Hybrites and water baths

Testosterone, Prostate Health Index and Sex Hormone Binding Globulin (SHBG), which is used for calculating the Free Testosterone. Other assays can be added, including Alpha-Fetoprotein, Carcino embryonic Antigen (CEA), Dehydroe piandrosterone-Sulfate(DHEA-S), Estradiol, Follicle Stimulating Hormone (FSH), beta HCG Quantitative (HCG), Luteinizing Hormone (LH), Parathyroid Hormone (PTH), Progesterone, Prolactin, and Vitamin D. Other meaningful tests for urology practice s can be added if test volumes justify them.

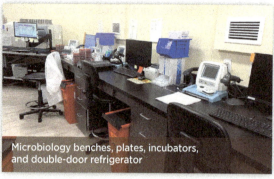

Microbiology benches, plates, incubators, and double-door refrigerator

▶ *Microbiology*

Urine cultures and sensitivities can either be performed by manual means or automated, depending on the group's volume and types

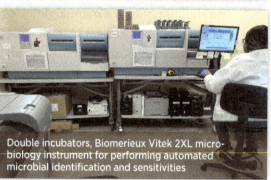

Double incubators, Biomerieux Vitek 2XL microbiology instrument for performing automated microbial identification and sensitivities

of specimens plated. Both methods will require plating of the suspected organism(s) on primary plates, for instance, on TSA 5% SB and CNA 5% SB/EMB bi-plates, which need to stay refrigerated until brought to room temperature for use. Processing 2,000 cultures per month would require a double-door refrigerator; volumes larger would potentially need a triple-door refrigerator for plate storage.

Incubators. Sufficient space is needed for incubators that will hold primary plates as well as the larger plates, if using Mueller Hinton agar for sensitivities. It is recommended to have at least two incubators for rotation of reading schedules and for backup measures in case of sudden volume increases, emergency, or equipment failure.

Basic reagents used to classify organisms as gram negative or gram positive include indole, oxidase, hydrogen peroxide and staph latex kits. Additional growing media may be required, such as slants, broths, and other selective agars. Rapid kits are cost effective manual panels that aid in the identification of common urinary tract pathogens, medically important Enterobacteriaceae, and other selected oxidase-negative, Gram-negative bacilli.

Automated innovative microbiologic platforms are available that deliver rapid and accurate identification and antibiotic susceptibility testing (AST), with often decreased turnaround times as compared to standard sensitivities. Some organisms can result in as little as five hours. These systems receive software updates for antibiotic break points and have customizable alerts. Antibiograms tailored to physician, location, or care center can give providers additional information needed for monitoring resistance trends.

Assessments are either internal or external and comprise a large portion of the quality assessment program. Assessment of quality is integral to achieving it. It is the means to determine the effectiveness of the Quality Management System.

▶ Internal Assessments

Safety Audit

Performing an annual internal safety audit is a great way to assess and document whether the laboratory is in compliance with general safety and housekeeping; personal protective equipment availability and use; safety training and documentation; blood-borne pathogens; chemical hygiene; electrical;, eye wash/shower stations; fire; and waste management requirements. This can be accomplished with a checklist that summarizes each requirement and performed on a quarterly basis.

Routine Self-Assessment

During the off year from the accreditation inspection or survey, a self-inspection that utilizes the same tools and checklists as the professional inspectors or surveyors is recommended, even if it is not required. It is also recommended that the persons performing the testing be involved in the self-inspection process to aid administration in identifying any deficiencies that can be corrected prior to the actual inspection.

Initial and Biannual Linearity/Validations

Initial validations studies are often performed by the manufacturer from whom the equipment is purchased. This service should be included in pre-purchase discussions as it is not always guaranteed. In the clinical laboratory, it is imperative that validations are performed in a timely fashion, and any new test methods or IHC stains added to the test menu in pathology are also validated.

Quality Indicators

Quality indicators set by the laboratory are used to benchmark and monitor quality and performance on a continual basis. These are selected by administration and can be changed at will as errors trend.

Some common items to monitor:
- Test volumes
- Rejected specimens
- Missed tests/ordered wrong test
- Turnaround times
- Corrected reports
- IT errors

Statistical Reporting

A quarterly report should be printed to include volumes for cytology, FISH, histology, and diagnostic rates by provider and location. This is reviewed by the medical director and provided to the clinical staff.

Monthly QA Report

Each month, the quality assessment activities are documented and compiled for the previous month to be evaluated, reviewed, and signed by the laboratory manager, QA specialist, and medical director. This should be done separately for both the clinical and the pathology labs and process maintained in a binder for annual review and proof of a sound quality assessment plan.

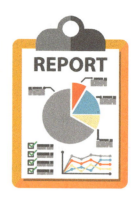

▶ *External Assessments*

Routine Accreditation Assessments

The College of American Pathologists (CAP), Agency for Health Care Administration (AHCA), or appropriate state agency, is the accrediting agency that will conduct a biennial inspection of the pathology laboratory. COLA® is most commonly used for inspection and accreditation in the clinical laboratory. Each testing specialty will be reviewed with a targeted checklist of requirements. If any deficiencies are cited, they need to be corrected onsite or within a specified time frame, with documentation proving corrective measures have taken place. Performance of a peer inspection of another laboratory similar in size and specialty is a requirement of CAP.

Proficiency Testing

The American Proficiency Institute (API) and American Association of Bioanalysts (AAB) offer comparable proficiency testing programs that are accreditation approved. CAP also offers proficiency testing for the clinical and pathology laboratories; however, it is cost effective to use CAP solely for the pathology laboratory and either API or AAB for the clinical laboratory.

Samples with known values are sent to the laboratory on a quarterly basis and compared to peer laboratory results nationwide. Enrolling in a proficiency program is mandatory, and performance results are reported to CLIA and state agency, if applicable. Biannual Non-GYN Cytology Proficiency Program Federal CLIA and state laboratory regulations stipulate that if a proficiency testing program is not available for a particular analyte, the laboratory must develop an internal proficiency program for verification of the individual who performs the test. Twice annually, the pathologist will receive "Proficiency Slide Sets" from the external lab pathologist. A copy of the case log will be provided to each reading pathologist and reports verified within two degrees of diagnosis to be acceptable.

Biannual Tissue and IHC Proficiency Program

Choosing to either participate in a commercial proficiency program for histological tissue or creating an internal program where at least two cases per year are submitted for external diagnostic comparison would satisfy the proficiency program requirements.

Pathologist External Consult Correlation

Documentation is maintained for correlation for every consultation requested, whether it is a consultation ordered by the pathologist to assist with diagnosis or ordered for a second opinion by the ordering physician of the patient. Any major discrepancies are noted and discussed with the ordering physician to determine whether to send the case out to a third-party for resolution.

CLIENT SERVICES

▶ Client Services Manual

The client services section of the QMS should mirror what is provided to clients in the directory of services that is distributed. The client is anyone who utilizes the laboratory services. This could include medical assistants, nurses, and providers. As a start, a client services manual should include copies of the clinical and pathology requisitions with details on how to fill them out, patient demographics sheets, and insurance policy information.

A laboratory supply request list should be provided along with instructions on how to place orders for supplies. Instructions should also cover the precise specimen container needed, including the correct colored tubes/additives for whole blood and serum specimens, collection details, labeling, processing, storage, and transport requirements. Also, to be included is information about which fixative to use for collecting histology and cytology/FISH specimens, and how to obtain an adequate sample for testing.

▶ Courier Service

Planning the logistics of courier services can be intimidating, but with a well-thought-out plan and dedicated couriers, this component is easily accomplished. When choosing between in-office couriers and outsourcing this service, consider staffing costs, vehicle purchases and depreciation, required maintenance, and insurance costs. The easiest route is outsourcing to a courier company with an impeccable reputation. Factor in the number of pickup locations, size and quantity of lockboxes needed, scheduled pickup times, and unscheduled calls for emergency supplies. Couriers will need dedicated coolers that are validated to maintain required temperatures for biological specimens. Biohazardous training is required for these positions, as well as knowledge of transporting biohazardous specimens and managing related accidents in transit.

A client satisfaction survey should be sent periodically throughout the year to assess that the lab is providing excellent service to clients. This form is included in the quality assessments and elicits feedback that is valuable to identify opportunities to improve or add services.

With molecular microbiology, identification of resistance genes and historical data (antibiograms) are being used to give suggested antibiotic treatment. This is quicker than traditional methods but may not be as accurate since specific antibiotics are not tested against the exact organism causing the infection.

An alternative approach is to identify organisms by PCR or NGS, reference antibiograms and then perform individual microbe sensitivities using an automated microbiology platform.

With traditional culture, sensitivities are performed when uropathogens are present in significant amounts, usually >10^5 colony count.

With PCR/NGS concentration thresholds (bacterial loads) are usually divided into <10^5, 10^5, 10^7 and >10^7, or a low, medium, and high concentration and antibiotic therapies are given based on "research based recommendations", some of which, sources and documentation are unknown and not regulated. These methodologies also recommend treatment for concentrations <10^5 organisms, which would not be given with traditional culture methodology, which begs the questions of levels of pathogenicity and antibiotic stewardship.

Traditional sensitivity testing is performed on each individually isolated organism. There exist methodologies of antibiotic testing in a "pooled" setting mimicking the polymicrobial environment with shared resistance and shared metabolites of multiple organisms resulting in stronger resistance when in the collective state.

PCR and NGS identification of urinary tract pathogens can be brought in-house independently or a third-party reference laboratory can assist in setting up instrumentation, performing testing validation and training personnel.

Issues to consider when evaluating these technologies include:

1. Is it a significant improvement over the existing test (will it help patients)?
2. Is it supported by current literature or NCCN guidelines?'
3. Is it FDA approved (not always necessary)?

Issues to consider when adding a new technology to the laboratory:

1. There should be a trial period where the test is sent out to a reference laboratory to see if clinicians support and order the test.
2. Is the test reimbursed by Medicare and private payers?
3. Are current employees capable of performing these tests?

In summary, these are the basic components required for developing an outstanding laboratory, tailored to a urology group's needs. There are multiple reference resources for further details. Discussion with other urology groups who have been though the process of setting up a laboratory is also helpful.

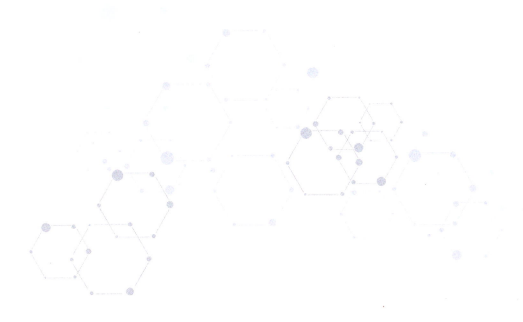

[1] CLSI. Quality Management System: A Model for Laboratory Services; Approved Guideline – Fourth Edition. CLSI document GP26-A4. Wayne, PA: Clinical and Laboratory Standards Institute; 2011.

[2] CLSI/NCCLS. A Quality Management System Model for Health Care; Approved Guideline – Second Edition. CLSI/NCCLS document HS01-A2. Wayne, PA: NCCLS; 2004.

[3] QMS: A Model for Laboratory Services GP26-A4, Motschman, Rhamy, Walsh, Lab Guidelines and Standards, January 2012. Lab Medicine, Volume 43 Number 1.

[4] Guidelines for Developing a Quality Management Plan, John Hopkins University, Doc 10-14, Version 1.0.

[5] CAP, www.cap.org, Accessed August 17, 2016.

[6] COLA, www.cola.org, Accessed August 19, 2016.

[7] Lab University, Quality Management Systems, www.labuniversity.org, Accessed August 25, 2016.

[8] Maruniak C, Maruniak N, Willets C. Advanced Urology Institute QMS. 2015.

[9] Garcia LS, ed. in chief. Clinical Laboratory Management, 2nd ed., Santa Monica, CA: American Society for Microbiology, LSG & Associates. ASM Press; 2014.

[10] A Head-to-Head Comparative Phase II Study of Standard Urine Culture and Sensitivity Versus DNA Next-generation Sequencing Testing for Urinary Tract Infections; Rev Urol. 2017;19(4):213-220

Terms and Tests Used in Pathology and Clinical Laboratory System

To understand the inner workings of a pathology/clinical laboratory system, it is important to understand the terms and tests being used in that system.

▶ Anatomic Pathology

Anatomic Pathology is a medical specialty that is focused on the diagnosis of diseases based on the macroscopic, microscopic, biochemical, immunologic, and molecular examination of organs and tissues.

▶ Histology/Histopathology

Histology is the study of cells and tissues under a microscope. These specimens have been sectioned (cut into a thin cross section with a microtome), stained, and placed on a microscope slide. Histopathology is the microscopic study of diseased tissue to identify cancers and other types of disease states. The study of these tissues is usually performed by a pathologist who provides a diagnostic assessment of the tissue and issues a report to the surgeon or clinician. The patient's treatment is guided by the pathologist's report.

▶ Cytology

Cytology or cytopathology is the study of single cells or small clusters of cells for the purpose of diagnosis of diseases. Cytology usually involves tests on body fluids, with the most common for urology being urine, although sputum and fluids such as spinal, pleural, pericardial, or ascites can be evaluated as well. Papanicolaou (PAP) smears are also included in cytology.

FISH

Fluorescence in situ hybridization (FISH) is a test that looks for changes in the genetic material in a person's cells. These genes may provide information as to how a particular tumor may behave and/or respond to certain therapies. From that analysis, the pathologist can help determine proper diagnosis and treatment options. The most common use for FISH in urology is the UroVysion® test done on cells found in urine. The UroVysion® FISH test is performed in conjunction with cytology and is more sensitive than cytology alone in diagnosing bladder cancers.

CLINICAL TESTING

▶ Testosterone (Free & Total)

A testosterone test checks the level of male hormone (androgen) in the blood. Testosterone affects overall development and sexual features in both men and women. For men, testosterone is produced by the testicles and in women by the ovaries, but for both men and women, small amounts are made by the adrenal glands.

In men, testosterone levels typically peak around the age of 40 and then gradually decrease over time. Most of the testosterone in the blood is bound to a protein called sex hormone binding globulin (SHBG) or albumin. Testosterone that is not bound is called "free" testosterone and can be checked if a man or a woman is having sexual function issues. Other issues such as hyperthyroidism or some kidney diseases may be checked if SHBG levels are changing.

▶ PSA Testing

Prostate-specific antigen, or PSA, is a protein produced by cells of the prostate gland. The PSA test measures the level of PSA in a man's blood. Traditionally, a PSA level of under four (4) ng/mL has been considered "normal," although prostate cancer can develop at levels less than four (4) ng/ml. As a result of recent studies, PSA values of between 2 and 3.5 ng/mL are being considered at risk, depending on the patient's age.

▶ Urine Cultures and Sensitivity

A urine culture is a test to find and identify organisms, such as bacteria or fungi that may be causing a urinary tract infection (UTI). Normally, the urine in the bladder is sterile and does not contain any bacteria or other organisms. Sometimes bacteria can enter the urethra and cause an infection, requiring a urine culture for identification and treatment. A urine sample is cultured to foster bacteria growth. If there are no new organisms detected, then the test is deemed to be negative; conversely, if growth does occur sufficient to indicate an infection, then the culture is positive. Sensitivity testing will be used to select a specific antibiotic to treat those infections.

The practice should develop an ad hoc committee or assign a key physician to work with the administrative team/lab director to address key items prior to opening or expanding a urology-specific laboratory.

KEY POINTS

- **When planning and designing the floor plan,** it is important to understand the use of Lean design principles for routing the flow of specimens through processes to eliminate wasted steps and time.

- **All laboratory employees should** undergo a pre-employment drug screening and baseline testing for Hepatitis B and HIV.

- **There are multiple types of waste in the laboratory** that need to be appropriately sorted and discarded.

- **The Quality Management System** is the set of documents and records for the laboratory to be compiled in a binder and easily accessible on the practice's internal website.

- **Each department should have its own manual** detailing step-by-step listing each reagent, calibrator, quality control material, and other supplies used in a testing process.

- **The optimal Laboratory Information System** is a singular platform that can support clinical, microbiology, pathology, and molecular pathology.

- **When shopping for equipment,** it is wise to compare at least three brands, makes, and/or models.

- **Availability of dependable and reliable test kits and supplies** is essential to the seamless operation of the laboratory.

- **Internal and external assessments** can help ensure safety and compliance.

- **The client services section of the QMS** should mirror what is provided to clients in the directory of services that is distributed.

- **When choosing between in-office couriers and outsourcing this service,** consider staffing costs, vehicle purchases and depreciation, required maintenance, and insurance costs.

Nicholas A. Maruniak, MD

Dr. Maruniak is the Pathologist and Laboratory Director for Advanced Urology Institute, a group of more than 40 urologists based in Florida. He has practiced pathology for 30 years, with the past 20 years dedicated to specializing in urologic pathology and working directly with groups of urologists.

Adam J. Cole, MD

Dr. Adam J. Cole attended the University of Arkansas in Fayetteville and graduated with honors with a bachelor's degree in microbiology. He also holds a master's degree in health science from Duke University. He concluded his medical training with a residency in pathology at the University of Arkansas for Medical Sciences. Dr. Cole is a Board-Certified Pathologist with a Genitourinary and Molecular Pathology focus.

E. Scot Davis, BA, MPA, MBA, CMPE

Scot serves as Chief Executive Officer of Arkansas Urology. With more than 20 years in physician practice management serving in a variety of executive roles, he has developed an expertise in physician recruitment, joint-venture arrangements, compensation modeling and operational efficiency. Scot is a member of the Arkansas Medical Group Management Association and the American Medical Group Association and earned the Certified Medical Practice Executive designation from the American College of Medical Practice Executives in 1999.

Stephanie Evans, BS, MT

Stephanie Evans joined the staff of Arkansas Urology in July of 2015 as Clinical Director of Lab & Pathology. She brings 16 years of laboratory experience with previous positions at the Arkansas Heart Hospital, Baptist Health, and the Central Arkansas Radiation Therapy Institute. Stephanie is a Certified Medical Technologist with the State of Arkansas. She received an Associate of Science in Medical Laboratory Technology in 2001 from Arkansas State University and a bachelor's degree in Medical Technology from the University of Arkansas for Medical Sciences in 2008.

Candy M. H. Willets, MT (AAB)

Candy Willets is the Laboratory Manager for Advanced Urology Institute, a group of more than 40 urologists based in Florida. She has many years of experience in laboratory medicine working with hospital facilities, outreach programs, and specialty group practices.

CHAPTER 18

Genomic and Hereditary Testing in Prostate Cancer: Implications for the Urology Practice

Christopher J.D. Wallis, MD, PhD, FRCSC
Raoul S. Concepcion, MD, FACS

Due to the availability of next generation sequencing (NGS), data continues to emerge on the incidence of both germline and somatic mutations in DNA repair genes that increases the risk for the development of prostate cancer. These pathogenic alterations have significant clinical implications in the diagnosis and management of advanced and high-grade disease. This chapter provides an overview of the mutations that are highly associated with prostate cancer, as well as the rationale for developing a robust testing program in a urology practice.

Watson and Crick first described the double helix structure of DNA in 1953, and subsequently, awarded the Nobel Prize in 1962 for their monumental work. Initial efforts to sequence the nucleotide base pairings of short fragmented DNA segments were very labor intensive, requiring years of lab time with a correspondingly high price. A major advance came in 977[1] with the development of the Sanger chain termination technique, which dramatically accelerated the process and became the foundation for NGS.[1] The Human Genome Project (HGP) was conceived in the 1980's as an international collaborative effort. The goal was to completely map the 3 billion plus nucleotides that make up a human's DNA. After multiple iterations and with Congressional funding, a five-year final plan was articulated and written jointly in 1998 by the United States Department of Energy and the National Institute of Health to complete the project by the ambitious date of 2003.[2] In what would amount to a genetics arms race between competing public and private interests, the project was hailed a success in 2001, a full two years ahead of the deadline.

As a result of this effort, the impact and benefits derived are innumerable. Beyond its obvious implications to potential improvements in patient care, from an economic perspective it has been estimated that the accrued benefit from the $3.5 billion-dollar investment to fund the HGP has approached $800 billion since its inception![3] Several improvements to the original Sanger methodology and the first semi-automated sequencers resulted in more rapid and faster sequencing times during the 1980s and 90s. Current or third generation NGS platforms refer to deep, high-throughput, and parallel DNA sequencing from multiple sources with analysis. Besides whole genome sequencing (WGS), it can also be used for sequencing of the entire transcriptome (RNA-seq), as well as whole exome (coding proteins) and candidate or target genes. The ability to develop this "panomic" profile, including DNA, RNA and protein, has been transformational. As the cost of NGS has come down, we have now tested hundreds of thousands of patients. The result has been a much deeper insight into associations of mutational variants and how they may correlate with certain disease phenotypes.

Genomics versus Genetics

Modern day cancer genomics, made possible by NGS, is the complex analysis of the patient's genes, their interaction with other genes, and the environment that may result in unregulated cell growth and cancer formation. Fundamentally, cancer is a genetic disease and there are mutations that occur in two major classes of genes: tumor suppressors and oncogenes. Mutations that result in inactivation of the former or activation of the latter will cause disruption of the genetic code and increased susceptibility to cancer formation. Prostate cancer genomics has been relatively dormant until recent years. But as a result of NGS, which is now more affordable with rapid turnaround, more and more patients are undergoing testing in both the localized and advanced prostate cancers, especially those diagnosed with metastatic castration resistant prostate cancer (mCRPC). We are gaining a better understanding to identify the drivers of these tumors. The development of large data sets will prove to be valuable, especially for men who have been exposed to multiple lines of therapy.

In contrast to genomics, genetic testing is the evaluation of a patient's inherited genetic make-up that is predicated on their personal cancer history, familial history of known cancers (especially in first degree relatives), and medical history. Historically speaking, urologists have recognized that men of African American descent and those with a paternal family history of prostate cancer were more susceptible and at a higher risk of developing the disease. Detailed family cancer histories, however, were not part of our intake questions, unlike our colleagues that manage well-documented family cancer syndromes, such as HBOC (Hereditary Breast and Ovarian Cancer) or Lynch (hereditary non-polyposis colorectal cancer, uterine, ovarian, gastric, upper tract urothelial) syndrome. While we have long been aware of the increased familial susceptibility to the development of prostate cancer, it is only recently been discovered that men with metastatic or lethal disease may have inherited germline mutations, very much akin to women with breast cancer.

One of the earliest observations that an environmental exposure could lead to the development of cancer was published in 1775 by Sir Percivall Potts.[4] In his epoch paper, he observed an increased prevalence of erosive sores on the scrotum of young men who worked as chimney sweeps in London, which, if left untreated, ultimately gave way to cancers of the scrotum. The working hypothesis was that soot and coal tar remained trapped in the rugal folds of the scrotum. Combined with the lack of poor hygiene, common in that time period, and a prolonged latency of 20-plus years, came the eruption of "sootwarts," which would ultimately transform into cancer of the scrotum. This occupational exposure was the first to attribute malignant changes to external factors and resulted in historic legislation at the time of The Chimney Sweepers Act of 1788.

These "external factors," which we now label as carcinogens, are well recognized by urologists, albeit not so commonly in prostate cancer. In patients with newly diagnosed urothelial cancer of the bladder, we have been trained to inquire about a personal history of cigarette smoking, as well as work-related exposure to a number of potentially detrimental environmental elements, such as aromatic amines, arsenic, and aniline dyes to name a few. But how do these irritants, analogous to the soot from chimneys, ultimately result in tumor development and carcinogenesis? Do they in fact "cause" cancer, or is the incidence markedly increased in those who are for some reason more susceptible?

Understanding and elucidating the underlying genetic basis of carcinogenesis has been the holy grail for cancer researchers, for both the scientific understanding of disease pathophysiology and potential therapeutic implications. Perhaps the best example of the therapeutic implications of understanding carcinogenesis come from CML (chronic myeloid leukemia) where the identification of the "Philadelphia chromosome."[5] This aberrant fusion gene, which encodes the breakpoint cluster region-proto-oncogene tyrosine-protein kinase (BCR-ABL) oncogenic protein with persistently enhanced tyrosine kinase activity,[5] led to the development of targeted therapy in the form of imatinib mesylate (Gleevec, Novartis, Switzerland), a BCR-ABL tyrosine kinase inhibitor.[6] This proved to be a revolutionary treatment not simply due to the efficacy of the treatment, but also because the underlying defect (BCR-ABL fusion protein) is highly prevalent, being found in more than 90% of all patients with chronic myeloid leukemia. In contrast, to date in prostate cancer, the most prevalent underlying genetic defects have been identified in less than one-fifth of patients. Despite this, prostate cancer is among the most heritable cancers.[7]

Adequate patient management may include current cancer treatment, identification of future risks to other malignancies, and family counseling. It is also crucial for health care providers to understand both modern genomics and the role of genetic testing, given they are dependent on each other. Intrinsic to this is having a basic working understanding of the fundamentals, what genes and pathways are implicated, and the platforms utilized that are currently available.

Somatic Versus Germline Testing

Prostate cancer is a clinically heterogenous disease with variability in progression once diagnosed, ranging from the very indolent that may require no therapy to those that present with de novo metastasis. There have been several key genomic mutations that have been consistently identified in prostate cancer patients, both hormone naïve and in mCRPC. These include gene fusion/chromosomal rearrangements (TMPRSS2-ERG), androgen receptor (AR) amplification, inactivation of tumor suppressor genes (PTEN/PI3-K/AKT/mTOR, TP53, Rb1) and oncogene activation (c-MYC, RAS-RAF).[8] More significantly, defects in DNA repair appear to be central in increasing one's susceptibility to malignant transformation.

The human body is constantly monitoring for insults and errors that affect the cell cycle and threaten our survival. In general, DNA damage can be classified into two main categories: endogenous/internal or exogenous/external. Examples of the former include replication errors, DNA base mismatch and methylation. Exogenous incursions are a result of our interaction with the environment, which may involve ionizing radiation, UV radiation or chemical agents. Once the damage or alteration has been detected, a very robust DNA damage repair (DDR) response is recruited to begin the restorative process to ensure the cell cycle can continue unimpeded and, most importantly, without errors. This can be thought of as a two-step process. The initial phase is to excise the damage to the native DNA, which acts as a template for both replication/division and transcription. Ultimately this results in protein production via translation. Such pathways include homologous recombination repair (HRR), base excision repair (BER), nucleotide excision repair (NER), and mismatch repair (MMR). Each has its own set of genes and enzymes that will facilitate the process. Once the damaged area has been excised and purged, the second step involves the actual repair of the DNA strand so it can then resume its activities. This too, can be thought of as having two main categories: single stranded break repair (SSBR) versus double stranded break repair (DSBR). While the mechanisms of the two pathways are well beyond the scope of this manuscript, in general, the PARP1 (Poly [ADP-ribose] polymerase 1) enzyme plays a vital role in SSBR, while the BRCA 1/2 (BReast CAncer gene 1 and 2) and ATM (Ataxia-Telangiectasia Mutated) genes are heavily recruited in DSBR, in which HRR is the most understood.[9]

The importance of having a working understanding of these concepts is that over the past few years, new data, again in large part as a result of NGS, has emerged that identification of mutations in these genes not only increase the risk of development of prostate cancer, but in fact in certain patients may be inherited, similar to breast cancer. While the actual incidence of these inherited or germline mutations are low (< 2-6%) in localized disease as shown within existing data sets, men with more aggressive phenotypes, vis a vis, metastatic disease and those dying of prostate cancer, may have a much higher incidence. This appears to be independent of race or family history of prostate cancer. These mutations include DDR genes involved in MMR (MLH1/MSH2/3/6, which are implicated in microsatellite instability/MSI), SSBR (PARP1) and HRR (ATM, BRCA 1/2).[10]

It is critical to patient management that we determine whether these mutations are inherited (germline) or acquired (somatic). Germline mutations are changes in DNA that are present in the reproductive cells of the patient (sperm or ovum), and thus, passed from generation to generation and will be identified in EVERY cell of the body. Therefore, germline testing can be conducted with just a swab from the mouth, saliva, or blood from the patient. There are many companies in the United States that currently offer germline testing. Genetic testing through NGS in a diagnostic laboratory is mandatory to obtain the most comprehensive analysis and report. In contrast, there are many direct to consumer tests (DTC) currently marketed to patients. The testing platforms deployed by many of these companies are much less robust and often include a limited number of known genetic mutations in their panels. For example, there are thousands of identified BRCA mutations that have been identified, but only a handful may be tested in some of these DTC testing kits. This can lead to an unacceptable number of false negative studies and should not be used for clinical decision-making.

Acquired or somatic mutations can be defined as any alteration in DNA that occurs after conception. These can occur in any cell of the body (except the reproductive cells) and usually result from the exogenous exposures we discussed earlier. Therefore, somatic testing requires NGS of cells extracted from the tumor itself and cannot be performed with a saliva or blood sample. This should be differentiated from genomic testing on tissue that looks at a predefined genetic signature (not the entire genome or exome) associated with cancers to determine potential presence or absence and possible aggressiveness.

Genomics and Prostate Cancer

In 2019, there were an estimated 174,650 newly diagnosed prostate cancer cases in the United States and a cancer specific mortality of 31,620 that was directly attributable to the disease. This breaks down to 5.2% of all cancer deaths.[11] Over the past decade, we have become more cognizant of the fact that all prostate cancer cases do not require treatment intervention. Based on histopathologic criteria, active surveillance (AS) is an appropriate initial therapy for select patients. Thus, there is a need to be more judicious on which patients truly should undergo prostate biopsy in efforts to detect "significant" disease. Several newer therapies, all mechanistically different, and treatment regimens have been approved for management of advanced prostate cancer in both the metastatic castration sensitive (mCSPC) and mCRPC patient types. A unique dynamic progressive model estimates the incidence of the latter two subsets may approach 42,970 patients in 2020.[12] Unfortunately, despite the availability of superior agents, optimal sequences or combination of these oncolytics has yet to be determined as there are no predictive biomarkers to inform the provider of the most ideal initial line of therapy (LOT) and future LOT as patients progress. Even more challenging, these newer and soon-to-be-approved therapies are targeted for molecular drivers of prostate cancer. Thus, several clinical challenges across the spectrum of prostate cancer currently face the urologic provider:

 What testing beyond PSA (prostate specific antigen) and DRE (digital rectal exam) can be used to determine which patient is at risk for aggressive disease and should undergo prostate biopsy?

 For the patient with newly diagnosed prostate cancer, who is the optimal candidate for AS versus active treatment (AT), whether that be surgery or radiation?

 For the patient with mCSPC or CRPC disease, how can we best determine the initial and subsequent LOTs, given the limitations of the monotherapy registration trials?

 How do we best counsel patients and their families as to the relative risks of cancer development?

Historically, we have risk-stratified patients based on histopathologic and radiographic features, including Gleason grading, number and percentage of cores involved at the time of biopsy, extracapsular/surgical margins, and presence/volume of metastasis on imaging studies. Our traditional thinking of cancer management, as well as clinical trial development, is based on the organ of origin and not the molecular drivers of the tumors. In order to deliver true precision medicine, there is a need to develop and utilize biomolecular markers to inform appropriate decision making.

Somatic Testing in Prostate Cancer

As discussed, somatic testing involves assessment of the genetic and genomic characteristics of the prostate cancer cells themselves. Thus, testing is performed on the prostate tissue sample, which has some reimbursement challenges. Numerous somatic, genetic, and epigenetic (a change in gene expression without a change in genotype) changes are associated with prostate cancer carcinogenesis. These may occur at many levels, including somatic copy number alterations, structural rearrangements, point mutations, single nucleotide polymorphisms (SNP's), microRNAs, and methylation changes.[13] Use of these tests, and the specific nature of the test employed varies across the disease spectrum.

Many molecular and genetic factors have been examined in an attempt to provide more meaningful prognostication for patients with prostate cancer. As with nomograms, there are many commercially available molecular biomarkers, which have been developed to aid in prostate cancer diagnosis, prognosis, and the provision of post-surgical radiotherapy. These tests have been commercially available for quite some time and have been previously reviewed.[14, 15] While these tests have value in specific clinical scenarios, an extensive review of both their indications and underlying data is beyond the scope of this chapter.

However, it is worth noting that, despite their value, there are many limitations to the molecular factors, which have been examined thus far. Frequently, there are systematic errors in the design and execution of the discovery studies.[16] First, many biomarkers are developed without a clear clinical or research question, which they seek to address. This is reflected in the wide variety of outcomes reported in the studies assessing the available tests. Further, the majority have been developed using pathological findings at the time of prostatectomy or biochemical recurrence as the endpoint.[1] More clinically relevant research questions include (1) distinguishing patients with clinically-significant prostate cancer and a low or indeterminate PSA level from those with clinically-insignificant disease or benign prostatic hyperplasia; (2) distinguishing between disease destined to progress from that which will have an indolent course; and (3) identifying patients with metastatic disease, prior to radiographic evidence. In addition, most biomarkers have been tested

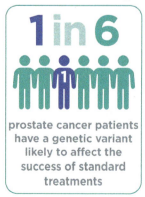

1 in 6 prostate cancer patients have a genetic variant likely to affect the success of standard treatments

among patients who have undergone radical local treatment and extrapolated these data for men undergoing active surveillance, where the primary is still present. Finally, there is a significant publication bias in biomarker development studies with selective non-reporting.

In addition to these panels, somatic testing for specific gene variants may be undertaken. For the most part, this approach is employed in patients with advanced disease with the goal of identifying particular actionable targets. For example, mutations in HRR or MMR genes and identification of MSA high vs low status may suggest treatments are more likely to be beneficial. In addition to genetic testing of tumor tissue, assessment of circulating tumor cells (CTCs) may offer important information. For example, testing of AR-V (androgen receptor variant) status can be performed using CTCs and may be predictive.

Germline Mutations in Prostate Cancer

Over the past decade and as a result of NGS, significant strides have been made to identify the key molecular pathways in prostate cancer. **Table 1** is a listing of the common genomic alterations that have been identified.

Pritchard and colleagues were among the first to demonstrate the value of assessing inherited genetic changes in prostate cancer. Among 692 patients with metastatic prostate cancer, they examined the prevalence of mutations in 20 DNA-repair genes. Mutations were identified in 82 men (11.8%) with significant geographic heterogeneity, treated at the University of Washington, and 18.5% in patients treated at Memorial Sloan Kettering.

TABLE 1 Common genomic alterations in advanced prostate cancer

GENE	ALTERATION TYPE
ETS Transcription factors	Rearrangement
Androgen Receptor	Mutation/Amplification
PTEN	Loss
RB1	Loss
PIK3A	Mutation/Amplification
MYC	Amplification
AURKA	Amplification
AKT	Mutation
RAF	Rearrangement/Mutation
KRAS	Mutation/Rearrangement

Adapted from: Kumar-Sinha C, Tomlins SA, Chinnaiyan AM: Recurrent gene fusions in prostate cancer. Nat Rev Cancer 8:497-511, 2008

This potentially reflects referral biases. Subsequently, Castro et al. found a prevalence of germline DNA damage repair gene mutations of 16.2% in patients with metastatic castrate resistance prostate cancer.[18]

TABLE 2: Top 10 germline variants among patients with prostate cancer undergoing genetic testing

Mutated gene	Prevalence in entire cohort	Prevalence among men with mutations
BRCA2	4.74%	24.3%
CHEK2	2.88%	14.1%
ATM	2.03%	9.6%
MUTYH	2.37%	8.2%
APC	1.28%	6.4%
BRCA1	1.25%	4.5%
HOXB13	1.12%	4.5%
MSH2	0.69%	3.4%
TP53	0.66%	3.3%
PALB2	0.56%	2.7%

Adapted from: Nicolosi P, Ledet E, Yang S, et al. Prevalence of Germline Variants in Prostate Cancer and Implications for Current Genetic Testing Guidelines. JAMA Oncol 2019; 5(4):523-528

However, these data were limited to patients with advanced prostate cancer. In a diverse cohort of 3,607 men with prostate cancer, at various stages of the disease trajectory,[19] germline variants in 620 patients (17.2%), of which BRCA1/2 comprised only a small proportion. The 10 most commonly identified variants are listed in **Table 2**.

Germline genetic testing provides both prognostic information, and potentially guides specific therapeutic decisions. In patients with metastatic castrate resistant prostate cancer in the PROREPAIR-B cohort, Castro et al. found that germline BRCA2 mutations specifically were associated with significantly worse prostate cancer specific mortality (17 months compared with 33 months, hazard ratio 2.11, p-value – 0.033). Also of note, an aggregate assessment of ATM, BRCA1, BRCA2, or PALB2 was not associated with prostate cancer specific survival (different in survival 10 months, p = 0.264)[18]. Discussion of the role of genetic testing in treatment decisions is discussed on the next page.

While commonly identified germline mutations may be actionable in other disease states, they are relatively uncommon in prostate cancer. Nicolosi and colleagues found that actionable mutations were identified in 1.74% of their study cohort with a diverse patient population. In previous analyses, Robinson et al. reported clinically actionable pathogenic germline mutations in 8% of 150 patients with metastatic castrate resistant prostate cancer. This contrasts with clinically actionable aberrations in the androgen receptor in 63% of patients, and aberrations in other cancer-related genes in 65%.[20] Perhaps it is not surprising that actionable underlying germline mutations would be more common in a cohort with more advanced prostate cancer.

Who to Test – Guideline Recommendations

There are two main reasons to undertake genetic testing for patients with prostate cancer: first, to guide their treatment where significant prognostic or therapeutic information can be derived from genetic testing and, second, to guide counselling of relatively, including siblings and children.

Genetics has become an integral part of Prostate Cancer care as evidenced by partnerships between pharmaceutical and genetic testing companies. Consequently, it is critical that physicians be aligned with NCCN guidelines and consistent with the clinical care pathways within their own practice. Reasonable adherence to an established pathway ensures that all patients are receiving all appropriate services and that monitoring methods have been established and are being followed.

Some large groups have found success by centralizing patient navigation by disease state, by incorporating pathways into the EMR, and/or by assigning an advanced practice provider to ensure the physician, the patient navigation team, and the patient are remaining compliant with the pathway and with that specific patient's care plan.

The advanced practice provider (APP) can discern nuances in care not necessarily captured by data-mining software and can effect clinical changes to the course of treatment by discussing additional genetic testing, other ancillary services, and the overall plan of care with the treating urologist. This work can be accomplished by integrating the APP into the prostate cancer committee or clinical pod or by assigning periodic review activities to an APP versed in genetics associated with specific types of cancer (prostate, bladder, etc.).

Recently, the American Society of Clinical Oncology (ASCO) released their guideline on the role of molecular biomarkers in localized prostate cancer, focusing solely on somatic molecular biomarkers. The National Comprehensive Cancer Network (NCCN) provides recommendations across the disease spectrum and incorporates both somatic and germline recommendations.

The NCCN guidelines highlight the first step in a genetic assessment of a patient's prostate cancer risk is a thorough personal and family history. Among patients with localized disease, recommendations regarding both germline testing and molecular somatic tumor testing depend on clinicopathologic risk groups (**Table 3**). In the August 2019 update, the NCCN guideline panel also focused on advanced prostate cancer, which they divided into patients with regional disease (node-positive non-metastatic disease; any T stage, N1, M0) and metastatic disease (any T stage, any N stage, M1). In both groups, the NCCN guideline panel recommended germline testing with consideration for molecular and biomarker analysis of the tumor.

Risk Group	Clinicopathologic Characteristics	Germline Testing	Molecular/biomarker Testing of Tumor
Very Low Risk	All of: -T1c -GGG1 -PSA <10ng/mL -<3 positive cores AND <50% involvement per core -PSA density <0.15ng/mL/g	Recommended in patients with family history OR intraductal pathology	Not recommended
Low Risk	All of: -T1-T2a -GGG1 -PSA <10ng/mL	Recommended in patients with family history OR intraductal pathology	Can consider in patients with life expectancy >10 years
Intermediate-Favorable	Any ONE of (IRFs): -T2b-T2c -GGG2 -PSA 10-20ng/mL AND < 50% cores positive	Recommended in patients with family history OR intraductal pathology	Can consider in patients with life expectancy >10 years
Intermediate-Unfavorable	Any of: -2 or 3 IRFs -GGG3 ->50% biopsy cores positive	Recommended in patients with family history OR intraductal pathology	Not routinely recommended
High	Any of: -T3a -GGG4 or 5 -PSA >20ng/mL	Recommended in all patients	Not routinely recommended
Very High	Any of: -T3b or T4 -Primary Gleason pattern 5 ->4 cores GGG4 or 5	Recommended in all patients	Not routinely recommended
Regional	-N1M0 disease	Recommended in all patients	Consider testing for DNA repair defects, DNA mismatch repair defect, or microsatellite instability
Metastatic	-M1 disease	Recommended in all patients	Consider testing for DNA repair defects, DNA mismatch repair defect, or microsatellite instability

TABLE 3: NCCN risk categories and corresponding recommendations regarding germline and molecular testing

Note: GGG = Gleason Grade Group; IRF = intermediate risk factors
Adapted from: NCCN Clinical Practice Guidelines in Oncology: Prostate Cancer - Version 1.2019. 2019.

The panel suggests consideration of the use of tumor-based somatic molecular assays for localized prostate cancer patients ONLY in those risk stratified with low risk/LR or favorable intermediate risk/F-IR. This is based on data that demonstrates these molecular assays can provide additional prognostic information beyond that provided by risk groupings utilizing clinicopathologic data, such as the NCCN or CAPRA risk groups. The rationale is that intervention is likely not warranted among patients with LR or F-IR disease who have limited (less than 10 years) life expectancy and it is unlikely that additional information derived from molecular testing would change therapeutic decision. Therefore, molecular testing should only be considered in LR or F-IR patients with a minimum of 10 years life expectancy. Similarly, therapeutic decisions are unlikely to change on the basis of molecular testing results in patients with very low risk/VLR disease, where AS is almost certainly the preferred option, and those with unfavorable intermediate risk/U-IR, high risk/HR, and very high risk/VHR disease for whom active treatment with curative intent is likely warranted in all but the most comorbid of patients.

In patients with regional or metastatic prostate cancer, somatic tumor testing may also be considered on the basis of the observation that nearly 90% of men have potentially actionable mutations at the tumor level, while only a relatively small proportion of men would have actionable germline mutations (approximately 9% of patients with mCRPC, according to the NCCN). In these patients, testing may be undertaken for somatic HRR gene mutations (for example, BRCA1, BRCA2, ATM, PALB2, FANCA, RAD51D, and CHECK2) and for MSI or MMR.[20]

A family history of prostate cancer is strongly predictive of a man's risk and one must distinguish hereditary versus familial cases. The strongest risk is associated with hereditary prostate cancer, which is a small subset of all prostate cancers with Mendelian transmission of susceptibility genes.[21] To be considered hereditary prostate cancer, a family must have three affected generations, three first-degree relatives affected, or two relatives diagnosed prior to age 55[21]. In men with familial prostate cancer, a clear hereditary pattern is not demonstrated, but family history is still critical. Men with one first-degree relative previously diagnosed with prostate cancer have a risk of prostate cancer diagnosis that is two to three times that of individuals without a family history.[22] In addition, the number of affected family members and their age at diagnosis are related to an individual's risk of prostate cancer.[23] Thus, assessment of family history relevant to prostate cancer risk includes not only an assessment of the family history of prostate cancer but should also include inquiry to other genetic syndromes including Lynch and HBOC syndrome.

Ductal and intraductal pathology identified histopathologically may be associated with an increase in genomic instabilities, particularly with respect to MMR genes.[24] The NCCN panel felt that data for intraductal pathology was more convincing than for ductal pathology and recommends germline testing for patients with intraductal pathology, regardless of conventional risk classification.

Thus, in addition to routine somatic testing in patients with regional and metastatic disease, among patients with localized disease, the NCCN guideline panel advocates genetic testing for all patients with HR and VHR localized disease with a relevant family history, intraductal histology, or Ashkenazi Jewish ancestry.

With respect to germline testing, the NCCN guidelines recommend assessment of several germline variants, which are known to be associated with prostate cancer and may affect treatment options (**Table 4**). This testing may be undertaken on a gene-by-gene basis or as part of a prostate cancer risk multi-gene panel (MGP) commercially offered by many companies. Assessment of other, non-actionable genetic variants may be relevant in some circumstances where it may affect patient counseling. For example, testing for HOXB13 mutations does not provide directly actionable information to guide therapeutic decisions. However, it may provide important information on prostate cancer risk that could be valuable in counseling, given the increased frequency of the G84E mutation in those patients diagnosed at an early age (< 55 years old) and a positive FH.[25]

TABLE 4: Recommended germline variants for assessment during germline testing	
Category	**Examples**
Mismatch repair (Lynch syndrome)	MLH1, MSH2, MSH6, and PMS2
Homologous recombination repair genes	BCRA1, BRCA2, ATM, PALB2, and CHECK2
Adapted from: NCCN Clinical Practice Guideslines in Oncology: Prostate Cancer - Version 1.2019. 2019.	

In 2017, the Philadelphia Prostate Cancer Consensus Conference was convened to define the role of genetic testing in inherited prostate cancer.[26] The strongest conclusion of the expert panel was that appropriate patients, which include those with suspected hereditary or familial prostate cancer and those with a FH of suspected HBOC or Lynch syndrome, should be engaged in shared decision making to encourage genetic testing and counseling. The genes that were most critical to be tested were BRCA1, BRCA2, ATM, HOXB13 and DNA MRR (**Table 5**). In discussions regarding prostate cancer screening and early detection, the panel strongly felt that BRCA2 mutations should be considered; men with more advanced disease includes the addition of BRCA1 and ATM.

Variants of Unknown Significance (VUS)

Genetic testing yields results, for the most part, that are unambiguous and that a gene mutation is present or absent. However, the reporting of the significance and association of that mutation relative to a disease state can be quite variable. Given that the coding sequence for a particular gene has been defined and the sequencing machines are fairly similar, what is considered "positive" or deleterious versus "negative" or favorable/no mutation relative to disease risk is predicated on the number of patients tested.

As described in the prior section, several genes have been identified and associated with an increased susceptibility risk for prostate cancer. MGPs are becoming more and more utilized, but the makeup of these panels is not uniform. A recent analysis looking at various commercially available MGPs shows the average number of genes tested is 12 (range 4 – 16). BRCA 1, BRCA 2 are included in all the panels, but 20% did not include HOXB13 or MMR genes.[27] The clinical experience and number of patients tested with BRCA1/2 is more extensive relative to other genes.

TABLE 5: Associated Cancer Risk and Action

GENE	PCa RISK	MECHANISM
ATM	Elevated	DNA damage response
BRCA1	~ 20%	DNA damage repair
BRCA2	~ 20%	DNA damage repair
CHEK2	Elevated	DNA repair
EPCAM	Up to 30%	Upregulate c-MYC
HOXB13	Up to 60%	AR repressor
MLH1	Up to 30%	DNA repair
MSH2	Up to 30%	DNA repair
MSH6	Up to 30%	DNA repair
NBN	Elevated	DNA repair
PMS2	Up to 30%	DNA MMR
TP53	Unknown	Tumor Suppressor
PALB2	Preliminary	Tumor Suppressor
RAD51D	Preliminary	DNA repair

Based on data in Nicolosi, et al ASCO Abstract 5009 2017 Chicago

More and more mutations continue to be discovered, but the significance to the patient has yet to be determined until more and more samples are processed. These discoveries, classified as VUS (Variants of Unknown Significance) represent a grey area in which there is a change in the genetic sequence, but it is still unknown presently if this change is associated with a deleterious or favorable prognosis. Among women with breast cancer, detection of a VUS is more common than identification of known pathogenic variants.[28] While ongoing work seeks to better delineate the importance of these VUS, the involvement of a genetic counselor is key to helping patients navigate this uncertain situation.

What to Do After Testing

All testing should be actionable. In patients for whom somatic molecular tumor characterization was performed for risk stratification in localized disease, shared decision making should be undertaken to assess the next steps in management. This may include prostate biopsy; repeat biopsy; initial treatment of their primary tumor or post-prostatectomy treatment decisions; integrated information derived from the molecular test; and standard clinicopathologic data.

In patients with a high index of suspicion for germline mutations, consideration should be made for pre-test genetic counseling. For those who do not receive pre-test counseling, referral for genetic testing should be undertaken in those with identified germline variants. Particularly, patients with identified mutations in BRCA1, BRCA2, ATM, CHECK2, or PALB2 should receive a genetic counseling referral to assess for the potential of HBOC. Similarly, those with identified MSI high status or defects in DNA MMR, genetic counseling referral should be undertaken to assess the potential of Lynch syndrome.

In addition to genetic counseling, identification of germline or somatic defects may have important treatment and therapeutic implications. A recent study looked at over 1,100 patients on AS. Using a 3 gene (BRCA1, BRCA2, ATM) risk panel, they found those who harbored the mutation were at a higher risk for pathologic upgrading than those who were non-carriers.[29] Thus, despite histopathologic criteria, AS may not be optimal in select patients.

In patients with advanced prostate cancer, identification of underlying germline mutations may guide treatment selection to determine the most appropriate next LOT (Line of Therapy), particularly for those who have progressed through multiple lines of prior therapy, including AR signaling agents. Patients with identified MSI high status, defects in DNA MMR genes, or CDK-12 biallelic loss, may in fact respond to checkpoint inhibition therapy.[30] Pembrolizumab (Merck and Co., NJ), an FDA approved PD-1 inhibitor, is the first immunotherapy, which won approval in a tumor-agnostic manner and is not based on organ type. Further, patients with mutations in HRR genes (including BRCA1/2, CHEK2, and Fanconi's anemia genes) may be better suited for treatment with the poly (adenosine diphosphate [ADP]–ribose) polymerase (PARP) inhibitors, many of which are in ongoing phase 3 trials with expected approval in 2020. Finally, patients with DNA repair defects may have increased sensitivity to platinum-based chemotherapeutics.[31] Given the uncertainty regarding optimal treatment selection and pending approval of current agents in trial, the NCCN prostate cancer guideline panel recommends clinical trial enrollment for all men with prostate cancer and identified DNA repair gene mutations.

Operational Challenges and Issues

Given the nature of most urology practices in the Unites States, the number of prostate cancer patients being diagnosed and routinely followed continues to mount annually. We have entered an age of precision medicine where patient management will hinge on modern day genomic testing. Admittedly, it will be challenging to incorporate an evidence-based genetic testing program with the ever-changing guidelines, rapid expansion of data, and anticipated approval of more therapeutic agents. However, many would argue that failing to develop one is negligent and a disservice to our patients. Here are four key components that are foundational to a successful initiative:

 Patient identification. The guidelines continue to evolve, but they do spell out which patients are appropriate candidates for testing. How every practice chooses to find these patients is a challenge and hopefully next generation electronic health record (EHR) systems will be able to assist.

 Education. Providers and practices will need to understand the role and implications of testing, whether that is in the area of risk identification/stratification, pharmacogenomics, cascade testing, or clinical decision making.

 Genetic counseling. Current estimates suggest that the number of certified genetic counselors in the U.S. is approximately 5,000, and much of their focus has been centered in the neonatal population and rare disease space. Those who focus primarily on oncology are a small but growing number. Access, whether it be pre-or post-testing, is a challenge and concern, given the number of patients across all tumor types who are indeed candidates. To meet this demand, it will be important that alternative delivery models are developed.

 Partnering with a certified NGS testing lab that provides quality accurate reporting to patients and providers, as well as educational support.

Relative to education, practices should provide information to their patients on The Genetic Information Nondiscrimination Act (GINA) of 2008.[32] In a nutshell, it protects Americans from discrimination based on their genetic information when obtaining both health insurance and employment. It does not, however, offer protection in cases of life, long-term care, or disability insurance and does not apply to employers with less than 15 employees.

Conclusions

Urologists and urology practices will need to begin incorporating comprehensive genomic testing, just as we embraced PSA testing back in the 1990's. A recent survey conducted amongst 52 single specialty independent urology community practices identified the following three issues to incorporate and develop a comprehensive testing program.[33]

> 1 Medical/legal liability for unaddressed identified mutations.
>
> 2 Reimbursement concerns and cost of testing.
>
> 3 Complexity and time involved entering a complete family history and pedigree into the EHR.

None of these, however, are insurmountable if the practice commits to enhancing and delivering precision medicine for our prostate cancer patients.

1. Sanger F, Nicklen S, Coulson AR: DNA sequencing with chain-terminating inhibitors. Proc Natl Acad Sci USA. 1977; 74:5463–7.
2. Roberts L. Controversial From the Start. Science 2001; 16 Feb: 1182-1188.
3. Hood, L., Rowen, L. The Human Genome Project: big science transforms biology and medicine. Genome Med 5, 79 (2013).
4. Brown, J. R.; Thornton, J. L. (1957). Percivall Potts and Chimney Sweepers' Cancer of the Scrotum. British Journal of Industrial Medicine. 14 (1): 68–70.
5. Kang ZJ, Liu YF, Xu LZ, et al. The Philadelphia chromosome in leukemogenesis. Chin J Cancer 2016; 35:48.
6. An X, Tiwari AK, Sun Y, et al. BCR-ABL tyrosine kinase inhibitors in the treatment of Philadelphia chromosome positive chronic myeloid
7. Lichtenstein P, Holm NV, Verkasalo PK, et al. Environmental and heritable factors in the causation of cancer – analyses of cohorts of twins from Sweden, Denmark, and Finland. N Engl J Med 2000; 343(2):78-85.
8. Rubin MA, Maher CA, Chinnaiyan AM: Commongene rearrangements in prostate cancer. J Clin Oncol 29:3659-3668, 2011
9. Kunkel TA, Erie DA. DNA Mismatch Repair. Annu Rev Biochem. 2005; 74:681-710.
10. Pritchard CC, Mateo J, Walsh MF, et al. Inherited DNA-Repair Gene Mutations in Men with Metastatic Prostate Cancer. N Engl J Med 2016; 375(5):443-53.
11. Siegel, R.L., Miller, K.D. and Jemal, A. (2019), Cancer statistics, 2019. CA A Cancer J Clin, 69: 7-34.
12. Scher HI, Solo K, Valant J, Todd MB, Mehra M (2015) Prevalence of Prostate Cancer Clinical States and Mortality in the United States: Estimates Using a Dynamic Progression Model. PLoS ONE 10(10): e0139440.
13. Wallis CJ, Nam RK. Prostate Cancer Genetics: A Review. EJIFCC 2015; 26(2):79-91.
14. Alford AV, Brito JM, Yadav KK, et al. The Use of Biomarkers in Prostate Cancer Screening and Treatment. Rev Urol 2017; 19(4):221-234.
15. Kornberg Z, Cooperberg MR, Spratt DE, et al. Genomic biomarkers in prostate cancer. Transl Androl Urol 2018; 7(3):459-471.
16. Prensner JR, Rubin MA, Wei JT, et al. Beyond PSA: the next generation of prostate cancer biomarkers. Sci Transl Med 2012; 4(127):127rv3.
17. Martin NE, Mucci LA, Loda M, et al. Prognostic determinants in prostate cancer. Cancer J 2011; 17(6):429-37.
18. Castro E, Romero-Laorden N, Del Pozo A, et al. PROREPAIR-B: A Prospective Cohort Study of the Impact of Germline DNA Repair Mutations on the Outcomes of Patients With Metastatic Castration-Resistant Prostate Cancer. J Clin Oncol 2019; 37(6):490-503.
19. Nicolosi P, Ledet E, Yang S, et al. Prevalence of Germline Variants in Prostate Cancer and Implications for Current Genetic Testing Guidelines. JAMA Oncol 2019; 5(4):523-528.
20. Robinson D, Van Allen EM, Wu YM, et al. Integrative clinical genomics of advanced prostate cancer. Cell 2015; 161(5):1215-1228.
21. Potter SR, Partin AW. Hereditary and familial prostate cancer: biologic aggressiveness and recurrence. Rev Urol 2000; 2(1):35-6.
22. Bratt O. Hereditary prostate cancer: clinical aspects. J Urol 2002; 168(3):906-13.
23. Gronberg H. Prostate cancer epidemiology. Lancet 2003; 361(9360):859-64.
24. Isaacsson Velho P, Silberstein JL, Markowski MC, Luo J, Lotan TL, Isaacs WB, Antonarakis ES.Prostate. 2018 Apr;78(5):401-407. doi: 10.1002/pros.23484. Epub 2018 Jan 25.
25. Pilie PG, Giri VN, Cooney KA. HOXB13 and other high penetrant genes for prostate cancer. Asian J Androl. 2016;18(4):530–532.
26. Giri VN, Knudsen KE, Kelly WK, et al. Role of Genetic Testing for Inherited Prostate Cancer Risk: Philadelphia Prostate Cancer Consensus Conference 2017. J Clin Oncol 2018; 36(4):414-424.
27. Aldubayan SH. Considerations of multigene test findings among men with prostate cancer - knowns and unknowns. Can J Urology. Oct, 2019; 26(52):14-16.
28. van Marcke C, Collard A, Vikkula M, et al. Prevalence of pathogenic variants and variants of unknown significance in patients at high risk of breast cancer: A systematic review and meta-analysis of gene-panel data. Crit Rev Oncol Hematol 2018; 132:138-144.
29. Carter, H. Ballentine et al. Germline Mutations in ATM and BRCA1/2 Are Associated with Grade Reclassification in Men on Active Surveillance for Prostate Cancer. European Urology, Volume 75, Issue 5, 743 - 749.
30. Wu YM et al. Inactivation of CDK12 Delineates a Distinct Immunogenic Class of Advanced Prostate Cancer. Cell. 2018 Jun 14;173(7):1770-1782.
31. Humeniuk MS et al. Platinum sensitivity in metastatic prostate cancer: does histology matter? Prostate Cancer Prostatic Dis. 2018 Apr;21(1):92-99.
32. https://www.genome.gov/about-genomics/policy-issues/Genetic-Discrimination
33. Concepcion RS. Germline testing for prostate cancer: community urology perspective. Can J Urology. Oct 2019;26(52): 50-51.

KEY POINTS

- **The Human Genome Project** not only aims to improve patient care. Economically, the estimated accrued benefit from the $3.5 billion-dollar investment to fund the project has approached $800 billion since its inception!

- **It is critical to patient management** that we determine whether these mutations are inherited (germline) or acquired (somatic).

- **Somatic testing** involves assessment of the genetic and genomic characteristics of the prostate cancer cells themselves, thus, testing is performed on the prostate tissue sample.

- **Germline genetic testing** provides both prognostic information, and potentially guides specific therapeutic decisions. While commonly identified germline mutations may be actionable in other disease states, they are relatively uncommon in prostate cancer. The NCCN guidelines recommend assessment of several germline variants, which are known to be associated with prostate cancer and may affect treatment options.

- **The main reasons to undertake genetic testing for patients with prostate cancer** is to guide their treatment where significant prognostic or therapeutic information can be derived from genetic testing; and to guide counselling of relatively, including siblings and children.

- **The NCCN guidelines** highlight the first step in a genetic assessment of a patient's prostate cancer risk is a thorough personal and family history. A family history of prostate cancer is strongly predictive of a man's risk and one must distinguish hereditary versus familial cases.

- **Admittedly, it will be challenging to incorporate an evidence-based genetic testing program with the ever-changing guidelines, rapid expansion of data, and anticipated approval of more therapeutic agents.** However, many would argue that failing to develop one is negligent and a disservice to our patients.

Christopher J.D. Wallis, MD, PhD, FRCSC

Dr. Wallis is a Urologic Oncology Fellow and Instructor in Urology at Vanderbilt University Medical Center. He obtained his Doctor of Medicine from the University of British Columbia, his Doctor of Philosophy in Clinical Epidemiology & Health Care Research from the Institute of Health Policy, Management & Evaluation at the University of Toronto, and completed his clinical residency in Urology at the University of Toronto affiliated hospitals.

Raoul S. Concepcion, MD, FACS

Dr. Concepcion is the current Director of The Comprehensive Prostate Center and also a Clinical Associate Professor, Department of Urology at Vanderbilt University Medical Center. He is a founding Board member and Past President of LUGPA.

CHAPTER

The Basics of Developing an Ambulatory Surgery Center (ASC)

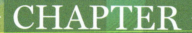
Michael W. Holder, MBA

There are many factors to consider when building an ambulatory surgical center (ASC). This chapter will highlight the more important components, but, by intent, the information is not exhaustive.

Initially, one must recognize the major benefits an ASC offers patients. These include, a higher quality of medical care than is typical compared to other sites of service, turnaround times that are often better than hospital-run ASCs, substantial savings to the patient and insurance company, often in the 30-40% range, because the urologists control equipment purchases. In addition, the physician experiences a quantum leap in efficiency, which is perhaps the one factor that has compelled most urology groups to proceed with developing an ASC.

Rules and Regulations

After the need for a facility in the community has been identified, and prior to construction, one must be knowlegeable of all applicable state and federal rules and regulations regarding the building of an ASC. As an example, in the state of Texas one can review the website **www.dshs.texas.gov/facilities/asc,** which guides the user through the rules and regulations, as well as the licensing requirements of an ASC. This is a very helpful guideline to ensure nothing is missed. Texas also has an ASC application that must be submitted at the appropriate time to start the process for applying for a state license. It is important to plan for enough time to understand and fulfill all the state and federal requirements necessary to become an ASC. There are also several national ASC trade associations, such as the American Association of Ambulatory Surgery Centers, that have many resources to offer. These will be discussed later in the chapter.

Single Vs. Multi Specialty

Before moving forward, one must decide whether to become a single specialty urology ASC or multi-specialty ASC. There are many advantages to adding multiple specialties, including diversifying the risk with more partners, less individual investment, and an opportunity for greater utilization, and therefore, a diversified revenue stream. The urology practice must look at the compromise to the ASC's capacity and utilization by including other specialties. One way to proceed is to build a single specialty urology ASC. After the center is in operation and utilization and capacity is understood, management can reassess a move to a multi-specialty facility.

Construction

Before starting construction, the practice may wish to contact several urology-specific ASCs as reference points. The LUGPA community can be a valuable resource during the planning process. Touring successful ASCs offers management the opportunity to ask questions regarding the design and layout, management, supplies, employees, anesthesia and outside contractors, insurance contracts, accreditation, software systems, etc.

The next decision is whether to hire an architect, an ASC consultant, or ASC management company to direct the design and building of the ASC. There are companies that provide a turnkey operation to start an ASC. If an architectural firm is hired, it is important to make sure it has experience and a firm grasp of local, state, and federal Medicare codes as well as knowledge of all rules and regulations in the healthcare industry. An architect must also have extensive experience working in the desired geographical region. For example, someone who usually builds on the bedrock of mountainous terrain may not understand the nuances of sandy or clay foundations. The importance of finding a good and trustworthy architect, consultant, or management company cannot be stressed enough.

Joint Ventures

Some groups have found it strategic to enter into a joint venture with a hospital, multispecialty clinic, or a healthcare system. The pros and cons of this decision depend on local politics and geography. Benefits to joint ventures include better relationships with commercial payers and higher volumes. However, when entering into a joint venture, it is crucial to ensure that both parties' goals align and are agreed upon, and that they are clear about who will manage the ASC (which could be a third-party management company). The joint venture will also need to determine if a change in licensure or classification is required by the state, and be in compliance in regards to receiving referrals per the Anti-Kickback statue.

Importance of a Pro Forma Financial Statement

Equally important is the process of developing a business plan and pro forma financial statements that project the future status of the company and detail projected volume, revenue, expenses, and income potential compared to the capital expenditures and accrued debts of building an ASC. This project is a major commitment. Not only are good and trustworthy figures required in the pro forma financial plans, but each scenario, for example, a single or multi-specialty ASC, needs to be thoughtfully explored. Financial projections should also include the total number of employees that will need to be hired, what equipment the physicians will require, and the cost of supplies. An ASC gets reimbursed by appropriate coding of the service provided using Current Procedural Terminology (CPT®) codes; therefore, the cost of staff and supplies is very important. If these costs are not understood, it could mean the difference between a profit and a loss.

During the development of the business plan, one must determine which cases can be brought to the ASC. Procedures that are typically performed in the clinic can be sent to the ASC for improved patient safety and higher-quality standards. For example, a significant benefit to the practice and the patient is a comprehensive sterilization process with sophisticated sterilization equipment in place at the ASC as compared to the clinic. Treatment rooms at the ASC can be used to accommodate clinic procedures like vasectomies, cystoscopes, and prostate biopsies. For procedures that do not require general anesthesia, the layout and staffing differs from the rest of the ASC. Moving these procedures out of the clinic to the ASC demonstrates to the community and payors the practice's commitment to a higher level of quality.

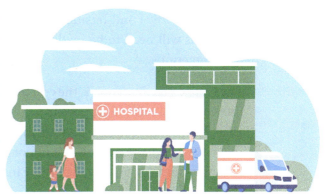

Those considering an ASC must identify the historical percentage of outpatient surgeries they feel confident in taking to the new ASC. There are financial benefits to retaining some procedures in the clinic or at the hospital. If the practice is engaged in a standing lithotripsy partnership, then a business analysis should be done to consider the impact of dissolving the partnership and purchasing a lithotripter and C-arm to provide extracorporeal shock wave lithotripsy (ESWL) at the ASC. Another option is to dedicate one operating room solely for cystoscopies with specialized equipment, such as a fixed fluoroscopic cystoscopy table.

Depending on the requirements stated in the latest state and federal regulations, there is also the possibility of keeping patients overnight in the ASC for a 23-hour observation period.

The pro forma should document the volume of procedures by month, identify which type of room they require (operating or treatment room), and detail the expected reimbursement of each compared to the historical reimbursement. It is important to be aware of the potential difference in the professional fee if clinical procedures are moved to an ASC. According to the Medicare fee schedule, the professional fee with an ASC, may be smaller, while the ASC facility fee may be increased in some CPT codes. Therefore, it is important to know not only what one will receive in revenue for the identified volume of procedures, but also the amount of revenue lost on the professional fee side.

Even though it is not possible to provide an exhaustive list of procedures offered in ASCs, many centers offer laparoscopic procedures as well as neuromodulation—one of the most beneficial surgeries for the ASC. To offer neuromodulation in an ASC setting, a solid process should exist to identify costs, patient insurance, preauthorizations of the procedure, and due diligence in the coding, billing, and collection cycle.

Once one has a good understanding of projected volume and revenue, it is time to move to the expense side of the equation, which can present many pitfalls. First, a good estimate of the total number of employees is important. This includes management, RNs, OR technicians, radiology technicians, instrument sterilization staff, front office and business office staff, janitors—or any combination of these. Decisions will need to be made whether one wants to hire or contract out some of these functions.

The second consideration is the cost of supplies and equipment. It is important to keep the supply cost as low as possible. Two ideas to accomplish this include partnering with a Group Purchasing Organization (GPO) or price shopping between suppliers. In an ASC, implants represent a major supply expense and should be "carved out" for reimbursement on any managed care insurance contracts. One must have an excellent grasp of reimbursement vs. the cost of supplies for each procedure. Since costs and reimbursements can change yearly, these numbers should be continually analyzed and monitored to keep supply costs as low as possible.

Other areas to be addressed are rent, taxes, purchased outside services, and contracts. One must also note the usual mainstay expenses like insurance, utilities, interest expense, equipment leasing, any sub-categories of the expenses, and miscellaneous expenses that may arise. Again, the due diligence of researching the true expenses of the whole organization will pay off in the end. The pro forma financial statements, very useful and meaningful tools, will be revisited many times in the future, especially to compare actual financial and volume numbers to the numbers that were estimated on the pro forma. As previously noted, the LUGPA community and ASC trade organizations can be very useful in this stage of development.

Corporate Structure, Investors, and Partnership Agreement

The next area that demands additional time and attention is the new ASC's corporate structure, potential investors, and the creation of a partnership agreement. One way to structure the ASC is to create two new companies, the first one a property group to purchase land and build the building; the second an operating company to run the day-to-day ASC. While it is possible to have different investors in the real estate and the operating company, a simpler structure is to keep the same investors in both. Another reason to create the two companies is the opportunity to open the possibility of investment in the future with other specialties without compromising the current clinic partnership.

The creation of new corporations and the development of a new partnership agreement may result in the bulk of initial legal expenditures. One area of the partnership agreement for the ASC that requires additional attention is the "Buy/Sell" portion of the agreement. This outlines the requirements of becoming a partner and what actions will constitute the need to sell one's share. One must hire an experienced healthcare attorney who understands the needs of the partnership and can navigate the Anti-Kickback Statute (AKS), the Physician Self-Referral Law (Stark Law), and other federal laws. Language becomes critical when one is buying into or selling a partnership interest.

Once the decision is made on the corporate structure, the "heavy lifting" or critical decisions should be completed by experienced healthcare attorneys. Partnership agreements are one area where it is helpful to spend additional funds to ensure the details are correct. A little extra expense in setting up these agreements will save much as the ASC grows and matures. One way to save a little on legal expenses is to engage two different attorneys—a less expensive, more junior healthcare attorney to do the bulk of the agreement, and the second attorney, an expert in physician-owned surgical centers, to review the fine details of the agreement.

The financing of the ASC has not been previously discussed, but it is worth mentioning. There are many options to secure financing and many creative ways to finance. A popular choice is using an existing bank relationship to negotiate a financing agreement to meet the investors' needs. To gain a full understanding of financing options, it is helpful to discuss this with an accountant to make the best decisions and to maximize tax benefits.

The Role of the Architect and Contractor

As noted earlier, hiring an experienced architect is essential to the process of building the ASC. A trusted architect should be included in onsite visits to other ASCs to provide expert opinions on the best options in building an ASC. The architect can also collaborate on providing insight into the "flow" of the ASC, both from a patient and employee perspective. Once the site visits are completed, the architect can create initial drawings of the ASC. Multiple weeks will be necessary to complete this step so that the physicians, administrators, and seasoned employees have time to carefully review the detailed designs for moving people and materials through the building.

Besides hiring an expert architect, one must obtain bids from several experienced general contractors in the medical field to build the ASC. Once a general contractor is identified, the contractor will work closely with the architect and the owners, or partners, on each aspect of building the ASC.

To keep these relationships as smooth as possible, one contract option is a Guaranteed Maximum Price (GMP). This cost-type contract compensates the contractor for the actual costs, plus, it stipulates a fixed fee subject to a ceiling price. The advantage of this type of contract is it caps the total amount of cost the ASC could incur. The GMP also puts the responsibility of cost overruns on the contractor, unless change orders occur. A change order would only be communicated by the architect, with everyone's approval of said change. A pitfall of construction is too many change orders, which can add extra cost to the project and extend the time to completion. Due diligence in the beginning can mitigate the overutilization of change orders during the building process.

Another effective tool that the architect can employ is value engineering. Once the GMP is established, it is helpful to conduct a meeting with the architect, general contractor, and all the sub-contractors to look at any value engineering ideas for cutting or saving costs. Not every idea may be used, but often several opportunities to cut more cost off the GMP are identified.

Building an ASC creates a busy and hectic atmosphere. One should prepare for daily to weekly meetings to discuss the details of the building process with the architect and general contractor. With multiple decisions to make and so many moving parts, a dedicated project manager to oversee the project is helpful. If there is not room in the budget for such a person, then a cohesive team that includes the architect and general contractor is advised.

If possible, the chosen general contractor should have extensive experience building healthcare facilities, ASCs, and/or surgical hospitals. Their expertise in navigating city, state, and federal codes is invaluable. There are many nuances to building an ASC and successfully addressing code requirements. The contractor should be able to handle that level of detail, track each code requirement, and have the expertise to successfully address each code.

The general contractor also controls the building schedule. While most jobs run longer than expected, with communication and measured effort, it is possible to complete the building on time.

One last caveat: do not underbuild, which is a common occurrence with physician-run projects. The reasons are many. Obviously, the cost of the ASC is at the top of that list. When an analysis is done comparing the cost of later additions, there is no doubt the best advice is to err on the side of too much space. Keeping code requirements tight is honorable, but sometimes something as simple as adding an extra inch in hallway width can avoid frustrations later.

Even with seasoned architects, builders, and advisors, ASCs are frequently built without sufficient space for clerical work. Of course, the shift to electronic health records (EHR) created problems for centers that were already built without the proper layout for this change; for new ASCs, sufficient clerical work spaces should be part of the initial planning. Even with forethought, it is rare for physicians to say they have too much space. Finally, in planning the ASC, a 10-year plan for growth and expansion should be incorporated. It would be shortsighted to fail to provide adequate OR space (and all accompanying areas) in the initial planning stages.

Location, Location, Location

Obviously, the ultimate efficiency comes with an ASC that is located on the same campus as the physician's office. If not, the location should be the top priority in deciding where to build, lease, or purchase an ASC. Patient accessibility should be considered, but the highest priority is to be in close proximity to surgeons' clinics and to hospitals where the surgeons work and where patients would be transferred. The target area may already have a building that can be modified or updated to accommodate an ASC; there may even be an ASC available to lease or buy.

If the choice is made to purchase land and build an ASC, then the architect can be utilized to help identify the correct amount of land necessary. An architect can also help identify the ideal shape and size of the land to be bought.

Management of the ASC

Another important variable to consider is the management of the new ASC once it is up and running. This person or team has many responsibilities and should have some level of expertise in how an ASC is managed. There are also management companies that are willing to manage the ASC for a fee.

Often, the ASC will need to create all new policies and procedures for which the management team will be responsible. State rules and regulations can serve as a guide to ensure that nothing is left out. The management team will also be responsible for hiring all staff, staff training, documenting staff certificates, facility licenses, physician credentialing, and other facility needs that may arise. Other responsibilities include creating the facility's patient forms, and setting up the EMR and Practice Management systems, and the process of coding, billing, and collecting of monies on procedures. In addition, the management team must identify facility equipment needs, choose outside contractors, secure transfer agreements with local hospitals, complete licensure applications, and decide on hours of operation, to name just a few responsibilities.

The ASC management team or management company, if that is the preferred route, should be identified early in the ASC planning process and participate when the pro forma and architectural plans are prepared. The person chosen to act as a director or administrator of the ASC should be involved at least six months prior to its opening. This time frame is dependent upon the level of effort needed to identify and complete all preparatory tasks. The administrator should receive a list of daily deadlines and tasks to help move the project forward to ensure the ACS's timely opening.

The group should also consider electing a medical director from its ranks. This is a large time commitment and cannot be casually assigned. The medical director will attend local and national meetings, be involved in credentialing, oversee utilization and quality, and will often be called upon to counsel peers. Because of the breadth of this job, it should be a compensated position.

Insurance Contracting

The group must decide whether the ASC will be "in-network" or "out-of-network" with commercial insurance companies. The current trend is starting to shift from an "out-of-network" model to an "in-network" model. An out-of-network model is viable in the short-term, but the in-network model is better off in the long run and is easier on schedulers and patients.

Communications should begin with major insurance companies to secure managed care in-network contracts before the ASC opens. Although insurance companies may seem interested to hear about the new ASC, the contracts will not immediately be forthcoming. From the time of ASC's opening, it may take 6 to 14 months to negotiate and execute the in-network contracts, and it may be helpful to include a one-year review with contracting payors. After the savings inherent in the ASC design have been demonstrated, the insurance companies often offer more favorable contracts.

The negotiation process with insurance companies takes time and requires patience. Considering that an ASC is reimbursed by CPT® codes, and in most cases through the ASC grouper system, one must continue to revisit the initial pro forma financial statements, especially the volume figures. It is important to work diligently with each insurance company to negotiate the highest possible ASC grouper rates, but also to identify 10 to 15 major CPT® codes for the highest volume procedures to carve-out for better reimbursement. As stated earlier, it is also important to negotiate carve-outs on specific implants and high price medications. Medicare does not use the ASC grouper system, but rather a CPT® code fee-for-service reimbursement model. A staff member who is knowledgeable about the procedures offered and its coding is very helpful to the practice. And, physician partners will require periodic training to understand the nuances of coding, which are unique in this environment.

Accreditation and Medicare Number

The final area to address is accreditation and Medicare participation. With any ASC, it important to choose the correct accreditation company. There are several accreditation companies to consider, two of which are: Accreditation Association for Ambulatory Health Care (AAAHC) and American Association for Accreditation of Ambulatory Surgery Facilities (AAAASF). AAAHC utilizes a Medicare "deemed status" program to achieve accreditation and receive the Medicare number within the same audit time period.

For example, if AAAHC is chosen, the administrator should work diligently prior to the facility's opening to create all the policies and procedures necessary to fulfill AAAHC's protocols and approval systems. One useful idea is for the administrator to attend an AAAHC annual meeting prior to opening the ASC to gain contacts and greater insight into the AAAHC's policies and procedures. These contacts can be beneficial in helping the administrator to learn what is required to pass the initial AAAHC audit and then become Medicare deemed status approved.

Once the facility is open and 10 cases are complete, the state and AAAHC should be contacted to audit the facility. At this point, the state has the greenlight to visit unannounced to audit the facility and its policies and procedures as a last checkbox prior to the state's licensure. When the state arrives, it is a good idea to have the architect, general contractor, and sub-contractors available to answer questions about Life Safety Code (fire protection requirement) issues. AAAHC has six weeks from the submission of the first 10 cases to show up for a surprise audit of the facility, policies, and procedures. Upon completion of this audit, it will take a couple more weeks for the accreditation company to send confirmation of accreditation. If Medicare deemed status was chosen, then the Medicare number approval happens concurrently with AAAHC confirmation.

Even though AAAHC is the source and guide for creating and maintaining internal policies and procedures, one also needs to understand the expectation of the Centers for Medicare & Medicaid Services (CMS) and the state. CMS has a program called Ambulatory Surgical Center Quality Reporting (ASCQR) that is a pay-for-reporting, quality data program. Under this program, the ASC needs to report quality of care data for standardized measures to receive the full annual update to the annual payment rate. CMS's goal with this reporting is to improve healthcare outcomes, quality, safety, efficiency, and satisfaction for patients.

This program includes eight possible requirements as listed:

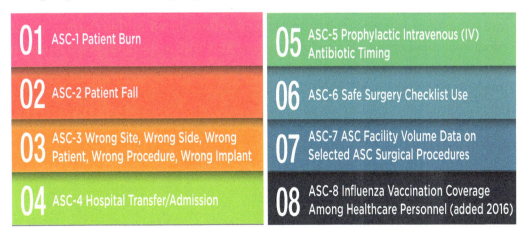

In some states, such as Texas, state reporting is completed quarterly online through the Texas Health Care Information Collection (THCIC). The state requires ASCs to report on several items, namely ASC volume, charges, patient demographics, diagnosis and procedure codes, hospital transfers, and percent of commercial insurance.

AAAHC not only requires comprehensive policies and procedures to be written; more importantly, it audits whether the ASC follows them. For example, within the facility's policy and procedures is a list of equipment and maintenance logs that require daily, weekly, monthly, quarterly, and annual inspections. These inspections must be documented, dated, and signed according to the identified schedule in the policy and procedures. Therefore, it is important for staff to know and understand the requirements set forth and to strictly follow them.

Unfortunately, out-of-network claims, can take at least 90 days to complete. Once a Medicare number is obtained, one still must go through the Medicare process and paperwork of obtaining a provider transaction access number (PTAN) number for billing purposes. This process can take three or more months. Even though Medicare patients can go to the ASC once a Medicare number is received, the facility cannot bill Medicare procedures/surgeries until the PTAN number is finalized. This is a good time to mention that a bank line of credit is important to fund the first four to six months of the ASC expenses.

Conclusions

Adding an ASC to the practice portfolio is a decision that each practice should consider, whether it partners with a local, larger health system or hospital, or builds a single specialty urology or multi-specialty ASC. To recap, the major benefits of an ASC for the patient are: improved patient quality of care; lower risk of infection; greater efficiency throughout the process; lower cost to both the patient and the insurance company; better patient outcomes; and an overall greater level of patient satisfaction. With the patient experience at the forefront, building an ASC is a rigorous process as referenced in this chapter. One cannot go it alone and must use experienced and trusted individuals and companies to successfully complete all actions listed in this chapter. Finally, successfully opening an ASC is a long-term venture with many unexpected issues and costs that can arise; therefore, the process requires a strong foundation of physicians/investors who understand each step.

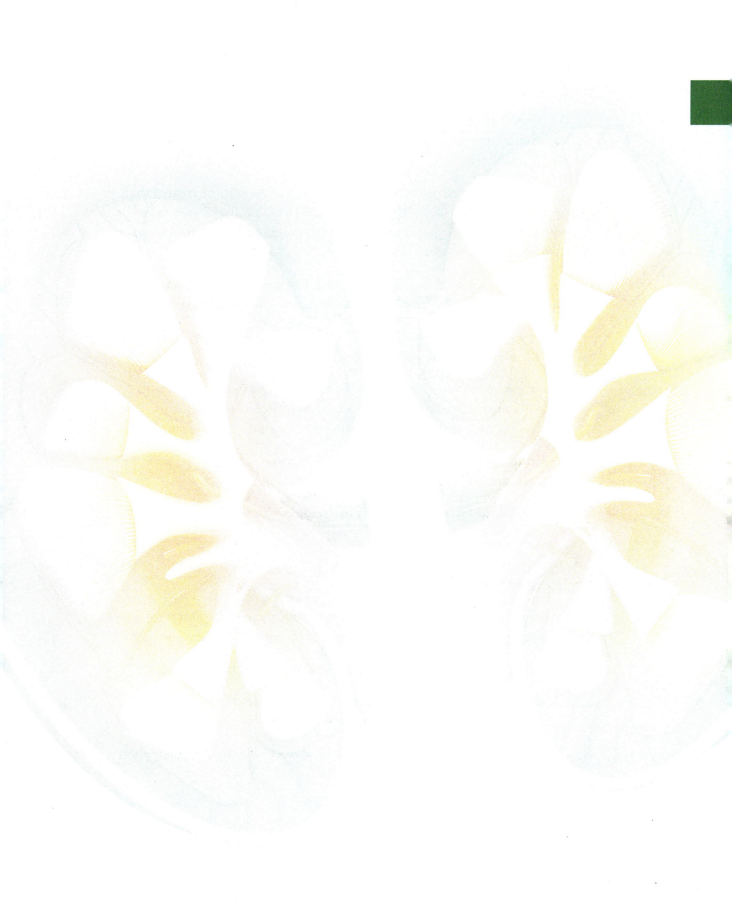

KEY POINTS

- **When** considering an ASC, recognize patient benefits, which include a lower risk of infection, greater efficiency, lower cost, better patient outcomes, and a greater level of patient satisfaction.

- **Decisions** need to be made between a single-versus a multi-specialty ASC, and whether to enter a joint venture with a hospital, multispecialty clinic, or healthcare system.

- **A business plan** and pro forma financial statements must be created that project the future status of the company and detail projected volume, revenue, expenses, and income potential compared to the capital expenditures and accrued debts of building an ASC.

- **The pro forma** should document the volume of procedures by month, identify which type of room they require, and detail the expected reimbursement of each.

- **All applicable** state and federal rules and regulations must be understood before building an ASC.

- **A good** estimate of supplies and the number of employees is important, including management, RNs, OR techs, radiology techs, instrument sterilization staff, front office and business office staff, and janitors.

- **Time** must be dedicated to solidify the ASC's corporate structure, potential investors, and the creation of a partnership agreement.

- **Location** should be the top priority in deciding where to build, lease, or purchase an ASC.

- **Hiring** an experienced architect and general contractor are essential to the process of building the ASC.

- **Often, the ASC** will need to create all-new policies and procedures for which the management team or hired management company will be responsible.

- **The group** should consider electing a medical director from its ranks.

- **The group** must decide whether the ASC will be "in-network" or "out-of-network" with commercial insurance companies.

- **With any ASC**, it important to choose the correct accreditation company.

Michael W. Holder, MBA

Michael "Whitt" Holder serves as Chief Executive Officer of Amarillo Urology Associates and AUA Surgical Center. He has more than 25 years of experience in various industries in accounting, operations and management. In addition to a B.S. in Accounting and an MBA in Healthcare Management, he also is a certified Lean Six Sigma Black Belt and Master Black Belt.

CHAPTER 20
In-Office Dispensing

Christopher Setzler, MBA, CMPE
Simi Banipal, BS, RHIT

According to some studies: more than 30 percent of prescriptions do not get filled. In-office dispensing (IOD) delivers medications to patients at the point-of-care. The prescription can be prescribed, filled, and billed during outpatient, surgical center, and intensity-modulated radiotherapy (IMRT) visits.

An IOD eliminates the process during which patients leave the practice with a written prescription or e-prescribed directive for which a third-party retail pharmacy must fill, provide instructions, and bill. It is much more efficient and convenient for patients to be able to fill their prescriptions at the practice. It can save them commute time and help them avoid long lines and additional wait times. This results in improved quality of care and increased patient satisfaction.

These benefits and operations must function within the proper environmental and structural factors, as dispensing can carry a level of risk. Success relies heavily on compliance, staff structure, contracting, software, and provider adherence. Additionally, operationalizing IOD begins and is dictated by the dynamics of the practice, leadership, and monitoring.

INITIAL STEPS

There are many medical practices of different specialties in the United States that have incorporated in-office dispensing. From the start, it is important to understand that in-office dispensing is a different operation/function than medical care delivery, but does have some similarities that can be incorporated into already established operations. Before exploring in-office dispensing, one must develop a relationship with a consultant or group that is already dispensing or has extensive knowledge of dispensing. Developing relationships is key to providing an initial overview of the process and, later to potentially providing services. Urology groups should partner with companies that have established a track-record of well-informed operational guidance and urologic-specific knowledge of in-office dispensing processes. The partner must continue to provide practices with information and guidance as changes and updates occur.

Along with developing relationships with consultants, it is important to perform and analyze proper financial and cost projections. Many of the drugs that are dispensed by urologists are advanced prostate cancer drugs, overactive bladder medications, and hormone replacement therapies. It is helpful to review the drugs that the practice plans to dispense and know their margins for commercial and Medicare Part D plans. Start with running reports on diagnosis frequency and produce volume projections on possible dispensing candidates within the practice management system. Producing this data as well as providing physicians with education on medications to be dispensed in-office is a crucial part of the implementation process.

In many instances, it is imperative to create teams or champions to manage the physicians' willingness to fully participate in in-office dispensing. A long-term strategy must be developed to produce compliance, benchmarks, and oversight. Creating and structuring an IOD may require committees to review and interpret information and data to develop strategies for rollout, communication, standards, and penalties for non-compliance.

After performing the proper financial analysis and projections for creating an IOD, it is essential to have a thorough legal review of federal, state and local laws, regulatory bodies, and state pharmacy boards. The committee that is managing the IOD process must also have complete understanding of the federal government's in-office ancillary service exception and Anti-Kickback Statute (AKS) rulings and know how these laws and legislation apply to the practice's legal, financial, and operational structure. There are many law firms that specialize in interpreting these laws in context of the practice's structure.

STATE REGULATIONS

State regulations are much more focused than federal regulations. Each state dictates how an in-office dispensary is owned and operated. Most states allow practitioners rather than pharmacists to dispense medications to their patients. Within that majority, there are some states that restrict dispensing practitioners to the MD or DO level, excluding physician assistants and nurse practitioners. It is important for practice staff to understand the specific state's view on interpretation of in-office dispensing and related regulations.

State regulations also can incorporate or defer to state medical or pharmacy board regulations regarding non-pharmacist dispensing operations. Some of these regulations can detail operational hours, closed versus open-door (limiting services to patients within the practice versus open pharmacy services to the public), delivery limitations, storage requirements, etc.

Some states also require applications for a state license to dispense at each individual site versus providing a global license to cover the practice's entire operation. This requirement can be challenging for an organization that has multiple delivery points and multiple locations.

Local counties and insurance contracts also can have requirements and restrictions. In some instances, a local tax is enforced on all non-governmental transactions, which requires proper tracking and reporting. Inevitably, an in-office dispensary will be visited by a regulatory body and/or a pharmacy benefit provider to perform a financial and operational audit, so diligence and planning must be a priority.

NETWORKS

Dispensing network design is somewhat like the design of medical provider networks in that it requires participation and functions mainly on a third-party payer system. The networks mostly consist of commercial insurance payers, pharmacy services administrative organizations (PSAOs), and pharmacy benefit managers (PBMs). PBMs are third-party administrators of pharmacy benefits for Medicare, commercial payers, and other collective groups. In many instances, PBMs will manage pharmacy benefit design, formularies, and claims administration. Currently all Medicare Part D benefits are administered through PBMs, which makes them the largest pharmacy benefit providers.

PSAOs are designed to provide access to networks of health insurance plans and PBMs that are not directly contracted with the practice's IOD. Included with network access are negotiated reimbursements, formularies, and structured contracts. PSAOs normally invoice the dispensary directly and do not generate revenue from the payers. The urology practice pays the PSAO for access, and the invoice is based on size, access, and region.

CREDENTIALING/CONTRACTING

Once the practice receives approval from a regulatory standpoint and understands the networks, it then can contract and credential. First one must apply for a National Council for Prescription Drug Programs (NCPDP) number, which is required by most payers, PSOAs, and PBMs. The NCPDP is the leading body for producing standards for the electronic exchange of pharmacy benefits. The application process is like Electronic Data Interchange (EDI) for medical claims. The NCPDP will issue an identification number that health plans utilize to process pharmacy claims. The NCPDP also provides a great deal of current information on the payer processes, health plans, and advocacy (**www.ncpdp.org**).

The contracting and credentialing process is very similar to credentialing with payers in the medical business. The applications require much of the same information as provider credentialing. Required information includes medical or pharmacies licenses, legal structure, and malpractice and general practice information. In many instances the PSAO will require the practice to fill out a universal application that will manage all the credentialing associated with that particular PSAO's plans and access. The practice needs to provide the information and keep it up to date.

Most of the required information for credentialing is produced by the practice's "Pharmacist in Charge" (PIC). State or pharmacy board requirements will help the practice to determine who will be the PIC. Whether the practice has a provider managing the dispensing or is required to become a pharmacy with a pharmacist dispensing, this individual must be appointed prior to credentialing. Some groups appoint two providers to serve as PIC to make certain vacation time is covered, since a PIC needs to be onsite and sign off on the dispensing. PBMs such as CVS Caremark™ and Express Scripts® require direct contracting and do not function within a PSAO.

OPERATIONALIZING

In-office dispensing is a completely separate ancillary operation within a practice and can be an extremely risky process if not properly managed. When implementing an IOD for patients, the practice must follow all regulations. The initial drug expenditures may be costly and similar to the medical delivery revenue cycle; there is lag time before getting reimbursed.

In designing the IOD, the practice must consider and refer to original volume projections to determine scale and staffing.

Urology groups that are geographically/strategically centralized have a distinct advantage. Those practices can place point-of-care dispensing where the patients can be processed as they leave the practice. There are challenges with groups that are not integrated or do not share the same location, as delivery and regulatory factors weigh heavily on the operation. For example, if most practice sites are within the same building or campus, patients can easily access the pharmacy prior to departure. Their provider can e-prescribe directly to the pharmacy (within their office), and the pharmacist/ PIC/ pharmacy tech can fill the prescriptions in one visit. Additionally, the management of compliance and supply chain is easier in this setting. Practices that are spread out geographically or regionally must adopt different communication strategies with patients and commit to sophisticated delivery operations.

CHOOSING A SOFTWARE SYSTEM

One of the key elements within operations is choosing a software system that is ideal for the practice. When choosing this system, there are multiple considerations, similar to the practice selecting an Electronic Health Records (EHR) system. Some of the considerations are workflow, access, patient eligibility, prior authorization, e-prescribing interfacing, pricing capabilities, rebate programming, warning labels, printing capabilities, reliability, and point-of-care capabilities. The dispensing software should manage the intake of e-prescriptions from the EHR. It should also manage the patient's demographics and bill the pharmacy benefits. Software systems must also provide reporting for financial and compliance purposes. The software will be the essential hub of operations for the IOD.

It is important to note that there are many software systems available for the IOD. The practice will need to pick the right program to fit the operation. A helpful website is **www.capterra.com/pharmacy-software**.

STAFFING

Staffing the practice's IOD is mostly reliant on size, structure, scope, and volume of dispensing. It also must comply with state requirements that dictate who can and cannot be part of the dispensing process, as mentioned earlier. To make the operation more efficient and cost effective, medical assistants or pharmacy technicians should be trained to handle the daily tasks of the pharmacy, while the pharmacist or the provider should focus only on prescribing tasks as regulated by the state.

In some practices, the pharmacy technician or medical assistant will process the e-prescriptions of the IOD. Most of these processes involve checking the patient's demographics for eligibility and prior authorization status and performing an initial review of the integrity of the script. The software should be able to produce a label with the appropriate information about the prescription along with directions. Once these functions are processed within the software, the script is ready for review by the PIC to verify pill count, medicine interaction with other drugs, and correct patient name on the container label.

The practice's EHR system allows the demographics to be easily transferred from the EHR into the dispensing software. There are many systems that can be interfaced with the practice's EHR to streamline information exchange and limit human error. Sometimes prescription drug benefit information is not entered into the EHR, so having a dispensing system that seeks this information is ideal. This can be a timely process, sometimes taking several days, which means that patients will not receive their medication at the point-of-care and may need to return to the site or have the medications shipped directly to their location.

Operations are optimal when the practice has both point-of-care dispensing and a secure and trackable delivery system. Ideally, the practice is able to determine benefit requirements quickly because the patient can provide the appropriate and needed information to fill the prescription. Also at each of the dispensing locations, copayments can be collected, and credit card information is archived in the software for refills. Questions about medicine directives can be addressed during the visit with the prescribing physician or PIC. If prior authorization is required, the practice can send the prescription via

FedEx®, UPS®, or US Mail. It is important to select a service that offers these options and has trackable receipt and signature confirmations. Delivery confirmation logs and the display of the patient receipt of medications are usually reviewed during audits.

To combat some of the geographic challenges, practices need to have properly equipped and trained staff and necessary technology at each location to process patients. Some IODs have prescriptions processed at a central location and then deliver the labels and directives through a networked printer at the point-of-care. Staff at the satellite location labels the medication, counsels the patient on directives, and collects any demographic information or copays.

The central location of the IOD houses the PIC, pharmacy tech, and software to manage the process. The central location is responsible for managing compliance of medicine delivery, receipt logs, and all questions from the provider or the patient.

ACCREDITATION

Many Pharmacy Benefit Managers (PBMs) are now suggesting in-office dispensaries have specialty pharmacy certification or accreditation in order to participate in their specialty networks and dispense specialty medications. Even though this is not a requirement at present, it is a good idea to review and implement the standards of best practices for IOD. This benefits the IOD to operationalize new and improved requirements which helps practices to provide the highest quality of patient care. Many of these accreditations provide helpful resources and process improvement measures to help educate staff and providers to deliver care to patients. It is important for dispensaries seeking to meet the requirements of payors as they continue to pursue network contracts. In-office dispensaries that undergo the accreditation process demonstrate compliance with standards that address pharmacy licensure, better patient care, patient and employee safety, medication adherence and ongoing quality improvements.

There are few approved accreditations out there that are available for in-office dispensing programs. Most states only require obtaining a single accreditation or association; however, there are some states that require getting two forms of accreditation. Best practice is to refer to your individual state's Board of Pharmacy to confirm the requirement process. Community Oncology Pharmacy Association (COPA) partners with the Accreditation Commission for Health Care (ACHC) to provide urology/oncology practices with a customized suite of specialty pharmacy accreditation offerings, including discounts on accreditation fees and education resources to their accreditation programs. By undergoing certified accreditation, dispensaries can demonstrate their commitment to providing the highest quality service by complying with strict national guidelines and industry best practices. This will help your dispensary to meet the same standards as commercial pharmacies as well as meet any additional requirements or restrictions set forth by PBMs.

COPAYMENTS AND PATIENT ASSISTANCE

It has become increasingly important to review the process of copayments and patient financial assistance. Many specialty medications require large out-of- pocket expenses incurred by the patient. Patient assistance foundations are available to provide funding if the patient qualifies. Most pharmaceutical companies also provide patient education and assistance for economically challenged patients. These programs help patients receive medication free of charge and outside of the IOD if they fall below the certain income levels. In many cases, the pharmacy tech can help manage the funding to ensure that patients get the access they need to medications, regardless of financial status.

COLLABORATION WITH PROGRAMS

The combination of an IOD and clinical pathways provide valuable information to enhance the practice's operations while managing patient populations. Also valuable is incorporating an analytics tool that can surface, categorize, and monitor patients throughout their episodes of care within the organization. This data is key in managing cost and potentially adding value for contract negotiations with payers or networks.

IOD services have also been proven to increase medicine adherence as well as clinical pathway processes. For example, practices have recently implemented a program to monitor patients on oral oncolytics. Ideally, a navigation team contacts patients monthly to ask several questions for status evaluation, which is then communicated to the prescribing provider. The status evaluation determines whether or not the patient is a candidate for additional therapies along the practice's pathways.

While the practice becomes more efficient through this process, patients also benefit as they become more compliant with medications and directives. As a result patients stay healthier; their costs decrease; and they experience better quality outcomes. Creating a solid communication vehicle that keeps in contact with patients from the onset of service delivery is key.

ECONOMICS

Due to changing reimbursement guidelines in dispensing, costs and reimbursements must be carefully monitored for the IOD to avoid losing practice income.

As outlined earlier, the medications are processed through patients' pharmacy benefits and/or Medicare Part D. Practice staff must be sure to review all fee schedules prior to dispensing or signing contracts with PSAOs, PBMs, or payers. It is also important to note that many of the margins are larger through Medicare Part D than Part B. What tends to be undervalued with Part D are the benefits resulting from patient satisfaction that create more complete patient care. Patients must also receive careful communication and consideration regarding the out-of-pocket costs associated with most of the medications.

When patients are challenged with paying their copayments or need additional navigation to get their medications, it becomes a process much like managing self-pay medical claims. The practice must have a process in place to properly manage these receivables as copay balances tend to be large and frequent.

The expenses in an IOD are largely dependent on the structure of the practice and the contracts in place. Costs may increase when regulations require a pharmacist instead of a practice physician to fill the role of PIC. The scale, structure, and delivery processes for dispensing that impact expenditures have been discussed in the "Operationalizing" section.

Additional costs should be measured by assessing the practice's contracts with pharmaceutical vendors. Understanding volume is critical when negotiating or reviewing different vendors. There are many group purchasing organization contracts that provide discounted pricing through volume or rebates, which will increase margins.

There may not be a better time for urology and oncology practices to consider adding an in-office dispensary to their operations. IOD can provide patients with access to key oral medications and open a new potential revenue stream for practices regardless of many external influences. With availability of generic medications, practices can take advantage of cheaper drug options for their patients. Margins on generics medications can be better than on brand name medications and patients can afford their out-of-pocket costs more than ever. In many instances copayment on the generic drugs at the retail pharmacy is more than the full cost of the same drug purchased in the in-office dispensary and for the most part, the patient is also willing to pay for them in cash. PBMs also use max allowable cost to reimburse multi-source generic medications so it is always better to shop your wholesalers to find the cheapest generic drug available to maximize the revenue. One should note, however, that generics often do not qualify for patient assistance programs

There are many government funded copayment assistance programs that are available to provide patient assistance for economically challenged patients. The assistance foundation programs provide out-of-pocket assistance if they fall below the certain income threshold. These foundations can provide copayment assistance to not only brand name drugs but also to generic drugs recipients.

ADHERENCE WITH ORAL ONCOLYTICS

"Improving adherence also enhances patients' safety." World Health Organization

Studies have shown that increasing the effectiveness of health interventions have significantly reduced the overall medical cost. Adherence is a process by which patients take their oral medications as prescribed by their physician. Adherence with oral drugs requires a continuous and dynamic process. There are many factors that lead to nonadherence to their complex therapies. We see many patients falling outside of adherence due to socioeconomic status and lack of education.

There are a lot of opportunities for in-office dispensaries to provide patient assistance with their medication. Practices can gain much more control to help their patients in managing patient medication compliance. Most pharmaceutical manufacturers also provide assistance and patient education for socially and economically challenged patients. Insured oncology patients on average pay about $4,800 out of pocket per year. These patients can receive copayment assistance from government funded foundations and can also get drug free of cost from outside specialty pharmacies or in-house IOD.

Practices must have a formal oral adherence program or set guidelines for documenting the prescribing of oral medications, patient education, monitoring for adverse effects and tracking patient adherence. The IOD champion team that normally consists of patient (nurse) navigators, medical assistants and pharmacy technicians are suitable for supporting oral oncolytic adherence programs within a practice. A long-term strategy must be developed for an ongoing commitment to quality improvement. Patient navigators or MAs can schedule touchpoints regularly to educate patients on medication adherence. Clinical and operational teams can be a great resource in monitoring for medication and adherence and financial toxicity. It is important for practices take these steps in order to be successful in an oral adherence program.

COST TO HEALTHCARE

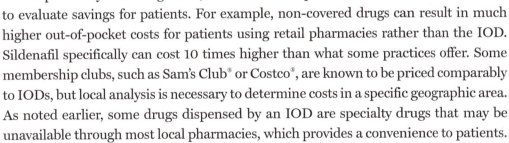

Before developing an IOD system, practices must perform local market research and review the scale of cost. Information on national chains, such as CVS pharmacy® and Walgreens®, and their mark-ups should be examined to evaluate savings for patients. For example, non-covered drugs can result in much higher out-of-pocket costs for patients using retail pharmacies rather than the IOD. Sildenafil specifically can cost 10 times higher than what some practices offer. Some membership clubs, such as Sam's Club® or Costco®, are known to be priced comparably to IODs, but local analysis is necessary to determine costs in a specific geographic area. As noted earlier, some drugs dispensed by an IOD are specialty drugs that may be unavailable through most local pharmacies, which provides a convenience to patients.

Specialty drugs tend to require more careful adherence and monitoring. Retail pharmacies cannot provide the monitoring and correspondence that is sometimes required with patients who take these medications. Patients who have not been appropriately informed by their pharmacy about medications may require additional—and preventable—healthcare services, which is a disadvantage for the patient and adds cost to the overall healthcare system. When the prescribing physician provides medications directly to the patient and the practice monitors adherence, better outcomes result, while overall costs are kept to a minimum.

CHALLENGES

Some of the challenges with managing IODs are the limited competition within the market and networks. Most of the pharmaceutical business appears to be with major PBMs such as Caremark, Optum Rx, and Express Scripts®. Credentialing and network access can be challenging if the PBMs limit IODs from completing credentialing and/or accessing certain networks that contain their patient populations.

A recent example of this challenge is CVS Caremark's™ interpretation of Medicare regulations that has allowed it to limit access for physician-owned dispensaries by stating that they are considered out of network. CVS Caremark™ is not only a PBM, but also has business lines in CVS/pharmacy® chains. In most practices, Medicare is one of the largest payers, which means that it will limit an IOD from dispensing to a majority of its patients or at least a significant portion. A practice would need to measure this impact and consider the economics of developing an IOD.

In closing, managing an in-office dispensary within one's practice can be a successful, yet daunting endeavor. Prescribing and delivering a patient's medication during a visit adds value to the patient-practice relationship.

This value can be found particularly with cancer patients where timeliness can be vital for optimal survival outcomes. Most retail pharmacies do not provide additional services such as direct-patient contact to check for adherence and for side-effects. In general, and outside of normal integrated delivery offerings, it is rare that a practice has opportunities to include ancillary services that can enhance quality for the patient population and foster positive economics. Much like pathology and IMRT, IODs can be integrated into delivery services and help manage practice processes while increasing communication with patients. As we move into a more measured environment, a properly functioning IOD can better equip a practice to control costs and produce better-quality metrics.

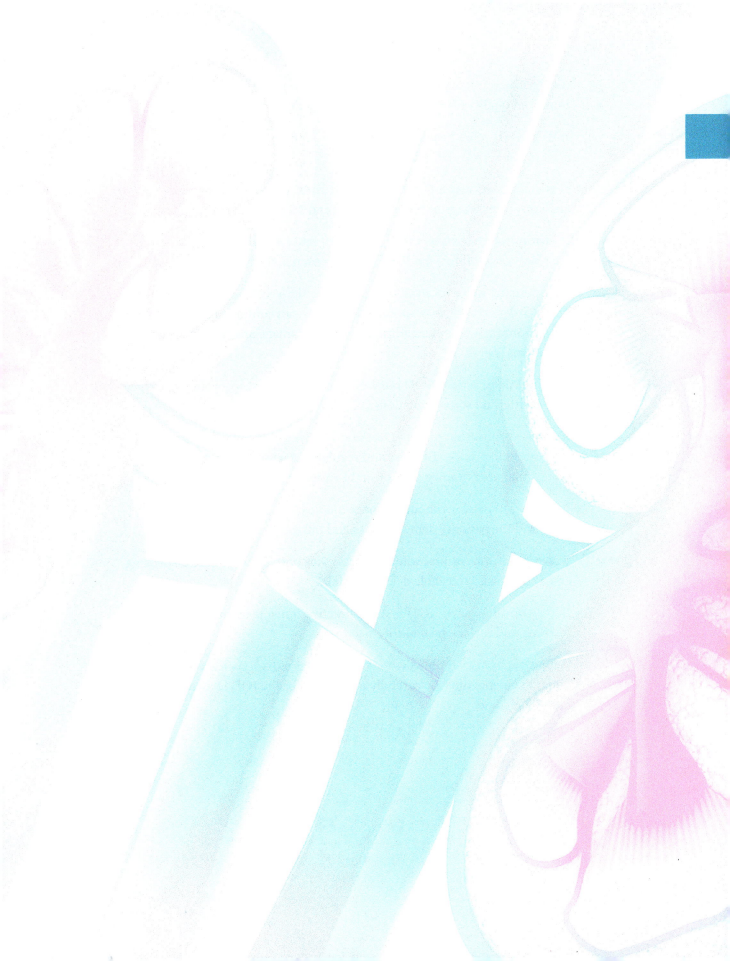

KEY POINTS

- **An in-office dispensary** can result in added convenience for patients, improved quality of care, and patient satisfaction.

- **IOD success** relies heavily on compliance, staff structure, contracting, software, and provider adherence.

- **It is helpful to review the drugs that the practice plans to dispense** and know their margins for commercial and Medicare Part D plans.

- **It is imperative to have a thorough legal review of federal, state, and local laws, regulatory bodies, and state pharmacy boards.**

- **A dispensing network design requires participation and function mainly on a third-party payer system,** which consists of commercial insurance payers, pharmacy services administrative organizations, and pharmacy benefit managers.

- **Staffing the practice's IOD** relies on size, structure, scope, volume of dispensing, and state regulations.

- **Urology groups that are geographically/strategically centralized have a distinct advantage.** Delivery and regulatory factors weigh heavily on groups that are not integrated or in the same location.

- **Dispensing software** should manage intake of e-prescriptions from the EHR and the patient's demographics and bill the pharmacy benefits.

- **Operations are optimal** when a practice has both point-of-care dispensing and a secure and trackable delivery system.

- **Before developing an IOD system,** practices must perform local market research and review the scale of cost.

- **Due to changing reimbursement guidelines in dispensing,** costs and reimbursements must be carefully monitored for the IOD to avoid losing practice income.

Christopher Setzler, MBA, CMPE and Simi Banipal, BS, RHIT

Chris Setzler is the President of UroMSO, a division of Specialty Networks, LLC.

Chris has over 25 years of experience in the healthcare space with expertise in: Revenue Cycle Management, Integrated Medical Delivery Systems, Patient Population Management, Medical Operations, Healthcare Analytics, and Technology.

Chris was formally the Chief Operating Officer of UroPartners. UroPartners, a Chicago-based independent medical group, is one of the largest Urology practices in the country. Previous to UroPartners, Chris was the founder and owner of Healthcare Provider Management (HPM). HPM focused on independent medical groups in the private sector and quickly became a leader in developing Private Medical Practices into successful and thriving organizations. Prior to HPM, Chris was the Administrator at Graduate Hospital Department of Medicine and Research Foundation.

Simi Banipal, B.S, RHIT

Simi Banipal, B.S, RHIT is the Director of In-Office Dispensary at Uropartners LLC, one of the largest urology practices in the country. She is responsible for managing the operations of Advanced Prostate Cancer Department at Uropartners. She is a healthcare management professional with over 12 years of experience in Revenue Cycle Management, Health Insurance, Operations Project Management and Coding Compliance. She is a certified coder, credentialed through American Health Information Management Association (AHIMA). Currently, she is pursuing her MBA post graduate degree in Healthcare Administration.

CHAPTER 2

Durable Medical Equipment: Operationalizing an In-House Catheter Service

Alan D. Winkler, MHSA, FACMPE

Identifying new ancillary revenue opportunities is critical to a medical practice's success. With consolidation of market forces, such as insurance carriers merging with retail pharmacy chains—physicians' margins on medications and imaging revenue will continue to decline. What once was protected as a physician office function is being extracted through a variety of initiatives by both the Centers for Medicare and Medicaid Services (CMS) and commercial carriers. Incorporating services, such as catheters, into the urology practice allows physicians to reinsert themselves in the continuum of care. It provides seamless service to patients while replacing dwindling income from other ancillary services.

Many urology practices assume the margin and market for ancillary services like catheters are not worth the practice integration effort. This is caused by confusion around durable medical equipment policies and the long-standing stronghold many national catheters have had in the market.

Intermittent catheters are paid by the CMS Durable Medical Equipment (DME) carriers; however, the catheters are considered under Medicare to be a Prosthetic Benefit. Durable means "reusable," and most catheters are single-use items. Catheters are designed to replace all or part of the function of a permanently inoperative or malfunctioning organ. Meeting criteria for coverage of intermittent catheters requires permanent urinary incontinence or retention. "Permanent" in Medicare terminology is a physical requirement lasting more than 90 days.

While several well-established national catheter companies provide a similar service, urology practices have the opportunity to further participate in the continuum of care, provide structured education for patients, and help ensure patient success with a catheter service. There are specific guidelines, which must be followed; however, once a system is put in place, staff members can easily provide exemplary service while the practice earns a reasonable return on its investment.

While specific costs and profit margin by individual product are proprietary, the economics of a catheter service easily justify the meticulous effort required to maintain operational logistics and compliance. Historical direct expense of 53% (salaries/benefits at 14%; supplies at 38%; occupancy at 1%) can translate to a gross distribution per year of up to $25,000 per partner per year. The service line grows slowly over the first few years, then stabilizes over the subsequent years with an average of 17-20 recurring patients per physician per month as patients are added and removed from the service line.

Under CMS regulations, patients must have a choice of DME suppliers. Although it is appropriate to outline the benefits of your practice providing the service, it should be made clear to the patient that he retains the right to select whatever supplier he prefers. Benefits of the practice providing the catheters include seamless and timely communication regarding modifications in usage and type of catheter. Remember, catheters require an order and your physicians and advanced practice providers are the ones placing the order. Respecting the patient's wishes is critical in terms of meeting regulatory requirements; however, most patients will choose convenience and effective care coordination when making healthcare decisions.

Since DME—in this instance, catheters and related supplies—is an integral part of a urology practice's treatment regimen, it may be simpler to treat the service just as you would any other practice-based service like x-ray, CT, cystoscopy, etc. Approaching the venture from the inherent ancillary perspective also facilitates managed care contracting, billing/collections, etc. Most importantly, it provides for integrated clinical care, which better meets the needs of the patient by streamlining points of contact.

Integrating the ordering process within your EMR system via Order Sets just as you do with other ancillary services such as CT, KUBs, etc. makes the ordering process inside the practice simpler than it is through separate paper forms required by outside DME companies. Having your DME division process insurance authorizations for internal referrals, including submitting required medical records, further incentivizes the physicians and medical assistants to appropriately promote your practice's DME service. If the medical assistant or nurse must handle all aspects of the external referrals (submitting records, completing forms), he is more likely to promote the established benefits of coordinated care offered by your DME division if his role ends at submitting the order.

The historical assumption of medical practices has been that ancillary services like this require separate incorporation. This simply is not true. This is an ancillary service, not a separate business. If a practice were to establish a separate corporation for DME, such as a Limited Liability Company (LLC), it must follow the Department of Health and Human Services Office of Inspector General's Safe Harbor "60/40 Investors Rule." It) requires that 60% of the value of the investment interests that relate to that specific health-related service or product must be held by those who: are not in a position to make or influence referrals; furnish items or services to the entity; or otherwise generate business for the entity. In effect, this means at least 60% of the business generated in the DME/catheter business must come from outside your group of investors.

> The first 60-40 rule, known as the "60-40 investor rule," requires that no more than 40 percent of the investment interests of the entity be held by investors who are in a position to make or influence referrals to, furnish items or services to, or otherwise generate business for the entity.

This is a difficult threshold to meet. As an ancillary service functioning under the same Tax ID number and same provisions of other ancillary services within the medical practice, the 60/40 rule does not apply.

Professional liability risk for catheters is no higher than it is for any other urologic service, so there is no compelling reason to establish a separate corporation to protect against undue risk. Start-up costs for the service are minimal, so there is no need for external investors. Treat the catheter service line just as you do any other ancillary and avoid the most challenging aspects of the venture.

EXTERNAL ACCESS

Under CMS regulations, patients have a right to choose the provider of their care—hospitals, physicians, DME, catheters, etc. If a patient indicates a preference, it must be respected. For example, if the patient's aunt used a national catheter provider and she wishes to do the same, you must respect the patient's wishes and cooperate with that provider to establish service. However, that cooperation typically extends no further than providing an appropriate order and the supporting documentation, as well as any follow-up medical chart documentation needed to continue the service. It does not mean that company has a right to come onsite and market its services to other patients.

A practice is under no obligation to allow any outside company to market onsite to its patients. Catheter companies have no right to demand access to your providers or to your patients. Just as a practice may choose to limit access to pharmaceutical and/or medical device sales representatives, it has a right to refuse access to catheter companies.

Transparency is key in proving that your practice is compliant. You may choose to include a listing of other catheter service providers and their 1-800 phone number on your web-site, which is accessible by patients. You may choose, instead, to post a notice or create a rack card advertising your in-house catheter service, but mentioning that the patient has a right to select any catheter provider he wishes. It is advisable to change vendors only when requested to do so by the patient or caregiver and to document that request. In other words, when you open a catheter service, do not automatically move all patients from existing external providers to your service. Allow the service to grow organically and function as one of the options a patient may select.

OPERATIONALIZING THE SERVICE

When the practice identifies a patient who needs catheters, the EMR template may be constructed as a series of questions:

Has the patient cathed in the past? YES

Does the patient have a specific catheter supplier he prefers to use?

YES Fax an order to that company along with progress notes. The company then bears the responsibility of contacting the patient and arranging for the service. The medical practice is not responsible for verifying insurance coverage for the external company.

NO Introduce your practice's DME service and ask if he would like to use your service for the catheters. The use of a simple marketing "rack" card may provide contact information. The order is placed via the electronic medical record, and the in-house catheter service accesses the patient's medical record, contacts the insurance carrier, and contacts the patient with delivery date/cost information. The practice's clinical staff typically are not involved once a complete and accurate order is processed by the provider.

Has the patient cathed in the past? NO

1 Introduce your practice's DME service and ask if he would like to use your service for the catheters. The use of a simple marketing "rack" card may provide contact information. The order is placed via the electronic medical record, and the in-house catheter service accesses the patient's medical record, contacts the insurance carrier, and contacts the patient with delivery date/cost information. The practice's clinical staff typically are not involved once a complete and accurate order is processed by the provider.

2 Remind the patient that additional catheter companies' contact information appears on your website and is available via web search if he prefers.

3 Secure patient's preference.

Modifications may be made to prior order catheters to ensure that neither the patient nor his insurance carrier pays for catheters that will not be used. This is doable since the practice's DME service contacts the patient each month to determine remaining supply address any concerns or questions, and has immediate access to the patient's electronic medical record.

BILLING FOR CATHETERS

Although there are specific guidelines for when catheters are covered, the actual set of billable codes is surprisingly small:

> **A4351** Intermittent urinary catheter; straight tip, with or without coating, each
>
> **A4352** Intermittent urinary catheter, coude (curved) tip, with or without coating, each
>
> **A4353** Intermittent urinary catheter, with insertion supplies
>
> **A4332** Lubricant, individual sterile packet, for insertion of urinary catheter with sterile technique

DOCUMENTATION REQUIREMENTS

While documentation requirements are similar between carriers, it is important to review specific requirements under carrier policies. For Medicare, items must be reasonable and necessary for the diagnosis or treatment of illness or injury. A patient's record must include the following:

- The treating provider's office records, which typically will be the urology practice's generated chart note and order,

- Any relevant hospital, nursing home, and/or home health agency records, and

- Records from other healthcare professionals and/or test results, which establish a need for the service.

Since CMS requires documentation be maintained for seven years, it is important that the record clearly establishes the patient's diagnosis, duration of condition, clinical course of care, prognosis, and functional limitations. CMS does not deem supplier-produced records as part of a patient's medical chart, so a practice should not depend on the distributor's/supplier's documentation to establish medical necessity or substantiate service provision.

At a minimum, the documentation relating to the DME order must include the following:

- Detailed written order, which includes the patient's name, the prescribing provider's name, and the date of the order. The order must support both the initial need and the continued use of the item.

- Under Section 6407 of the Affordable Care Act, payment also is contingent on the treating (prescribing) physician having had a face-to-face encounter examination with the patient within six months of writing an order for certain items of DME. Oddly enough, the provider who conducted the examination does not have to be the prescriber for the DME item; however, the prescriber must verify that the in-person exam occurred within the six months prior to completion of the written order.

- Electronic documentation/signature acceptable. The order is invalid without a written or electronic signature.

- Certificate of Medical Necessity currently is not required for catheters; however, audit rates are high, so it is best to check the Local Coverage Determination (LCD) policies for specific DME carrier requirements.

- Beneficiary authorization is documented.

- Proof of delivery.

    - An Advance Beneficiary Notice of Noncoverage (ABN) is issued if non-coverage is suspected/known prior to delivery. It must be issued prior to dispensing an item. You cannot routinely issue ABNs just to cover yourself in the event of a denial. If CMS (Medicare) does not ever allow the item, no ABN is needed. If Medicare might otherwise pay for the item, but you do not expect Medicare to allow it, an ABN is necessary. For example, when a patient insists on receiving more catheters than Medicare allows, or if the patient's period of usage is less than required by Medicare, but the patient insists on the service being billed to Medicare, you can issue an ABN which states, "Medicare does not pay for this item or service at quantities more than xx." ABNs are not effective for more than one year. Extensive ABN resources are available at: https://bit.ly/CMSmedicare and on the Medicare Learning Network at: https://bit.ly/CMSOutreach.

- Supporting documentation for any specific modifiers used.

- Commercial carriers, such as Blue Cross Blue Shield and United Health Care typically follow Medicare guidelines for coverage. For example, United Health Care's Guideline Number MPG359.04, approved on May 8, 2019, states:

    "When urological supplies are furnished in a physician's office, they may be billed only if the beneficiary's condition meets the definition of permanence. (In this situation, the catheters and related supplies are covered under the prosthetic device benefit.) If the beneficiary's condition is expected to be temporary, urological supplies may not be billed. (In this situation, they are considered as supplies provided incident to a physician's service, and payment is included in the allowance for the physician services.) When billing for urological supplies furnished in a physician's office for a permanent impairment, use the place of service code corresponding to the beneficiary's current place of residence; do not use POS 11, office."

Always check online for specific coverage limitations and documentation requirements for commercial carriers, as some benefits may vary by specific employer group plan.

CORRECTIONS TO MEDICAL DOCUMENTATION

All changes to original documentation must clearly identify what was originally in the record, in addition to any amendment, correction, or reason for delayed entry. All entries must reflect the date and author. Paper chart entries should have a single line to strike through what is being changed. The signature or the initials of the author of the change should be accompanied by the date of the change. Stamped signatures are not acceptable. Electronic entries require the same attention to detail, allowing an auditor to reconstruct the original order/documentation and all subsequent addendums/changes.

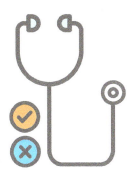

For Medicare, attestation statements may be submitted after the fact unless the carrier's policy states a signature must be in place prior to the provision of the service/item. It is imperative that LCD policies be reviewed prior to opening a DME service. Periodic review of the applicable LCDs is recommended.

Who May Order DME Services?

- Physicians

- Advanced Practice Providers, such as a nurse practitioner (NP), a Physician Assistant (PA), or a Clinical Nurse Specialist (CNS).

A new order is required when there is a change in the product or quantity.

RECURRING ORDERS REQUIRE THE SUPPLIER TO:

- Since urological supplies are consumable, you must document the quantity of the supply item remaining for use by the patient, and determine if that supply will be almost exhausted by the next delivery date. Automatic shipments are not permitted. You must contact the patient no sooner than 14 calendar days prior to dispensing.

- Not deliver items sooner than 10 calendar days prior to the end of the current product's scheduled/prescribed usage period.

▶ Proof of Delivery

As the supplier, you are required to demonstrate proof of delivery by documenting the following items:

- Patient's name and address.

- The delivery service's package ID number, supplier invoice number, or by an alternative means, which ties the DME supplier (urology practice) with the delivery service's (such as USPS, UPS, DHL, etc.) records.

- Shipping date (CMS does allow this to be the date the shipping order/label is created or the date the item began its transit to the patient.)

- Delivery date.

- Quantity delivered.

COMPREHENSIVE ERROR RATE TESTING (CERT)

CMS contracts with independent medical review companies to retrospectively audit DME claims for compliance with Medicare guidelines. These CERT entities will review a sampling of DME claims and will assist in educating the provider of recurrent errors. CERTs do have the ability to initiate recoupments for overpayments or initiate payments for underpaid claims. CERT data is used to report error rates for fee-for-service claims on an annual basis. These rates do not necessarily suggest fraudulent activity, but rather activity which resulted in inappropriate payment.

DME services are among the most highly audited services paid by Medicare, so it is imperative that a group have a clear understanding of the guidelines, have internal monitoring/auditing processes in place, and allocate appropriate resources to deal with regular audits from CMS and private insurance carriers. The high audit rate should not discourage practices from providing DME services; however, it should inform those practices of the importance of knowing and carefully following the guidelines published by each carrier.

CERT errors may be appealed, and each region's CERT auditing company can provide the specifics of its auditing and appeal processes. Because CERTs audit all types of DME services, one should understand that many of its efforts are around the larger cost items such as Oxygen, PAP and PAP supplies, Prostheses, and Ostomy supplies.

If CMS or a CERT contractor identifies a high error rate or billing practices that appear to be inconsistent with similar providers, a Target Probe and Educate (TPE) process may be initiated in which 20-40 claims per provider or type of service are reviewed. Providers then are offered individualized education based on the results of the review.

TPE activities are not intended to be punitive but rather instructive. DME providers should view these TPE activities as opportunities to correct recurrent errors before a full-scale audit is triggered.

MEDICARE COVERAGE GUIDELINES

Understanding Medicare's coverage guidelines is essential. While you should check Local Coverage Determination policies for variations in the general Medicare guidelines, the requirements outlined below have remained unchanged for many years.

- **To qualify for catheters** under Medicare guidelines, patients must have:

  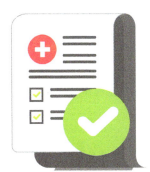

  - **Permanent urinary incontinence (R32) or urinary retention (R33.9)** for greater than 90 days documented in the chart notes.

  - Been **trained on self-catheterizations** or have an appointed person trained on self-catheterizations AND

- **The patient must be in retention.** Stricture is not enough in itself.

- **EMR** notes must reflect Continuous Intermittent Catheterization that is on the catheter supply form.

- **Prescribe catheters to reflect their use:** bid = 60 per month; qid = 120 per month. The "times per day" should reflect the quantity per month (3 x daily = 90; 4 x = 120).

- **Medicare** allows for a new catheter every time a patient catheterizes with a limit of 200 per month. More than 200 may be provided with established medical necessity. However, the typical patient will require far fewer than 200. The prescribing provider should determine the actual number needed based on the patient's condition, and the medical documentation must clearly explain why a large number are needed.

  - The patient or caregiver must request refills of urological supplies before they are dispensed. The practice is not allowed to automatically dispense a quantity of supplies on a regular schedule, even if the patient has indicated a desire for the dispensing provider to do so. Since the practice is required to check with the patient prior to each catheter order, most have integrated a practice of asking about urological supply needs during the same phone call.

- **Straight Tip Catheters** – Practices should include the option "With Lube Only" on the order form. "Insertion Supplies" refers to the sterile supply pack and should not be used with a normal catheter order.

- **Coude Tip Catheters** – The profit margin on coude catheters is larger than for straight catheters; however, practices should provide coude catheters only to those patients requiring them. The supporting chart notes must state why the patient cannot pass a straight tip catheter (i.e., "due to BPH/obstruction" or "due to urethral stricture").

- **Closed System Catheters** – Two documented UTI's while practicing sterile cathing technique within a 12-month period are required unless the patient resides in a nursing facility, is a post- transplant patient, or has HIV/AIDs. When closed system catheters are ordered, the order should specify "With Insertion Supplies."

The order for all catheters must match the numbers of catheterizations needed per day, the diagnosis of retention/incontinence, and the permanence of the condition being greater than 90 days.

SUPPLY ORDER FORMS

Certain elements are required on all supply order forms for them to be compliant under Medicare and most commercial carrier guidelines. The form must specify:

- The patient's name

- Description of the item (16Fr Coude Tip Cath or 12Fr Straight Tip Closed Kit Cath)

- Frequency (number of caths per day)

- Length of Need (Must be at least 90 days; 99=Lifetime)

- Physician signature with date (Cannot be a signature stamp. Electronic signatures are acceptable.)

SERVICE GROWTH

One should expect a slow but steady growth trend if a practice chooses to grow its DME/catheter business organically by adding patients incrementally as the need arises and as the patients select the practice as the provider. Reasonable projections suggest a practice with a patient visit volume of 100,000 visits per year to add roughly 500 catheter patients per year. While this may seem inconsequential, it is important to remember that the patient base is ordering catheters monthly so one patient may represent 2,400 catheters per year. A monthly patient base of 350 represents sales of almost 70,000 catheters per month.

Be patient as the service grows. Be attentive to providing exemplary service. Be precise in record keeping. Remain focused on accurate billing and attentive to filing appeals when services were provided according to the carrier's guidelines. Many times, the service with the greatest benefit to the patient also benefits the medical practice.

CONCLUSION

As healthcare integrates across the care continuum, the urology practice should be ready to carefully evaluate and intentionally implement new ancillary service lines, which improve service to our patients and augment efforts to grow the revenue base. Office visits and minor procedures may keep the doors open, but they cannot sustain a practice in a time of cost increases and a stagnant reimbursement environment. Add in the challenges of a dwindling pool of available urologists, and the impetus for change is clear.

Urology practices interested in expanding services into durable medical equipment through initiation of a catheter division should carefully construct a plan of action which is built on exemplary patient service while remaining vigilant about regulatory and contractual compliance.

Identifying new revenue opportunities means identifying new ways to provide compassionate, timely, and needed services for our patients. DME can be part of that plan.

KEY POINTS

- **Structure the service simply and efficiently,** leveraging existing staff and space where appropriate while ensuring a clear understanding of and commitment to regulatory requirements.

- **Create EMR templates and order sets** which streamline the processing of orders while still offering patients choice.

- **Document the underlying need for the services being provided** and follow CMS (Medicare/Medicaid/Government Payer) guidelines for coverage, as well as being aware of variations required by the managed care carriers.

- **Set up an effective communication and tracking system** to ensure patients are provided only with the services they need and that those services are provided in a timely, cost-efficient manner.

- **Focus on key provisions such as patient contact** prior to filling a recurring order, capturing/retaining proof of delivery documents.

- **Be patient.** Catheter services grow organically over time. Do it right the first time, and ensure you retain the customer and the business over time.

ABOUT THE AUTHOR

Alan D. Winkler, MHSA, FACMPE

With thirty-nine years of experience in healthcare, Alan D. Winkler has served as the Executive Director of Urology San Antonio, P.A. since October 2012. Alan holds a master's degree in Health Services from the University of Arkansas for Medical Sciences and has worked in private and corporate settings with physicians of many specialties. Alan is a Fellow in the American College of Medical Practice Executives (MGMA ACMPE) and served on its board of directors for nine years, concluding as its chair. Mr. Winkler currently serves on the LUGPA Board of Directors.

CHAPTER

Developing a Radiation Oncology Center

Patrick R. Aldinger, RT, (R) (T)
Stephen M. Beach, PhD, DABR
Terry FitzPatrick, MPA

Urology groups that have adopted the approach of caring for a man throughout his lifetime after a diagnosis of prostate cancer have found that radiation therapy is an important piece of the treatment continuum. Radiation Centers are expensive to develop, which tends to make groups hesitant moving forward, but given appropriate volumes they are good long-term investments. A medical group-owned radiation oncology center allows the group to control the quality of care provided to the patient, is a significant source of revenue for the practice, and allows the patient to remain connected within the practice throughout the course of treatment. Additionally, with the number of treatments needed, having the service within the practice is more convenient for the patient.

CENTER STAFFING

A standard staffing ratio for one linear accelerator center would be a radiation oncologist, medical physicist, dosimetrist, registered nurse or certified medical assistant, receptionist, and biller. A minimum of two radiation therapists are needed (per LINAC), but ideally three are necessary for full coverage, with two therapists working on the machine at all times, while the third therapist typically acts as the lead or chief therapist.

THE RADIATION ONCOLOGIST

The primary role of the radiation oncologist (RO) is to oversee the care of the patient in the radiation setting. The RO typically will consult with a patient (60-90 minutes) for radiation therapy, brachytherapy, or Xofigo® administration. If the patient decides to proceed with radiation therapy, the RO will order fiducial placements and/or SpaceOAR® implant (if necessary) along with a CT scan. The CT scan is used to create the personalized radiation therapy plan for the patient, and the RO will contour tumor volumes on this scan and other pertinent aspects specific to the patient's plan. A prescription is created by the RO that supports the amount of radiation each patient shall receive. The RO is responsible for proper documentation of all consults, prescriptions, orders, etc.

All patients who receive external beam radiation therapy should have a weekly visit with the RO. During this visit (10-15 minutes), the RO discusses the patient's general health, any side effects he or she may have, and determines if radiation treatments shall resume as prescribed. The RO also reviews daily/weekly images (port films or CBCT images) to ensure accurate radiation delivery.

The radiation oncologist will consult with patients receiving Xofigo® treatments, typically for about 60-90 minutes. If the patient is viewed as a good candidate for the drug and consents to treatment, the RO will prescribe Xofigo® and provide proper documentation. When Xofigo® is administered, the physicist plays a significant role in ordering and verifying the dosage, while the RO performs the drug administration and documents appropriately.

MEDICAL PHYSICIST

The medical physicist's primary commitment is to the patients' treatment accuracy and their safety. The physicist will perform weekly, monthly, and annual quality assurance tests (QA) on the linear accelerator to verify that the proper dose will be delivered to the patient. During treatment planning, the physicist works in conjunction with the RO and dosimetrist to create a plan that maximizes effectiveness while sparing healthy tissue. Once a radiation treatment plan is complete, the physicist performs a QA examination of the patient's personal treatment plan on the linear accelerator; this is done prior to the patient coming in for treatment to confirm machine output matches the computer plan.

Typically, the physicist also acts as the clinic's radiation safety officer who monitors and maintains records of the staffs' exposure to radiation as well as maintains and enforces onsite procedure/protocols involving radiation.

The medical physicist oversees and modifies, when necessary, items located in Data Administration and Radiation Therapy Administration within the Radiation Oncology Electronic Medical Record (ARIA or IMPAC). With Xofigo®, the medical physicist is responsible for maintaining the hot lab, calibrating the dose, assaying the dose, assessing the release-ability of the now radioactive patient, assessing the room post procedure, and facilitating the storage of radioactive materials and any radioactive waste generated by a Xofigo® administration.

DOSIMETRIST

The dosimetrist works directly under the radiation oncologist and uses software programs (e.g. Eclipse or Pinnacle) to create the radiation treatment plan for the patient based on the radiation oncologist's (RO) prescription.

The patient's safety and minimizing radiation exposure to healthy tissue and organs is of utmost importance to the dosimetrist. Upon completion of the RO and medical physicist-approved treatment plan, the dosimetrist then builds QA plans for the medical physicist to evaluate and run on the treatment machine. Proper billing and documentation are completed by the dosimetrist in the patient's chart throughout the planning process.

RADIATION THERAPISTS/LEAD THERAPIST

The radiation therapists' (RTs) primary commitment is to deliver accurate radiation treatments to the patient and assure his or her safety. The RTs warm up the linear accelerator on a daily basis and run the medical physicist- prescribed QA using the DailyQA™3 array (from SunNuclear or equivalent) and the MIMI phantom cube (from Standard Imaging or equivalent), prior to starting treatments for that day.

When a patient decides to pursue radiation treatments, the therapists perform the CT scan necessary to create a radiation plan. For an onsite CT scanner, radiation therapists also perform morning QA. When the patient's plan is complete and approved by both the RO and medical physicist, the RT schedules the patient for treatments on the LINAC. Once the patient is scheduled, the chart is reviewed to assure all is in order for treatments to take place. The RTs deliver daily radiation treatments to the patient, while conducting daily image management, and documenting appropriate billing. At the end of the day, the charges for the day are then exported to the billing department for review.

The RTs maintain the patient portal software and offer guidance to the patient as needed. Data administration modifications and updates are managed by the RTs. Quarterly Media-Span or equivalent updates are completed to maintain up-to-date medication lists and possible interactions. RTs also gather Meaningful Use data when it is due and prepare it for submission along with Physician Quality Reporting System material.

CERTIFIED MEDICAL ASSISTANT AND/OR NURSE

The certified medical assistant (CMA) or nurse is responsible for gathering the medical records necessary for the radiation oncologist to carry out the consult with the patient. This task includes entering the data in the radiation oncology electronic medical record (EMR) to meet both clinical and meaningful use standards. The CMA or nurse takes patients—both new consults and those scheduled for ongoing treatments—to the exam rooms and administers patient assessment for RO review. CMAs or nurses also perform the patients' blood work and administer hormone therapy injections. The CMA or nurse regularly reviews patient medications and maintains an up-to-date list in the radiation oncology EMR.

RECEPTIONIST

The receptionist is typically the first person in the radiation center who the patient encounters. Therefore, it is of the utmost importance for the first impression to be caring, sincere, and professional. The receptionist organizes and schedules the patient for consults, fiducial placements, and/or SpaceOAR® implant (if necessary), CT simulations, and any other procedure that may pertain to radiation therapy. The receptionist also receives all telephone calls that come into the facility and routes them to correct staff.

BILLING STAFF

Billing staff oversees billing and coding functions of the center. They ensure services are preauthorized, work with patients to understand their insurance coverage, develop payment plans as necessary, and answer patient questions regarding payments and insurance. They work with the lead therapist to export daily charges generated from procedures, treatments, and consults. Billing staff also keeps billing procedures up to date with current changes in the Centers for Medicare and Medicaid Services' reimbursements and makes sure that proper charges are being applied. In addition, billing staff members work with insurance companies when a claim is denied.

STANDARD BUILDING LAYOUT

When designing a radiation oncology facility, the key aspect is a vault to house the medical grade linear accelerator (LINAC), which requires a significant amount of shielding. Working with a qualified Medical Physicist or Health Physicist the vault is normally constructed out of poured concrete of the proper thicknesses. For example, any wall surface that the direct radiation beam could strike is upwards of 8 feet thick of solid poured concrete while the remaining walls are 5 feet thick. There could be substantial cost savings if the vault is located in a basement as the dirt surrounding the vault is normally adequate for shielding purposes. The roof of the vault is also shielded with poured concrete, the thickness of which will depend upon the surrounding buildings' height, proximity, and occupancy. If the vault is located above the first floor of a building or has a basement below, then the same shielding requirements apply to the floor. There must be a control area near the vault where therapists manage the treatment machine, and it houses the multiple computers and monitors utilized by the therapists. In addition to having the vault, CT simulations are needed. Some medical practices that already have a CT scanner may choose to do the CT simulations at the existing CT scanner; others choose to have a CT scanner at the radiation center to perform CT scans onsite. If one chooses to perform the CT scans onsite, a control room and shielded CT vault to house the scanner are required. A restroom connected to the CT vault is also advised. Additional facility aspects include: a waiting area, both in the reception area and near the vault (for gowned patients), a minimum of three exam rooms, multiple changing rooms, a nursing station, staff offices, ample storage space, and plenty restrooms for patient use as they are usually treated with full bladders.

The layout of the building typically has the front waiting area and the receptionist's desk (office space) controlling the flow of patients to the rest of the facility. The nurse's station is normally next in the flow of patient movement and is bordered by the exam rooms. Restrooms are near this area for waiting room and exam rooms. The shielded vaults (both LINAC and CT simulator) are typically at the rear of the facility and the flow of patients at this point is strictly controlled by the therapists. The patient changing rooms should be located very close to the vaults and normally have locking doors to house the patient's valuables while they are treated. Restrooms near the treatment vault and changing rooms are pertinent. Staff offices typically include at least 5 offices: Radiation Oncologist, Medical Physicist, Dosimetrist, Lead Therapist/building administrator, and billing staff. Office space for these staff is really at the discretion of the architect, however one particular element should be present in the offices of the Radiation Oncologist, Medical Physicist, and Dosimetrist and that is the ability to completely darken the office space while work is done with the patients' CT data sets (similar to requirements for Radiologists as they read films). Other aspects of the building should include an IT closet for housing the servers and computer equipment required along with storage rooms for radiation equipment (Vac-Lok bags, positioning equipment, etc.). It may also be necessary to build a hot lab for the preparation and verification of the Xofigo dose for administration if your center will be providing this service.

ISSUES TO CONSIDER BEFORE BUILDING A RADIATION CENTER

When considering whether or not to build a radiation center, a medical practice should be prepared to make a significant capital investment—up to $5 million, depending on a variety of factors, including facility size, land values, equipment required, and construction costs.

WHAT EQUIPMENT IS NEEDED?

Any specific equipment models and/or vendors named in the following section are for illustrative purposes only. Naming specific models is not an endorsement or recommendation.

➡ *Equipment Leasing*

Medical equipment leasing can substantially lower the upfront cost of developing a radiation oncology center. In the long run, the group pays more than it would in purchase financing. But the upside is that leasing makes it easier to turn over equipment and upgrade to the latest models. What is more, the IRS treats operating leases as monthly payments for the expense of doing business. This decreases a practice's income, which could reduce taxes owed.

➡ *Linear Accelerator (LINAC) and Vault Room*

The most critical piece of equipment for the radiation center is a LINAC. It is housed in a shielded vault as designed by an approved medical physicist or health physicist. The LINAC should be dual photon energy and multiple electron energy capable. The dual photon energies (high and low mega-voltage beams) allow for a better treatment plan tailored to each patient's unique geometry and tissue composition than that provided by a single energy LINAC. The ability to treat with electrons broadens the center's ability to treat more patients with different types of cancer.

The LINAC must come equipped with a beam defining multi-leaf collimator (MLC). This is a computer-controlled set of tungsten "leaves" that are arrayed in two opposing banks of leaf sets mounted on the exit port of the accelerator structure. The individual MLC leaves either block or allow radiation through their positions depending upon the patient's treatment plan. The industry standard is 120 leaves, 60 on each side.

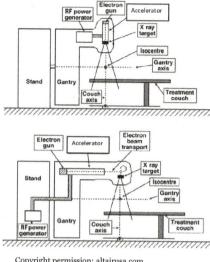

Copyright permission: altairusa.com

If necessary, other options allow for finer detail in the radiation beam output such as a micro-MLC where the tungsten leaves are thinner. (These are often utilized in brain radiosurgery treatments). MLCs are usually purchased with a software license from the LINAC vendor. The ability to have the MLCs deliver intensity modulated radiation therapy (IMRT) treatments is key to being able to deliver precise and high-dose radiation treatment plans.

▶ Imaging Options

With the purchase of the LINAC, the clinic will need to choose how it will image patients to be able to target the specific location of the cancer. Most common and least expensive is imaging with the treatment beam via an electronic portal imager device (EPID). This allows for snapshots of the patient anatomy in the treatment position, usually taken from orthogonal angles to determine 3D shifts. The other common, yet more expensive option of linear accelerator by Varian Medical Systems (a radiation oncology treatment and software vendor) is the addition of a kiloVoltage X-ray tube and associated imaging panel (mounted on the LINAC structure, but at 90 degrees from the treatment beam), referred to as the onboard imager or OBI. The kiloVoltage imaging will allow for superior soft tissue imaging, as well as the option to use it as a cone beam computed topography (CBCT) for daily positioning of the patient.

Yet another option for treatment site tracking and monitoring is the 4D localization system known as Calypso®. Calypso uses electromagnetic tracking beacons (three) that are placed into the prostate and monitored via radiofrequencies during a patient's treatment. If treatment site movement is detected outside the set tolerances, the therapists are alerted and can stop the treatment beam and make adjustments

The treatment vault will need to be outfitted with a closed-circuit camera system with at least two in-room cameras and an audio/intercom system for the radiation therapists to communicate with the patient who is inside the vault during treatment. Positional lasers calibrated to converge on the "isocenter" of the LINAC are also necessary. An in-room radiation detector that will visually alert those outside the vault when radiation is present within will need to be in place. If the LINAC is not set up to be on city water, a chiller is necessary to maintain appropriate LINAC water temperature as dictated by the LINAC vendor.

Using the LINAC will require a service contract with the LINAC manufacturer or third-party vendor. Prior to treating patients, there will need to be a full commissioning of the LINAC by an approved medical physicist, either by a consulting medical physics group or by the onsite physicist.

In order to complete the commissioning by the onsite physicist, the following items are needed:

- A scanning water tank with minimum of 40 cm sides
- Scanning software for the water tank
- Laptop to run the water tank
- Calibrated multiple channel electrometer
- Calibrated 0.6cc Farmer type therapy class ion chamber, such as the PTW model n30013 or equivalent
- Two calibrated small volume ion chambers, such as the PTW 31010 0.125cc ion chamber or equivalent
- Calibrated micro-point ion chamber such as the 0.007cc Exradin model (A16) ion chamber or equivalent
- Calibrated PTW pinpoint ion chamber or equivalent
- Calibrated thermometer
- Calibrated barometer (corrected for altitude etc.)
- Calibrated hand held radiation survey meter
- Calibrated handheld neutron radiation survey meter

Other necessary pieces of equipment include an ion chamber/diode array for the daily morning warm-up measurements made by the radiation therapists, along with a agreement to maintain its relevance.

Also required are imaging phantoms to maintain the image quality of the portal imaging system and onboard imaging (OBI) system. This includes an *MV* phantom, kV phantom and phantom for daily verification of IGRT (QC-3, QCkV-1, and MIMI phantoms respectively). In addition, associated software for tracking image quality to allow for other monthly and annual testing of the accelerator is also necessary.

In order for the physicist to maintain the output of the LINAC, some supplies from the commissioning list will be needed (Farmer type ion chamber, electrometer, thermometer, and barometer, all calibrated by the appropriate standards lab), in addition to a diode array, such as the MapCheck®2 system by SunNuclear or an equivalent ion chamber array to check for planar fluency. Software support and a service contract will be necessary to maintain relevance of the software that runs the diode/ion chamber array.

CT Simulation

The CT simulation room will need to be shielded as specified by the state or Nuclear Regulatory Commission, with a shielding survey to illustrate to the licensing entity that the scanner room is adequately shielded.

The following equipment is required for the CT simulation room:

- A multi-slice CT scanner (large bore preferably)
- Positional lasers for marking "isocenter" on the patient
- Thin tabletop pad for palliative patients
- Prone belly board
- CT couch insert that matches the LINAC's flat table top upon which the patient is treated

Additional equipment includes patient immobilization devices (vacuum positioning cushions, vacuum for the bags, neck sponges, knee wedges, pillows, wingboard, tattoo supplies, radiopaque "bb" markers, head and neck mask material, heated water tank or hot air oven for head and neck masks), contrast material and Lidocaine Urojets, penis clamps, antiseptic solution to clean clamps, cart to hold supplies, and pillows/sheets/pillow cases.

PROVIDING ELECTRON TREATMENTS

To provide electron treatments, it will be necessary to have either predefined Cerrobend electron field blocks or the ability to construct them onsite (block room). If using a block room, a Cerrobend heating tank, fume hood, stock Cerrobend, cutting/filing tools, block trays, and a cooling/vibrating table are required.

ITEMS TO CONDUCT DAILY ACTIVITIES

Following are other notable items necessary for a radiation center to conduct daily activities:

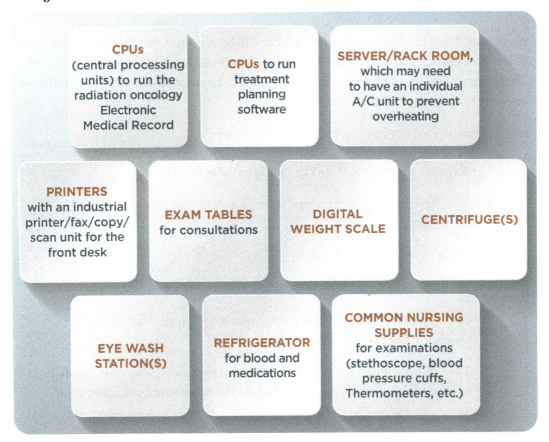

Brachytherapy is done primarily in an ambulatory surgery center; therefore, the equipment needed for a radiation center is minimal.

XOFIGO® ADMINISTRATION

Xofigo® administration requires a room designated to be the "hot lab," where constant exposure to low levels of radiation will not be an issue to surrounding rooms. It also requires a Radioactive Materials license with provisions for the use of Ra-223 as an unsealed brachytherapy treatment, issued either by the Nuclear Regulatory Commission (NRC) or the state, depending upon Agreement State status for the clinic's location.

The appropriate radioactive check sources will be required for the quality assurance and calibration of hot lab equipment; these will usually consist of:

- Cs-137 (nano-Curie size) rod source
- Eu-152 (nano-Curie size) rod source
- Co-57 (micro-Curie size) e-vial source
- Cs-137 (micro-Curie size) e-vial source
- Ba-133 (micro-Curie size) e-vial source

A one-time Ra-223 (micro-Curie size) source will be required for the initial calibration of the dose calibration setting that will be used for assaying patient treatments, and a Tc-99m source from the local radio-pharmacy will be needed every three months for linearity testing of the dose calibrator.

Other supplies for Xofigo® administration include:

- A Dose Calibrator (CRC-R from Capentic or equivalent)
- NaI (Sodium Iodide) well type wipe detector (CRC-55t from Capentic or equivalent)
- Work bench or counter space
- Leaded glass L-shield for the work bench
- Enough lead bricks to shield the equipment from any radioactive sources in the room
- Two calibrated handheld Geiger Muller survey meters (two are needed so that one can always be present while the other is out for calibration)
- Calibrated handheld ionization chamber survey meter, calibrated to read out in dose

- Various disposable items, such as wipe sample swabs, absorptive chucks, one-time use gowns, gloves, etc.

- Storage containers to hold radioactive items generated by the treatment process, so that they may decay in storage (10 half-lives) prior to disposal in the facility garbage.

SERVICES TO OFFER AT A RADIATION ONCOLOGY CENTER

External beam radiation therapy (EBRT), is the primary service provided in a radiation oncology center. EBRT is delivered with a linear accelerator (LINAC) ***using image-guided radiation therapy (IGRT)***.

IGRT and the LINAC should have no less than intensity-modulated radiotherapy (IMRT) capabilities. To perform IGRT, the radiation oncologist must locate implanted fiducials and/or soft and bony anatomy via cone beam computed tomography (CBCT), planar x-ray radiography, B-mode acquisition and targeting (BAT Ultrasound), or radiofrequency beacon tracking. Respiratory gating can be used for thoracic area treatments.

Tomotherapy, also called helical tomotherapy (HT), is a form of IMRT but differs from LINACs in that radiation is delivered slice-by-slice in a pinpointed fashion as the patient moves through the bore. Therefore, there is no need to reposition the patient during treatment.

Brachytherapy, involves inserting radioactive implants, generally called seeds, directly into the prostate, and is performed by radiation oncologists and urologists.

Xofigo® (Ra-223) infusions are also commonly offered. The process involves injecting an alpha emitting radionuclide into the bloodstream of metastatic prostate cancer patients. Xofigo® binds with minerals in the bone to deliver radiation directly to bone tumors, limiting the damage to the surrounding normal tissues.

SpaceOAR® hydrogel is an absorbable gel that is injected between the rectum and prostate. It allows for increased dose to the tumor area, while minimizing or eliminating damage to the rectum. The gel remains intact for about three months then breaks down and is absorbed by the body after roughly six months. This procedure is performed via a needle and ultrasound guidance and can be done by either a Urologist or Radiation Oncologist on an outpatient basis. Local anesthesia is used along with a sedative or Nitrous Oxide.

TrueBeam® is an advanced linear accelerator that is newer to the market. It can be used as an all-inclusive linear accelerator with the newer technologies already installed (i.e. CBCT, RapidARC®, etc.).

CyberKnife® is another device that can be used to deliver external beam radiation. When referring to the treatment of prostate cancer, the CyberKnife equipment delivers the required radiation dose to the prostate with sub-millimeter precision, thereby minimizing the radiation delivered to the bowel and urinary tract. Also, CyberKnife can deliver the desired dose in a matter of five treatment fractions compared to the traditional/conventional external beam radiation treatment timeframe of 40-45 fractions. The lack of adoption of CyberKnife in the outpatient setting has been due to the relatively high cost of the equipment.

Hypofractionation and ultrahypofractionation are methods of delivering high doses of external beam radiation in a shorter timeframe. This may be a good option for a patient, depending on a patient's risk of disease, location to a treatment center and other factors.

With a conventional intact prostate, the patient, would receive around 45 treatment fractions for their course of treatment. With hypofractionation the same total dose could be achieved in 25-30 fractions, while ultrahypofractionation can achieve the total dose in as little as 5 treatments. The verdict is still out as to whether this should be implemented as common practice as these methods of treatment are relatively new.

Typical services provided for EBRT prostate treatments:

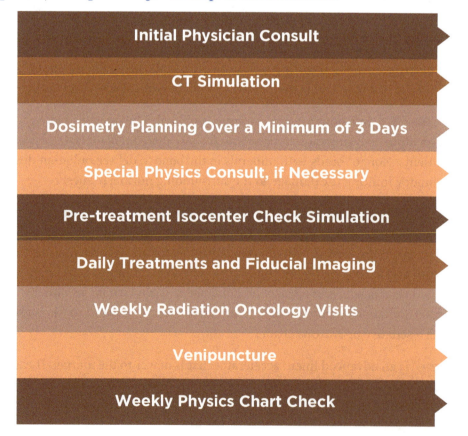

Typical services provided for brachytherapy of the prostate:

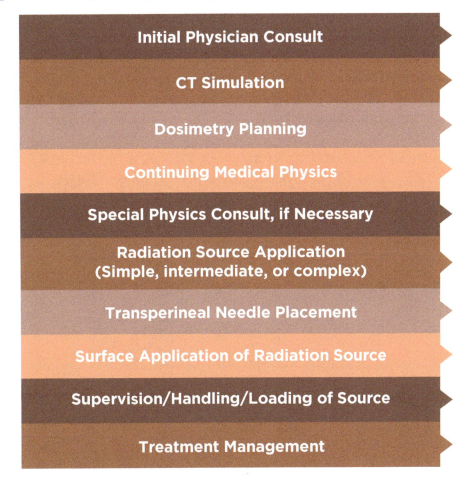

Typical services provided for Xofigo® administration:

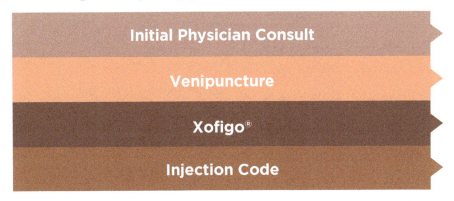

PROJECTED REIMBURSEMENT AND CHARGES

Radiation therapy treatments are covered by Medicare, Medicaid, and commercial insurance carriers; however, preauthorization requirements do exist and vary by carrier. Reimbursement rates for commercial insurances vary by region and local market rates, and charge codes may vary depending on the complexity of the exam/procedure being completed. Below are examples of reimbursement rates based on CMS 2020 fee schedule for Noridian Jurisdiction F.

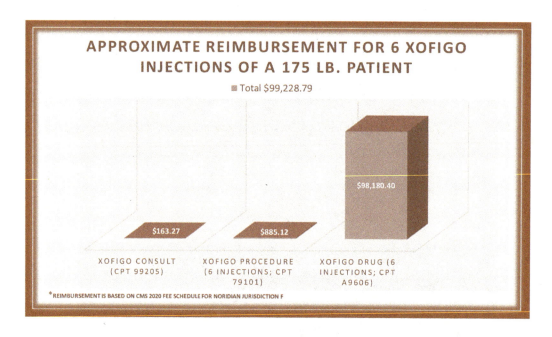

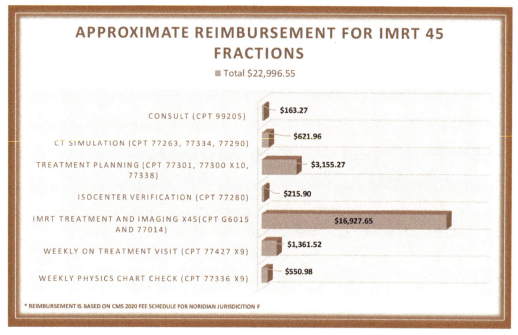

PATIENT WORKFLOW AND QUALITY CONTROL

Following is a standard patient workflow for prostate cancer external beam radiation:

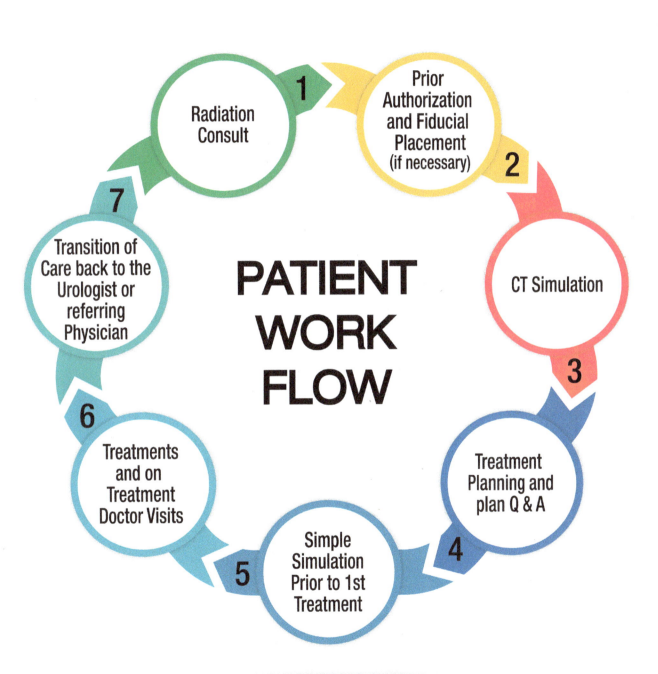

1. The patient will be referred to the radiation oncologist and placed on the schedule for a consult within a two-week window.

2. If proceeding with radiation and the insurance company gives prior authorization, the fiducial placement is scheduled within 7-10 business days, unless hormone treatment is used; then typically six weeks post hormone treatment (fiducial placement step can be omitted if necessary, fiducial placement and/or SpaceOAR procedures can also be scheduled at this.

3. CT simulation is performed at least 7 days post fiducial placement and/or SpaceOAR to allow for healing and stable placement

4. Treatment planning and plan quality assurance (QA) is done within 7-10 business days upon the doctor's treatment approval. If the treatment plan passes QA, the patient is placed on the treatment schedule in a 15-20 minute time block.

5. Prior to the patient's first radiation treatment, he or she is brought into the center for a "trial run" of the treatment plan (Simple Simulation 77280) to ensure all is in place and proper administration is carried out during treatments.

6. Once per 5 fractions, the patient will stay and visit with the radiation oncologist for weekly treatment management (77427), which usually takes 10-15 minutes.

7. Upon completion of radiation treatments, the patient is then referred back to the urologist or referring physician, and a 30-day follow-up with the radiation oncologist can be scheduled on an as-needed basis.

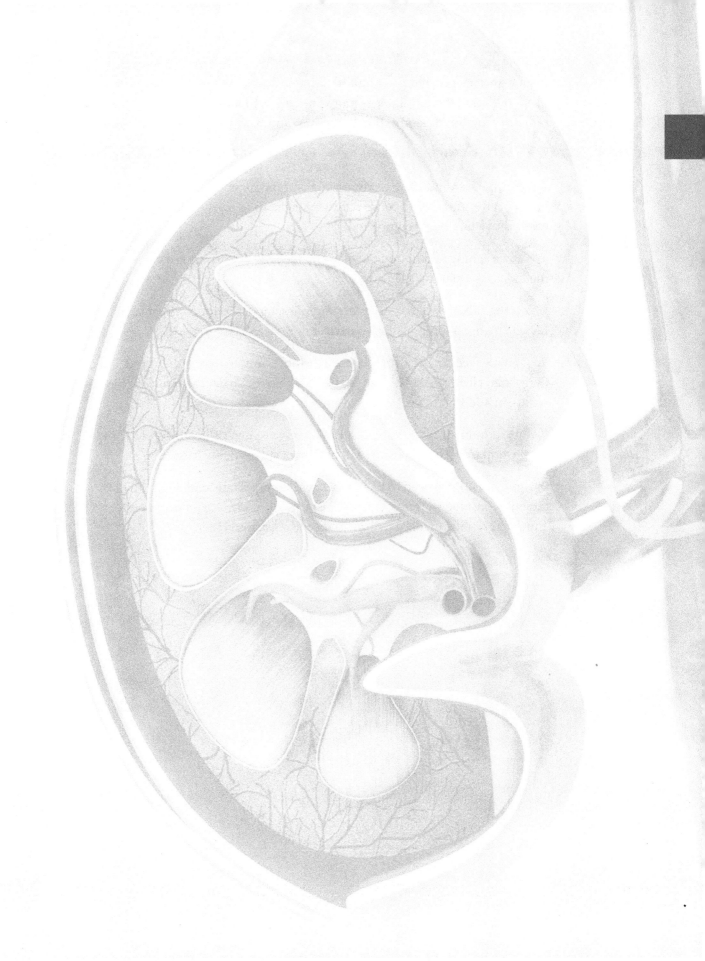

KEY POINTS

- **Common services** offered at a radiation oncology center include external beam radiation therapy, image-guided radiation therapy, intensity-modulated radiotherapy, tomotherapy, brachytherapy, and Xofigo® (Ra-223) infusions.

- **A Radiation Center** can cost up to $5 million to build.

- **Reimbursement** rates for commercial insurances vary by region and local market rates, and charge codes may vary depending on the complexity of the exam/procedure being completed.

- **When** designing a radiation oncology facility, the key aspect is a vault to house the Linear Accelerator (LINAC).

- **Using** the LINAC will require many supplies and a service contract with the LINAC manufacturer or third-party vendor.

- **To provide** electron treatments, it will be necessary to have either predefined Cerrobend electron field blocks or the ability to construct them onsite (block room), in addition to necessary equipment.

- **Xofigo®** administration requires a Radioactive Materials license and a "hot lab," so constant radiation exposure will not affect surrounding rooms.

- **Patient workflows** need to be in place with appropriate staff, including a radiation oncologist, radiation therapists, medical physicist, dosimetrist, nurse or certified medical assistant, receptionist, and biller.

Patrick R. Aldinger, RT, (R) (T)

Patrick R. Aldinger, RT (R) (T) is the Site Manager and Lead Therapist at the Oregon Urology Institute (OUI) Radiation Oncology Center in Springfield, Oregon. Patrick has been with the OUI Radiation Center since 2009 and previously worked at a hospital-based radiation oncology center as a Radiation Therapist and Medical Dosimetry Apprentice. Patrick started his education by receiving his B.S. in Radiographic Science from Idaho State University, followed by a B.S. in Radiation Therapy from Weber State University. Patrick maintains board certification through the American Registry of Radiologic Technologists in Radiography and Radiation Therapy, as well as being licensed with the Oregon Board of Medical Imaging.

Stephen M. Beach, PhD, DABR

Stephen M. Beach, PhD, DABR, RSO is the staff Medical Physicist for the Oregon Urology Institute and has overseen all the radiation therapy treatments in the Radiation Oncology department since early 2008. With over 14 years of clinical experience in various clinical settings, he serves as the quality assurance manager of all physics related calculations and simulations within the department. Dr. Beach received his Bachelor of Science in Radiation Health Physics with a Minor in Physics and an option in pre-med from Oregon State University in 1999. He then went on to earn his Master of Science and Doctor of Philosophy degrees from the University of Wisconsin - Madison in 2001 and 2005 respectively. Dr. Beach was certified in Therapeutic Radiation Physics by the American Board of Radiology in 2010. He also serves as the Radiation Safety Officer for the clinic.

Terence G. FitzPatrick, MPA

Terence G. FitzPatrick, MPA, serves as the Administrator of the Oregon Urology Institute (OUI), a 22-provider urology medical group in Springfield, Oregon. He has more than 35 years of experience in the management of medical groups, with the last 11 at OUI. Terry has a B.S. in Recreation Administration from Fresno State and a master's degree in Public Administration, Health Service Option, from the Universityof Southern California.

CHAPTER

Establishing an Advanced Prostate Cancer Clinic in the Urology Office

Bryan A. Mehlhaff, MD
Christopher M. Pieczonka, MD

Advanced prostate cancer, defined as metastatic or castration resistant prostate cancer or both, continues to be a rapidly advancing field of diagnostics and treatment. While this is good news for patients with a prostate cancer diagnosis, the challenge of optimal patient management is growing exponentially. Since the first writing of this chapter, new imaging modalities have become available and an older one has essentially disappeared. Previously available medications have expanded indications; new categories of therapy have emerged; newer medications have been added; and an older class of medications has finally been relegated to the trash heap. In addition, advances in our understanding of genetics has crept into our guidelines and pathways. To help identify and manage the treatment of patients, there is increasing use of data analytic tools.

It was true before, and more so today, developing an Advanced Prostate Cancer Clinic (APCC) is essential. The survival advantage data with treatment in some areas of advanced prostate cancer is so significantly improved that variance from these treatment pathways will soon become a violation of standards of care (if this has not happened already).

The necessary steps in setting up an APCC has not changed. With a physician champion, a patient navigator, and staff to complete the operational tasks, the APCC can successfully provide care that is current, state-of-the-art, and financially viable in urology offices, regardless of group size. What is more, the APCC can be physical or virtual, depending on the nature of the urology practice.

The importance of "buy-in" of the entire group and agreement among the providers to refer patients into an APCC remains unchanged and cannot be overemphasized. Building an APCC without also directing or preferably mandating patients' care via an APCC pathway results in poor care. It also puts an APCC at financial risk.

APCC LOGISTICS

At some point in the continuum of care, advanced prostate cancer patients review their disease progression with the APCC care team; a care plan is developed; and patients are assigned to an intra-office referral to a champion physician or physicians. Identification of these patients requires system developments to review those at risk of developing metastasis and/or castration resistant prostate cancer (CRPC). Initially, a new APCC clinic requires identification of patients on androgen deprivation therapy (ADT) followed by identification of the subset of patients with rising prostate-specific antigen (PSA) levels. Data analytic programs are now available as an overlay to our EMRs to assist with this identification and allows reports to be based on various search criteria.

Currently, any patients starting ADT should be evaluated by the APCC, and many should have their ongoing care incorporated and managed by the APCC. This is a change from previous whereby some groups developed either a "bone health clinic" or had the referral setpoint be CRPC only.

CHANGING LANDSCAPE

Since this chapter was last written there has been a paradigm shift in what defines advanced prostate cancer. This can be divided into two categories: New diagnosis hormone sensitive metastatic prostate cancer and biochemical recurrence.

> **Metastatic hormone sensitive prostate cancer (mHSPC), also called metastatic castration sensitive prostate cancer (mCSPC), has been the topic of numerous studies:**
>
> | | |
> |---|---|
> | **CHAARTED** | ADT alone vs. ADT plus taxotere chemotherapy |
> | **LATITUDE** | ADT alone vs. ADT plus abiraterone |
> | **TITAN** | ADT alone vs. ADT plus apalutamide |
> | **ARCHES** | ADT alone vs. ADT plus enzalutamide |

Each of these studies has shown a survival advantage of roughly 18 months of the combination therapy over ADT alone. The authors feel this data is compelling enough to establish a standard of care where starting ADT alone in a patient with metastatic hormone sensitive prostate cancer borders on malpractice. This creates a greater impetus to identifying and routing patients into a well-organized APCC.

Since the United States Preventative Services Task Force (USPSTF), began advising against screening for prostate cancer, the number of new prostate cancer diagnoses has decreased. Simultaneously, there has been a radical shift towards active surveillance in appropriate low risk prostate cancer patients. Not surprisingly, however, the incidence of prostate cancer development has not changed. Prostate cancer still occurs; we are simply diagnosing an increasing number of patients later in their disease course. In the absence of rational, effective screening, the diagnosis of prostate cancer in many cases looks much like it did in the pre-PSA era: symptomatic, metastatic, higher volume prostate cancer at initial diagnosis. In the recent past, studies have shown this group of patients has a 5-year survival rate of 29% versus a 5-year survival rate of 100% in patients diagnosed with early stage prostate cancer. At Oregon Urology Institute, we have seen an exponential rise of such patients: In 2017, we saw 11 patients; in 2018, we saw 34 patients; and in 2019, we saw more than 60 patients. This is a pattern duplicated in every group across the country.

These new mHSPC prostate cancer patients should now be managed within the APCC. Treatment should include initiation of ADT with either docetaxel or one of the Next

Generation Hormonal Agent's (NHA). Consideration should also be given to adjuvant radiation therapy to metastatic sites that are symptomatic or worrisome for future complications. In addition, in patients with lower volume metastatic volume, consideration can also be given to treating the primary lesion with definitive metastasis directed radiation as well.

BIOCHEMICAL RECURRENCE

Historically, after patients were treated with definitive therapy, such as either surgery or radiation therapy, they were put on androgen deprivation therapy if PSA recurrence was noted. This is called biochemical relapse. There is currently no FDA approved treatment, for this specific condition has been associated with an increased risk of mortality. In fact, many urology offices have a legacy cohort of patients who would have started androgen deprivation therapy many years ago.

One interesting way to further evaluate patients with biochemical relapse is to consider PET/CT scanning using one of the newer agents. There has been up until recently usage of PET/CT scanning using sodium fluoride as the radiopharmaceutical agent, which shows excellent evidence of bony metastatic disease; however, this particular radiopharmaceutical has never been approved by Medicare for reimbursement. More recently in the United States, Fluciclovine F18 has been developed and has been found to be quite sensitive and specific for the detection of lower volume of metastatic disease, both soft tissue and bony, that was previously found on both bone scan as well as CT scanning. This is also an excellent treatment modality to make sure radiation failure patients have a potential diagnosis made to assess for local recurrence rather than being treated with long-term systemic disease inappropriately when there would be a chance for salvage cryotherapy or salvage prostatectomy.

We believe that the APCC clinic should set up imaging guidelines to help assess when imaging should be performed for patients who have biochemical relapse to try and assess whether metastatic disease is present. One commonly used mechanism to help guide imaging techniques and the frequency and timing of imaging are the RADAR 3 guidelines.

Patients with biochemical relapse alone, who are referred to the advanced prostate cancer clinic will likely have androgen deprivation therapy withheld until there is documented metastatic disease. There are three specific reasons for this: First, patients who have all the metastatic disease could benefit from radiation to the low-volume metastasis site. In the event that the patient who had biochemical relapse was treated with androgen deprivation therapy without assessment of metastasis status; we might lose an option to treat these patients with radiation therapy, which has a trend towards overall survival. Second, the current NCCN guidelines now talk about the possibility of metastasis guided biopsy. There are a variety of commercially available companies that will do precision guided recommendation based on metastasis tissue. This would be inclusive of assessment for mismatch status or tumor mutational burden, which potentially would allow the patient to begin pembrolizumab. Pembrolizumab now has approval to treat any patient with solid tissue malignancy who is found to have either mismatch repair or increase in tumor mutational burden. Third, once patients are defined as metastatic, they will carry the diagnosis of metastasis with them for life. This is a binary discussion point when patients are looped into the advanced prostate cancer descriptive terms–either metastatic or nonmetastatic. A different way to explain this might be that when a patient is treated with androgen deprivation therapy and/or some of the newer hormonal agents without assessment of metastatic status, it might delay or preclude the usage of certain therapies that can be utilized in the metastatic setting only, e.g. sipuleucel-T or radium 223.

Thus, the authors believe that patients who have biochemical relapse should not begin androgen deprivation therapy. The patients with biochemical relapse should be imaged frequently to assess once metastatic disease is present. If metastatic disease is present, then any available therapies for mHSPC prostate cancer could be utilized. There are, however, a group of legacy patients who have already begun androgen deprivation therapy who may not have obvious metastatic disease. These patients who have progression in PSA without any obvious evidence of metastatic disease are called Non-metastatic Castration-Resistant Prostate Cancer (nmCRPC) patients. It now appears as though the testing for inherited genomic mutation should be performed on all patients who have metastatic disease or intraductal carcinoma. This is a new recommendation according to the NCCN for germline testing. Patients with high and very high risk clinically localized prostate cancer, regardless of family history as well as lower risk patients with positive family history (or those of Ashkenazi Jewish ancestry), should be tested for underlying genomic disease as well. This is important because there is impending approval of both olaparib as well as rucaparib for patients who have deleterious DNA repair gene changes, either at the genomic level or in their tumor biopsy itself. The initial approval for these medicines will be in the post chemotherapy and novel hormonal agent failure setting, however, some poly ADP ribose polymerase (PARP) inhibitors are now considered first line therapy in some metastatic breast cancer patients. PARP inhibitors are well-tolerated with neutropenia, thrombocytopenia, and anemia, with nausea and vomiting being the most troublesome side effects. Ongoing clinical studies are using PARP inhibitors with other NHA and other therapies to assess for synergistic benefit.

NEW THERAPIES FOR ADVANCED PROSTATE CANCER

A successful APCC requires urologists to stay abreast of imaging modalities and the latest approvals in agents to treat metastatic prostate cancer.

After a lengthy period of few significant advancements in metastatic prostate cancer therapies, the arrival of new agents has been both exciting and challenging for clinicians to incorporate into their patients' care plans. An APCC within the urology practice is an effective way to care for patients amidst the advent of these new therapies.

Since 2009, eight new therapies have been approved for the treatment of metastatic prostate cancer. These therapies include a wide range of action mechanisms, significant improvements in overall survival, and tolerable side effect profiles. In addition, treatment of metastatic prostate cancer with ADT is commonplace in urology offices since the introduction of injectable castration agents.

While newer therapies enable urologists to continue to manage and treat patients, the challenge is in coordinating the array of treatment options available into a comprehensive care pathway for individual patients. Best practice patterns for coordination of treatment function best with a physician champion who is facile in the indications and use of these newer treatments. In some communities, this may be a medical oncologist specializing in urologic oncology and possibly may require an outside referral by the urologist.

More commonly, this type of specialist is not locally available. Rather than outsourcing this care, many practices choose to have a physician champion within the APCC.

Physician Champion

An APCC's physician champion is essential for coordinating the array of treatment options into a comprehensive care pathway for a patient. He or she should have interest in—even a passion for—the science, development, and indications for use of the new ADT therapies. Utilizing just one novel hormonal agent and not also offering other therapies in the APCC pathway leads to poor management and possibly poorer outcomes for the patient. Not every patient should be treated with every agent. The indications for each treatment option create a "therapeutic window" of indications/ exclusions that, without active screening and management, may lead to missed treatment opportunities due to disease progression.

The specialization of a physician champion is like acquiring the skills needed to be proficient at complicated urologic surgeries, such as cystectomy or complex pelvic reconstruction, etc. Not every physician should be performing all complex surgeries, nor should every urologist feel adept in advanced therapeutics for prostate cancer.

Nurse Navigator

A nurse navigator is essentially the patients' concierge who helps them "navigate" through the care process. The role of navigator may be a nurse or nurse practitioner, but can also be filled by a physician assistant, research staff, or someone else involved in the APCC. Duties also may be divided among more than a single individual.

Navigators also can effectively follow a protocol for identifying potential patient candidates in various categories for studies and referring them to the APCC.

CLINICAL CHAMPION
Urologist or Oncologist

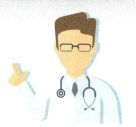

- Special interest, training and passion for learning latest information regarding advanced prostate cancer
- Understands the benefits and risks of each treatment
- Develops a treatment pathway with group consensus for patient care plans
- Organizes a system for patient identification disease states for inclusion in the APCC
- Review outcomes, update pathway with new information and treatments, and continuously advocate for best patient care

Operational Champion

The APCC also needs an operational champion to accomplish infusion programs, such as Provenge®, Keytruda®, Xofigo® and other therapies in the APCC. While a physician champion will direct care of patients, and a navigator will assist with patient identification and enactment of the care plan, an operational champion (usually group administrator) provides leadership to make the APCC function successfully.

NURSE NAVIGATOR CHAMPION

- Familiar with the operations of the practice
- Embraces role as patient advocate to ensure successful initiation and assists with administration of Xofigo® therapy
- Works with clinical champion to identify appropriate Xofigo® patients
- Coordinates the setup, clinical procedure, scheduling, and treatment of patient
- Assists patient in navigating the Xofigo® process, including communication with Xofigo® Access Services
- Explains procedure and potential benefits and risks of Xofigo® to the patient
- Builds a partnership with Xofigo® Access Services

INJECTION CHAMPION
Radiation Oncologist or Nuclear Medicine Physician

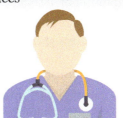

- Willing to invest in creating/maintaining hot lab services
- Trained and licensed to handle and administer radio-pharmaceuticals—usually a radiation oncologist or nuclear medicine physician
- Understands the clinical benefits and risks of Xofigo® and clearly explains them to patients
- May be an existing member of your staff or an individual your practice contracts with for services
- Advocates for Xofigo®

CHEMOTHERAPY IN THE UROLOGY OFFICE

Urologists can administer chemotherapy in the urology office; however, it requires some infrastructure and clinical support. Some urologists give chemotherapy without a medical oncologist on staff. Other urology groups incorporate the services of a medical oncologist into the APCC. The oncologist may visit the urologist office on a scheduled basis or other groups may employ the oncologist within the urologist office.

With recent studies demonstrating the utility of giving chemotherapy upon the initial diagnosis of hormone sensitive metastatic prostate cancer (mHSPC) and with the use of chemotherapy in later stage M1CRPC, it is important to create a plan for the delivery of cytotoxic therapy to these patients. However, recent data from ASCU GU 2020 shows a significant QoL improvement in usage of abiraterone vs docetaxel in this disease space confirming the smaller window for docetaxel in the HSPC disease space. This therapy can be included in the urology APCC, or a referral to an oncologist with experience treating advanced prostate cancer may be required. Usually, ADT is continued throughout CRPC. When chemotherapy is initiated, it should be determined whether a patient should continue Zytiga® or Xtandi®, as the potential for interaction and metabolism issues with these drugs in combination with chemotherapy has yet to be fully studied.

BONE HEALTH PROGRAM

Evidence has shown hazards to ADT, especially over the long term. Decrease in bone mineral density is a known side effect, with possible development of osteopenia/osteoporosis.[1] The APCC needs to incorporate a bone health program to evaluate and mitigate this risk.

Some patients may have pre-existing bone mineral density (BMD) deficiencies that will only worsen with ADT. At initiation of ADT, a baseline DEXA (Dual-energy X-ray absorptiometry) scan, or alternatively, a CT bone density, should be completed, and calcium and vitamin D3 levels should be checked and treated accordingly.[2] Low calcium and vitamin D3 levels require correction. Daily supplementation of both calcium and vitamin D3 is recommended for all patients on ADT.[2] Normally, 1,200 mg of calcium and at least 800 IU of vitamin D3 is recommended to start.

Use of antiresorptive agents should be employed. Most offices are using zolendronic acid (Zometa®) by IV infusion or subcutaneous injection of denosumab (Prolia®). For example, use of Prolia® is indicated for patients on ADT for cancer treatment-induced bone loss (CTIBL),[3] which includes many patients in a typical urology office. Prolia® use in patients with documented decrease in bone mineral density (BMD) is a standard of care and supported by numerous guidelines.[1] Imaging should also follow a protocol for patients on continued ADT, repeated at least every two years.[4]

A good bone health program also leads to better identification of patients with progression of their prostate cancer and indicates a possible need for other therapies directed at their disease later in the care pathway. Approximately 80% of metastases will be to the bone.[5] As the disease progresses into the bone, patients are candidates for monthly denosumab.

(Xgeva®). Though the risk is low,[3] calcium levels need to be checked monthly to ensure that hypocalcemia does not develop. Risk of hypocalcemia with Prolia® is lower. Both versions of denosumab can also cause osteonecrosis of the jaw. A dental evaluation should be done before initiation of these agents. One very other important consideration is to maintain integrity of usage of Xgeva in particular. When there is abrupt cessation of Xgeva, it can lead to osteoclastogenesis causing very rapid bone demineralization.

Initially, most patients with advanced prostate cancer have castrate-sensitive disease and respond well to the initiation of ADT with a significant drop in PSA levels and, often, radiographic regression of known metastatic disease. Over time, most patients on ADT will show PSA levels rise and/or clinical or radiographic progression. This is the definition of Castrate Resistant Prostate Cancer (CRPC).

A rise in PSA alone on ADT without known metastasis is known as, non-metastatic CRPC, or M0 CRPC, and the nurse navigator follows these patients. The navigator for the APCC can join efforts with entities that have a research coordinator who understand different inclusion/exclusion criteria of specific studies and can guide patients accordingly.

Metastatic prostate cancer is often occult, potentially under-diagnosed in approximately one-third of patients.[6] A diagnosis of metastasis-positive CRPC, M1 CRPC, now avails the patient to the full array of treatment options in the APCC. Historically, urologists would frequently order imaging in search of metastases in reaction to a change in the patient's condition, new pain, or clinical deterioration. This often diagnosis an advanced degree or some amount of metastatic disease. Also, in the past, a diagnosis of M1 CRPC led to only a few treatment options, sometimes only palliative or treatments with poorly tolerated side effects.[7] Currently, the urologist needs to approach metastatic prostate cancer differently.

AN ARRAY OF TREATMENT OPTIONS

Today, we have several treatment options available, each with significant improvement in patient survival, and tolerable side effects, making identification of M1 disease more imperative. Numerous studies suggest that earlier identification of M1 CRPC leads to better survival outcomes than later identification. For example, in the PROCEED registry

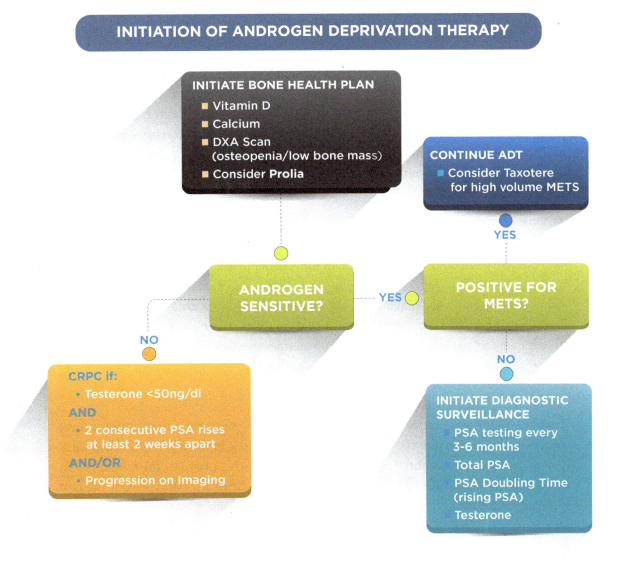

that looked at the real-world survival in patients treated with sipuleucel-T, those treated with a PSA <5.27 ng/ml had a survival of 47.7 months. This is substantially better than what was reported in the original pivotal trials with sipuleucel-T and probably represents some synergy with usage of other agents after initial immunotherapy.

Therefore, the APCC needs to have protocols in place for the nurse navigator to follow to proactively image patients with or without symptoms in search of metastatic disease. The RADAR 3 guidelines included in the table on page , as well as additional guidelines regarding NGI, should be adopted by the APCC.

With the diagnosis of M1 CRPC, the patient now needs a comprehensive approach to developing a care plan that incorporates the appropriate advanced therapies. As 80% of CRPC patients will develop bone metastasis, these patients are at risk for bone complications or skeletal related events (SRE), defined as fracture, spinal cord compression or the need of bone radiation or surgery. Bone complications result in significant morbidity for the patient and significant costs of treatment.

Proactive management can be preventative. Again, use of antiresorptive therapies, such as zolendronic acid (Zometa®) or denosumab (Xgeva®) is indicated for the prevention of skeletal related events.[5] In a head-to-head trial, Xgeva® showed statistical superiority to Zometa®. Xgeva® administration is simpler, with a monthly subcutaneous injection rather than IV infusion every 3-6 weeks and requires no monitoring or dose adjustment for renal function. Again, attention to bone health and management of bone metastases also enhances identification of advanced disease and treatment with other concomitant therapies.[3, 5]

The M1 CRPC patient is potentially eligible for sipuleucel-T immunotherapy, abiraterone (Zytiga®), enzalutamide (Xtandi®), radium 223 (Xofigo®), chemotherapy, and external beam radiation treatment. In the absence of many combination or sequencing trials to date, this potential eligibility requires the APCC to develop a care pathway tailored to the individual patient that utilizes the best evidence available currently. This is challenging with overlapping indications of treatments, each approved in trials that mostly compare to placebo. With unique mechanisms of action of these therapies, there is also the potential for additive survival benefits. When compared to older placebo controlled trials demonstrating a median survival of the M1 CRPC patient of approximately 18 months, more recent studies show survival of nearly 36 months.[7, 8] With the doubling of life expectancy of the advanced metastatic prostate cancer patient, these results are a testament to the revolutionary advancement in the care of these patients. Unfortunately, in communities without a comprehensive program for management of the advanced disease state, many patients receive neither optimal care nor the best survival outcomes.

Provenge®

A physician champion with the APCC needs to consider all treatment options for the individual M1 CRPC patient. Provenge® is shown to improve patient survival. In fact, the National Comprehensive Cancer Network indicates Provenge as first line therapy for patients with newly diagnosed asymptomatic or minimally asymptomatic M1 CRPC.[9] Provenge® is an autologous cellular immunotherapy that has been available since 2010. The product does not change PSA levels, and there is no specific monitoring needed for this treatment.[10]

The regimen of treatment includes an apheresis cell collection followed three days later by infusion of the Provenge activated cells. This is repeated in two weeks and again in four weeks. There is currently no approval for additional Provenge treatments after a set of three apheresis/infusions.[10] The treatments require a nurse or other qualified person to give IV therapy, a space with a chair for the patient, and a protocol for treatment of usually relatively mild infusion-related reactions, such as fever and chills. The therapy is completed within a month, and other therapies can follow subsequently (or sometimes previously or concomitantly).

It is important to note that if the patient has a fewer than 6-12-month life expectancy, this is probably not the optimal therapy consideration.

Additionally, if patients take narcotics for cancer-related pain, they probably would be considered to have symptomatic disease and are likely outside the indication for this treatment. There is, however, recent information from the Proceed clinical registry, which reflected roughly 2,000 patients in the real-world setting who had received Provenge therapy. The survival benefit found in those patients is much better than what was reported in the Impact study and no significant change in safety signals.

Androgen Receptor Blockers
The Use of Antiandrogens

Urology groups with an APCC need to make certain that all providers are utilizing the APCC uniformly. This usually includes a deviation in practice pattern for many providers who, for example, may have traditionally referred patients to a medical oncologist as soon as a patient fails initial LHRH or develops CRPC. These patients should now be channeled via intra-office referral to the APCC or physician champion.

In another example, patients who develop CRPC should not begin a first-generation antiandrogen, such as bicalutamide. This is a major change in both AUA and NCCN guidelines. This is also a major change for many physicians as the treatment with bicalutamide as a secondary hormonal maneuver has been a part of many training programs and clinical practice for many years. Recent studies have shown that this therapy often results in a decrease in the patient's PSA but does not improve survival.

This brings to light one fundamental difference between first-generation antiandrogens (e.g., bicalutamide) and second-generation antiandrogens (e.g., enzalutamide). The first-generation drugs are not pure antagonists and with time will exhibit agonist activity. This is the basis of the PSA decrease response seen with the cessation of first-generation antiandrogens. It is advised that in patients with either a rising PSA or progression on ADT and CRPC, these first-generation drugs are not to be used in this setting.

To solidify this argument, there has been recent information published comparing the usage of first-generation antiandrogens, such as bicalutamide with enzalutamide, which is one of the second-generation antiandrogens. This was done in a randomized controlled fashion through the TERRAIN study and showed a benefit in overall survival for patients using enzalutamide versus bicalutamide.

There are now three different FDA approved second-generation antiandrogens: Enzalutamide, apalutamide, and darolutamide. Enzalutamide has the oldest approval for prostate cancer and appears to be approved in the widest clinical setting for advanced prostate cancer. The original approval for enzalutamide was for post chemotherapy patients with CRPC, which quickly transitioned to enzalutamide usage in patients who are chemotherapy naïve with CRPC. The most recent indications for enzalutamide are inclusive of patients who have nonmetastatic castrate resistant prostate cancer. The recent ARCHES study showed an improvement in rPFS, and the ENZAMET study showed an improvement in OS in patients who were newly diagnosed with metastatic prostate cancer mHSPC.

Apalutamide is very chemically similar to enzalutamide and also has approval for nonmetastatic castrate resistant prostate cancer as well as mHSPC. The drugs have a reasonably similar side effect profile however it appears as though there might be a slightly higher risk of neurocognitive sideeffects with enzalutamide whereas a rash happens fairly frequently with apalutamide.

The newest medicine is darolutamide, which at this point, appears to be a fairly niche product. The only approved indication for darolutamide is for nmCRPC. This is the third antiandrogen and is chemically quite different than the two agents previously mentioned. It appears that because of its large molecular size, it is less likely to cross the blood-brain barrier, and reportedly has significantly fewer neurocognitive side effects than the two agents previously mentioned. Recent data shows that there is a significant survival advantage with daralutamide, enzalutamide and apalutamide have all shown a survival benefit as predicted in the nmCRPC patient.

Darolutamide, according to the FDA approved labeling indication, cannot be used in metastatic disease, which makes this challenging because of the availability of newer imaging techniques. The patients who have traditionally been defined as metastatic for clinical protocols have been based on bone scan or CT scan, which were traditionally required as enrollment for study criteria. However, recently with the advent of the Axumin® scan, we are finding metastatic disease much earlier, which raises the suspicion that nonmetastatic castrate resistant prostate cancer is a misnomer and does not really exist. To bolster that argument, a recently published abstract presented at the American Urological Association in 2020, looked at a cohort of 100 patients who would have met the criteria for enrollment in the SPARTAN study that used apalutamide for nmCRPC. Upon PSMA screening, 98% of those patients were found to have metastatic disease.

Abiraterone

Since the last time that this chapter was written, Zytiga® has gone off patent and is now available generically, though the medicine is still quite expensive. The usage of abiraterone in many urology practices has been less than the antiandrogens because of the need for blood work monitoring. The usage of this agent functions to prevent the intracellular production of testosterone as well as the adrenal production of testosterone in a man who being treated with androgen deprivation therapy. There is currently FDA approved indication for usage of this medicine for both metastatic castrate resistant prostate carcinoma as well as mHSPC.

One of the important reasons for the usage of this medicine in the APCC must deal with the need for routine blood work. These patients require biweekly blood work for the first several months after initiation of the medicine as well as monthly blood work essentially for as long as they take the medicine. The typical side effects from this medicine would include hypertension and fluid retention in the legs. However, the blood work is really performed to look for occult hepatotoxicity as well as hypokalemia. Too often it is seen that patients begin this medicine without the concomitant blood work, which could lead to a legal problem in the event the patient had either hepatotoxicity or hypokalemia.

More recently, a formulation of abiraterone has become available called Yonsa®. This version represents a micro-polymerize version of abiraterone that can now be taken on an empty stomach, which is much easier from a patient compliance standpoint. Yonsa uses methylprednisolone rather than prednisone to minimize the mineralocorticoid type side effects seen with the usage of the sip 17 inhibitors. The authors have also seen insurance companies try to force physicians into using generic abiraterone purposely with food as a 250 mg dosing to control cost. Although there is some data to suggest that the absorption is the same, the authors caution against this.

Urologists have long been familiar with the use of older androgen receptor blockers and steroid synthesis inhibitors. Newer medicines, Zytiga® and Xtandi®, are oral therapies acting on the androgen receptor pathway, the principle mechanism that stimulates prostate cancer cells to grow and proliferate. Zytiga® is an androgen synthesis inhibitor, and Xtandi® is an androgen receptor pathway inhibitor.[8,11] Both treatments require four oral pills to be taken daily. They have similar indications for the M1 CRPC patient, with studies in both the pre- and post-chemotherapy patient. There are certain restrictions and parameters with each. This sometimes makes one medicine more appropriate for an individual patient.[13,14] Both drugs have attractive, however, different side effect profiles. Which drug to choose is often a physician's choice, so an understanding of both drugs, side effects, monitoring, and other aspects is essential.

As patients progress with advanced prostate cancer, they are typically seen in the office frequently, ranging from every three months to monthly. Sometimes these patients are already coming in for monthly Xgeva® injections. ADT therapy is continued throughout, as is periodic monitoring of PSA, testosterone, calcium, and vitamin D3 levels. Monitoring of PSA levels alone to determine persistent response to therapy is not always sufficient, and perhaps a minimum repeat imaging schedule of every six months is prudent. The schedule can include a repeat CT scan and bone scan; however, a repeat of an Axumin PET/CT scan may be appropriate if this imaging test was initially used to first diagnose metastasis.[4]

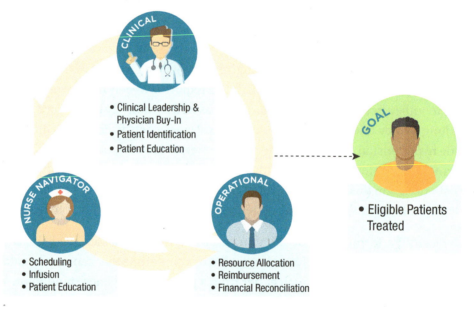

Increase of PSA Levels

Evidence of radiographic progression may be an indication to change therapy or to possibly consider adding another therapy. An increase in PSA level alone, without other clinical or radiographic evidence of progression, should not prompt a change in therapy. In the trials for each of the oral NHA's, progression is defined as clinical or radiographic progression, not a rise in PSA.[13,14] Therefore, increases in PSA should prompt repeat imaging and evaluation of the patient, but may not necessarily mean oral therapy is to be discontinued.

In fact, there are many examples in other Metastatic Castration Resistant Prostate Cancer mCRPC clinical trials that show the inconsistency between PSA reductions and achieving overall survival in those clinical trials. Over a seven-year period, there have been six new therapies studied in mCRPC that have shown a statistically significant reduction in PSA, but not in overall survival; thus, the FDA did not approve those agents.

There are no definitive head-to-head trials to guide the use of one NHA over another. There is some debate about whether there is a benefit to the patient's treatment with the second agent after progression of disease on the first. The duration of the second oral therapy will typically be less than the first one, possibly proportional in time to the duration of therapy of the first drug. In other words, if the patient progressed quickly on the first agent, there may be limited utility of trying the second. Again, changing therapy only because of an increase in PSA should be avoided.

NHAs are distributed through specialty pharmacies. Due to the high cost of these oral medications, the drugs may require prior authorization under most insurances, and patients will need assistance with copays and out-of-pocket expenses. A drug adherence program for patients is also essential. Zytiga® must be taken on any empty stomach and requires oral prednisone to minimize side effects. Prednisone is also a common concomitant medication for patients on any NHA to improve patient's complaints of fatigue, decreased energy, and mood changes.[13]

Radium 223 (Xofigo®)

Radium 223 (Xofigo®) is a radiopharmaceutical indicated for the treatment of symptomatic bony metastatic prostate cancer. Like calcium and earlier radiopharmaceuticals, when given via IV, Xofigo® goes to the bone and tends to bind preferentially to areas of greatest metabolic activity in bone, typically areas of metastasis.[14] Different from prior radiopharmaceuticals, which release beta and some gamma particles, Xofigo® releases alpha particle radiation.

The alpha radiation results in relatively greater double stranded DNA breaks leading to cell death, decreased distance of radiation travel, and reduced myelosuppression. Xofigo® also gives patients a significant survival advantage, which is different than other radiopharmaceuticals that provide palliation only.

Xofigo® therapy is tolerated with a side effect profile that typically is easily managed in the outpatient setting. The treatment consists of six-monthly IV infusions with dosage calculated based on the patient's weight.[14] Complete blood count (CBC) should be monitored one week prior to each infusion.

Identification of patients eligible for Xofigo® requires finding patients with at least two bony metastatic lesions and symptoms. The symptoms related to their disease could be identified as bone pain, but could also be less energy, decreased ability to perform daily activities, and others.

One risk of Xofigo® is late identification of the patient's disease progression and delayed initiation of therapy. It is important for a navigator to actively find Xofigo® patients. Often these patients are on oral Zytiga® or Xtandi® and seem to be doing well, but often progress to a more advanced disease very quickly while the clinician is waiting for the patient to complain of pain rather than identifying other symptoms that may also indicate progression. Since Xofigo® is given over six months, late identification may result in the patient not getting all six treatments due to progression, decreasing blood counts, and other symptoms.

One important factor to identify is whether a patient who is taking Xofigo® could continue on either one of the antiandrogens or abiraterone. There will be ongoing clinical studies to help answer the safety of this particular combination as recent literature showed a potential increased risk of mortality with the usage of Xofigo®, specifically with abiraterone (albeit this was a trial that did not allow for bone tropic support in patients who were otherwise asymptomatic with their bony metastatic disease). As a result, the package insert now specifically precludes the usage of Xofigo® with abiraterone, although the same caution does not appear to apply on the package insert to the antiandrogens.

Operational Champion Important for Xofigo®

The operational piece of Xofigo® is important and will require oversight of an operational champion. He or she must ensure there is space for a "hot lab;" consider licensure and equipment; and make sure administration of the treatment is performed under an Authorized User, typically a radiation oncologist, nuclear medicine doctor, or other physician with credentials to handle a liquid, unsealed source of radiation. Each state has different rules and requirements for licensure to handle Xofigo®, and approval can take variable amounts of time.

Once the treatment area is set up, the IV injection is given over one minute, repeated monthly, for a total of six treatments. Patients can have palliation of bone metastasis related pain, but the principle indication is increased survival of the patient.

In clinical trials, Xofigo® was administered along with the best standard of care available at the time. Although NHAs were not available during this time, use of Xofigo®, in addition to either of these oral medications, can be effective at controlling potential symptomatic skeletal related events due to the bony metastatic disease. This may lengthen the duration of treatment possible with NHAs before progression necessitates discontinuation of the oral medication.

In the case of Xofigo®, there is no published evidence that indicates earlier treatment is better. However, Xofigo® is dosed according to the patient's body weight and not based on overall tumor burden. Therefore, there is some thought that dosing a patient with a lower overall metastatic burden may be more beneficial than waiting until the tumor burden is quite high.

One way of evaluating the tumor burden is to use technetium-based bone scans, but this can often underestimate the tumor burden. Alkaline phosphatase is a marker for bone turnover. Patients with increased alkaline phosphatase levels have a higher burden of disease. This can be a biomarker used to observe Xofigo response as the pivotal clinical study did not show a statistically significant decrease in PSA for patients treated with Xofigo relative to control. Thus, adding routine alkaline phosphatase levels to the battery of blood work done on the patient in the APCC is recommended.

CHEMOTHERAPY WITH DOCETAXEL OR CABAZITAXEL

Chemotherapy with docetaxel or second line cabazitaxel has been pushed to the later stages of prostate cancer given the relative shorter associated survival advantages and increased risk of side effects. However, there is a role for chemotherapy for M1 CRPC, especially in certain classes of patients with genetic variants of prostate cancer.[15,16] There has been interest recently in the usage of docetaxel in the newly diagnosed patient with metastasis who is hormone naïve. The patients who benefit most from this approach are patients with high volume disease. There is also recent literature to support the usage of cabazitaxel with an improvement in overall survival seen in patients who have failed novel hormonal agent with the usage of cabazitaxel as the second line therapy showing improvement in overall survival.

Excluding bone health treatments, all the aforementioned therapies are associated with improved survival and should be utilized instead of first- generation antiandrogens. Also, important to recognize are therapies, such as Provenge and Xofigo, do not typically change PSA levels, but have been proven to improve survival. These are examples of nuances in treatments that the APCC provider understands and encounters daily, while the general urologist may not readily recognize them.

CRPC OUTPATIENT TREATMENT

Some groups, with prior approval of their providers, utilize navigators to identify patients as soon as they develop CRPC and immediately refer the patient to the APCC. Also, all metastatic prostate cancer patients should be treated under the APCC. The update to this chapter indicates that all patients with ADT should be referred to the APCC. This allows the right patient to see the right provider and likely get the right treatments at the right time in their disease course. In the future, with the measurement of patient outcomes and the cost of care efficiency, these care pathways may become part of alternative payment models. With active management within the APCC, these patients are often treated as outpatients and avoid hospitalization. Although some are concerned about the high cost of these treatments, the APCC care pathway makes significant savings possible by keeping these patients out of hospitals and ICUs.

THE IN-OFFICE DISPENSARY

The urology office can take over the responsibilities of the specialty pharmacy by becoming an in-office dispensary. State specific regulations should be followed, as in-office dispensaries are prohibited in some states. The dispensing pharmacy can be incorporated into a patient's care and monitoring plan. Along with adjudicating claims for the medication, the office is also assuming the responsibility of monitoring the patient for proper dose administration, side effects, possible drug-drug interactions, and contacting the patient each month before the medication is refilled. This is another point of contact with the patient that can enhance the patient's care and identify a possible need for new/additional evaluation or therapies.

The office dispensary can be centrally located, and prescriptions can be mailed to patients in many states. Some states require patients to pick up medication from the office, which may involve transporting it to satellite offices from the central office. The drug is ordered into the dispensary as needed for each patient, and therefore, no inventory of medication is kept.

Finally, a provider needs to provide medication-specific counseling to the patient, which is required when one picks up any drug from a pharmacy.

This discussion of dosing, potential side effects, and precautions needs to be documented in a patient's chart.

FINAL WORDS ON THE APCC

Unfortunately, to date, these therapies for prostate cancer are not curative.

The best that can be hoped for is that patients in the APCC enjoy a slowing or stabilization of their disease, with maximal maintenance of their quality of life. Patients always seem to have future life events (e.g., a grandchild's graduation, marriage, or the birth of a great grandchild) that they would like to reach. Their personal timetable may guide the treatment plan.

Patients may need assistance with management of pain or require accommodations or help in the home. A discussion of palliative care or referral to hospice should be a part of office visits as the patient progresses into later stages of disease. Established contacts with the organizations that provide these services is helpful so referral can be ready when the patient reaches that point in disease progression. Some groups also make use of chronic care management codes to provide these services. Briefly, this involves monthly documented telephone calls to the patient by nursing staff to evaluate patient status and possible needs. The goal is to minimize use of the emergency department or admission to the hospital.

Finally, the care of a patient in the APCC is very rewarding. Patients appreciate the comprehensive nature of care that an APCC provides. They notice the coordination of care and often find comfort and hope in the understanding that there are numerous treatment options for their advanced stage or metastatic cancer. The APCC may also lead to a culture of excellence and pride in staff who begin to share in the care of an APCC patient and feel they are making a positive impact in patients' lives. At the same time, the frequent contact with APCC patients often leads to an intimate knowledge of their family and personal life. For this reason, support for staff members may be needed when a patient reaches the end of life.

REFERENCES

1. Gralow JR, Biermann JS, Farooki A, et al. NCCN Task Force report: bone health in cancer care. J Natl Compr Canc Netw. 2013;11(suppl 3): s1-s50.
2. Lupron Depot® [package insert]. AbbVie Inc. North Chicago, Illinois.
3. XGEVA® (denosumab) prescribing information, Amgen.
4. Crawford ED, Stone NN, Yu EY, et al. Challenges and Recommendations for Early Identification of Metastatic Disease in Prostate Cancer. Urology 81: 664-669. 2014.
5. Lipton A, Fizazi K, Stopeck AT, et al. Superiority of denosumab to zoledronic acid for prevention of skeletal-related events: a combined analysis of 3 pivotal, randomised, phase 3 trials. Eur J Cancer. 2012; 48:3082-3092.
6. Yu EY, Miller K, Nelson J, et al. Detection of previously unidentified metastatic disease as a leading cause of screening failure in a phase III trial of zibotentan versus placebo in patients with non-metastatic, castration resistant prostate cancer. J Urol. 2012; 188:103-109.
7. Tannock IF, de Wit R, Berry WR, et al, for the TAX 327 Investigators. Docetaxel plus prednisone or mitoxantrone plus prednisone for advanced prostate cancer. N Engl J Med 2004;351: 1502-12.
8. Beer TM, Armstrong AJ, Rathkopf DE, et al, for the PREVAIL Investigators. Enzalutamide in metastatic prostate cancer before chemotherapy. N Engl J Med. 2014;371(5):424-433.
9. National Comprehensive Cancer Network (NCCN) Guidelines - Prostate Cancer Version 2.2016.
10. Kantoff PW, Higano CS, Shore ND, et al; for the IMPACT Study Investigators. Sipuleucel-T immunotherapy for castration-resistant prostate cancer. N Engl J Med. 2010;363(5):411-422.
11. Rathkopf DE1, Smith MR2, de Bono JS, et al. Updated interim efficacy analysis and long-term safety of abiraterone acetate in metastatic castration-resistant prostate cancer patients without prior chemo- therapy (COU AA-302). Eur Urol. 2014 Nov;66(5):815-25.
12. Xtandi® [package insert]. Northbrook, IL: Astellas Pharma US, Inc.
13. Zytiga® (abiraterone acetate) Tablets [prescribing information]. Horsham PA, Jansen Biotech, Inc.
14. Xofigo® (radium Ra 223 dichloride) injection [prescribing information]. Whippany, NJ: Bayer Health- Care Pharmaceuticals Inc.; March 2016.
15. Tannock IF, de Wit R, Berry WR, et al, for the TAX 327 Investigators. Docetaxel plus prednisone or mitoxantrone plus prednisone for advanced prostate cancer. N Engl J Med 2004;351: 1502-12.
16. de Bono JS, Oudard S, Ozguroglu M, et al, for the TROPIC Investigators. Prednisone plus cabazitaxel or mitoxantrone for metastatic castration-resistant prostate cancer progressing after docetaxel treatment: a randomized open-label trial. Lancet 2010;376: 1147-54.
17. Shore, Neal, Tutrone, Ronald, Mariados, Neil, Nordquist, Luke, Mehlhaff, Bryan, Harrelson, Stacey, for eRADicAte: an Open Label Phase Two Study of Radium Ra 223 dichloride with Concurrent Ad- ministration of Abiraterone Plus Prednisone in Castration-Resistant (Hormone-Refractory) Prostate Cancer Subjects with Symptomatic Bone Metastases.

Lupron References:

1. Lupron Depot® [package insert]. AbbVie Inc. North Chicago, Illinois.

Denosumab References:

1. XGEVA® (denosumab) prescribing information, Amgen.
2. Gralow JR, Biermann JS, Farooki A, et al. NCCN Task Force report: bone health in cancer care. J Natl Compr Canc Netw. 2013;11(suppl 3): s1-s50.
3. Lipton A, Fizazi K, Stopeck AT, et al. Superiority of denosumab to zoledronic acid for prevention of skeletal-related events: a combined analysis of 3 pivotal, randomised, phase 3 trials. Eur J Cancer. 2012; 48:3082-3092.
4. Bekker PJ, Holloway DL, Rasmussen AS, et al. A single-dose placebo-controlled study of AMG 162, a fully human monoclonal antibody to RANKL, in postmenopausal women. J Bone Miner Res. 2004; 19:1059-1066.
5. Keizer RJ, Huitema ADR, Schellens JHM, Beijnen JH. Clinical pharmacokinetics of therapeutic monoclonal antibodies. Clin Pharmacokinet. 2010; 49:493-507.
6. Lewiecki EM. Denosumab: an investigational drug for the management of postmenopausal osteoporosis. Biologics. 2008; 2:645-653.
7. Mould DR, Green B. Pharmacokinetics and pharmacodynamics of monoclonal antibodies: concepts and lessons for drug development. BioDrugs. 2010; 24:23-39.
8. Sutjandra L, Rodriguez RD, Doshi S, et al. Population pharmacokinetic meta-analysis of denosumab in healthy subjects and postmenopausal women with osteopenia or osteoporosis. Clin Pharmacokinet. 2011; 50:793-807.
9. Stopeck AT, Lipton A, Body J-J, et al. Denosumab compared with zoledronic acid for the treatment of bone metastases in patients with advanced breast cancer: a randomized, double-blind study. J Clin Oncol. 2010; 28:5132-5139.
10. Henry DH, Costa L, Goldwasser F, et al. Randomized, double-blind study of denosumab versus zoledronic acid in the treatment of bone metastases in patients with advanced cancer (excluding breast and prostate cancer) or multiple myeloma. J Clin Oncol. 2011; 29:1125-1132.
11. Fizazi K, Carducci M, Smith M, et al. Denosumab versus zoledronic acid for treatment of bone metastases in men with castration-resistant prostate cancer: a randomised, double-blind study. Lan- cet. 2011; 377:813-822.

Provenge® References:

1. Provenge® [prescribing information]. Seattle, WA: Dendreon Pharmaceuticals; 2014.
2. Kantoff PW, Higano CS, Shore ND, et al; for the IMPACT Study Investigators. Sipuleucel-T immunotherapy for c astration-resistant prostate cancer. N Engl J Med. 2010;363(5):411-422.
3. Schellhammer PF, Chodak G, Whitmore JB, et al; Lower Baseline Prostate-specific Antigen is Associated With a Greater Overall Survival Benefit from Sipuleucel-T in the Immunotherapy for Prostate Adenocarcinoma Treatment (IMPACT) Trial. Urology 81: 1297-1302. 2013.

Xtandi® References:

1. Xtandi® [package insert]. Northbrook, IL: Astellas Pharma US, Inc.
2. Beer TM, Armstrong AJ, Rathkopf DE, et al, for the PREVAIL Investigators. Enzalutamide in metastatic prostate cancer before chemotherapy. N Engl J Med. 2014;371(5):424-433.
3. Scher HI, Fizazi K, Saad F, et al. Increased survival with enzalutamide in prostate cancer after chemotherapy. N Engl J Med. 2012;367(13):1187-1197.

Zytiga® References:

1. Zytiga® (abiraterone acetate) Tablets [prescribing information]. Horsham PA, Jansen Biotech, Inc.
2. Rathkopf DE1, Smith MR2, de Bono JS, et al. Updated interim efficacy analysis and long-term safety of abiraterone acetate in metastatic castration-resistant prostate cancer patients without prior chemotherapy (COU-AA-302). Eur Urol. 2014 Nov;66(5):815-25
3. de Bono JS, Logothetis CS, A Molina, et al. Abiraterone and Increased Survival in Metastatic Prostate Cancer. N Engl J Med. 2011;364(21):1995-05.

Xofigo® References:

1. Xofigo® (radium Ra 223 dichloride) injection [prescribing information]. Whippany, NJ: Bayer HealthCare Pharmaceuticals Inc.; March 2016.
2. Parker C, Nilsson S, Heinrich D, et al. Alpha emitter radium-223 and survival in metastatic prostate cancer. N Engl J Med. 2013;369(3):213-223.
3. Supplementary appendix to Scher HI, Fizazi K, Saad F, et al; AFFIRM Investigators. Increased survival with enzalutamide in prostate cancer after chemotherapy. N Engl J Med. 2012;367(13):1187-1197. Supplementary appendix available at: http://www.nejm.org/doi/ suppl/10.1056/NEJMoa1207506/suppl_file/nejmoa1207506_appendix.pdf.
4. Fizazi K, Scher HI, Molina A, et al; COU-AA-301 Investigators. Abiraterone acetate for treatment of metastatic castration-resistant prostate cancer: final overall survival analysis of the COU-AA-301 randomised, double-blind, placebo-controlled phase 3 study [published correction appears in Lancet Oncol. 2012;13(11): e464]. Lancet Oncol. 2012;13(10):983-992.
5. Tannock IF, de Wit R, Berry WR, et al; TAX 327 Investigators. Docetaxel plus prednisone or mitoxantrone plus prednisone for advanced prostate cancer. N Engl J Med. 2004;351(15): 1502-1512.

KEY POINTS

- **An APCC is becoming necessary for urology groups to survive.**

- **An APCC needs a physician champion, nurse navigator, and operational champion.**

- **A successful APCC requires** urologists to stay abreast of imaging modalities and the latest approvals in agents to treat metastatic prostate cancer.

- **A physician champion with the APCC** needs to consider all treatment options for the individual M1 CRPC patient.

- **The many treatment options available** make identification of M1 disease imperative as early identification can lead to better survival outcomes.

- **Urologists can administer chemotherapy in the urology office** with infrastructure and clinical support.

- **The urology office can take over the responsibilities of the specialty pharmacy** by becoming an in-office dispensary.

Bryan A. Mehlhaff, MD

Originally from Oregon, Dr. Mehlhaff attended Beloit College in Wisconsin followed by medical school at Oregon Health Sciences University. After completing a General Surgery and Urology residency at Albany Medical Center, he joined the Department of Urology as an Assistant Professor.

For the past 18 years, he has practiced in Eugene, Oregon. At the Oregon Urology Institute (OUI), as Medical Director of Research, he oversees numerous clinical trials in advanced prostate cancer and benign prostate conditions. At OUI he has developed a comprehensive bone health and advanced prostate cancer clinic. Dr. Mehlhaff is also a managing partner of OUI. He continues currently as a Board member of the Oregon Urology Society.

Christopher M. Pieczonka, MD

Dr. Pieczonka has been at the forefront of advanced prostate cancer care since the beginning of the decade. He has an interest in advancing the implementation of advanced prostate care by urologists and actively participates in many of the advanced therapeutic trials in this disease space.

CHAPTER

The Next Advance In Comprehensive Urologic Oncology Care: Establishing A Comprehensive Bladder Cancer Clinic (CBCC)

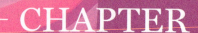

Sandip M. Prasad, MD, MPhil

For several decades, novel therapies have not been available for use by urologists managing either non-muscle invasive bladder cancer (NMIBC) or muscle invasive bladder cancer (MIBC). Hence, treatment strategies have remained the same, despite multiple large, randomized, prospective clinical trials that have evaluated the use of intravesical, surgical and systemic therapies.

In recent years, significant advances have been developed to aid in the diagnosis, staging, treatment and follow-up of bladder cancer that can now be incorporated into clinical practice. The challenge for many urology groups is identifying a team of experts in bladder cancer and centralizing care for a condition that has historically been treated at the individual urologist level for NMIBC or referred to a "cystectomist" or medical oncologist for more advanced disease. In addition, the national shortage of available Bacillus Calmette-Guerin (BCG) intravesical therapy provides an additional incentive for optimizing delivery of therapies for this disease. However, caring for bladder cancer patients in all stages of their disease can be a source of professional and financial satisfaction if performed in a rigorous and high-quality fashion.

The success of urology practices in creating an Advanced Prostate Cancer Clinic (APCC) provides the incentive for establishing a Comprehensive Bladder Cancer Clinic (CBCC). Like setting up an APCC, this effort requires a thorough evaluation of existing services and clinical practices, choosing which therapies to insource or outsource, and developing a business plan and pro forma. Later in this chapter, we will review the most recent changes in evaluation and management of bladder cancer that drive the need for centralization and practice standardization, which may improve guideline compliance and patient outcomes. First, we will discuss logistical challenges and solutions to build a modern, data-driven and financially viable clinic.

Metastatic Bladder Cancer Management in the CBCC

Historically, urologists have deferred the management of metastatic bladder cancer to medical oncologists. While most urology practices will likely continue to refer advanced bladder cancer patients, others have embraced the idea of delivery of immunotherapy by the practice now that it has been approved in NMIBC. It is clear that immunotherapy has and will continue to change the treatment paradigm for bladder cancer. Prior to 2016, there was only one FDA-approved regimen for locally advanced or metastatic bladder cancer; in the following year, five checkpoint inhibitors (atezolizumab, avelumab, durvalumab, nivolumab, and pembrolizumab) were approved. These treatments can be given every two-three weeks in clinic through peripheral IV and have a favorable short- and long-term safety profile.

Not all CBCCs will have an interest in treating with immuno-oncolytics (IOs) and there may be pressure for these treatments to remain based in the hospital or in the hands of medical oncology. Urologists should recall that the same discussions occurred across the clinical spectrum. This can serve as an attractive tool for patient referral and retention and offers another clinical area to create a Center of Excellence.

How to Get Started

LUGPA has developed resources to help practices initiate the process of developing a CBCC. Prior to postponement secondary to the coronavirus pandemic, an Advanced Bladder Cancer Workshop was scheduled in conjunction with the Bladder Cancer Advocacy Network (BCAN) to help practices implement IO therapies in their practices. This workshop focused on developing an interprofessional team, management of immune-related adverse events specific to IOs, and logistical and financial considerations for implementing IOs and other bladder cancer therapies in the community setting.

Figure 1 summarizes the initial steps in establishing a CBCC. First, successful LUGPA practices have created a CBCC after agreement from the partnership regarding the importance of and commitment to comprehensive care of bladder cancer patients. In addition to the key steps outlined previously in this chapter (identifying clinical champions, creating practice infrastructure, and establishing the culture), we have found that central review of all high-risk NMIBC and all MIBC by bladder cancer clinical champions is critical to ensure consistent and quality care. In our practice, care of these patients is transferred to one of the bladder cancer clinical champions for consultation, pre-treatment lab work and staging, and subsequent management. Administration of IOs and management of immune-related adverse events are also best performed under the direct supervision of these clinical champions. In-service for clinic staff and reimbursement specialists are also key prior to initiating IO treatment. **Appendix 1** outlines a sample clinical policy that may be of help to practices looking to begin their CBCC.

Once a CBCC has been established, the physician champions will need to identify locations to perform specialized care. For IO administration, we have found that integrating these into the physical space for the APCC (where infusions of medications like Provenge® are likely already performed and lab monitoring for oral medications for advanced prostate cancer are routinely collected). For new enhanced technologies such as blue-light cystoscopy with Cysview®, CBCC champions need to identify the locations where this will be performed as there are financial considerations for use of this technology. There is a significant capital expenditure for the acquisition of a dedicated cystoscopy tower, light source and camera (e.g. KARL STORZ D-light C Photodynamic Diagnostic System®) that may obviate performing this in the office and may be better situated in a hospital and ambulatory surgical center setting. Currently, there is also no separate CPT code for blue light cystoscopy (although there are complexity adjustments for 2 of the 7 applicable cystoscopy CPT codes in the hospital outpatient setting) which does not adequately reimburse the investment in some instances, such as in the ambulatory

Figure 1: Key Steps to Starting a CBCC

PHYSICIAN BUY-IN

- Is there commitment to comprehensive care of NMIBC and MIBC?
- Do partners want to participate in the start-up costs and clinical commitment?
- Are partners willing to transfer care of high-risk NMIBC and MIBC to clinical champions?
- Are there multiple providers willing to serve as clinical champions?

PRACTICE INFRASTRACTURE

- Are there existing mechanisms to internally identify and refer candidate patients (e.g. central pathology review, data mining)?
- Is there a central physical location for administration of therapies with appropriate facilities (e.g. a hood, IV pumps)?
- Have reimbursement specialists developed a protocol for co-pays and out-of-pocket expenses prior to initial infusion?
- Have the clinical champions (physicians and nursing staff) developed a clinical protocol (see **Appendix 1**)?

PRIOR TO LAUNCH

- Has a navigator (mid-level or nurse) been established to lead the CBCC team?
- Are there standing orders prior to and following each infusion or treatment for adequate monitoring?
- Have all clinical providers been educated on rapid identification (in the office or on call) and management of IO-related AEs?
- Has a monthly meeting schedule with clinical champions, navigator, practice manager and reimbursement staff been scheduled?

surgical center. In addition, Cysview® is not unpackaged from the procedure payment when administered in an ASC. Multiple urology advocacy groups are working on ameliorating the above reimbursement issues to account for the additional resources required to provide Finally, there are logistical concerns to integrating blue light cystoscopy into some practice settings as it does require intravesical instillation of the photosensitizer at least 1 hour prior to cystoscopy, which may impede workflow in certain settings. We have found, however, that all the above issues can be managed with defined protocols and consolidation of blue light cystoscopy to one or two practice settings across the entire group.

Epidemiology

Urothelial carcinoma of the bladder (UCB) is the fifth most common cancer in the United States, with an estimated 81,000 new cases resulting in 17,980 deaths in 2020. This has increased over the past decade when an estimated 70,530 new cases resulted in 14,680 deaths.[1] It is a heterogeneous disease, with a dichotomy at presentation between superficial lesions (70% of newly diagnosed tumors), which recur but are generally not associated with mortality, and muscle-invasive lesions (30% of incident tumors), which are associated with poor survival.[2] Approximately 50% of newly diagnosed cases are in-situ lesions, 35% localized, 8% regional, and 4% distant. A strong relationship exists between stage at diagnosis and survival, with in-situ, localized, regional, and distant disease having 97%, 73%, 36% and 6% 5-year survival rates, respectively.[ii] UCB has the highest lifetime treatment cost of all cancers,[3] with estimated expenditures of approximately $187,000 per case and, in 2010, a cost of approximately $4 billion to treat.[4] This is a result of long-term survival in the majority of patients, frequent disease recurrence and the requirement for lifelong cancer surveillance.

NMIBC Management In The CBCC

Optimal management of patients with NMIBC per American Urological Association (AUA)/Society for Urologic Oncology (SUO) guidelines include accurate stratification with complete visual resection of the bladder tumor(s) at the time of transurethral resection (TURBT) with use of intravesical immunotherapy or chemotherapy.[5] Assignment of accurate risk stratification at the time of each occurrence/recurrence is critically important to determine the recommended frequency and intensity of surveillance with cystoscopy and imaging (**Figure 2**).

This may include the use of blue light cystoscopy (BLC) and narrow band imaging (NBI) to increase detection and decrease recurrence. Despite these evidence-based guidelines, there is significant variation in practice pattern in the management of NMIBC.[6,7,8] Given the low rates of compliance with these guidelines, establishment of a formal bladder cancer program provides an opportunity to develop protocols and pathways to improve guideline-concordant care in the areas on the next page.

Figure 2: Follow-Up Schedules for Cystocopy, Imaging, and Urine Testing In Patients with NMIBC

LOW RISK Non-Muscle Invasive Bladder Cancer

TEST	YEAR						
	1	2	3	4	5	5 - 10	>10
CYSTOSCOPY	3, 12		ANNUALLY			AS CLINICALLY INDICATED	
UPPER TRACT AND ADOMINAL PELVIC IMAGING	BASELINE IMAGING	AS CLINICALLY INDICATED					
BLOOD TEST	N/A						
URINE TEST	N/A						

INTERMEDIATE RISK Non-Muscle Invasive Bladder Cancer

TEST	YEAR						
	1	2	3	4	5	5 - 10	>10
CYSTOSCOPY	3,6,12	EVERY 6 MONTHS	ANNUALLY			AS CLINICALLY INDICATED	
UPPER TRACT AND ADOMINAL PELVIC IMAGING	BASELINE IMAGING	AS CLINICALLY INDICATED					
BLOOD TEST	N/A						
URINE TEST	URINE CYTOLOGY 3,6,12	URINE CYTOLOGY EVERY 6 MONTHS	ANNUALLY			AS CLINICALLY INDICATED	

HIGH RISK Non-Muscle Invasive Bladder Cancer

TEST	YEAR						
	1	2	3	4	5	5 - 10	>10
CYSTOSCOPY	EVERY 3 MONTHS		EVERY 6 MONTHS			ANNUALLY	AS CLINICALLY INDICATED
UPPER TRACT IMAGING	BASELINE IMAGING AND AT 12 MONTHS	EVERY 1 – 2 YEARS					AS CLINICALLY INDICATED
ABDOMINAL PELVIC IMAGING	BASELINE IMAGING	AS CLINICALLY INDICATED					
BLOOD TEST	N/A						
URINE TEST	URINE CYTOLOGY EVERY 3 MONTHS CONSIDER URINARY UROTHELIAL TUMOR MARKERS (Category 2B)	URINE CYTOLOGY EVERY 6 MONTHS				ANNUALLY	AS CLINICALLY INDICATED

At the most favorable end of the clinical spectrum of NMIBC, management is fairly straightforward and is best left in hands of all urologists. Low-grade, superficial lesions tend to be more of a nuisance than a real threat. While they pose an extremely low risk of progression, they frequently recur and require long-term monitoring.[9] As with low risk prostate cancer, active surveillance of low grade tumors has been studied with low reported rates of disease progression.[10,11] However, even for non-muscle invasive disease there exist wide ranges for risk of recurrence (15-70%)[12] and progression (7-40%).[13,15] Therefore, optimizing the urologist's tools of non-invasive testing with biomarkers and diagnostic cystoscopy are critical in providing high-quality genitourinary care.

Biomarkers

Advances have been made in the use of biomarkers to aid in diagnosis and surveillance of bladder cancer. Historically, the gold standard has been urinary cytology, despite its low sensitivity for the majority of tumors.[14] Over 30 urinary biomarkers have been developed for bladder cancer, although only BTA, NMP-22, UroVysion® FISH and ImmunoCyt® have been approved by the FDA. All these biomarkers generally have low-sensitivity and are primarily utilized in the setting of atypical cytology and following BCG therapy. Newer tests employ novel technologies that incorporate genomics, metabolomics, inflammatory markers and epigenetics. These tests have improved sensitivity and specificity but have limited comparative testing. **Figure 3** summarizes several of the most commonly utilized biomarkers.

Figure 3: Selected Urinary Biomarkers for Bladder Cancer

Available commercial kits performance and characteristics

Name	FDA Approval/ CE Mark	Present in EAU guidelines 2019	Sample	Starting Material	Technology	Type of biomarker assessed	Purpose	Overall Performance	References
Cytology	Yes	Yes	Urine	Exfoliated cells	Giemsa and H&E staining	Cell Phenotype	Diagnostic and Surveillance	Sensitivity = 38% Specificity = 98%	Christopher GT Blick et al. 2016
uCyt+	Yes/NA	No	Urine	Exfoliated cells	Immunofluorescence	Antigen/Metabolites	Surveillance	Sensitivity = 73% Specificity = 66%	He, H et al. 2011
NMP22	Yes/Yes	Yes	Urine	Exfoliated cells	Elisa	Peptides	Surveillance	Sensitivity = 40% Specificity = 99%	Mowatt, G. et al 2010
CellSearch	Yes/Yes	No	Plasma/ serum	CTCs	Immunomagnetic enrichment	Proteins	Surveillance	Sensitivity = 35% Specificity = 97%	Zhang, Z, et al. 2017
UroVysion	Yes/Yes	Yes	Urine	Exfoliated cells	FISH	DNA (Aneuploidies)	Diagnostic	Sensitivity = 72% Specificity = 83%	Hajdinjak, T et al. 2008
BTA stat/ BTA Track	Yes/NA	No	Urine	Exfoliated cells	Dipstick immunoassay	Proteins	Diagnostic and Surveillance	Sensitivity = 70% Specificity = 75%	Glas, A. S., et al. 2003
CxBladder	No/No	No	Urine	Exfoliated cells	RT-qPCR	RNA (messenger RNA)	Diagnostic	Sensitivity = 82% Specificity = 85%	O'Sullivan, P et al. 2012
Xpert Detection	No/Yes	No	Urine	Exfoliated cells	RT-qPCR	RNA (messenger RNA)	Diagnostic	Sensitivity = 76% Specificity = 85%	Valenberg, FJP, V., et al. 2017
Uromonitor	No/Yes	Yes	Urine	Exfoliated cells	Real-time PCR	DNA (tumor cell DNA)	Surveillance	Sensitivity = 74% Specificity = 93%	Batista, R. et al. 2019

Cystoscopy and TURBT

As all members of a urology practice typically surgically manage NMIBC, optimizing the quality and practice of bladder cancer identification, resection and risk-stratification is one of the most significant challenges in establishing practice-wide protocols and behaviors in a bladder cancer program. This mandates the "buy-in" of the entire group and agreement about management. Education about the reason behind potentially practice-altering modifications in a condition that most urologists have treated their entire careers is critical to achieve success in a CBCC.

Advances in optimal imaging techniques have improved disease identification and the completeness of resection at the time of TURBT and are now broadly available for use in the office, ambulatory surgical center, and hospitals. The AUA/SUO guidelines note that BLC should be offered and NBI may be considered in patients with NMIBC at the time of TURBT to increase detection and reduce recurrence. BLC is performed with the use of hexaminolevulinic acid (CysView®), which is an FDA-approved optical imaging agent instilled in the bladder prior to cystoscopy that preferentially accumulates in cancerous cells. This enhances the contrast between normal and malignant urothelial cells when viewed under blue light illumination. Fluorescing tumors are then easier to detect and more completely seen, optimizing resection. BLC does require a specialized camera (both rigid and flexible scopes are available) and light source, but an adaptor has been developed to use with most endoscopes. BLC has been shown to increase detection of CIS by 32% and all tumors by 42% with no change in false-positive rates.[15] In addition, BLC has been shown to reduce disease progression in multiple studies and on meta-analysis.[16] NBI improves the discrimination between more vascularized tumors from normal urothelium and has been shown to identify up to 12% more tumors versus conventional white light cystoscopy.[17]

Incorporating advanced optimal imaging techniques into a CBCC facilitates accurate pathologic staging and complete resection of UCB. Under-staging secondary to inadequate tumor resection can lead to inappropriate disease management and can significantly delay the diagnosis of muscle invasive disease and application of appropriate treatment. This cannot be accomplished without obtaining muscularis propria in the TURBT specimen. Multiple studies have identified an increased risk of upstaging at the time of cystectomy in patients who did not have muscularis propria in the original resection specimen.[18] Furthermore, a repeat TURBT should be performed in all high-risk NMIBC, even if muscularis propria was reported and uninvolved in the original specimen. Upstaging to MIBC at the time of repeat TURBT has been reported to range up to 32%.[19] In addition, repeat resection is important to maximally remove all macroscopic and microscopic disease, thereby maximizing the benefit of intravesical therapy if indicated.

Accurate Risk Stratification

Figure 4 summarizes the updated risk stratification for NMIBC from the AUA/SUO. Adherence to risk stratification reporting is low, and the complexity of calculating and communicating this risk has been implicated in its clinician support.[20] Education of providers as to the critical aspects to capture in reporting of UCB during cystoscopy may improve risk stratification adoption, as well as the use of other implementation science methods.[21]

Stage is clearly a risk factor for recurrence and progression, with Ta disease being significantly less likely to do either than T1.[22] Stage alone, however, based on transurethral resection is not adequate for accurate risk stratification. The clinical course is highly variable even within T1 disease, with progression to MIBC ranging from 15%-50%.[23] In a study of almost 1,300 patients who were diagnosed with T1 or Ta disease who underwent early cystectomy without neoadjuvant chemotherapy, 46% had muscle-invasive disease in the cystectomy specimen.[24] This variability highlights the importance of other pathologic factors that play an important prognostic role alongside stage.

Alongside stage, pathologic grade has historically been considered an important factor in disease progression. While low-grade disease has a less than 10% risk for progression, the rate triples to over 30% for high-grade UCB.[25, 26] In addition to high-grade disease, Alongside stage, pathologic grade has historically been considered an important factor in disease progression. While low-grade disease has a less than 10% risk for progression, the rate triples to over 30% for high-grade UCB.[25, 26] In addition to high-grade disease, the most important prognostic factor for both recurrence and progression was the concomitant presence of CIS. In addition to increasing the risk of recurrence and progression to muscle-invasive disease in patients with NMIBC,[27] CIS is a strong predictor of finding muscle invasion at the time of early cystectomy for non-invasive disease (20%).[28] The presence of multiple (versus single) lesions at the time of TURBT almost doubles the risk for both recurrence and progression.[29] Similarly, compared to patients with < 3cm

Figure 4: Risk Stratification from NCCN Guidelines

LOW RISK	INTERMEDIATE RISK	HIGH RISK
- Low grade (LG) solitary Ta< 3cm - Papillary urothelial neoplasm of low malignant potential	- Recurrence within 1 year, LG Ta - Solitary LG Ta>3 cm - LG Ta, multifocal - High Grade (HG) Ta, < 3cm - LG T1	- HG T1 - Any recurrent, HG, Ta - HG Ta, >3 cm (or multifocal) - Any carcinoma in situ (CIS) - Any BCG failure in HG patient - Any variant histology - Any Lymphovascular invasion - Any HG prostatic urethral involvement

tumors, those with lesions > 3cm have twice the risk of disease progression. The presence of lymphovascular invasion at TURBT also carries a poorer prognosis and an increased risk for progression.[30, 31]

While the risk associated with each pathologic feature can be described independently, in clinical practice it is rare to find any of the above in isolation. A sample post-TURBT op note template is provided in **Figure 5** and can be easily incorporated into any electronic medical record post-operative visit note for a bladder cancer patient to capture the above clinical risk factors to facilitate assignment of risk stratification.

The goal of surveillance is to prevent progression to a higher stage, without performing unnecessary, costly, and potentially morbid interventions. Predicting exactly which patients will recur and progress—and therefore require more intensive care—must be individualized and remains more of an "art" than "science." This balance is captured in the NCCN recommendations for risk-stratified follow-up for NMIBC in **Figure 5**.

One benefit of crafting a protocol for risk-stratified surveillance is that appropriate radiographic surveillance of the upper tract can be recorded, and tools can be devised to prompt for radiography at the appropriate interval and intensity.[32]

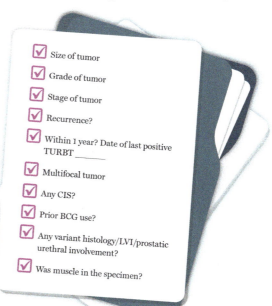

Figure 5:
Sample Template for Post-TURBT Office Visit Note to Facilitate Risk Stratification

Risk Category for This Patient: HIGH

LOW RISK	INTERMEDIATE RISK	HIGH RISK
■ Low grade (LG) solitary Ta< 3cm ■ Papillary urothelial neoplasm of low malignant potential	■ Recurrence within 1 year, LG Ta ■ Solitary LG Ta>3 cm ■ LG Ta, multifocal ■ High Grade (HG) Ta, < 3cm ■ LG T1	■ HG T1 ■ Any recurrent, HG, Ta ■ HG Ta, >3 cm (or multifocal) ■ Any carcinoma in situ (CIS) ■ Any BCG failure in HG patient ■ Any variant histology ■ Any Lymphovascular invasion ■ Any HG prostatic urethral involvement

Intravesical therapy

One area of focus for the CBCC should be to develop guideline-based protocols for the management of high-risk NMIBC bladder cancer (15% of all NMIBC), given its tendency to progress and metastasize without appropriate management. While intravesical therapy should not substitute for complete surgical resection of all visible disease as noted above, it does serve as an important adjuvant therapy for disease prophylaxis. Intravesical immunotherapy and chemotherapy reduce both disease recurrence and progression as demonstrated by multiple randomized trials examining several agents, with BCG demonstrating superiority to mitomycin C. The national shortage of BCG has emphasized the importance of selecting which patients may best benefit from induction and maintenance BCG to optimize the use of this limited resource. In our practice, centralized pathology review is performed following each TURBT and a determination is made centrally regarding the recommendation for induction, maintenance, and re-induction BCG or chemotherapy. We have found that centralizing the decision-making of our use of intravesical therapy has improved guideline compliance and increased the number of patients undergoing adjuvant intravesical treatment.

In treatment-naïve patients with high-risk NMIBC, the AUA recommends induction BCG and at least one year of maintenance intravesical therapy with either BCG or 6-12 months of maintenance intravesical chemotherapy. In patients who have failed BCG either through lack of response or recurrence within 5 years, intravesical treatment strategies are contingent upon time to recurrence. Repeat intravesical therapy should be used cautiously in place of radical therapy after non-muscle invasiveness is confirmed by repeat TURBT. Treatment beyond two courses is not recommended given the poor rates of success (<20%),[33] and management of BCG failure is both a clinical conundrum for many urologists and an opportunity for referral into the CBCC.

Historically, valrubicin was the only FDA-approved agent for BCG failure but its use was limited due to low complete response rates (18% at 6 months and 10% at 12 months).[34] However, there are more than 20 active clinical trials evaluating BCG-unresponsive (see **Table 1**) NMIBC with the recent FDA approval of intravenous pembrolizumab (Keytruda®) for BCG-unresponsive CIS who are ineligible for or refuse cystectomy.

TABLE 1
FDA DEFINITION OF BCG-UNRESPONSIVE DISEASE
Failed 2 course of induction BCG (5 of 6 instillations) and at least 2 of 3 maintenance instillations
Persistent HG disease at 6 months
Persistence or progression to T1 after induction BCG

Additional intravesical therapies such as Vicinium® (single-protein drug fused with E.coli endotoxin) and Instiladrin® (gene therapy that expresses human interferon alpha-2b inside tumor cells) are in FDA submission, and novel combinations of chemotherapy and vaccines also are under active study. Given the rapidly changing therapeutic landscape in BCG-unresponsive NMIBC and the desire to avoid the morbidity of cystectomy in these patients, the CBCC would be the ideal place for referral of these complex patients following BCG failure.

MIBC MANAGEMENT IN THE CBCC

Radical cystectomy is the standard of care for MIBC. In most groups, management of MIBC is referred either to academic centers or to urologic oncologists within the practice for management. It is critical that these surgeons are part of the CBCC as they typically serve as the bladder cancer "experts" in the practice. There are opportunities for improvement in MIBC management; we will review these here.

Neoadjuvant chemotherapy and immunotherapy

A recent meta-analysis of over 35,000 patients undergoing radical cystectomy demonstrated that only 17% utilized neoadjuvant chemotherapy (NAC) despite level one evidence regarding its survival benefit.[35] Multiple prospective randomized trials have been performed, which demonstrate a small but durable 5% to 6.5% benefit of neoadjuvant platinum-based combination chemotherapy on survival at 5 years.[36] The decision to forgo NAC should be an intentional one, and a potential cystectomy candidate should be reviewed in the CBCC for NAC eligibility.

Both clinical tools and biomarkers can aid CBCC physicians in determining the best candidates for NAC. NAC is most efficacious in patients who have specific pathologic (MIBC, LVI, bulky tumor or micropapillary, small cell or urothelial histology with squamous or glandular differentiation), radiographic (perivesical stranding, hydronephrosis or enlarged or suspicious pelvic lymph nodes), or clinical (palpable pelvic mass, favorable performance status) features.[37,38] The Decipher Bladder™ genomic test was derived from over 46,000 genes in the Cancer Genome Atlas project and classifies a bladder tumor into four molecular subtypes, which predict response and survival outcome to NAC. This "precision medicine" approach allows the CBCC provider to determine which patients may benefit from NAC and which should proceed to immediate cystectomy.

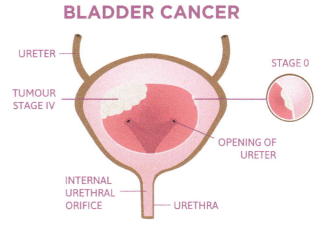

Unfortunately, approximately 50% of patients with MIBC are cisplatin-ineligible. For these patients, neoadjuvant immunotherapy with checkpoint inhibitors, such as pembrolizumab appear to be safe[39] and several phase 3 studies are underway using these agents as monotherapy or in combination with chemotherapy in the neoadjuvant setting.

Bladder-sparing protocols

In appropriately selected patients, bladder-sparing tri-modal therapy (TMT) with complete TURBT and chemoradiation should be offered to patients with MIBC with favorable pathologic features. These include RT2 disease, solitary tumors, no lymphadenopathy, no multifocal CIS or nonurothelial histology, and no hydronephrosis.[40] Radiotherapy or chemotherapy alone is both inferior to chemoradiation in this setting and neither should be offered as a primary modality.[41]

There is an important role for the CBCC to help advocate for TMT, especially in the elderly and racial minorities. Almost half of patients 65 years or older with MIBC receive no or non-aggressive treatment for their MIBC despite positive oncologic outcomes (2-year OS of 94% and 2-year DFS of 73%) with TMT. It is important that TMT does not become the default for management of MIBC in a practice if there are no providers who perform radical cystectomy. There are no randomized data comparing the outcomes of TMT to extirpative surgery, and so each patient with MIBC should be presented in the CBCC with an individualized treatment plan. If appropriate for cystectomy, these patients should be referred to other community-based or academic practices performing these procedures.

APPENDIX 1
Comprehensive Bladder Cancer Clinic (CBCC)
Clinical Policy for IO administration and associated care

Policy: To safely administer and manage IO (currently, only Keytruda®) infusions and associated care.

Procedure:

Day of consult/enrollment:

1. Review/enroll patient and appropriate care team:

   ✓ Review Keytruda® mechanism of action (Refer to Merck's, *A Treatment Guide for Keytruda®*, page 4.)

   ✓ Merck's Keytruda® Patient Support Booklet with wallet card

   ✓ Merck Access Program

   ✓ Merck's Key + You

   ✓ Your practice's Keytruda® Consent Form

   - Patient, witness, and physician must sign consent form
   - Give signed copy to patient
   - Send signed original to stat scanning to EHR

2. Obtain/document baseline ROS assessment, Merck's ROS Assessment form.

3. Obtain/document baseline vital signs: BP, HR, temp, O2 saturation.

4. Assess/document baseline ECOG score.

5. Send completed Merck Access information to Front Office Specialist (FOS) for processing.

6. Front Office Specialist must obtain approval from practice manager prior to placing medication order.

7. Upon RCM approval, order medication from Purchasing Manager (delivery should be no more than 2 days prior to scheduled infusion.).

8. When medication is received, store under refrigeration. *Do NOT freeze.

APPENDIX 1
Day of Infusion:

1. FOS registers patient and accepts all co-pays and/or OOP expenses prior to infusion.

2. CBCC RN accepts patient from FOS and verifies patient by two forms of ID name/DOB.

3. Obtain/document ROS assessment, Merck's ROS Assessment form.

4. Obtain/document vital signs: BP, HR, temp, O2 saturation.

5. Assess/document ECOG score.

6. CBCC RN will enter standing lab order and draw labs: *Enter test logbook per protocol.

   - ✓ Stat CBC (if UA lab) *Notify CBCC provider of abnormal results stat
   - ✓ CMP
   - ✓ LDH
   - ✓ T4
   - ✓ TSH
   - ✓ Cortisol

7. If patient is of childbearing years and negative history of hysterectomy, CBCC RN will perform pregnancy test. Document results.

8. Give patient opportunity to ask any additional questions or discuss any concerns.

9. Notify CBCC provider immediately of any ROS/vitals/ ECOG changes, results of pregnancy test, and/or patient concerns.

10. Provider performs EOV and will notify CBCC RN to proceed or not to proceed with infusion.

11. If CBCC provider orders to proceed, CBCC RN will establish venous access per protocol.

12. CBCC RN will prepare medication for infusion by diluting Keytruda® solution from two (2) vials (Keytruda® vial = 100mg/4mL) into 250mL bag of Normal Saline 9% IV solution. *Ensure to inject only 8mL of solution for infusion; vial may have overfill. Waste unused drug per protocol.

13. Store diluted solution at room temperature for no more than 6 hours from the time of dilution. If refrigerated, you may store for no more than 24 hours. *Do not prepare solution until CBCC provider and patient have confirmed to proceed with infusion.

14. CBCC RN will complete label and place on prepared medication bag. Include patient name, name of medication, dose, date, and time prepared, and the preparing CBCC RN's initials on label.

15. CBCC RN will ensure IV is patent with blood return and administer the infusion solution over 30 minutes through an IV line with a 0.2 to 5 micron in-line or add-on filter. *Do NOT co-administer other drugs through the infusion line.

16. CBCC RN will monitor patient throughout infusion and offer warming device as needed.

17. In case of infusion reaction, refer to page 12 of CTCAE Infusion Reaction protocol and notify CBCC provider stat.

18. Upon completion of infusion, flush IV line with 5cc of Normal Saline. CBCC RN will discontinue IV access and discharge patient to appropriate caregiver.

19. CBCC RN will complete appropriate documentation in EHR as per protocol for billing purposes and CBCC provider sign-off.

20. CBCC RN will reconcile test logbook as per protocol, review lab results, and notify CBCC provider of any changes or abnormal labs; will follow through with any additional orders given.

21. CBCC RN or CBCC Nurse Navigator will contact patient on days 3 and 10 post-infusion to follow-up on tolerance by documenting a phone encounter and will include:

    ✓ ROS assessment, Merck's ROS Assessment form

    ✓ ECOG score

    ✓ Notify patient of labs drawn at previous infusion

    ✓ Notify CBCC provider immediately of any ROS/ECOG changes, and/or patient concerns

    ✓ Instruct patient on any next step necessary, as per CBCC provider instructions

    ✓ Arrange for labs to be drawn on day 10 post-infusion

22. At 2 weeks post-infusion (i.e. 1 week pre-infusion), the patient will be seen by the CBCC provider for an OV to review labs and to assess SE (e.g., rash, fatigue, diarrhea, nausea, cough/SOB) in person prior to the next infusion.

Standing Imaging Orders:

1. CBCC FOS and/or RN may initiate Imaging orders on the following dates:
   - ✓ 9 weeks after first infusion
   - ✓ Then every 6 weeks for the first year
   - ✓ Then every 12 weeks thereafter
1. Patients presenting with pulmonary changes
   - ✓ AP/LAT chest
   - ✓ ± Chest CT
1. Patients with pituitary changes
   - ✓ Head MRI

Other Standing Orders:

1. Patients with Endocrine changes -> Refer to Endocrinologist

REFERENCES

1. Siegel, R.L., Miller, K.D.& Jemal A. Cancer statistics, 2020. CA Cancer J Clin 202; 70, 7-30.
2. Altekruse, S.F. et al. (National Cancer Institute, Bethesda, MD).
3. Riley GF, Potosky AL, Lubitz JD, et al. Medicare payments from diagnosis to death for elderly cancer patients by stage at diagnosis. Med Care 1995; 33:828-41.
4. Mariotto AB, Yabroff KR, Shao Y, Fe et al. Projections of the cost of cancer care in the United States: 2010-2020. J Natl Cancer Inst 2011; 103:117-28.
5. Chang SS, Boorjian SA, Chou R, Clark PE, Daneshmand S, Konety BR, Pruthi R, Quale DZ, Ritch CR, Seigne JD, Skinner EC, Smith ND, McKiernan JM. Diagnosis and Treatment of Non-Muscle Invasive Bladder Cancer: AUA/SUO Guideline. J Urol. 2016 Oct; 196(4):1021-9.
6. Skolarus TA, Ye Z, Montgomery JS, et al. Use of restaging bladder tumor resection for bladder cancer among Medicare beneficiaries. Urology 2011; 78:1345-9.
7. Karl A, Adejoro O, Saigal C, et al. General adherence to guideline recommendations on initial diagnosis of bladder cancer in the United States and influencing factors. Clin Genitourin Cancer 2014; 12:270-7.
8. Hollenbeck BK, Ye Z, Dunn RL, et al. Provider treatment intensity and outcomes for patients with early-stage bladder cancer. J Natl Cancer Inst 2009; 101:571-80.
9. Pruthi, R.S., Baldwin, N., Bhalani, V. & Wallen, E.M. Conservative management of low risk superficial bladder tumors. Journal of Urology 179, 87 90 (2008).
10. Pruthi RS, Baldwin N, Bhalani V, et al. Conservative management of low risk superficial bladder tumors. J Urol 2008; 179:87-90.
11. Tiu A, Jenkins LC, Soloway MS. Active surveillance for low-risk bladder cancer. Urol Oncol 2014; 32:33.e7-10.
12. Allard, P., Bernard, P., Fradet, Y. & Tetu, B. The early clinical course of primary Ta and T1 bladder cancer: a proposed prognostic index. Br J Urol 81, 692-8 (1998).
13. Kurth, K.H. et al. Factors Affecting Recurrence and Progression in Superficial Bladder-Tumors. European Journal of Cancer 31A, 1840-1846 (1995).
14. Bladder cancer. Kaufman DS, Shipley WU, Feldman AS. Lancet. 2009 Jul 18; 374(9685):239-49.
15. Daneshmand S, Patel S, Lotan Y, et al. Efficacy and Safety of Blue Light Flexible Cystoscopy with Hexaminolevulinate in the Surveillance of Bladder Cancer: A Phase III, Comparative, Multicenter Study. J Urol. 2018;199(5):1158-1165.
16. Gakis G, Fahmy OJ. Systematic review and meta-analysis on the impact of hexaminolevulinate-versus white-light guided transurethral bladder tumor resection on progression in non-muscle invasive bladder cancer. Bladder Cancer. 2016;2:293-300.
17. Burger M, Grossman HB, Droller M, et al. Photodynamic diagnosis of non–muscle-invasive bladder cancer with hexaminolevulinate cystoscopy: a meta-analysis of detection and recurrence based on raw data. Eur Urol. 2013; 64: 846-854.
18. Badalato, G., Patel, T., Hruby, G. & McKiernan, J. Does the presence of muscularis propria on transurethral resection of bladder tumour specimens affect the rate of upstaging in cT1 bladder cancer? Bju International (2010).
19. Cumberbatch, Marcus G.K. et al. Repeat Transurethral Resection in Non–muscle-invasive Bladder Cancer: A Systematic Review. European Urology, Volume 73, Issue 6, 925 – 933.
20. Downs TM et al. Can we improve non muscle invasive bladder cancer guidelines adherence with smarter risk stratification? J Urol 2018; 200: 706-8.
21. Schroeck, F. R., Smith, N., & Shelton, J. B. (2018). Implementing risk-aligned bladder cancer surveillance care. Urologic oncology, 36(5), 257–264.
22. Kiemeney, L.A., Witjes, J.A., Heijbroek, R.P., Verbeek, A.L. & Debruyne, F.M. Predictability of recurrent and progressive disease in individual patients with primary superficial bladder cancer. J Urol 150, 60-4 (1993).
23. Chang, S.S. & Cookson, M.S. Non-muscle-invasive bladder cancer: The role of radical cystectomy. Urology 66, 917-922 (2005).
24. Svatek, R.S. et al. Discrepancy between clinical and pathological stage: external validation of the impact on prognosis in an international radical cystectomy cohort. Bju International 107, 898-904 (2011).
25. Torti, F.M. et al. Superficial bladder cancer: the primacy of grade in the development of invasive disease. J Clin Oncol 5, 125-30 (1987).
26. Kwak, C. et al. Initial tumor stage and grade as a predictive factor for recurrence in patients with stage T1 grade 3 bladder cancer. Journal of Urology 171, 149-152 (2004).
27. Althausen, A.F., Prout, G.R., Jr. & Daly, J.J. Non-invasive papillary carcinoma of the bladder associated with carcinoma in situ. J Urol 116, 575-80 (1976).
28. Masood, S., Sriprasad, S., Palmer, J.H. & Mufti, G.R. T1G3 bladder cancer--indications for early cystectomy. Int Urol Nephrol 36, 41-4 (2004).
29. Sylvester, R.J. et al. Predicting recurrence and progression in individual patients with stage Ta T1 bladder cancer using EORTC risk tables: a combined analysis of 2596 patients from seven EORTC trials. Eur Urol 49, 466-5; discussion 475-7 (2006).
30. Streeper, N.M. et al. The significance of lymphovascular invasion in transurethral resection of bladder tumour and cystectomy specimens on the survival of patients with urothelial bladder cancer. Bju International 103, 475-9 (2009).
31. Cho, K.S. et al. Lymphovascular Invasion in Transurethral Resection Specimens as Predictor of Progression and Metastasis in Patients With Newly Diagnosed T1 Bladder Urothelial Cancer. Journal of Urology 182, 2625-2630 (2009).
32. Allen, Brian C. et al. ACR Appropriateness Criteria® Post-Treatment Surveillance of Bladder Cancer. Journal of the American College of Radiology, Volume 16, Issue 11, S417 - S427

33. Grossman, H.B. et al. Neoadjuvant chemotherapy plus cystectomy compared with cystectomy alone for locally advanced bladder cancer. N Engl J Med 349, 859-66 (2003).

34. Dinney CP, Greenberg RE, Steinberg GD. Intravesical valrubicin in patients with bladder carcinoma in situ and contraindication to or failure after bacillus Calmette-Guerin. Urol Oncol. 2013; 31:1635-1642.

35. Liu W. The utilization status of neoadjuvant chemotherapy in muscle-invasive bladder cancer: a systematic review and meta-analysis. Minerva Urol Nefrol 2020 (epub ahead of print)

36. Neoadjuvant chemotherapy in invasive bladder cancer: update of a systematic review and meta-analysis of individual patient data advanced bladder cancer (ABC) meta-analysis collaboration. Eur Urol 48, 202-5; discussion 205-6 (2005).

37. Scosyrev, E. et al. Do mixed histological features affect survival benefit from neoadjuvant platinum-based combination chemotherapy in patients with locally advanced bladder cancer? A secondary analysis of Southwest Oncology Group-Directed Intergroup Study (S8710). BJU Int (2010)

38. Wheat, J.C. & Lee, C.T. Contemporary management of muscle invasive bladder cancer, in Marshall FF (ed.): AUA Update Series Lesson 34. Linthicum, MD: American Urological Association, 2010, Volume 29, 338-347.

39. Briganti A, Gandaglia G, Scuderi S, et al. Surgical safety of radical cystectomy and pelvic lymph node dissection following neoadjuvant pembolizumab in patients with bladder cancer: Prospective assessment perioperative outcomes from the PURE-01 trial [published online January 3, 2020]. Eur Urol. doi: 10.1016/j.eururo.2019.12.019

40. Premo, C., Apolo, A. B., Agarwal, P. K., & Citrin, D. E. (2015). Trimodality therapy in bladder cancer: who, what, and when? The Urologic clinics of North America, 42(2), 169.

41. James ND, Hussain SA, Hall E, Jenkins P, Tremlett J, Rawlings C, Crundwell M, Sizer B, Sreenivasan T, Hendron C, Lewis R, Waters R, Huddart RA, BC2001 Investigators. Radiotherapy with or without chemotherapy in muscle-invasive bladder cancer. N Engl J Med. 2012 Apr 19; 366(16):1477-88.

42. Mohamed HAH, et al. Trimodalities for bladder cancer in elderly: Transurethral resection, hypofractionated radiotherapy and gemcitabine. Cancer Radiother 2018; 22: 236-40

43. Lerner SP, Dinney C, Kamat A, et al. Clarification of bladder cancer disease states following treatment of patients with intravesical BCG. Bladder Cancer. 2015;1:29-30.

44. NCCN guidelines in bladder cancer, version 3.2020

45. Batista, R et al. 2020. Biomarkers for Bladder Cancer Diagnosis and Surveillance: A comprehensive review. Diagnostics (Basel: Switzerland), 10(1).

KEY POINTS

- **Drug development and approval in bladder cancer therapeutics** over the past 5 years have added to the complexity and options for urologists to use in the treatment of the disease.

- **There is tremendous heterogeneity of practice patterns** through the spectrum of disease, leading to overuse of treatments in low-risk patients and underuse among high-risk patients.

- **Establishing a Comprehensive Bladder Cancer Clinic (CBCC)** to aid in the management of non-muscle invasive bladder cancer (NMIBC), muscle invasive bladder (MIBC) and even metastatic bladder cancer can improve resource utilization, optimize oncologic outcomes and be financially successful.

- **Adoption of centralized review and decision-making** may improve the availability, efficacy and quality of management of all stages of bladder cancer.

- **The designation of a bladder cancer clinical champion is critical** to navigate the developments in diagnosis, treatment and surveillance of this disease.

Sandip M. Prasad, MD, MPhil

Sandip Prasad is a member of Garden State Urology and serves currently as the director of Genitourinary Surgical Oncology at Morristown Medical Center/Atlantic Health System in New Jersey. He has published over 60 peer-reviewed journal articles and book chapters and serves as an associate editor for Urology Practice and Current Urology Reports and as an editorial reviewer for nine specialty journals in urology.

CHAPTER 25

Women's Pelvic Health Centers

David C. Chaikin, MD
Michael Ingber, MD

As large urology groups continue to integrate and mature, there is great interest in organizing subspecialty service lines. Many LUGPA groups have been able to establish centers of excellence, including clinics in advanced prostate cancer, bone implications of prolonged hormone ablation in prostate cancer, pediatrics, stone disease, and women's pelvic health. This chapter will concentrate on women's pelvic health.

The practicing urologist has traditionally cared for women with stress urinary incontinence and overactive bladder. Urologists would often refer more complicated patients, especially those with pelvic prolapse, to more specialized urology or gynecology clinics. A patient who was unwilling or unable to travel to a more specialized clinic would often have to live with their problem. In 2013, as a response to increased interest by gynecologists in the field and the desire to formalize training for the care of these patients, The American Board of Urology added a subspecialty certification in Female Pelvic Medicine and Reconstructive Surgery (FPMRS). Now, several years later, most large urology groups have subspecialized FPMRS urologists or gynecologists. Additionally, large groups have had a chance to integrate, consolidate and organize strategic plans to provide efficient and comprehensive urologic care. These facts should lead the LUGPA groups to establish women's pelvic health centers of excellence.

Why We Need Women's Pelvic Health Centers of Excellence

Federal healthcare legislation is changing the landscape for how providers get paid. Traditional fee-for-service care is being replaced by Merit Based Payment System (MIPS). We expect commercial payers across the United States to follow suit. As this occurs, groups are realizing an opportunity to have better data for more targeted decision making, performance information to guide and identify areas for improvement, and the ability to enhance market position. We believe as this occurs, there will be fewer complications, improved outcomes and a better patient experience.

Developing a Women's Center can allow groups the ability to position their physicians as specialists in the field. Additionally, developing a women's pelvic health center of excellence will give a practice the ability to demonstrate, with measurable data, a commitment to patient care. It will also help capture and retain more patients. Traditionally, a woman went to see a urologist with bladder complaints that may include incontinence, pain, recurrent urinary tract infections, urinary urgency, and frequency or the feelings of vaginal bulging. She may pick a particular urologist based on patient, physician, or insurance referral or reputation. The urologist she picked may or may not have a particular interest or expertise in female pelvic health. The urologist will oftentimes try to treat the patient's complaints. He/she may place a sling if she is complaining of stress incontinence, but may not pay attention to how much prolapse she has. The urologist may give medications for her urinary urgency and frequency, but may not provide more advanced therapies or be thorough enough with follow up. It is well known that medication compliance is extremely poor, particularly with overactive bladder, when patients are not under the care of a dedicated female urologist, or part of a women's health program where follow up can be monitored and structured. Chancellor reported that 73% of women discontinued their medication in the first year of treatments.[1] D'Souza revealed that 92% of patients discontinued their medication within two years.[2] With such a significant drop off in patients taking medication long term, there is usually an associated drop-off in patient follow up. It is clear there are a few key elements that can make a women's health clinic successful: a dedicated physician team, a navigator, and appropriate pathways and education.

In general, there are a myriad of reasons for the lack of follow up by female patients in urology practices besides efficacy of treatment or medication side effects. The patient may feel she has hit the end of the road in terms of options. She may have heard about a friend who had a bad complication from surgery or that she just doesn't think her problem is bad enough for expensive therapy that doesn't work well. She may think that her incontinence is part of aging and she should have to live with it, or that sex is just painful and she should just deal with it! Perhaps she was never educated about more advanced therapies like Botox® and sacral modulation. With the recent FDA advisory warning on vaginal mesh and consequent television commercials outlining their legal rights, patients are far more reluctant to seek treatment for incontinence or prolapse. If they do, it is helpful for women to see the appropriate physician who can educate them on the topic and discuss the options.

No matter the reason, this is exactly why LUGPA groups should consider a dedicated women's health center of excellence. A woman needs to know there are conservative measures for prolapse such as a pessary. She needs to know there are successful ways to treat overactive bladder if medications don't work. She needs to know the facts behind using mesh for sling and prolapse surgery, and that there are effective non-mesh surgical options for both conditions. She needs to know that incontinence and prolapse are not things she has to live with.

We strongly believe that by using a focused approach, women will be better informed and have better outcomes and higher satisfaction. If groups choose to ignore the reality of these problems, they will likely lose these patients to groups that have instituted these changes, or even worse, to competing clinics.

Getting Started

In order to establish a women's pelvic health center of excellence, some basic guidelines should be followed. First and foremost, strong physician leadership and full support by the group is critical in order to succeed. Next, the group should decide which patients they want to include: all female patients with a bladder complaint or only the ones considering advanced therapies for overactive bladder. Our suggestion is to consider referring women to a center of excellence if they have a refractory overactive bladder, or are experiencing any form of incontinence (stress and urge) not responding to initial treatments, or voiding dysfunction secondary to a neurologic condition or complex bladder dysfunction. Patients with pelvic organ prolapse should be referred or "moved" as well, however, this requires this level of specialty care be represented within the practice by either a FPMRS-certified physician or a urologist with extensive experience in reconstructive surgery. Lastly, depending on available trained providers, patients with bowel-related complaints, such as accidental bowel leakage, or incomplete defecation can also be referred to the clinic.

Identifying Your Population

Once the LUGPA group has made the decision to move forward, formed a team, and identified the type of patients to be included, it's time to run some reports on different populations that exist in the practice. Subcategorizing and batching all patients with a diagnosis of overactive bladder symptoms, pelvic floor prolapse, stress Incontinence, and recurrent urinary tract infections should be accomplished. Another patient group of interest might be those who have had advanced therapies for OAB such as Percutaneous Tibial Stimulation (PTNS), Botulinum toxin (Botox®), or sacral neuromodulation (Interstim & Axonics). These reports of different patient populations will help you understand exactly how many patients exist in the practice in these areas. In turn, the practice will have a clearer picture as to what areas have low volume and need growth. The group could use existing benchmarks to compare how many women have undergone a therapy and decide if that would be an area of growth that would be desired. Understanding the population of patients from the start will help the team identify needs for advanced providers, and establish a baseline to measure the clinic's growth and shifts in therapies and treatments (see **Figure 1**). Much of this data is easily obtained from practice management systems as well as medication files.

FIGURE 1
Items for Data Collection/Per Patient:

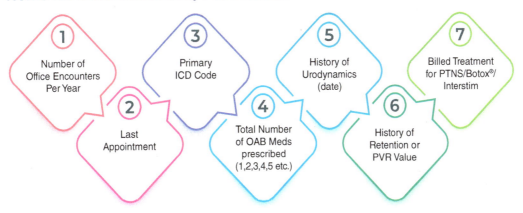

When Should a Women Be Referred

Oftentimes, the question is asked when to make the referral to a women's pelvic health center. Most LUGPA urologists are comfortable and want to treat women as part of their practice. Furthermore, with the uncertainty of healthcare, most providers are not looking to close their practice to a large segment of the population. We have found distinctive places within a pathway to make a referral. For example, in the authors' practice, all of our urologists treat all women with overactive bladder. Our OAB bladder patients will stay with their physician for conservative therapies, such as pelvic muscle rehabilitation and medical treatments. Once the physician orders urodynamics, we interpret that as a part of the patients' treatment; they are failing conventional therapy and are interested in further treatment. Urodynamics is performed and the patient is then referred or "moved" to our Women's Pelvic Health Center. There, physicians with knowledge and training in interpreting urodynamics can assess the patient and make a recommendation. In the case of refractory OAB, the patient may be counseled on advanced therapies like Botox®, PTNS, or Neuromodulation. Other times, occult stress urinary incontinence, or stress-induced urgency may be found, where the patient may warrant an outlet-related procedure, such as a suburethral sling. With that approach, many more patients will have a better understanding of their options and will receive the best treatment for them. We have found this active approach is more successful than the passive approach of waiting for the physician to refer the patient. Another option would be to engage the patient from the outset with a treatment plan, in writing or on the practice's website, that shows them the pathway—when they meet certain "failure" criteria, they will be referred to the Women's Pelvic Health Center.

Women's Pelvic Health Team

In order to set up a successful clinic, members of the clinic should have a genuine interest in treating the female patient and her problems. Groups need to identify these physicians upfront and others need to acknowledge their expertise. Oftentimes, not every member of a LUGPA group should be included. This will ultimately help create the referral pathway needed to provide specialized care that is often not offered to patients in groups where pathways and specialists are not aligned.

Governance of the center is essential. The center should name both a medical director and a center coordinator. These are often different members. The next step is to identify the center's panel of members. The panel should include a general urologist from the group, a nurse navigator, a FPMRS surgeon or female urology specialist, a behavioral health specialist, and a physical therapist with specialty-training in female and male pelvic health. In addition, because pelvic floor dysfunctions are sometimes complicated and involve bowel dysfunction, it is imperative that the panel also include a colorectal surgeon or gastroenterologist well-versed in treating accidental bowel leakage and other defecatory dysfunctions. The colorectal surgeon should be familiar with defecography testing and surgical repair. Other potential panel members may include a psychologist, a nutritionist, and even a health coach. The panel should meet regularly to discuss challenging cases and to ensure the center is running properly.

The Role of the Nurse Navigator

Nurse navigators are essential to the management and growth of the women's pelvic health center. The navigator should be familiar with each pathway step. Physician time and effort is needed to educate navigators about medications that are used, treatments offered and surgical options available. Providing them with basic reporting and analytic tools so they can begin to identify patients within the practice that fit available therapies will be very helpful. This can be impactful for not only patients, but also the practice.

Generating lists of patients in need of follow up or re-evaluation can be a gateway for a navigator to reach out to patients. Some examples of how nurse navigators are currently used in LUGPA groups include tracking the progression of patients who are in a pelvic floor rehabilitation program for overactive bladder. Initiating phone calls for follow up on medication efficacy and tolerance can be a key strategy for the navigator to keep overactive bladder patients on track and in the practice. It is well-known that a significant number of patients drop out of a practice after failing their first overactive bladder medication. As patients fail their medications, the navigator can be there to educate and schedule them for office visits or urodynamics. After third-line therapies are offered, navigators can follow up with patients who have undergone these treatments to ensure proper follow up and care. For example, the navigator can ensure that patients who undergo Botox® injections have proper appointments to assess efficacy and verify that they are not in retention. Navigators can confirm follow up for sacral neuromodulation procedures for device interrogation and to maximize battery life.

The navigators act as a point of contact and often provide direction when patients are confused about expectations or start to lose hope. Additionally, some navigators assist in insurance precertification, something that many private payers require for third-line therapies for overactive bladder. A navigator who is familiar with the patient's situation can be their best advocate when seeking approval for more complex therapies. Finally, navigators can be very effective in reducing patient dissatisfaction or drop-out and can have significant impact on the growth of the clinic. The role of the navigator can be flexible, but their contribution is often a key component to a successful program.

Call Center

A centralized call center is a useful adjunct for establishing a successful Women's Pelvic Health Center. The initial phone call is the first interaction the patient has with the practice, and by engaging the patient from the get-go, the commitment to providing the highest possible quality of care is demonstrated to the patient. A dedicated call center can use a screening questionnaire to direct the patient to an appropriate staff member.

The first contact can show the patient the commitment to excellence. A patient can be sent registration forms, an introductory packet that includes some basic information about the pelvic health center, questionnaires and, when appropriate, instructions for completing a bladder diary. The questionnaires and diary can be completed prior to the first visit or subsequent visit either on paper or on an app in the patient portal, website, or mobile device. Symptom specific questionnaires added to the general medical and surgical history forms can include specific questions related to global pelvic floor function. Quality of life questionnaires useful in the OAB population include the AUA symptom score,[4] OAB questionnaire(OAB-q),[5] OAB symptom score,[6] Urogenital Distress Inventory-Incontinence Questionnaire[7] or the MESA questionnaire.[8] We strongly believe that women with overactive bladder, stress incontinence and/or pelvic prolapse should have a voiding diary and/or pad test as part of their evaluation and treatment.

Recently, we began using a mobile app (via an iPhone or Android phone) called weShare® URO (Symptelligence Medical, LLC, Franklin MA). The application is comprised of disease-specific validated questionnaires (Lower Urinary Tract Symptom Score, AUA Symptom Score4, Patient Global Impression of Improvement) and bladder diaries that are completed in real time by the patient. Based on the answers to the questionnaires and diary, a "WeScore" is calculated and displayed in a one-page summary that quantitates the severity of the patient's symptoms. The symptoms are divided into five subscores that represent five ICD-10 diagnostic categories—voiding dysfunction (e.g., urethral obstruction due to prolapse), storage problems, overactive bladder, incontinence, and nocturia. In addition, an overall bother score is displayed (**Figure 1 A and 1 B**).

This approach has many advantages. First, it engages the patient from the outset and demonstrates the center's commitment to excellence. Second, it is the first step in triage and ensures that the patient receives an appropriate referral and that the physician has sufficient information on the first visit to formulate a diagnostic and treatment plan. Finally, serial questionnaires and diaries serve as a scorecard to monitor treatment efficacy (**Figure 1 A and 1 B**), and as discussed below, the weShare database has been used as the substrate for developing lower urinary tract symptom phenotypes and clinical pathways.

Outsourcing data collection to the patient also has economic benefits. Not only does it saves administrative costs, the app also provides the physician and practice with the resources to optimize reimbursement and, where appropriate, utilize remote patient monitoring as a source of income. Finally, the composition data generated by weShare can be used to help formulate appropriate reimbursement methods based on MIPS and APM requirements.

FIGURE 1 A
Lower Urinary Tract Symptom Score

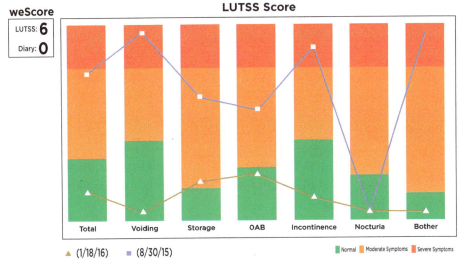

Here is an example of the one page summary. A. The colored graph displays the total LUTSS and the six subscores. The higher the score, the worse the symptoms. A score in the red represents the worst possible symptoms; green the least (normal). The blue line (square boxes) represents the scores prior to surgical treatment of urethral stricture. The brown line (triangles) shows the scores nearly 5 is months post operatively (yes, women get urethral strictures). Serial monitoring of the LUTSS score before and after treatment documents treatment efficacy. In this case, her LUTSS fell from 42 to 6 and all of her symptoms were abated.

FIGURE 1 B

Bladder Diary		
Diary Date	1/18/16	8/30/15
Voided Volume (ml)		
24 Hours	1470	1031
Daytime	1277	657
Nighttime	193	374
# Voided		
24 Hours	5	10
Daytime	5	7
Nighttime	0	3
Maximum Voided Volume	400	153
# Incontinent Episodes	0	0
# Urgency Voids	0	0
# Difficult Voiding Episodes	0	10
Nocturnal Polyuria Index	0.13	0.36
Urge Void Correlation	0.48	2.44
Urge Void Correlation	0.88	-0.28

The bladder diary corroborates the symptom score analysis. Postoperatively, she went from 10 to 5 daytime voids, 3 to zero episodes of nocturia, and from 10 to 0 episodes of difficulty voiding. Moreover, her bladder capacity increased from 153 mL to 400 mL.

Diagnostic Testing/Aids

It is imperative for a center of excellence to adopt standardized diaries and a process to utilize them across the entire practice. All physicians should be collecting this data as they make clinical decisions to assist in the diagnosis and treatment of women with bladder dysfunction.

A woman's pelvic health center should be able to noninvasively determine urine flow patterns (uroflow), as well as post-void residual (PVR by bladder scan) for its patients. The clinic should have a dedicated urodynamic lab and staff. Having a dedicated staff for urodynamics helps to create consistency, reliability, and predictability. The panel could consider a separate lab just for women or use the lab for both men and women with different entrances. The staff should feel they are part of the team and involved in communication with the patient.

Video urodynamics is also an option that can be added. Video urodynamics is especially helpful in identifying the cause and site of urethral obstruction, the mechanism of stress incontinence, bladder disease in patients with neurologic disease, and women where a fistula or urethral diverticulum is suspected (AUA/SUFU Guidelines, 2012). The use of fluoroscopy does require additional space and expertise (e.g., X-ray tech), but can be helpful to help answer the most difficult questions. We believe the physician should be involved in the urodynamic evaluation in real time.

Procedures

Any physician working in a women's pelvic health center should be well-versed in doing a detailed pelvic examination, and be fully competent with performing cystoscopy. Procedures functioning as an adjunct to any pelvic muscle rehabilitation program, such as manometry and electromyography (EMG) are essential. In addition, it is not uncommon for a FPMRS surgeon to perform other procedures in the office such as colposcopy and vulvar biopsies in order to diagnose common vulvar dermatoses, such as lichen sclerosus et. Depending on training in vulvodynia, many may offer treatments, such as pudendal nerve blocks and Botox® injections to the pelvic floor for high tone pelvic floor dysfunction. Lastly, there are a number of office surgical procedures that should be offered to meet the needs of patients coming to these types of clinics (see **Figure 2**).

FIGURE 2

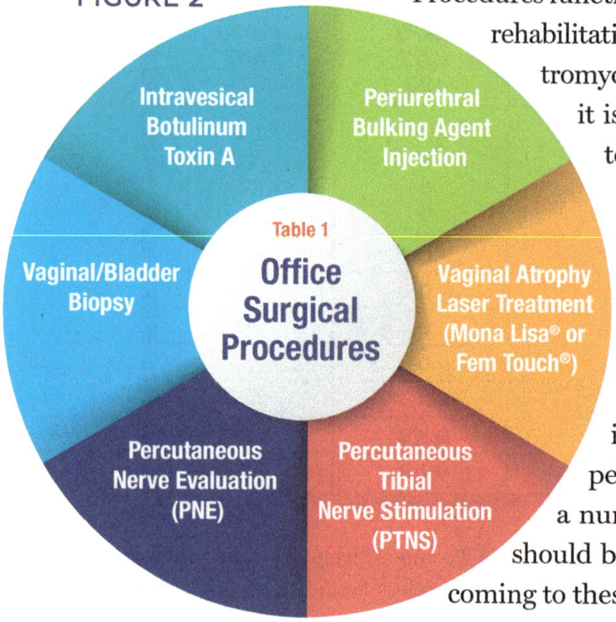

Table 1 — Office Surgical Procedures:
- Intravesical Botulinum Toxin A
- Periurethral Bulking Agent Injection
- Vaginal Atrophy Laser Treatment (Mona Lisa® or Fem Touch®)
- Percutaneous Tibial Nerve Stimulation (PTNS)
- Percutaneous Nerve Evaluation (PNE)
- Vaginal/Bladder Biopsy

Quality

Determining and maintaining quality is paramount for any health center. This is especially important with the change in the federal landscape for how providers are getting paid. In order to improve quality, the center should establish clinical pathways of care that would enable all physicians to treat each patient with accepted standards of care. A women's pelvic health center should measure outcomes through patient satisfaction surveys, retrospective and prospective studies.

Clinical Pathways

We believe establishing clinical pathways is critical for a LUGPA group to be effective. The clinical pathway needs to have the support and understanding of the entire group. If only a few physicians choose to adhere, the center will struggle. The panel should set a goal to establish a pathway for each condition in female urology. This would include recurrent urinary tract infections, overactive bladder, urinary and bowel incontinence, pelvic prolapse, pelvic pain syndromes and neurogenic bladder, and urethral masses. Pathways may vary from practice to practice.

Standardizing care will lead to better outcomes and more predictable growth for the practice. If there is no structured care model, analyzing data and making changes to improve patient care will be difficult. Similarly, if everyone in the practice is treating patients differently, then it's likely that outcomes will be vastly different. As quality of care becomes more important in fee reimbursement, this could lead to a significant decline in reimbursement.

The clinical pathway should be circulated to all supporting staff so they are familiar with the protocols. Additionally, staff can help explain the next step to each patient to help them through the process. Recently, The Society of Urodynamics, Female Pelvic Medicine, and Urogenital Reconstruction (SUFU) published a clinical pathway for Overactive Bladder. **http://sufuorg.com/docs/oab/sufu-oab-flyer.aspx**. Lightner et al demonstrate how a clinic can use the OAB pathway to treat women.[3]

The members of the Women's Pelvic Health Center could determine the ideal place to "move" a women who desires further treatment for her symptoms. Another example of an incontinence pathway used for incontinence can be seen in **Figure 3**.

A completely different approach to clinical pathways has been proposed based on phenotypes described by Blaivas et al. One example is the overactive bladder pathway depicted in **Figure 4**. Three primary phenotypes have been developed based on the 24-hour urinary output and maximum voided volume from the bladder diary – polyuria (13%), normal (80%), and oliguria (7%). Each of these phenotypes takes the patient down a different diagnostic and treatment pathway.

This approach has many advantages. First, it engages the patient from the outset and demonstrates the center's commitment to excellence. Second, it is the first step in triage and ensures that the patient receives an appropriate referral and that the physician has sufficient information on the first visit to formulate a diagnostic and treatment plan. Finally, serial questionnaires and diaries serve as a scorecard to monitor treatment efficacy (see **Figure 1 B**), and as discussed below, the weShare database has been used as the substrate for developing lower urinary tract symptom phenotypes and clinical pathways.

Outsourcing data collection to the patient also has economic benefits. Not only does it saves administrative costs, the app also provides the physician and practice with the resources to optimize reimbursement and, where appropriate, utilize remote patient monitoring as a source of income. Finally, the composition data generated by weShare can be used to help formulate appropriate reimbursement methods based on MIPS and APM requirements.

FIGURE 3
Urinary Incontinence Pathway

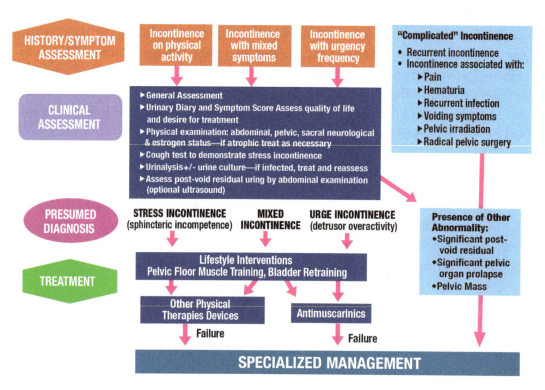

Initial management of urinary incontinence in women as recommended by ICI 2001 (adapted from Abrams P, Andersson KE, Artibani W, Brubaker L, Cardozo L, Castro D, et al. and the Members of the Committees. 2nd International Consultation on Incontinence Recommendations of the International Scientific Committee: Evaluation and Treatment of Urinary Incontinence, Pelvic Organ Prolapse and Faecal Incontinence. In: Abrams P, Cardozo L, Khoury S, Wein A, editors. Incontinence, 2nd edn. Plymouth: Plymbridge Distributors Ltd; 2002. p. 1094–5.)

FIGURE 4 Overactive Bladder Pathway

Remote Monitoring LUTSS & Bladder Diary

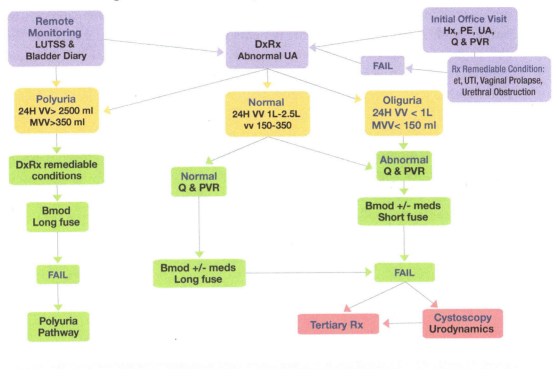

- **A** Behavioral therapies
- **B** Medication 1 (anticholinergic)
  - navigator follow up call to patients in 1-2 weeks
  - patient follow up with physician in 4-6 weeks
- **C** Medication 2 (beta-agonist/anticholinergic)
  - navigator follow up call to patient in 1-2 weeks
  - patient follow up with physician in 4-6 weeks
- **D** Urodynamics
- **E** Progress to 3rd line therapy
  - PTNS/Botox®/Interstim

The pathway is derived from OAB phenotypes based on the LUTSS, 24-hour bladder diary, Q and PVR. The overactive bladder pathway is based on phenotypes derived from bladder diaries and the LUTSS questionnaire, which may be completed prior to the initial office visit (remote monitoring) or requested at the time of the office visit and completed prior to the next visit. Three primary phenotypes have been developed based on the 24-hour urinary output and maximum voided volume from the bladder diary (polyuria, normal and oliguria). Each of these phenotypes takes the patient down a different diagnostic and treatment pathway.

24H BD = 24 hour bladder diary; Bmod = behavior modification, DxRx = diagnose and treat, LUTSS = lower urinary tract symptom score; Hx = focused history; OAB = over active bladder; PE = focused physical exam; PVR = estimation of post void residual urine; in Q = uroflow; UA = urinalysis, UTI = urinary tract infection.

MARKETING/OUTREACH

Community outreach should be an important part of any female health center. Several times a year, the panel should offer innovative, educational programs for patients. The center should provide the interested patients with written material describing the philosophy of the center, its members, and the types of conditions treated. In addition, this information as well as the patient-friendly clinical pathway should be available on your website. These programs offer an opportunity for patients to hear the most recent techniques and strategies for treating their conditions. In addition, it allows the patients to come and see the center and meet those involved in patient care. It also provides the patient an opportunity to compare the services provided by the center to other physicians in the community. Popular topics that can educate patients and effectively grow your practice include: advanced therapies in overactive bladder, new procedures for stress incontinence surgery, and options in treating pelvic organ prolapse.

1. (Chancellor MB et al. *Clin Ther.* 2013;35(11):1744-1751)

2. D'Souza AO et al. *J Manag Care Pharm.* 2008;14(3):291-301

3. Lightner DJ, Agarwal and Gormley EA. The Overactive Bladder and The aua Guidelines: A Proposed Clinical Pathway for Evaluation Management in a Contemporary Urology Practice. J Urol 2016. Vol. 3 399-405

4. Lepor H, Williford WO, Barry MJ et al: The efficacy of terazosin, finasteride or both in benign prostatic hyperplasia. Veterans Affairs Cooperative Studies Benign Prostatic Hyperplasia Study Group. N Engl J Med 1996; 533

5. Coyne K, Revicki D, Hunt T et al: Psychometric Validation of an Overactive Bladder Symptom and Health related Quality of Life Questionnaire: The OAB-q. Qual Life Res 2002;11:563

6. Blaivas JG, Panagopoulos G, Weiss JP et al.: Validation of the Overactive Bladder Symptom Score. J Urol 2007; 178:543

7. Uebersax JS, Wyman JF, Shumaker SA et al.: Short Forms to assess life quality and symptom distress for urinary incontinence in Women: the Incontinence Impact Questionnaire and the Urogenital Distress Inventory. Continence Program for Women Research group. Neururol Urodyn 1995; 14:131

8. Herzog AR, Diokno AC, Brown MB et al.: Two-year incidence, remission, and change patterns of urinary incontinence in noninstitutionalized older adults. J Gerrontol 1990;45:M67

KEY POINTS

- **In 2013, the American Board of Urology** met a female patient population need by adding a subspecialty certification in Female Pelvic Medicine and Reconstructive Surgery (FPMRS).

- **Today most large urology groups** have subspecialized FPMRS urologists or gynecologists.

- **Additionally, large groups have had a chance to integrate**, consolidate and organize strategic plans to provide efficient and comprehensive urologic care.

- **Developing a women's pelvic health center of excellence** will give a practice the ability to demonstrate, with measurable data, a commitment to patient care, and boost patient volume.

- **Key elements that can make a women's health clinic successful:** a dedicated physician team, a navigator, and appropriate pathways and education.

- **Women need to know that incontinence and prolapse** are not things they have to live with; a women's health center of excellence can provide them with better outcomes and higher satisfaction.

- **Begin by forming a team,** and identify the type of patients to be included, and identify your population.

- **Name a medical director and center coordinator** and identify the center's panel of members.

- **Nurse navigators** are essential to the management and growth of the women's pelvic health center.

- **A dedicated call center** can use a screening questionnaire to direct the patient to an appropriate staff member (consider weShare URO).

- **Adopt standardized diaries** and a process to utilize them across the entire practice.

- **The panel should set a goal** to establish a pathway for each condition in female urology.

- **Community outreach** should be an important part of any female health center.

David C. Chaikin, MD

Dr. David C. Chaikin is the Vice President of Garden State Urology in Morristown, New Jersey. Dr. Chaikin received his Bachelor's Degree in biology from the University of Illinois in Champaign, Illinois, before continuing his education at Albert Einstein College of Medicine in Bronx, New York, with his MD. After obtaining his MD, Dr. Chaikin performed his internship in General Surgery and residency in Urology at Hospital of the University of Pennsylvania. He then had a fellowship in Female Pelvic Medicine and reconstructive surgery under the direction of Dr. Jerry Blaivas. Dr. Chaikin is board certified in Urology and Female Pelvic Medicine and Reconstructive Surgery. Dr. Chaikin is a member of the American Medical Association, American Urological Association, Society of Urodynamics, Female Pelvic Medicine and Urogenital Reconstruction, International Continence Society, and the New York Section of the American Urological Association. He is currently a member of the executive committee of the New Jersey Urological Society, and a board member of New Jersey Patient Care, and Access Coalition. In addition, Dr. Chaikin serves on the Board of Directors of LUGPA.

Michael Ingber, MD

Dr. Ingber trained at the Cleveland Clinic where he completed a two-year fellowship in Female Pelvic Medicine and Reconstructive Surgery. He was a clinical instructor at the Cleveland Clinic and received specialty training in the treatment of urinary incontinence, pelvic organ prolapse, female sexual dysfunction, and robotic and laparoscopic surgery. He part of the team which performed the world's first removal of a kidney through a single vaginal incision. Dr. Ingber is an innovator in minimally-invasive surgery, also performing the world's first reported single-incision "scarless" laparoscopic posterior uterine suspension in 2010.

Dr. Ingber is the medical Director of COR MedSpa, one of the first urology-run medical spas in the tri-State region. Dr. Ingber is a reviewer for eight major journals in the field of urology and urogynecology. He is an active member of the American Urological Association, International Urogynecology Association, Society for Urodynamics and Female Urology, and the International Society for the Study of Women's Sexual Health.

CHAPTER 26

Establishing a Medical Spa

David C. Chaikin, MD
Michael Ingber, MD
Anika Akerman, MD

As medical reimbursement continues to be under downward pressure, urologists are continuously evaluating additional necessary patient services that can generate new revenue. The advent of surgical centers, lithotripsy ventures, and radiation centers paved the way for non-traditional business opportunities for the general urologist. In 2017 alone, the medical spa business generated almost $4 billion and still has significant room for growth.[1] Urologists, with their high volume and diverse patient population, are poised to take full advantage of this industry. With increasing interest in both male and female sexuality, urology practices are well positioned to take advantage of new and innovative approaches for male erectile dysfunction and female sexual disorders. (See also Chapters 25 and 27)

HOW TO OPEN AND OPERATE A MEDICAL SPA

▶ What is A Medical Spa?

A medical spa, also known as a medispa or medspa, is a spa-like facility that offers elective procedures to improve physical appearance. These services are provided under the direction of a physician and a team of trained nurses and aestheticians. Medical spas may offer a plethora of treatments from cosmetic injections and facials, to body contouring and vaginal rejuvenation. There are hundreds of treatments available across the medical spa industry, but all of them follow the same general principle: pamper the patient! The most popular treatments in 2017 include chemical peels, Botox, and Dermal Fillers (Allergan, Irvine CA), and aesthetician services (hair removal, facials, and permanent makeup).[2]

Medical spas should create a welcoming and relaxed environment in which patients can receive cosmetic treatments and services. This indulgent feel contrasts with the usual trip to the doctor. Although your current urology practice should already aim to make patients feel prioritized and calm, most visits to a medical office are no "day at the spa." Medical spas offer a patient-centric experience. A medical spa allows patients to honestly discuss their desires and goals, not just their illnesses and symptoms.

A medical spa appointment may not feel like a traditional doctor visit. However, it is important for both the medical spa staff and the client to keep in mind that most services do constitute the practice of medicine and should be taken seriously.

▶ Why Open a Medical Spa?

In 2017 there were 4,200 medical spas in operation in the United States. The industry generated $4 billion in revenue, double the amount from 2012.[1] It is projected to double again by 2022 (**Figure 1**). The average medical spa generated $954,000 in revenue in 2017.[1] The industry is booming and there is still significant room for growth, with new and improved treatment modalities entering the market every year. In-office treatments that are non-surgical and less invasive than traditional surgical options are the current trend.

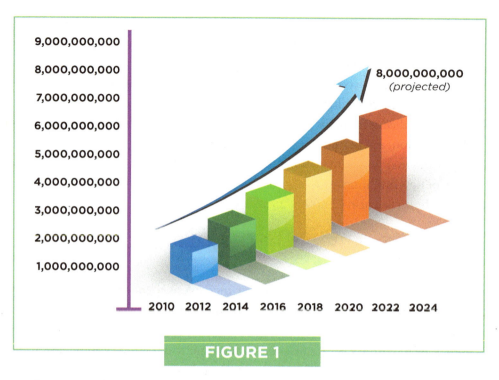

FIGURE 1

More than 85% of medical spa clientele are female [1]. However, the percentage of male medical spa consumers is on the rise as treatments and facilities are becoming more male-friendly and specialized marketing towards men has increased. Popular medical spa treatments for men include hair restoration, fat reduction, body sculpting, and hormone replacement therapy. With men as a rising sector in this industry, the revenue will be even more impressive.

While the industry is promising, opening a medical spa demands a large amount of capital and it takes some time to generate profit. Having a vague estimate of how much money you will need to open your medical spa is not good enough. Your financial picture should be thoroughly assessed and backed by accurate projections. When it comes to managing your medical spa, the worst thing that can happen is to suddenly run out of money. Developing, owning and operating a medical spa is a costly undertaking, and your budget should reflect the associated expenses.

Start-up costs can vary in different markets. In our market, start-up costs for basic medical spas are between $700,000 and $1,000,000. If physicians are going to open a medical spa, they must approach it as a small business venture and be committed to staying with it for a minimum of three years before they see any financial returns.

▶ *Know Your Market*

Most medical spa clients (52%) are middle-aged, between 35 and 54 years old. Another 30% are over the age of 55, generally considered the Baby Boomer generation.

Millennials, aged 18 to 34 years old, make up 17% of clients.[1] The Millennials will be the key generation in the years to come as they strive to preserve their youth, and as they move into their prime income-earning years. As far as geography, the largest number of medical spas are presently found in Texas, California and Florida.[1]

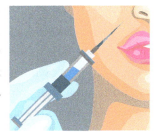

More patients, whether Baby Boomers or Millennials, are turning to medical spas to enhance their physical appearance and boost their confidence. While many may seek out dermatology or plastic surgery practices to obtain care, there remains a significant market opportunity for other medical specialties. In middle to upper-middle class demographic areas, we have the opportunity to provide a slightly lower-cost option with an even better overall patient experience.

▶ The Development Stage

The development stage of your medical spa is perhaps the most important step when it comes to operating a successful business. There are countless minute details that must be prioritized during this phase. Failing to do so could cause major financial setbacks for your medical spa.

First, choose a strong and memorable name for your medical spa. Branding and naming are perhaps the most important initial decisions you will make. Having a name that clearly depicts the business and is catchy is important. Ideally, the name is succinct rather than wordy and should exude beauty and class. Choosing the right name will boost your business. While many may choose to hire a consulting firm to aid in this decision, brainstorming with staff, friends, family members, and prospective clients may also help you make the best decision.

Once a name is chosen, the next step is to create a logo. The logo should reflect your business and its name. It should be attractive and simple. Be sure to choose colors that are pleasing because they will be seen across different media, signage, flyers, brochures, letterheads, etc. Many professional companies specialize in designing logos for businesses. You can tap into their experience and expertise to create a great-looking logo for your business.

Once a name and logo have been created, you will need to choose a location and do some research to differentiate your new practice from the established medical spas in the area.

▶ Choose Your Location

Before choosing a location, it is imperative to analyze the competition and perform a market feasibility study. Knowing this information will help you focus your marketing campaigns and give valuable insight into potential clientele.

Investigate what services the local competition offers, their current pricing, and who they are marketing to. Be sure to weed out and ignore any suspect or non-reputable operations. The goal is to compete with the best in-town physicians and their medical spas. Knowing what already exists and is available, versus what is lacking in your geographic area, will guide decision-making for the next steps: preparing your space and determining your services.

Several other factors will influence the location you select. First, make sure your city or town's zoning laws allow a medical spa. Medical spas are a relatively new business concept and many zoning boards do not understand what a medical spa is. This may lead to issues in getting zoning issues settled. A good way to avoid the hassle is to collect zoning data from other existing medical spas.[3]

Demographics, parking availability, street frontage, surrounding storefronts, and foot traffic are all factors to consider when selecting a location.

▶ Prepare Your Space

The build-out is the most expensive, time-consuming part of your project and typically the area about which physicians know the least.[3] The people on your development team are extremely important because if the facility is designed incorrectly, it will create problems. There are many firms that specialize in medical spa development. Some of these even offer turnkey services.

The initial experience at check-in sets the stage for the patient experience. The reception area of the medical spa should be open and inviting. Many medical spas have a display area close to the reception and check-out area, which serves as a centerpiece to showcase products offered for sale. If space permits, a private waiting room where patients can sit after check-in can provide the spa-like appearance that is unlike a traditional medical office. Here, you can offer coffee, tea, and water to patients. Patients can sit comfortably in a robe before their services, watch TV and relax. A consult room should be constructed close to the reception and waiting area. This can be a small room with a table and chairs, where the client can share his or her concerns before obtaining any services.

Treatment rooms are similarly constructed to medical office exam rooms. They should include plumbing for a small sink, electrical outlets for machines, enough space for a treatment table or chair and a provider space to work. While most medical spa equipment runs on a standard 120V and 60Hz outlet, other equipment may require a 240V outlet to be installed. Having a floor outlet available near the treatment table can avoid unnecessary cables across treatment rooms. Certain technology produces smoke, such as ablative laser therapies, and may require smoke evacuation technology or proper ventilation. Providers should ensure they follow proper local and state codes.

▶ Choose Your Services

Potential medical spa treatments are listed below in **Table 1**. Offering all these treatments is often not feasible for a new medspa. The goal should be to specialize in a few key treatments to start and strive to be the best in those areas. In time, additional services can be added.

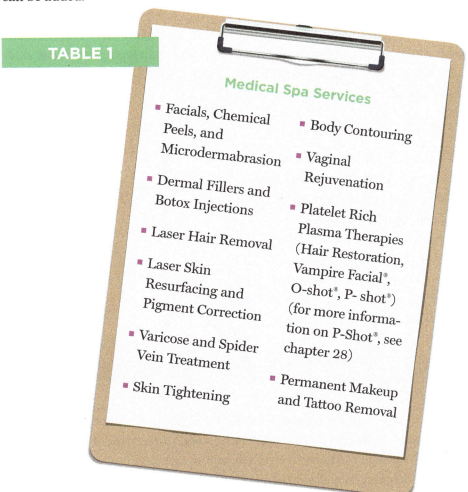

TABLE 1

Medical Spa Services

- Facials, Chemical Peels, and Microdermabrasion
- Dermal Fillers and Botox Injections
- Laser Hair Removal
- Laser Skin Resurfacing and Pigment Correction
- Varicose and Spider Vein Treatment
- Skin Tightening
- Body Contouring
- Vaginal Rejuvenation
- Platelet Rich Plasma Therapies (Hair Restoration, Vampire Facial®, O-shot®, P-shot®) (for more information on P-Shot®, see chapter 28)
- Permanent Makeup and Tattoo Removal

Even the most astute medical professionals in the cosmetic industry may have trouble keeping up with the latest, breaking technology and trends. The field is constantly changing and evolving. A consulting agency can be engaged to assist in deciding which therapies to offer and to aid in several other aspects of the opening process. This will be further discussed later in this chapter.

▶ Select the Right Staff and Training

The most successful medical spas are staffed with professionals who have prior experience in a medical setting as well as talent in achieving a pleasing aesthetic result.

Aestheticians with continued education certifications, registered nurses or nurse practitioners, and physician assistants who are trained in cosmetic procedures, should be hired to work with the physician. The aesthetic industry typically carries a high turnover rate. Help secure staff retention by creating a positive and friendly work environment and offering opportunities for continued learning and fair compensation with referral bonuses and commission.

Extensive training is not usually needed in order to break into the aesthetic field. Educational conferences will provide a broad overview on skin typing, key facial anatomy, skin health, laser techniques, and aesthetic treatments. Most equipment includes training specific to the purchased device.

▶ Ensure Safety to Your Patients and Follow State Laws

Safety is of utmost importance for a new medical spa. State laws vary on what procedures must be performed by a physician. Some states allow advanced practice providers, such as nurse practitioners or physician assistants to perform laser or radiofrequency procedures under the direct supervision of the physician. Others allow significant freedom for aestheticians to perform everything from basic facial aesthetic procedures to ablative laser treatments. Urologists should consult their state medical board as well as seek legal counsel to determine what is appropriate in their individual area. All risks of desired procedures must be disclosed and explained to the patient in detail. The space should be inspected regularly to ensure a sterile, safe environment, and specific strategies in case of emergency should be in place.

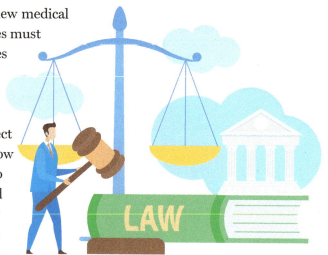

Commit to providing the highest quality service available and purchase or lease all medicines and equipment from authorized, reputable medical retailers and wholesalers.

▶ Creating a Unique Brand

Ensuring that the medical spa differs from other local practices will provide a competitive advantage that is of utmost importance. Medical spas that have been in business for a long time will have an edge, and therefore, it will take persistent effort to be competitive. Perform due diligence by analyzing nearby medical spas, taking note of what services they provide and what prices they offer. Then, develop a differentiation strategy that highlights the major differences between your spa and the competitors.

We chose to market based on the well-respected urologists at Garden State Urology who have provided urological services in the northern New Jersey region for many decades. Center of Rejuvenation (COR) MedSpa, a division of Garden State Urology, offers vaginal rejuvenation procedures like Mona Lisa Touch® CO_2 Laser (Hologic Inc, Marlborough MA), Votiva Radiofrequency Therapy (InMode Aesthetics, Lake Forest, CA), and "O-shot®" platelet-rich plasma (PRP) therapy for female sexual dysfunction, which ties our female urology practice to the medical spa. We also have specific treatments for men, including P-shot® PRP therapy for male sexual dysfunction, Coolsculpting® cryolipolysis for fat reduction (Allergan Inc., Irvine CA), and PRP for hair restoration. We see a majority of male patients in our urology practice, so we need to provide services that cater to men as well as women.

▶ Play to your strengths

As a urology practice, we serve 60,000 patients in Morris County, New Jersey, and the surrounding area. Having this patient population who already trust the urological providers in the practice provides a unique opportunity to market to a high-yield population. There are many simple ways to market to our existing patient base. We play video footage of our medical director discussing medical spa treatments in our waiting rooms. We also place posters for patients to read while waiting in each exam room, in addition to brochures containing medical spa service descriptions and information.

We include medical spa surveys with our general urology patient demographic and medical history intake forms. The survey asks prospects to select medical spa services they may consider trying. Those who fill out these surveys are contacted via telephone and are offered free consultations. Additionally, all patient email addresses from the urology practice are automatically added to our medical spa database so they can receive e-blasts containing medical spa updates, monthly specials, and new treatment releases.

▶ Marketing Your Medical Spa

The most challenging obstacle in creating a successful medical spa practice is effectively marketing the business. A medical spa is not a doctor's office and should not be treated as such. Generally, medical spas do not accept insurance, and the focus should not be on getting a bargain, but on the quality of services being offered.

Marketing efforts should demonstrate a commitment to safety, serenity, and luxury with professional pictures to show off your clean, modern spa, as well as your highly effective services (with before and after photos). It is imperative to have a forward-thinking marketing plan that takes a proactive, assertive approach to creating client traffic. This dedicated and ambitious strategy is crucial to success in the medical spa industry, even though physicians are not typically used to aggressive marketing practices to obtain patients.

The three steps to marketing spa services are communication, follow-up, and commitment.[3] We have worked to establish a list of patients and we continue to communicate with them by sending e-blasts informing them of upcoming promotions and events. We post and re-post social media content daily. When clients show interest on our website or through social media, we immediately follow up with a phone call within minutes to secure a visit. The faster we can respond, the more likely we are to keep their attention. This fast-paced, relentless level of commitment is necessary to be successful in this market.

Months before our opening day, we aligned with a consulting company that specializes in marketing medical spas. Companies like this can assist in the preliminary stages by thoroughly establishing your business foundation, management structure, operations, services offered, etc. All of this should be in place before your first client even walks in the door.

In addition to providing structure and guidance, a marketing/consulting company should offer web developers, paid search specialists, search engine optimization (SEO) managers, content writers, graphic designers, video and photography professionals, and media analysts. The marketing team should give you the support needed to start and grow your medical spa's online and social media presence.

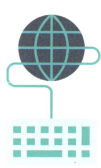

The most important aspect of your media content is your website. In this day and age, the digital presence of any business has become imperative. To stand out among your competitors, you need an engaging and attractive website that has the same look and feel across all devices and operating systems. We were able to give input and make adjustments by comparing our initial web design to the successful medical spa businesses we follow. Having a good search engine optimization practice will help drive traffic to your website from commonly used search engines.

▶ Social Media

Most urologists in an established practice likely do not have a Facebook page, nor would they typically have an Instagram profile. Opening a medical spa will force you, or at least your business, to have both. Simply having a page or profile is not enough. Social media is an important marketing outlet that can help you connect with your customers at a personal level, so posting and responding on these platforms is crucial. In fact, using the social media platforms to engage with your customers has become a way of life for businesses and most customers expect responses.

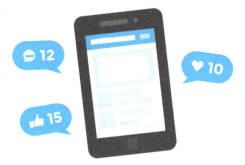

Facebook is powerful as more than a billion people have an account. Facebook marketing can be a full-time job in itself, so the physician cannot be relied upon to do all the social media posting. However, before and after photos, treatment videos, and other in-office content can be created by the physician and staff. Developing a personality for your page, inviting friends, families and colleagues to follow you, and creating high quality content is of utmost importance.

▶ Final thoughts

The medical spa industry is booming and the demand for medical spa services is at an all-time high. Opening a medical spa is costly, time-consuming and requires a great deal of attention to detail. However, with the right brand, location, team, marketing plan and support, a medical spa can become a lucrative venture for any physician (even a urologist). Always keep in mind, the goal is to create a serene, safe, and sterile environment for your patients to enjoy a spa-like experience under your care. Procedures must be executed safely, and pampering is a must! Prove to your potential patients that your medical spa is worth every penny and provide the highest level of service.

REFERENCES

1. AmSpa American Med Spa Association. 2017 Medical Spa State of the Industry Report. https://modernaesthetics.com/pdfs/0617_supp2.pdf. May/June 2017.

2. Boeckh, Aly. Top 5 Most Popular Medspa Treatments. https://www.americanmedspa.org/blog-post/1633466/283765/Top-5-Most-Popular-Med-Spa-Treatments. August 29, 2017.

3. American Spa Staff. 10 Steps to Developing a Successful Medical Spa. https://www.americanspa.com/medical-spa/10-steps-developing-successful-medical-spa. December 31, 2018.

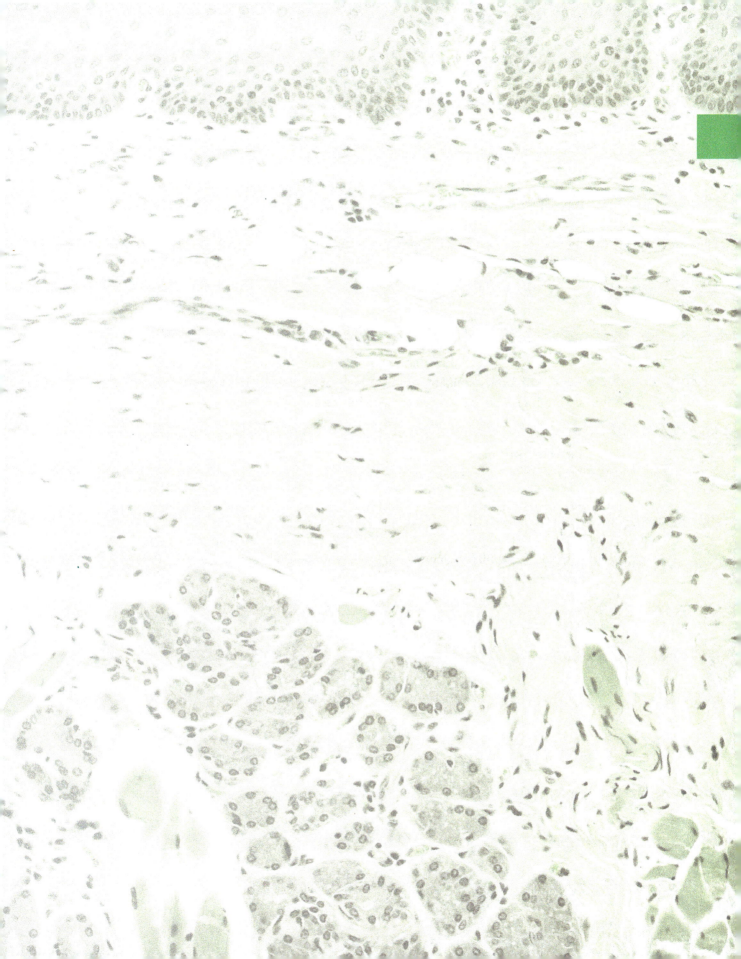

KEY POINTS

- **In 2017 alone, the medical spa business generated almost $4 billion** and still has significant room for growth.

- **Popular medical spa treatments for men** include hair restoration, fat reduction, body sculpting, and hormone replacement therapy.

- **The most popular treatments in 2017** include chemical peels, Botox, and Dermal Fillers (Allergan, Irvine CA), and aesthetician services, including hair removal, facials, and permanent makeup.

- Demographics, parking availability, street frontage, surrounding storefronts, and foot traffic are all **factors to consider when selecting a location.**

- **Urologists should consult their state medical board** as well as seek legal counsel to determine what is legally appropriate in their individual area.

- **Marketing efforts** should demonstrate a commitment to safety, serenity, and luxury with professional pictures to show off your clean, modern spa, as well as your highly effective services (with before and after photos).

- **The three steps to marketing spa services** are communication, follow-up, and commitment.

- **To stand out among your competitors,** you need an engaging and attractive website that has the same look and feel across all devices and operating systems.

- **Social media is an important marketing outlet** that can help you connect with your customers at a personal level, so posting and responding on these platforms is crucial.

David C. Chaikin, MD

Dr. David C. Chaikin is the Vice President of Garden State Urology in Morristown, New Jersey. Dr. Chaikin received his Bachelor's Degree in biology from the University of Illinois in Champaign, Illinois, before continuing his education at Albert Einstein College of Medicine in Bronx, New York, with his MD. After obtaining his MD, Dr. Chaikin performed his internship in General Surgery and residency in Urology at Hospital of the University of Pennsylvania. He then had a fellowship in Female Pelvic Medicine and reconstructive surgery under the direction of Dr. Jerry Blaivas. Dr. Chaikin is board certified in Urology and Female Pelvic Medicine and Reconstructive Surgery. Dr. Chaikin is a member of the American Medical Association, American Urological Association, Society of Urodynamics, Female Pelvic Medicine and Urogenital Reconstruction, International Continence Society, and the New York Section of the American Urological Association. He is currently a member of the executive committee of the New Jersey Urological Society, and a board member of New Jersey Patient Care, and Access Coalition. In addition, Dr. Chaikin serves on the Board of Directors of LUGPA.

Michael Ingber, MD

Dr. Ingber trained at the Cleveland Clinic where he completed a two-year fellowship in Female Pelvic Medicine and Reconstructive Surgery. He was a clinical instructor at the Cleveland Clinic and received specialty training in the treatment of urinary incontinence, pelvic organ prolapse, female sexual dysfunction, and robotic and laparoscopic surgery. He part of the team which performed the world's first removal of a kidney through a single vaginal incision. Dr. Ingber is an innovator in minimally-invasive surgery, also performing the world's first reported single-incision "scarless" laparoscopic posterior uterine suspension in 2010.

Dr. Ingber is the medical Director of COR MedSpa, one of the first urology-run medical spas in the tri-State region. Dr. Ingber is a reviewer for eight major journals in the field of urology and urogynecology. He is an active member of the American Urological Association, International Urogynecology Association, Society for Urodynamics and Female Urology, and the International Society for the Study of Women's Sexual Health.

Anika Akerman, MD

Dr. Ackerman trained at Duke University hospital and Columbia NY Presbyterian. She currently practices in Morristown, NJ and has special interest in female urology and sexual dysfunction.

Dr. Ackerman believes it is a great honor and privilege be a doctor, and especially to practice urology, where physicians have the opportunity to help patients improve very personal problems or symptoms. She aims to practice compassionate and cutting edge urology, and to treat every patient as if they were my own parent or sibling. She believes individualized care and an integrative approach serve the best platform for successful outcomes.

CHAPTER 27

Men's Health Clinics

Steven A. Kaplan, MD
Gregory R. Mullen, MD

Men's Health has many definitions. Previously, Men's Health focused mostly on diseases of the prostate and erectile dysfunction. Men were treated for these conditions by their urologists who historically focused only on the genitourinary tract without considering the effects of other organ systems. More recently, Men's Health has been redefined to cover a wider scope, which incorporates a more holistic approach. Combining the definitions proposed by Shabsigh and Minor, Men's Health can be viewed in four different categories:

01. Male-specific conditions such as prostate disease, male sexual dysfunction, and testicular diseases.

02. Diseases that are more prevalent in men compared to women, such as cardiovascular disease and most types of cancers.

03. Conditions whose risk factors and adverse outcomes are different in men compared to women, such as obesity.

04. Health issues for which men require different interventions than women in order to improve outcomes at an individual or population level, such as access to care (Shabsigh, 2003; Miner 2018)

GENDER DIFFERENCES IN HEALTH OUTCOMES

Men's Health is crucial to study because of disparities in health outcomes between men and women. According to the Centers for Disease Control and Prevention, the average life expectancy for American men is about 76 years, which is five years shorter than the life expectancy for American women (Arias, 2019). Not only do men live shorter lives than women do, but men also have higher morbidity rates across most diseases, notably cardiovascular disease and multiple cancers (White, 2014). Taken together, it is not surprising that a World Health Organization (WHO) report showed that men have a lower healthy life expectancy - the average number of years lived in good health - than women do (World Health Organization, 2019). Why do men live shorter, unhealthier lives? Some risk factors that contribute to men's poor health outcomes include risky lifestyle behaviors, limited utilization of healthcare, and insufficient access to care.

Taking lifestyle and risk behaviors into account, a 2016 WHO report showed that five times as many men smoked tobacco than women, and four times as many men consumed alcohol than women (World Health Organization, 2019). A review of the actual causes of death in the United States showed that tobacco was the number one preventable cause of death and that alcohol was the third most preventable cause of death (Mokdad, 2004). Getting men to live healthier, longer lives is incumbent upon making better choices and reducing harmful behaviors. Tobacco and alcohol aside, another WHO report showed that some of the difference in lifeexpectancy between men and women was due to violence and road injuries, both of which occur more frequently in men than in women. Furthermore, men are more likely to work in high-risk occupations such as construction, mining, and the military, all of which can contribute to higher rates of fatalities and injuries (The Lancet, 2019). Improving Men's Health begins with reducing these preventable risk factors. We must do better at counseling our male patients to quit smoking, limit their alcohol consumption, reduce violence, and practice workplace safety.

When examining healthcare utilization, we know men are lacking significantly. The National Health Interview Survey in 2018 estimated that almost 25% of American men had no visits to doctor's offices in the past 12 months, compared with only 12% of women (Villarroel, 2019). Men are also less likely to seek preventive healthcare than women. In 2016, about 80% of women had preventive care visits, whereas less than 50% of men had preventive care visits (Rui, 2016). Some of the most common barriers men cite as reasons for not seeking care include lack of time, lack of knowledge, fear, and painful screening procedures (Teo, 2016). This reluctance of men to actively participate in their health undoubtedly contributes to poor outcomes. A 2019 Cleveland Clinic survey reported that almost two-thirds of men will wait as long as possible to see their doctor if they have any health issue or injury (Cleveland Clinic, 2019). Delaying care until severe symptoms develop explains why, despite going to the doctor less often, men have higher hospitalization and mortality rates (Juel, 2008). As providers, we must do better to educate our male patients to seek care and to advocate for themselves. Men's poor utilization of healthcare is inextricably linked to men's limited access to healthcare.

There are a few theories as to why women access healthcare more frequently than men. One theory is that hospitals changed marketing strategies in the 1980s to target women who were felt to make household healthcare decisions and also utilize medical services more often than their male counterparts (Dearing, 1987; Weisman, 1995). Another theory is that around the same time, some perceived that women were underrepresented in medical research and argued that improvements be made (Mastroianni, 1994). Regardless of the reason, in 1990 the National Institutes of Health created the Office for Research on Women's Health, which ultimately led to the creation of the Centers of Excellence in Women's Health program. This program granted national funds to academic medical centers to be used to promote Women's Health (Milliken, 2001). These funds led to a boom in Women's Health research and the creation of dedicated Women's Health clinics. From 1970 to 2018, Nuzzo found that the term "women's health" appeared in the title or abstract of papers in PubMed 14,501 times, whereas "men's health" only appeared 1,555 times during the same time period (Nuzzo, 2019). Likewise, a 2015 study looking at gender specific health services among the top 50 "best hospitals" in America found that 49 of the 50 institutions advertised some form of a Women's Health clinic compared to only 16 of the 50 advertising a Men's Health clinic (Choy, 2015). In order to bridge the current gap in gender specific health outcomes, we must improve men's utilization of and access to quality, comprehensive healthcare.

ROLE OF THE UROLOGIST IN MEN'S HEALTH

Urologists are undoubtedly crucial to providing Men's Health care. Whereas most women transition their healthcare from pediatricians to obstetricians and gynecologists earlier on in life, many men go years without seeing a doctor. Often, the first symptoms that prompt men to re-enter the healthcare system later in life are lower urinary tract symptoms or erectile dysfunction (Kirby, 2005). Knowing the strong association between erectile dysfunction and the development of cardiovascular events, urologists must embrace the vital role they play in the early detection and prevention of potentially life-threatening events (Thompson, 2005). This change in emphasis over the past decade has refocused urologists' efforts away from dealing only with conditions of the genitourinary tract towards more holistic approaches that cater to all of Men's Health needs. The American Urological Association (AUA) created the Committee on Male Health in 2009. The Committee promoted a comprehensive approach to Men's Health that incorporates research, education, and community outreach, with emphasis on collaboration with other specialists in order to provide quality, comprehensive Men's Health care (Elterman, 2013). Recognizing that men ask fewer questions, have shorter visits, and are less likely to use preventive services than women, the AUA created an evidence-based Men's Health Checklist to facilitate discussions between urologists and patients about topics that might otherwise be missed during a routine visit (European Men's Health Forum, 2013). With the current trend in medicine, and urology in particular, towards larger group practices, patients may benefit from this model as they can be seen by multiple specialists during one visit. The advantage of this type of multidisciplinary healthcare cannot be understated and forms the basis for promoting comprehensive Men's Health clinics.

MEN'S HEALTH CLINICS

Ideally, Men's Health clinics offer multidisciplinary, comprehensive healthcare visits that address all Men's Health needs in one visit. Yet, not all Men's Health clinics offer multidisciplinary care. Many self-proclaimed Men's Health clinics only exist to replace testosterone and offer erectile dysfunction treatments (Von Drehle, 2014). Of 16 studied American Men's Health clinics, eight exclusively offered treatment for urologic conditions, while only four offered treatment for other medical conditions, such as cardiovascular disease, diabetes, and preventive care (Choy, 2015). The scarcity of comprehensive Men's Health clinics in the United States is due, in part, to the lack of a national Men's Health policy. Some legislators have attempted to address this. In 2003, a bill was introduced to create an Office for Men's Health, however, after three unsuccessful attempts, the bill died (Govtrak.us, 2020). Only four countries worldwide have national Men's Health policies: Australia, Brazil, Iran, and Ireland.

The Australian Government committed to Men's Health in 2010 by creating a national Men's Health policy. The goal of the policy was to support every man and boy in Australia to live long, fulfilling, and healthy lives. The policy identified six key priority areas including: optimizing health outcomes for men, promoting health equity between groups of men, creating strategies for health improvement for men at different life stages, focusing on preventive care, building evidence for future policy, and improving access to care (Australian Government, 2019). As a result of this policy, Men's Health clinics were created, which increased access to care and use of preventive services. In only five years, prostate cancer screening increased almost 10% (Australian Government, 2018). One of the successful Men's Health clinics in Australia is the Bendigo Men's Health Clinic. The clinic focuses on preventive health and workplace Men's Health initiatives. A dedicated Men's Health nurse practitioner coordinates the healthcare offered by the clinic. Initial clinic appointments typically last 45 minutes during which the nurse practitioner takes a comprehensive Men's Health assessment. This assessment includes a full medical history, evaluation of cardiovascular risk factors, determination of tobacco and alcohol use, screening for certain cancers, as well as mental and sexual health assessments. During this initial visit, the nurse practitioner also determines each patient's health education requirements and provides advice for patients on how to navigate the health system. At the end of this visit, each patient is given a folder with a copy of the health assessment, results of any tests, brochures containing health information, and a mutually agreed upon action plan (Strange, 2012). This clinic can serve as a model for other Men's Health clinics worldwide.

Despite the lack of a national Men's Health policy in the United States, several American academic centers have created Men's Health clinics in order to improve Men's Health. The first multidisciplinary Men's Health clinic in the United States opened at The Miriam Hospital in Providence, Rhode Island in 2008. Co-founded by urologist Dr. Mark Sigman and internist Dr. Martin Miner, this clinic focuses on providing clinical and psychological care for conditions that cause sexual dysfunction. The clinic also evaluates the relationship of sexual dysfunction to cardiovascular disease, and if necessary, leads to a cardiovascular workup and referral to a cardiologist (Hilton, 2014). Since then, many more Men's Health clinics have opened across the United States. The University of Utah opened its Men's Health clinic in 2013 with a mission to not only treat patients for sexual dysfunction and reproductive needs, but also to create a comfortable environment where men are willing to seek care and develop trusting relationships with Men's Health providers. As part of their model, men can schedule appointments without a referral. Based on the chief complaint, patients are given a particular appointment type with the appropriate providers. The clinic also offers extended evening hours and phone consultations to improve access to care (Taylor, 2018). As more Men's Health clinics open, certain similarities can be seen in aesthetics. The Iris Cantor Men's Health Center at New York Presbyterian Hospital predicated the concept of having a unified entry and exit portal encompassing Urology, Primary Care, Endocrinology, and Cardiovascular Disease. Men were able to have a one-stop center for a multidisciplinary educational, diagnostic, and therapeutic intervention. When NYU opened the Tisch Center for Men's Health in 2014, they based the model on its successful multidisciplinary, comprehensive Women's Health clinic. However, unlike the Women's Clinic, the Men's Health clinic was designed in such a way to specifically make men feel more comfortable discussing their health. The clinic was awarded overall Best of Competition in a 2014 healthcare interior design competition (Dinardo, 2014). In addition to constructing Men's Health clinics to be more inviting to men, clinics must develop clever marketing tools to attract male patients. When NYU opened their Men's Health clinic, one advertisement read, "It's the gentlemen's club your wife would approve of" (Hartocollis, 2014). Clinics with smaller budgets advertise by word of mouth, while others use outreach programs and community health talks (Hilton, 2014).

Creating a successful Men's Health clinic not only relies on garnering patients through advertising, but also requires financial backing, support from leadership, and collaboration with multiple providers including urologists, cardiologists, and primary care physicians. Moreover, a consistent branding vision abets continuity of vision. A 2015 study that looked at gender specific health services among the top 50 "best hospitals" in America found that of the 16 Men's Health clinics identified, six were staffed solely by urologists while another six were staffed by a variety of specialists in a multidisciplinary group setting (Choy, 2015). Studies comparing outcomes of Men's Health clinics staffed only by urologists to clinics with multidisciplinary teams are lacking, therefore, we must learn from the experiences of Women's Health clinics. Studies examining Women's Health clinics show that care at gender specific clinics is linked to higher patient satisfaction and use of preventive services when compared to care received at traditional medical practices (Anderson, 2002; Bean-Mayberry, 2003). Furthermore, providers working in multidisciplinary Women's Health clinics report having greater satisfaction due to increased collaboration and streamlining of care (Johnson, 2011). As more Men's Health clinics are created, it is important to consider the potential improvement in outcomes if these clinics are created as multidisciplinary, comprehensive health clinics.

Newer to the Men's Health arena are the direct-to-consumer digital healthcare companies, Hims and Roman, which were both founded in 2017. According to the Hims' website, the goal of the company is to provide men with "easier, more affordable access to the prescriptions, products, and medical advice they need. Especially about the "things they find hard to talk about" (Hims, 2019). Similarly, Roman's website states that their "mission is to improve the lives of men and their partners by making high-quality healthcare accessible and convenient" (Roman, 2020). These companies assert that they deliver healthcare more conveniently, discreetly, and inexpensively than traditional office visits (Perrone, 2019). Patients fill out questionnaires online, which are then reviewed by physicians who determine treatment plans. If a provider believes that a patient is not suited to be treated based on the digital encounter, the patient is referred for an in-person visit (Hilton, 2019). While these digital healthcare companies may improve access to more affordable care, the lack of face-to-face encounters and physical exams can lead to misdiagnosis and mistreatment.

The future of Men's Health is dependent on creating abundant multidisciplinary, comprehensive Men's Health clinics. Progress is already underway. In 2019, close to 50% of major hospitals had Men's Health clinics, up from about a third in 2015 (Landro, 2019). Prior to the development of a business plan for the creation of a successful Men's Health Clinic, there needs to be consensus among the various stakeholders regarding what and whom it will encompass, organization, revenue versus expenses, sustainability, and opportunities for growth. Regardless of clinical setting, there should be buy-in from leadership and the identification of partnerships with various subspecialists in cardiology, endocrinology, psychiatry, orthopedics, and dermatology, who are truly vested in the need for integration of thought, goals, and vision. Given the recent adaptations of various platforms in telemedicine and remote diagnostics, these will afford new opportunities to address and enhance the clinical management of male patients. Future clinics must work with men to identify and address barriers to care so that men start utilizing healthcare more frequently and appropriately. These clinics must consider operating with extended hours or have the capability to offer services like telemedicine in the workplace to increase access to care. Clinics need to consider hiring multiple specialists to allow all of Men's Health issues to be addressed in one visit. Furthermore, we must also develop a dedicated Men's Health curriculum to train existing and future providers about the unique aspects of Men's Health. Finally, research and legislation in Men's Health must increase. Only after we achieve all these goals will we start seeing measurable improvements in Men's Health outcomes.

REFERENCES

Anderson, R., Weisman, C., Scholle, S., Henderson, J., Oldendick, R., & Camacho, F. (2002). Evaluation of the quality of care in the clinical care centers of the national centers of excellence in women's health. *Women's Health Issues: Official Publication of the Jacobs Institute of Women's Health*, 12(6), 309-26. doi:10.1016/s1049-3867(02)00154-8

Arias, E., Xu, J.Q. (2019). United States life tables, 2017. National Vital Statistics Reports, 68(7). National Center for Health Statistics. Retrieved from https://www.cdc.gov/nchs/data/nvsr/nvsr68/nvsr68_07-508.pdf

Australian Government Department of Health. (2019). National Men's Health Strategy 2020-2030. Retrieved from https://www1.health.gov.au/internet/main/publishing.nsf/content/86BBADC780E6058CCA257BF000191627/$-File/19-0320%20National%20Mens%20Health%20Strategy%20Print%20ready%20accessible1.pdf

Australian Government Department of Health. (2018). The current state of male health in Australia. Retrieved from https://consultations.health.gov.au/population-health-and-sport-division-1/online-consultation-for-the-national-mens-health-s/supporting_documents/Evidence%20Review%20%20Current%20state%20of%20male%20health%20in%20Australia.PDF

Bean-Mayberry, B., Chang, C., McNeil, M., Whittle, J., Hayes, P., & Scholle, S. (2003). Patient satisfaction in women's clinics versus traditional primary care clinics in the veteran's administration. *Journal of General Internal Medicine*, 18(3), 175-181. doi:10.1046/j.1525-1497.2003.20512.x

Choy, J., Kashanian, J., Sharma, V., Masson, P., Dupree, J., Le, B., & Brannigan, R. (2015). The men's health center: Disparities in gender specific health services among the top 50 "best hospitals" in America. *Asian Journal of Urology*, 2(3), 170-174. doi:10.1016/j.ajur.2015.06.005

Cleveland Clinic. (2019). 2019 Cleveland Clinic MENtion It® Survey Results Overview. Retrieved from https://newsroom.clevelandclinic.org/wp-content/uploads/sites/4/2019/09/2019-Cleveland-Clinic-MENtion-It-Survey-Results-Overview.pdf

Dearing, R.H. (1987). Marketing to attract women. *Health Prog*. 68, 26–28.

DiNardo, A. (2014, October 2). Fine Tailoring At The Preston Robert Tisch Center For Men's Health. *Healthcare Design*. Retrieved from https://www.healthcaredesignmagazine.com/projects/ambulatory-care-clinics/fine-tailoring-preston-robert-tischc-center-mens-health/

Elterman, D., Kaplan, S., Pelman, R., & Goldenberg, S. (2013). How 'male health' fits into the field of urology. *Nature Reviews. Urology*, 10(10), 606-12. doi:10.1038/nrurol.2013.161

European Men's Health Forum. (2013). Men's Health and Primary Care: Improving access and outcomes. Retrieved from https://www.ecoo.info/wp-content/uploads/2013/11/mens-health-and-primary-care-emhf-roundtable-report.2013.medium-res.pdf

GovTrack.us, 2020. GovTrack.us. (2020). S. 1028—108th Congress: Men's Health Act of 2003. Retrieved from https://www.govtrack.us/congress/bills/108/s1028

Hartocollis, A. (2014, May 28). With Special Clinics, Hospitals Vie for Hesitant Patients: Men. *The New York Times*. Retrieved from https://www.nytimes.com/2014/05/29/nyregion/with-special-clinics-hospitals-vie-for-hesitant-patients-men.html

Hilton, L. (2019). Male patients ride online wave: Novel sites catering to men emerge, along with conflicting views about Internet-based care. *Urology Times*, 47(7).

Hilton, L. (2014). Urologists helping drive male-specific centers. *Urology Times*, 42(12).Hims. (2019). Retrieved from https://www.forhims.com/about

Johnson, P., Bookman, A., Bailyn, L., Harrington, M., & Orton, P. (2011). Innovation in ambulatory care: A collaborative approach to redesigning the health care workplace. *Academic Medicine: Journal of the Association of American Medical Colleges*, 86(2), 211-6. doi:10.1097/ACM.0b013e318204618e

Juel, K., & Christensen, K. (2008). Are men seeking medical advice too late? Contacts to general practitioners and hospital admissions in Denmark 2005. *Journal of Public Health*, 30(1), 111-3. doi:10.1093/pubmed/fdm072

Kirby, R. (2005). The urologist as the advocate of men's health. *BJU International*, 95(7), 929-929.

Landro, L. (2019, April 29). Why Men Won't Go to the Doctor, and How to Change That. *The Wall Street Journal*. Retrieved from https://www.wsj.com/articles/why-men-wont-go-to-the-doctor-and-how-to-change-that-11556590080

Mastroianni, A. C., Faden, R. R., & Federman, D. D. (1994). Women and health research: ethical and legal issues of including women in clinical studies. Vol. I. Washington, D.C.: National Academy Press.

Milliken, N., Freund, K., Pregler, J., Reed, S., Carlson, K., Derman, R., McLaughlin, M. (2001). Academic models of clinical care for women: The national centers of excellence in women's health. *Journal of Women's Health & Gender-Based Medicine*, 10(7), 627-36. doi:10.1089/15246090152563506

Miner, M., Heidelbaugh, J., Paulos, M., Seftel, A., Jameson, J., & Kaplan, S. (2018). The intersection of medicine and urology. *Medical Clinics of North America*, 102(2), 399-415. doi:10.1016/j.mcna.2017.11.002

Mokdad, A., Marks, J., Stroup, D., & Gerberding, J. (2004). Actual causes of death in the United States, 2000. *JAMA*, 291(10), 1238-45. doi:10.1001/jama.291.10.1238

Nuzzo, J. (2019). Men's health in the United States: A national health paradox. *The Aging Male: The Official Journal of the International Society for the Study of the Aging Male*, 1-11. doi:10.1080/13685538.2019.1645109

Perrone, M. (2019, June 5). Online Rx startups offer convenience but also raise concerns. *Associated Press*. Retrieved from https://apnews.com/ 18f50ba8671d44e592ac7c46a614cd22

Roman. (2020). Retrieved from https://www.getroman.com/our-story/

Rui, P., Okeyode, T. (2016). National Ambulatory Medical Care Survey: 2016 National Summary Tables. Retrieved from https://www.cdc.gov/nchs/data/ahcd/namcs_ summary/2016_namcs_web_tables.pdf

Shabsigh, R. (2013). A new multidisciplinary approach to men's health. *Journal of Men's Health*, 10(1), 1-2. doi:10.1016/j.jomh.2013.1500

Strange, P., & Tenni, M. (2012). Bendigo CHS Men's Health Clinic - improving access to primary care. *Aust Fam Physician*, 41(9), 731-733.

Taylor, K., & Hotaling, J. (2018). A Men's Health Clinic Exemplar: Experience at the University of Utah. In S. A. Quallich, M. Lajiness, & K. A. Mitchell (Eds.), Manual of Men's Health A Practice Guide for APRNs and PAs (pp. 243-260). New York, NY: Springer Publishing Company.

Teo, C., Ng, C., Booth, A., & White, A. (2016). Barriers and facilitators to health screening in men: A systematic review. *Social Science & Medicine*, 165, 168-176. doi:10.1016/j.socscimed.2016.07.023

The Lancet (2019). Raising the profile of men's health. *Lancet*, 394(10211), 1779-1779. doi:10.1016/S0140-6736(19)32759-X

Thompson, I., Tangen, C., Goodman, P., Probstfield, J., Moinpour, C., & Coltman, C. (2005). Erectile dysfunction and subsequent cardiovascular disease. *JAMA*, 294(23), 2996-3002. doi:10.1001/jama.294.23.2996

Villarroel, M.A., Blackwell, D.L., Jen, A. (2019). Tables of Summary Health Statistics for U.S. Adults: 2018 National Health Interview Survey. National Center for Health Statistics. Retrieved from https://ftp.cdc.gov/pub/Health_Statistics/NCHS/ NHIS/SHS/2018_SHS_Table_A-17.pdf

Von Drehle, D. (2014, July 31). Manopause?! Aging, Insecurity and the $2 Billion Testosterone Industry. Time. Retrieved from https://time.com/3062889/manopause -aging-insecurity-and-the-2-billion-testosterone-industry/

Weisman, C., Curbow, B., & Khoury, A. (1995). The national survey of women's health centers: Current models of women-centered care. *Women's Health Issues: Official Publication of the Jacobs Institute of Women's Health*, 5(3), 103-17.doi:10.1016/1049-3867(95)00038-6

White, A., McKee, M., De, S., De, V., Hogston, R., Madsen, S., . . . Raine, G. (2014). An examination of the association between premature mortality and life expectancy among men in europe. *European Journal of Public Health*, 24(4), 673-9. doi:10.1093/eurpub/ckt076

World Health Organization. (2019). World health statistics overview 2019: monitoring health for the SDGs, sustainable development goals. Retrieved from https://apps.who.int/iris/bitstream/handle/10665/311696/WHO-DAD-2019.1-eng.pdf

KEY POINTS

- **Men's Health is more than** erectile dysfunction and prostate disease.

- **Women live longer, healthier lives** and are more likely to see a doctor and use preventive services.

- **Research in Men's Health is lacking** and contributes to the scarcity of Men's Health clinics.

- **Urologists play a vital role** in promoting Men's Health.

- **Successful Men's Health clinics** offer multidisciplinary, comprehensive care.

About the Authors

Steven A. Kaplan, MD

Dr. Kaplan is Director of the Men's Wellness Program at Mount Sinai Health System and Professor of Urology at Icahn School of Medicine at Mount Sinai. During his time at Weill Cornell Medical College, he was responsible for the development of a new discipline within urology, Integrated Men's Health, and was Director of the Iris Cantor Men's Health Center.

Gregory R. Mullen, MD

Dr. Mullen is a urology resident at Icahn School of Medicine at Mount Sinai. His interests in urology include Men's Health and endourology.

CHAPTER

Urology Leadership In Erectile Dysfunction: Emerging Technologies

Judson Brandeis, MD

Sexual medicine has seen many revolutionary developments over the past 40 years. The invention of the penile implant, formulation of intracavernosal injection of vasoactive agents, and discovery and widespread use of PDE 5 inhibitors have given men the opportunity to become or remain sexually active at an age when previous generations were not. However, since the discovery of PDE 5 inhibitors, there have not been similar major advances. In a recent American Urological Association (AUA) point-counterpoint, Arthur Burnett, MD of Johns Hopkins University called shock wave therapy "the most exciting development in sexual medicine since PDE 5 inhibitors." Dr. Burnett, the AUA and the Sexual Medicine Society of North America do not currently recommend the use of shock wave therapy or potentially rejuvenating therapies like platelet-rich plasma and stem cells for the treatment of Erectile Dysfunction (ED) unless they are part of a research protocol.

Since urologists have not been aggressive about pursuing shock wave and regenerative treatments, alternative medicine practitioners have rushed to fill that void. My unpublished observations are that two-thirds of the medical practitioners that offer shock wave therapy and rejuvenating injection therapies to patients, are not urologists. In fact, I recently had a patient come to see me for a second opinion when his gastroenterologist wanted to give him a P-shot®.

Due to aggressive marketing, most laypeople use the term GAINSWave® instead of Low-Intensity Shock Wave Therapy and the term P-shot® instead of an intracavernosal injection of Platelet-Rich Plasma. GAINSWave® is a company in Florida that markets shock wave therapy for ED. The P-shot® is a term trademarked by Dr. Charles Runels, a family physician in Alabama who runs the Cellular Medicine Association and teaches training courses for the P-shot®, O-shot® and the Vampire Facelift®.

The American Urologic Association and the Sexual Medicine Society of North America both state that although there is significant evidence to support the efficacy of shock wave therapy in the treatment of Vasculogenic Erectile Dysfunction, shock wave therapy should be considered an investigational treatment. Perhaps this is the reason why the urology community has been so slow to adopt this technology. This reminds me of when I started using the da Vinci® robot for prostatectomies in 2002. The initial reaction of many of my colleagues, especially those in academia, was highly negative, but of course now the robot is ubiquitous. However, the complication rate during the early days of robotic surgery was unacceptably high leading to many unfortunate outcomes, whereas the complications of shock wave therapy and regenerative therapies are minimal.

The orthopedic community has been very enthusiastic about the use of platelet-rich plasma. The use of PRP and orthopedics has grown exponentially as has the clinical research. [Mehrabani] [Barnett] [Veronesi] [Catapano] [Cruciani] [Vilchez-Cavazos]

The dermatology community has also been prolific in the use of platelet-rich plasma, both for androgenic alopecia [Mao] as well as facial rejuvenation in combination with micro-needling. There is robust data supporting the use of platelet-rich plasma in both of these fields. [Hashim]

In contrast, the urology community has been very slow to embrace shock wave therapy as well as the use of platelet-rich plasma and stem cells, whether they are autologous or placental derived mesenchymal stem cells.

Urologists stand to lose both leadership and market share in the treatment of erectile dysfunction. The substantial growth of online pharmacies like Roman and HIMS threaten the referrals of these patients and eliminate urologists as the source of medical information. As experts in the male genitalia, both surgically and physiologically, urologists should reassert their leadership role in the investigation of and treatment with these emerging technologies. Any physician who has used these technologies will tell you that there are patients who clearly benefit, but certainly, not everyone improves. However, the development of optimal protocols, and the optimization of shock wave machines is still in its infancy, similar to the da Vinci robot in 2002.

EMERGING TECHNOLOGIES

Shock Wave Therapy for ED

Low-intensity extracorporeal shock wave therapy (SWT) is a non-invasive treatment for erectile dysfunction, which holds promise for the treatment of Vasculogenic Erectile Dysfunction. SWT is used throughout the world. The author has evidence that leads him to believe that at least 500 medical clinics are providing SWT to patients throughout the U.S. and that less than one third of these clinics are urologist-run. Initial research into the mechanism of action shows that shock waves stimulate neovascularization of tissue by causing activation of stem cells and the release of VEGF, which stimulates the growth of blood vessels, which ultimately improves blood flow to the penis. [Liu]

Focused shock wave therapy has been effective for the treatment of kidney stones for over 40 years. Over the past 20 years, shock wave utilization in orthopedics has increased and there are FDA cleared indications for the use of shock waves in orthopedics. The first time anyone published on the use of SWT for ED was in 2010. Vardi et al. found the theory behind this was that shock waves induce neovascularization.

Interest in SWT has been increasing in the past 10 years with numerous blinded and un-blinded studies investigating its effect on erectile function with and without the use of adjuvant therapy. Currently, multiple studies have proven efficacy on quality of life and blood flow outcomes using tools such as the IIEF-5 and penile duplex ultrasound. Still, no gold standard exists to guide treatment protocols in regards to treatment parameters, such as energy-flux density, number of pulses, treatment frequency, and length of

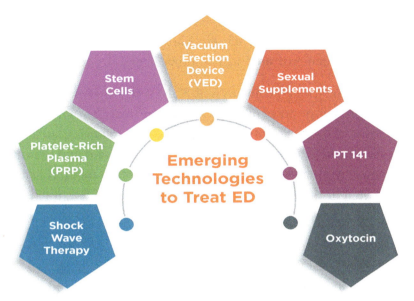

treatment. A further complication is the choice of outcome measurement applicable in SWT research. The wide variation in men's sexual medicine norms across religions and cultures make a singular standard outcome assessment difficult to identify. The most popular outcome measurements include EHS (Erection Hardness Score), the IIEF-EF (International Index of Erectile Function-Erectile Function), and penile duplex US.

In a recent systematic review and meta-analysis, Man et al. showed that higher number of shocks per treatment corresponded to a greater improvement in sexual quality of life improvement. They also noted a shorter treatment course corresponded to improved outcomes. Interestingly, more frequent treatment did not appear to improve erectile function significantly. The author's own study combining radial SWT 10,000 pulses weekly for 6-12 weeks and an oral nitric oxide booster led to a statistically significant improvement in SHIM score of 5.2 with a significant improvement in 70% of men.

Clinical improvement appears to differ by the severity of ED as well. Yee et al applied a treatment protocol of 1,500 total shocks per session delivered at 0.09 mJ/mm2 at 120 shocks/minute bi-weekly for three weeks. This was followed by a two- week period without treatment and finally two weeks of once-weekly treatment. In the sub-group analysis, men with severe ED (SHIM score: 5-7) demonstrated greater improvement from treatment than those with mild-to-moderate (SHIM score 12-21) ED.

The efficacy of SWT on the underlying pathophysiology of Vasculogenic Erectile Dysfunction is further evidenced by its effect in converting PDE-5 inhibitor non-responders to responders. [Kitrey] In a study of 58 men with moderate-to-severe ED who stopped using PDE-5 inhibitors due to lack of efficacy, Kitrey et al. utilized a treatment protocol of 12 sessions of 1,500 pulses at 0.09 mJ/mm2 with a frequency of 120 shocks/min over 9 weeks. Participants were exposed to PDE-5 inhibitors after treatment and evaluated by the Erection Hardness Scale (EHS) and IIEF-EF. After treatment, 54.1%

and 40.5% of the treatment group were able to achieve an erection sufficient for penetration and demonstrated improvement in erectile function, respectively. Comparatively, 0% of the sham group demonstrated such improvement.

SWT effects appear to be long-lasting as well. Kalyvianakois et al. conducted an RCT with an active treatment protocol of 1,500 shocks per treatment for 12 treatments at an energy intensity of 0.09 mJ/mm2 at 160 pulses/min, following subjects out to 12 months after treatment. They utilized penile triplex ultrasound and patient-reported outcomes, concluding improvement in the SWT group after 12 months. Notably, penile triplex ultrasonography demonstrated improvement in all SWT-exposed participants except one.

Shock wave therapy is a proven effective means of treatment for Vasculogenic Erectile Dysfunction. However many vital questions remain unanswered. Research is needed to standardize outcomes across the various treatment variables, including: the various types of shock wave devices (electromagnetic, electrohydraulic, piezoelectric), energy, and frequency, durration, and timing of treatment.

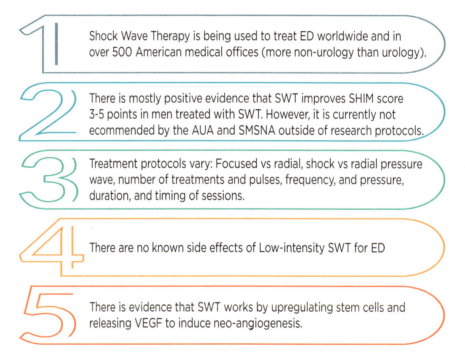

1. Shock Wave Therapy is being used to treat ED worldwide and in over 500 American medical offices (more non-urology than urology).

2. There is mostly positive evidence that SWT improves SHIM score 3-5 points in men treated with SWT. However, it is currently not ecommended by the AUA and SMSNA outside of research protocols.

3. Treatment protocols vary: Focused vs radial, shock vs radial pressure wave, number of treatments and pulses, frequency, and pressure, duration, and timing of sessions.

4. There are no known side effects of Low-intensity SWT for ED

5. There is evidence that SWT works by upregulating stem cells and releasing VEGF to induce neo-angiogenesis.

Platelet-rich plasma (PRP) for ED

PRP is the autologous transfer of whole blood that has been centrifuged with a separator agent to remove cellular products, leaving only plasma with a high concentration of platelets. [Sampson] PRP, as well as other platelet-derived therapies are growing in popularity in multiple fields due to the concentration of growth factors and regenerative potential for PRP. These growth factors play a role in many aspects of wound healing, such as cell proliferation and differentiation, chemotaxis, and angiogenesis. These qualities have garnered interest in PRP for curative treatment in Vasculogenic Erectile Dysfunction.

PRP is well established as an effective treatment in various medical situations, such as tendinopathies [Miller], burn care [Marck], androgenic alopecia [Mao], and even diabetes [Enderami]. In erectile dysfunction, PRP has had a number of preclinical studies and few clinical studies conducted.

Epifanova et al. conducted a three-armed trial evaluating the effect of PRP on peak systolic velocity, resistance index, IIEF-5, and sexual encounter profile. In those treated with PRP activated by 10% calcium chloride injected 3 times at weekly intervals, there was a statistically significant improvement in each outcome throughout follow-up. Men treated with PRP activated by 10% CaCl + PDE-5i demonstrated improvement in all domains with statistically significant p-values in PSV, IIEF-5, and SEP scores. Men treated with inactivated PRP also demonstrated statistically significant differences in IIEF-5 and SEP categories. Matz et al. demonstrated injections of PRP in men with ED with a maintained increase in IIEF-5 scores throughout 15 months of follow-up. Altogether, these studies reported few, if any side effects, indicating the safety of autologous PRP injection.

Despite widespread use in various branches of medicine, there are no standardized protocols for the production of PRP. [Dhurat] [Chahla] There is also a distinction to draw between PRP and PRP matrix: calcium chloride and thrombin may be added to the PRP to provide a gel matrix for the purpose of minimizing early washout of platelets from the site of injection [Gigante]. The use of differential nomenclature, single spin vs double spin technique, content and volume of PRP, as well as the skillful use of injection technique, can contribute to the overall efficacy of treatment [Everts]. Thus, when evaluating the literature, it is critical readers pay close attention to the description of PRP preparation and utilization.

CONCLUSIONS:

1. PRP stands for Platelet Rich Plasma. The P-shot® is a trademark name for PRP injection in the penis.

2. Platelets contain over 140 known growth factors. PRP is used in multiple fields including orthopedics and dermatology.

3. There have been very few papers written on the utilization of PRP in the penis.

4. PRP seems to be safe with no known side effects.

Stem Cells for ED

Stem cell therapy is another potential curative treatment approach to vascular erectile dysfunction.

Multiple human trials have demonstrated promise overall in the use of stem cells as restorative therapy for ED. Stem cells can be categorized based on the location they are derived from. Adult stem cells, from within matured organs, such as adipose tissue or the bone marrow, are clinically available and garnering great interest in human research. While differences between sources for stem cell cultivation are present (placental vs. embryonic), in-depth discussion of the nuance between all available forms of stem cells and treatment procedures is beyond the scope of this text.

Two studies conducted in men with post-prostatectomy erectile dysfunction reported beneficial results. Haahr. et al investigated the use of autologous adipose-derived regenerative cells isolated after liposuction in 17 men. Intracavernosal injection resulted in 8 of 17 men recovering from erectile function. When stratified by continence vs. incontinence, IIEF and EHS outcomes were significantly improved after six months in those who were continent compared to no improvement in those who were incontinent. Yiou et al. investigated the use of autologous bone marrow mononuclear cells in 18 total subjects across two stages of a phase 1/2 clinical trial. They also concluded significant improvement in IIEF and EHD scores compared to baseline without any side effects reported.

The angiogenic potential for stem cells in the treatment of Vasculogenic Erectile Dysfunction has been investigated in multiple studies in the past decade. Two stem cell studies conducted on the use of stem cells in diabetic men with erectile dysfunction reported benefit. Bahk et al. utilized human umbilical cord stem cells. After two months of follow-up, six of the seven participants in the experimental arm experienced morning erections compared to none at baseline. The three men assigned to the control group did not experience changes in penile rigidity. Al Demour et al. utilized autologous bone marrow-derived stem cells in four diabetic men with refractory ED. They reported a significant improvement in both IIEF-15 and EHD.

In a study of eight men reliant on injectable medication to sustain an erection, Levy et al. examined the use of placental matrix-derived mesenchymal stem cells. They reported a statistically significant increase in peak systolic velocity after the artificial induction of erection from a range of 23.1-49.3 cm/s to a range of 50.7 -73.9 cm/s. IIEF score changes were not statistically significant.

CONCLUSIONS:

1. Stem cells used in regenerative medicine come from three sources: adipose, bone marrow, and placental/umbilical.

2. There are very few studies on the use of stem cells in the penis. The completed small studies seem to show a beneficial effect.

3. Stem cells seem to work through a paracrine mechanism (personal communication with Anthony Atala).

4. Stem cells seem to be safe with no observed side effects.

Vacuum Erection Device (VED)

The first VED approved by the FDA was released in 1982 and has changed little over the course of time. Technologies differ slightly between devices, however, most include drawing blood into the penis through negative pressure in a cylindrical chamber. Units are either hand or battery operated.

Lin et al. proposed the VED increased arterial blood flow to the penis, which caused a reduction in hypoxia, and thus, a reduction in fibrosis and apoptosis at the penis. The result being protection of veno-occlusive mechanisms and improved erectile function outcomes. [Lin]

The most comprehensive study may be by Osbon et al. and the ErecAid™ system. In an update of 33,690 users, 95% of users reported an initial response with good erections. Studying the same device, Witherington et al. followed 6,902 men, demonstrating a 60% satisfaction rating and long-term usage.

VEDs have demonstrated beneficial effects in men undergoing radical prostatectomy. One trial randomized 109 men who had undergone radical prostatectomy and compared VED or observation for nine months starting four weeks after prostatectomy. It found 35% of VED users reported a decrease in penile length compared to 63% non-users. Kohler et al reported a similar benefit in comparing early VED users to late VED users. Of the early VED users, 12% reported penile length loss compared to 45% in the late VED users.

Qian et al. explored VED usage in the prevention of corporeal vaso-occlusive dysfunction and penile shrinkage in bilateral cavernous nerve crush in mice. They compared

VED in the setting of crush injury and no injury through a four-week period. The VED-treatment arm demonstrated superiority in penile shortening, peak intracavernosal pressure, and intracavernosal pressure drop rate, owing to increased smooth muscle/collagen ratios, decreased collagen I/III ratios, and perseveration of the integrity of the tunica albuginea. In spinal cord injuries, multiple studies have reported both efficacies in terms of increased sexual quality of life. Another study of 20 men found that 60% of men and 42% of their partners found that the device had improved their sexual relationship after six months. [Denil]

CONCLUSIONS:

1. In men who have lost erectile function, VEDs can restore and/or maintain penile length and health of erectile tissue.

2. 95% of men with ED are able to obtain an erection using a VED.

3. VEDs are relatively inexpensive, easy to use and have virtually no side effects.

SEXUAL SUPPLEMENTS

According to **medgadget.com**, the sexual enhancement supplements market is valued at $160 Million in 2018 and expected to reach $324 Million by 2025. Whether we agree with our patients taking supplements or not, many of them will purchase these over the counter medications. It is important for urologists to know the risks and benefits of the ingredients in these supplements.

Nitric oxide plays a pivotal role in the dilation of blood vessels and generation of penile erection, and levels tend to diminish steadily in men starting as early as age 30. Diminished levels of nitric oxide contribute to the development of multiple age-related diseases, including erectile dysfunction.

In endothelial cells, nitric oxide is synthesized from L-arginine by endothelial-nitric oxide synthase resulting in nitric oxide and L-citrulline. L-citrulline plays a key role in recycling L-arginine for repeated generation of nitric oxide. Surprisingly, previous research has established that L-arginine supplementation is not completely effective at increasing levels of nitric oxide. There are many reasons for this, including extraction via gastrointestinal and hepatic systems. Notably, the gastrointestinal tract also features high levels of arginase, which degrades orally ingested L-arginine. [Castillo] Alternatively, supplementation with L-citrulline has demonstrated increased plasma levels of L-arginine and increased nitric oxide bioavailability in murine and later human models. [Hartman][Schwedhelm][Suzuki]. This greater effect on nitric oxide generation can be attributed to the neutral amino acid lack of extraction by the GI tract and liver. [van de Poll] As a result, nitric oxide boosting supplements containing L-citrulline have been investigated for their use in cardiovascular disease [Bahri]. Ferrini et al. found that individually, L-citrulline supplementation at 0.9mg/ml resulted in a 2.8 fold increase in iNOS compared to controls.

Multiple studies have demonstrated L-citrulline to be effective in improving erectile function in murine models. [Shiota][Hotta] In humans, Shirai et al. demonstrated increased erectile function in men with PDE-5 inhibitors treated with a combination of L-citrulline and trans-resveratrol. Further, in a month-long study of 24 men, 1.5 g/d supplementation of L-citrulline was found to increase erection hardness scores compared to placebo. [Cormio]

Chang Rhim et al. conducted a systematic review and meta-analysis of the use of arginine supplementation in erectile dysfunction. Their results corroborated a beneficial effect of arginine on erectile dysfunction, however, treatment dosage varied from 1,500 to 5,000 mg.

The hepatic and intestinal clearance of arginine translate to a significantly higher dosage requirement for effect to be achieved. The adverse event rate in arginine-treated groups was also higher than in the placebo group (8.3% to 2.3%).

There are a number of other supplements that have not been as thoroughly researched as citrulline and arginine. Initial data suggests there may be a beneficial role for these supplements in quality men's sexual medicine. Tongkat ali is an herbal extract from Eurycoma longifolia, a plant found in Malaysian rainforests. Clinical research has demonstrated a daily dose of 300mg for 12 weeks resulted in a modest increase in IIEF score of 2.15 (95% CI: 1.03 to 3.27) compared to placebo. [Udani] Maca comes from the root of the Lepidium meyenii plant, found high in the Andes Mountains. In a 12-week study comparing 1,200 mg tablets of dehydrated Maca root twice a day (2,400 mg total per day) to placebo in men with erectile dysfunction, Maca-treated patients were found to have greater outcomes in both IIEF-5 and SAT-P scores. Horny goat weed has been tested in murine models and found to be associated with a positive neurotrophic effect and also a pro-nitric oxide synthesizing effect in the penis [Shindel].

There are a number of supplements that have purported men's sexual enhancement, the total list of which is too extensive for this chapter to cover. We list a number of supplements that have limited application in men's sexual medicine and/or peer-reviewed evidence of effect, yet may still be found by consumers. Yohimbe HCL has demonstrated beneficial effect in men's sexual medicine, however, the available formulations of Yohimbine have highly variables of quantities of the active ingredient and represent an unreliable source of supplement [Handbook]. DHEA is a prohormone used to increase testosterone. While it is involved in the synthesis of testosterone, supplementation with DHEA is inferior to supplementation with testosterone itself. Studies have shown DHEA may increase estrogen levels in men as well as testosterone. L-carnitine has been researched for its effect on endothelial function. Previous research has demonstrated its use as adjunctive treatment of Peyronie's disease to some effect. [Park] Used in combination with L-arginine and nicotinic acid, L-carnitine demonstrated improvement in IIEF-5 score in a group of men with erectile dysfunction and insulin-dependent diabetes compared to no treatment. [Gentile] Further, it demonstrated ability to increase sperm motility following oral administration 3g/day for 3 months. [Mongioi] Finally, Ginko biloba has limited human research conducted on its effect in sexual dysfunction. Wheatley conducted a 12-week study on the effects of 240mg of Ginko biloba compared to placebo. They did not find a statistically significant difference in sexual function outcomes.

CONCLUSIONS:

1. In the U.S., men spend in excess of $200 million a year on nutritional supplements in order to improve their sexual function.

2. Of the large number of supplements that are available, L-citrulline seems to have the best evidence for efficacy.

3. Tongkat Ali, Maca, Horny Goat weed, Yohimbine, DHEA, L-carnitine, and Ginko biloba are other compounds that are used as sexual supplements. The data is mixed.

PT141

PT-141, also known as Bremelanotide, is a synthetic heptapeptide melanocortin analog known to induce erection and increase sexual desire in men [Diamond]. It has been FDA approved for use in women with hypoactive sexual desire. Preclinical studies have demonstrated that PT-141 acts as an agonist at MC3 and MC4 receptors, which are members of the melanocortin receptor family. Unlike other members of the melanocortin receptor family (e.g., MC1-R, which is activated by alpha-MSH or MC2-R, which is activated by ACTH), MC3 and MC4 receptors are primarily expressed in the hypothalamus. [Gantz][Wessells]

Initially developed as a sunless tanning agent, PT-141 was discovered to induce erections in men. It was later developed as an intranasal agent for treatment of sexual dysfunction, however, testing was halted due to the adverse effect of increased blood pressure. [Ückert] Eventually, an injectable formulation was developed and found to produce significant improvements in multiple measures of female sexual dysfunction without the dangerous elevation in blood pressure. [Kingsberg] Currently, PT-141 has been developed as a self-administered, subcutaneous treatment for non-pregnant, premenopausal women with Hypoactive Sexual Desire Disorder. Marketed as Vyleesi, it acquired FDA approval in June of 2019.

In men, the association between nerve endings in the penis and the MC3R and MC4R in the hypothalamus was demonstrated by Molinoff et al. who found that when pseudorabies virus was injected into the corpus cavernosum, it was then detected in the hypothalamus via antiserum. One study found single intranasal doses of 7mg and 20mg were safe to administer to men with ED. The duration of increased rigidity from visual stimulation was higher with the larger dosing, with mean duration of >80% rigidity lasting 24 minutes. The average time to erectogenic onset was 30 minutes. The half-life of PT-141 was 2 hours with uncommon reports of adverse events; the most common AEs were flushing, and nausea with all reported AE's resolving without treatment or intervention. No serious adverse events were reported, including no significant changes in blood pressure or heart rate. [Molinoff][Diamond]

PT-141 is effective in increasing erections in men with mild-to-moderate erectile dysfunction. Its short-lived pharmacokinetic properties suggest the potential for use as an on-demand erectogenic medication. In addition to this, PT-141 has the effect of enhancing libido, though this is less well-studied in men.

CONCLUSIONS:

1. A peptide called PT-141, also known as Bremelanotide, has been shown to be effective in improving erectile function and libido in men. Even those who do not respond to PDE-5 inhibitors.

2. Bremelanotide is FDA approved in women for the treatment of hypoactive sexual desire.

3. PT-141 is administered as a subcutaneous injection. The most common side effect is nausea.

Oxytocin

The role of oxytocin in physiologic erection is well established in the sexual arousal and erectogenic response in men. Oxytocinergic neurons originate in the paraventricular nuclear project to the hippocampus, medulla oblongata, and spinal cord. Argiolas et al. used murine models to demonstrate that excitation of these neurons by dopaminergic agonism leads to penile erection. Oxytocin antagonism further served to inhibit erection. [Argiolas, 1995]

Following the observation that injection of oxytocin in the paraventricular nucleus and the hippocampus produced erection in murine models [Argiolas, 2005], Eckert et al. extracted penile blood from the corpus cavernosum and cubital vein during flaccidity, tumescence, and rigid erection in 25 men exposed to erotic stimulation. Radioimmunoassay revealed elevated oxytocin in the tumescent penis compared to the flaccid penis as well as in the rigid, erect penis compared to the tumescent stage.

Oxytocin may have further applications in sexual medicine. A case report by IsHak et al. demonstrated intranasal oxytocin administered intracoitally resulted in restoration of ejaculation in a treatment-resistant man with acquired male orgasmic disorder. [IsHak]

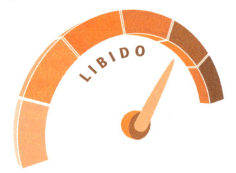

Similar research in women has also demonstrated improved sexual function in response to long-term intranasal administration of 32 IU of oxytocin compared to placebo. [Muin]

There is some evidence that Oxytocin is effective in improving libido, erection, and ejaculation.

PREMATURE EJACULATION

Premature ejaculation (PE) is the most common sexual disorder among men, with an estimated 30% across all age groups. [Montorsi] Prior to 2014, the definition of premature ejaculation (PE) varied considerably in literature. Lifelong PE was standardized in 2007 by the International Society for Sexual Medicine, however they were unable to provide a definition for acquired PE. In 2014, the ISSM's PE definition committee met again and established a unified definition for both forms of PE as male sexual dysfunction characterized by:

CONCLUSIONS:

1. Ejaculation that always or nearly always occurs prior to or within about 1 minute of vaginal penetration (lifelong PE) or a clinically significant and bothersome reduction in latency time, often to about 3 minutes or less (acquired PE);

2. The inability to delay ejaculation on all or nearly all vaginal penetrations; and

3. Negative personal consequences, such as distress, bother, frustration, and/or the avoidance of sexual intimacy. [Serefoglu]

Multiple treatments have been used in the treatment for premature ejaculation, including topical anesthetics, Tricyclic Antidepressants, Selective Serotonin Reuptake Inhibitors (SSRIs), centrally acting opiates, and PDE-5 inhibitors.

Topical anesthesia is well established as an effective and safe treatment for PE [Althof] and some are available over the counter. It is believed that by applying a local topical agent to the glans penis, the decreased sensitivity results in diminished stimulation of the sexual arousal pathways in the spinal cord and central nervous system.

Commonly, lidocaine is used in topical formulations, including sprays, such as Promescent®, Fortacin™, or Study-100, or in an emulsion, such as a eutectic mixture of local anesthetics, or EMLA cream, which is a mixture of lidocaine and prilocaine. A recent meta-analysis demonstrated an average increase in intravaginal ejaculation latency time (IELT) difference of 5.02 (95% CI: 3.03 – 7.00) after treatment with local anesthetics in a total of 954 subjects [Xia].

St. John's wort (Hypericum perforatum) is an herb with various medical properties that has been proposed as a treatment for premature ejaculation. One study assessed the safety and efficacy of 160mg of St. John's wort three times a day compared to placebo in 42 men with PE. In an analysis between groups, they concluded the average IELT time increased significantly in the treatment group (mean 349.09 seconds) compared to placebo (mean 99 seconds). However, in comparison to the pretreatment averages (70.23 and 67.50 seconds in treatment and placebo groups, respectively), did not demonstrate a statistically significant difference [Asgari].

A recent study compared the efficacy of on-demand use of 30mg paroxetine, 30mg Dapoxetine, 50mg Sildenafil, and a 30/50mg combination of Dapoxetine with sildenafil in a population of 150 men with premature ejaculation. All agents demonstrated improvement in intravaginal ejaculation latency time, although the combination of Dapoxetine and sildenafil demonstrated the greatest improvement from 38 to 266 seconds. Paroxetine demonstrated an increase from 39 to 174 seconds, Dapoxetine increased from 39 to 172 seconds, and sildenafil increased from 39 to 176 seconds. This pattern of improvement was mirrored in their secondary outcome of sexual satisfaction using the IIEF-5. [El-Hamd] Notably, while paroxetine and Dapoxetine are both SSRIs effective at treating PE, paroxetine is a daily medication with a prolonged side effect profile while Dapoxetine is licensed for on-demand treatment of PE.

One randomized controlled trial of 150 men comparing treatment of on-demand tramadol of 50mg and paroxetine of 20 mg to placebo. Patient-reported intravaginal ejaculation latency time and Premature Ejaculation Profile scores improved in all three groups. However, there was significant improvement in the tramadol-treated group compared to paroxetine and placebo. [Hamidi-Madani]

Another study analyzed the use of caffeine in a randomized, double-blinded trial of 40 men. Saadat et al. found 100mg of caffeine ingested 2 hours prior to intercourse resulted in an increase in IELT from 144 seconds pre-treatment to 312 seconds post-treatment and an increase in sexual satisfaction.

Tramadol is a centrally acting analgesic currently prescribed off-label for PE treatment. One study compared on-demand tramadol, sildenafil, paroxetine, lidocaine gel, and placebo in a group of 150 men who had PE for at least one year. They reported a significantly longer average IELT of 351 seconds compared to 67.2 seconds before treatment.

Topical lidocaine also demonstrated significant improvement (278 versus 54 seconds). Sildenafil demonstrated improvement from 58 to 228 seconds, and Paroextine improved IELT from 70 to 186 seconds. In comparison, the control group improved slightly from 61 to 81 seconds. [Gameel]. Another study compared tramadol at 25mg, 50mg, and 100mg in a group of men with an average IELT time of 2.82, 2.79, and 2.99 minutes, respectively. Among 300 randomized subjects, the average post-treatment IELT was 13.17, 23.43, and 36.49 minutes, respectively. Each of the three groups reported dose-dependent side effects of somnolence and pruritis, however, subjects in the 50mg and 100mg groups reported additional side effects, including dizziness, headache, and dry mouth. The 100mg-treated group additionally had reports of nausea and vomiting. [Eassa]

CONCLUSIONS:

1. Premature Ejaculation is likely the most common sexual issue that affects men ages 20-50.

2. Available options for the treatment of PE include delay sprays, numbing creams, herbal supplements based on St. John's wort, and SSRI anti-depressants.

3. Other agents that have been investigated for PE with mixed results include Tramadol, Sildenafil, and Caffeine.

Al Demour S, Jafar H, Adwan S, et al. Safety and potential therapeutic effect of two intracavernous autologous bone marrow derived mesenchymal stem cells injections in diabetic patients with erectile dysfunction: An open label phase I clinical trial. Urol Int 2018;101:358-365.

Althof SE, McMahon CG, Waldinger MD, et al. An update of the international society of sexual medicine's guidelines for the diagnosis and treatment of premature ejaculation (PE). J Sex Med. 2014;2:60–90.

Argiolas A, Melis MR. Central control of penile erection: role of the paraventricular nucleus of the hypothalamus. Prog Neurobiol. 2005 May;76(1):1-21.

Argiolas A, Melis MR. Oxytocin-induced penile erection. Role of nitric oxide. Adv Exp Med Biol. 1995;395:247-54.

Asgari, Seyyed & Falahatkar, Siavash & Hosseini Sharifi, Seyed Hossein & Enshaei, Ahmad & Jalili, Michael & Allahkhah, Aliakbar. (2010). Safety and Efficacy of the Herbal Drug Hypericum Perforatum for the Treatment of Premature Ejaculation. Urotoday International Journal. 03. 10.3834/uij.1944-5784.2010.06.21t4.

Bahk JY, Jung JH, Han H, et al. Treatment of diabetic impotence with umbilical cord blood stem cell intracavernosal transplant: Preliminary report of 7 cases. Exp Clin Transplant 2010;8:150-160. 14.

Bahri S, Zerrouk N, Aussel C, Moinard C, Crenn P, Curis E, Chaumeil JC, Cynober L, Sfar S. Citrulline: From metabolism to therapeutic use. Nutrition 2013:39;479-484

Balci M, Atan A, Senel C, Guzel O, Aslan Y, Lokman U, Kayali M, Bilgin O. Comparison of the treatment efficacies of paroxetine, fluoxetine and Dapoxetine in low socioeconomic status patients with lifelong premature ejaculation. Cent European J Urol. 2019;72(2):185-190. doi: 10.5173/ceju.2019.1855. Epub 2019 Jun 3.

Barassi A, Corsi Romanelli MM, Pezzilli R, Damele CA, Vaccalluzzo L, Goi G, Papini N, Colpi GM, Massaccesi L, Melzi d'Eril. Levels of l-arginine and l-citrulline in patients with erectile dysfunction of different etiology. Andrology. 2017 Mar;5(2):256-261. doi: 10.1111/andr.12293. Epub 2017 Feb 8.

Barnett J, Bernacki MN, Kainer JL, Smith HN, Zaharoff AM, Subramanian SK. The effects of regenerative injection therapy compared to corticosteroids for the treatment of lateral Epicondylitis: a systematic review and meta-analysis. Arch Physiother. 2019 Nov 13;9:12. doi: 10.1186/s40945-019-0063-6.

Bivalacqua TJ, Deng W, Kendirci M, Usta MF, Robinson C, Taylor BK, Murthy SN, Champion HC, Hellstrom WJ, Kadowitz PJ. Mesenchymal stem cells alone or ex vivo gene modified with endothelial nitric oxide synthase reverse age-associated erectile dysfunction. Am J Physiol Heart Circ Physiol. 2007 Mar; 292(3):H1278-90

Castillo L, Chapman TE, Yu YM, Ajami A, Burke JF, Young VR. Dietary arginine uptake by the splanchnic region in adult humans. Am J Physiol. 1993:265;E532-9

Catapano M, Catapano J, Borschel G, Alavania SM, Robinson LR, Mittal N. Effectiveness of platelet rich plasma injections for non-surgical management of carpal tunnel syndrome: a systematic review and meta-analysis of randomized controlled trials. Arch Phys Med Rehabil. 2019 Dec 7. pii: S0003-9993(19)31436-4. doi: 10.1016/j.apmr.2019.10.193.

Chahla J., Cinque M.E., Piuzzi N.S., Mannava S., Geeslin A.G., Murray I.R., Dornan G.J., Muschler G.F., LaPrade R.F. A call for standardization in platelet-rich Plasma preparation protocols and composition reporting: A systematic review of the clinical orthopaedic literature. J. Bone Joint Surg Am

Chang Rhim H, Kim MS, Park YJ, Choi WS, Park HK, Kim HG, Kim A, Paick SH. The Potential Role of Arginine Supplements on Erectile Dysfunction: A Systemic Review and Meta-Analysis. J Sex Med. 2019 Feb;16(2):223-234. doi: 10.1016/j.jsxm.2018.12.002.

Clavijo R, Kohn R, Kohn J, Ramasamy R. Effects of Low-Intensity Extracorporeal Shockwave Therapy on Erectile Dysfunction: A Systematic Review and Meta-Analysis. J Sex Med 2017;14:27-35.

Cormio L, De Siati M, Lorusso F, Selvaggio O, Mirabella L, Sanguedolce F, Carrieri G. Oral L-citrulline supplementation improves erection hardness in men with mild erectile dysfunction. Urology. 2011 Jan;77(1):119-22. doi: 10.1016/j.urology.2010.08.028.

Cruciani M, Franchini M, Mengoli C, Marano G, Pati I, Masiello F, Profili S, Veropalumbo E, Pupella S, Vaglio S, Liumbruno GM. Platelet-rich plasma for sports-related muscle, tendon and ligament injuries: an umbrella review. Blood Transfus. 2019 Nov;17(6):465-478. doi: 10.2450/2019.0274-19.

Denil J, Ohl DA, Smythe C. Vacuum erection device in spinal cord injured men: patient and partner satisfaction. Arch Phys Med Rehabil. 1996 Aug; 77(8):750-3.

Dhurat R, Sukesh M. Principles and methods of preparation of platelet-rich plasma: A review and author's perspective. J Cutan Aesthet Surg 2014;7:189-197

Diamond L, Earle D, Rosen R, Willett Molinoff P. Double-blind, placebo-controlled evaluation of the safety, pharmacokinetic properties and pharmacodynamic effects of intranasal PT=141, a melanocortin receptor agonist, in healthy males and patients with mild-to-moderate erectile dysfunction. Int J Impot. Res. 2004 16:51-59

Eassa BI, El-Shazly MA. Safety and efficacy of tramadol hydrochloride on treatment of premature ejaculation. Asian J Androl. 2013;15:138–42. doi: 10.1038/aja.2012.96.

El-Hamid M, Abdelhamed A. Comparison of the clinical efficacy and safety of the on demand use of paroxetine, Dapoxetine, sildenafil and combined Dapoxetine with sildenafil in treatment of patients with premature ejaculation: A randomised placebo controlled clinical trial. Andrologia 2018;50:12829

Enderami SE, Mortazavi Y, Soleimani M, et al. Generation of insulin-producing cells from human-induced pluripotent stem cells using a stepwise differentiation protocol optimized with platelet-rich plasma. J Cell Physiol 2017;232:2878-2886.

Epifanova M.V., Chalyi M.E., Krasnov A.O. Investigation of mechanisms of action of growth factors of autologous factors platelet-rich plasma used to treat erectile dysfunction. Urologiia. 2017:46–48.

Everts PA, Jakimowicz JJ, van Beek M, Schönberger JP, Devilee RJ, Overdevest EP, Knape JT, and van Zundert A. Reviewing the Structural Features of Autologous Platelet-Leukocyte Gel and Suggestions for Use in Surgery. Eur Surg Res. 2007. 39: 199–207.

Ferrini MG, Garcia E, Abraham A, Artaza JN, Nguyen S, Rajfer J. Effect of ginger, Paullinia cupana, muira puama and l- citrulline, singly or in combination, on modulation of the inducible nitric oxide- NO-cGMP pathway in rat penile smooth muscle cells. Nitric Oxide. 2018 Jun 1;76:81-86. doi: 10.1016/j.niox.2018.03.010. Epub 2018 Mar 16.

Fojecki G. L., Tiessen S., Osther P. J. S. (2017). Effect of low-energy linear shockwave therapy on erectile dysfunction-A double-blinded, sham-controlled, randomized clinical trial. The Journal of Sexual Medicine, 14(1), 106–112. doi:10.1016/j.jsxm.2016.11.307

Gameel T, Tawfik A, Abou-Farha M, Bastawisy M, El-Bendary M, El-Gamasy A. On-demand use of tramadol, sildenafil, paroxetine and local anaesthetics for the management of premature ejaculation: A randomised placebo-controlled clinical trial. Arab J Urol. 2013 Dec; 11(4): 392–397

Gantz I, Konda Y, Tashio T, Shimoto Y, Miwa H, Munzert G, Watson SJ, DelValle J, Yamada T. Molecular cloning of a novel melanocortin receptor. J. biol. Chem. 1993 268:8249

Gentile V, Antonini G, Antonella Bertozzi M, Dinelli N, Rizzo C, Ashraf Virmani M, Koverech A. Effect of propionyl-L-carnitine, L-arginine and nicotinic acid on the efficacy of vardenafil in the treatment of erectile dysfunction in diabetes. Curr Med Res Opin. 2009 Sep;25(9):2223-8.

Gigante A, Del Torto M, Manzotti S, Cianforlini M, Busilacchi A, Davidson PA, Greco F, Mattioli-Belmonte M. Platelet rich fibrin matrix effects on skeletal muscle lesions: an experimental study. J Biol Regul Homeost Agents. 2012 Jul-Sep; 26(3):475-84.

Gruenwald IE, Appel B, Vardi Y. The effect of a second course of low intensity shock waves for ED in partial or nonresponders to one treatment course. J Sex Med 2012;9:315.

Haahr MK, Harken Jensen C, Toyserkani NM, et al. A 12-month follow-up after a single intracavernous injection of autologous adipose-derived regenerative cells in patients with erectile dysfunction following radical prostatectomy:

An open-label phase I clinical trial. Urology 2018;121. 203.e6-13.

Hamidi-Madani A, Motiee R, Mokhtari G, Nasseh H, Esmaeili S, Kazemnezhad E. The Efficacy and Safety of On-demand Tramadol and Paroxetine Use in Treatment of Life Long Premature Ejaculation: A Randomized Double-blind Placebo-controlled Clinical Trial. J Reprod Infertil. 2018 Jan-Mar;19(1):10-15.

Hartman WJ, Torre PM, Prior RL. Dietary citrulline but not ornithine counteracts dietary arginine deficiency in rats by increasing splanchnic release of citrulline. J Nutr 1994:124;1950-60

Hashim PW, Levy Z, Cohen JL, Goldenberg G. Microneedling therapy with and without platelet-rich plasma. Cutis. 2017 Apr;99(4):239-242.

Hotta Y, Shiota A, Kataoka T, Motonari M, Maeda Y, Morita M, Kimura K. Oral L-citrulline supplementation improves erectile function and penile structure in castrated rats. Int J Urol. 2014 Jun;21(6):608-12. doi: 10.1111/iju.12362. Epub 2013 Dec 23.

IsHak WW, Berman DS, Peters A. Male anorgasmia treated with oxytocin. J Sex Med. 2008 Apr;5(4):1022-1024. doi: 10.1111/j.1743-6109.2007.00691.x. Epub 2007 Dec 14.

Kalyvianakis D., Hatzichristou D. (2017). Low-Intensity shockwave therapy improves hemodynamic parameters in patients with vasculogenic erectile dysfunction: A triplex ultrasonography-based sham-controlled trial. The Journal of Sexual Medicine, 14(7), 891–897. doi:10.1016/j.jsxm.2017.05.012

Kingsberg S, Clayton A, Portman D, Williams L, Krop J, Jordan R, Lucas J, Simon, J. Bremelantode for the treatment of hypoactive sexual desire disorder. Obs and Gyn 2019 134:5;899-908

Kitrey ND, Gruenwald I, Appel B, et al. Penile low intensity shock wave treatment is able to shift PDE5i nonresponders to responders: a double-blind, sham controlled study. J Urol 2016;195:1550-1555.

Levy JA, Marchand M, Iorio L, et al. Determining the feasibility of managing erectile dysfunction in humans with placentalderived stem cells. J Am Osteopath Assoc 2016;116:e1-e5.

Lindblom J, Schioth H, Larsson A. Autoradiographic discrimination of the melanocortin receptors indicate that the MC3 subtype dominates in the medial rat brain. Brain Res 1998 81-:161-171

Liu T, Shindel AW, Lin G, Lue TF. Cellular signaling pathways modulated by low-intensity extracorporeal shock wave therapy. Int J Impot Res. 2019 May;31(3):170-176. doi: 10.1038/s41443-019-0113-3.

Lu, S, Brandeis, J. "Shock Wave Erectile Enhancement Trial (SWEET) Study: A 41 site study on the use of shock wave therapy for the treatment of erectile dysfunction." 20th Annual Fall Scientific Meeting of Sexual Medicine Society of North America. 2019, Aug.

Man, L., & Li, G. (2017). Low-intensity Extracorporeal Shock Wave Therapy for Erectile Dysfunction: A Systematic Review and Meta-analysis. Urology. doi:10.1016/j.urology.2017.09.011

Mao G, Zhang G, Fan W. Platelet-Rich Plasma for Treating Androgenic Alopecia: A Systematic Review. Aesthetic Plast Surg. 2019 Oct;43(5):1326-1336. doi: 10.1007/s00266-019-01391-9

Marck RE, Middelkoop E, Breederveld RS. Considerations on the use of platelet-rich plasma, specifically for burn treatment. J Burn Care Res. 2014 May-Jun; 35(3):219-27.

Martyn-St. James M, Cooper K, Kaltenthaler E, Dickinson K, Cantrell A, Wylie K, Frodsham L, Hood C. Tramadol for premature ejaculation: a systematic review and meta-analysis. BMC Urol. 2015;15:6

Matz E.L., Pearlman A.M., Terlecki R.P. Safety and feasibility of platelet rich fibrin matrix injections for treatment of common urologic conditions. Invest. Clin. Urol. 2018;59:61–65

McMahon CG, Althof S, Waldinger MD, Porst H, Dean J, Sharlip I, Adaikan PG, Becher E, Broderick GA, Buvat J, Dabees K, Giraldi A, Giuliano F, Hellstrom WJ, Incrocci L, Laan E, Meuleman E, Perelman MA, Rosen R, Rowland D, Segraves R, International Society for Sexual Medicine Ad Hoc Committee for Definition of Premature Ejaculation. An evidence-based definition of lifelong premature ejaculation: report of the International Society for Sexual Medicine Ad Hoc Committee for the Definition of Premature Ejaculation. BJU Int. 2008 Aug; 102(3):338-50.

Mehrabani D, Seghatchian J, Acker JP.Platelet rich plasma in treatment of musculoskeletal pathologies. Transfus Apher Sci. 2019 Dec;58(6):102675. doi: 10.1016/j.transci.2019.102675.

Miller LE, Parrish WR, Roides B, et al. Efficacy of platelet-rich plasma injections for symptomatic tendinopathy: Systematic review and meta-analysis of randomised injection-controlled trials. BMJ Open Sport Exerc Med 2017;3:e000237.

Mohee A, Eardley I. Medical therapy for premature ejaculation. Ther Adv Urol. 2011 Oct;3(5):211-22. doi: 10.1177/1756287211424172.

Molinoff P, Shadiack A, Earle D, Diamon L, Quon C. PT-141: A Melanocortin Agonist for the Treatment of Sexual Dysfunction. Ann NY Acad Sci. 2003 994:96-102

Mongioi L, Calogero AE, Vicari E, Condorelli RA, Russo GI, Privitera S, Morgia G, La Vignera S. The role of carnitine in male infertility. Andrology. 2016 Sep;4(5):800-7. doi: 10.1111/andr.12191. Epub 2016 May 6.

Montorsi F. Prevalence of premature ejaculation: a global and regional perspective. J Sex Med. 2005 May;2 Suppl 2:96-102.

Muin DA, Wolzt M, Marculescu R, Sheikh Rezaei S, Salama M, Fuchs C, Luger A, Bragagna E, Litschauer B, Bayerle-Eder M. Effect of long-term intranasal oxytocin on sexual dysfunction in premenopausal and postmenopausal women: a randomized trial. Fertil Steril. 2015 Sep;104(3):715-23.e4. doi: 10.1016/j.fertnstert.2015.06.010. Epub 2015 Jul 4.

Park TY, Jeong HG, Park JJ, Chae JY, Kim JW, Oh MM, Park HS, Kim JJ, Moon du G. The Efficacy of Medical Treatment of Peyronie's Disease: Potassium Para-Aminobenzoate Monotherapy vs. Combination Therapy with Tamoxifen, L-Carnitine, and Phosphodiesterase Type 5 Inhibitor. World J Mens Health. 2016 Apr;34(1):40-6. doi: 10.5534/wjmh.2016.34.1.40. Epub 2016 Apr 30.

Qian SQ, Qin F, Zhang S, Yang Y, Wei Q, Wang R, Yuan JH. Vacuum therapy prevents corporeal veno-occlusive dysfunction and penile shrinkage in a cavernosal nerve injured rat model. Asian J Androl. 2019 Jun 25. doi: 10.4103/aja.aja_57_19. [Epub ahead of print]

Rosen RC, Allen KR, Ni X, et al. Minimal clinically important differences in the erectile function domain of the International Index of Erectile Function scale. Eur Urol 2011;60:1010-1016.

Saadat S, Ahmadi K, Panahi Y. The effect of on-demand caffeine consumption on treating patients with premature ejaculation: a double-blind randomized clinical trial. Curr Pharm Biotechnol. 2015;16(3):281-7.

Sampson S, Gerhardt M, Mandelbaum B. Platelet rich plasma injection grafts for musculoskeletal injuries: a review. Curr Rev Musculoskelet Med. 2008 Dec; 1(3-4):165-74.

Schwedhelm E, Maas R, Freese R, Jung D, Lukacs Z, Jambrecine A, Spickler W, Schulze D, Boger RH. Pharmacokinetic and pharmacodynamic properties of oral L-citrulline and L-arginine: Impact on nitric oxide metabolism. Br J Clin Pharmacol 2008:65;51-9.

Serefoglu EC, McMahon CG, Waldinger MD, Althof SE, Shindel A, Adaikan G, et al. An evidence-based unified definition of lifelong and acquired premature ejaculation: report of the second international society for sexual medicine ad hoc committee for the definition of premature ejaculation. Sex Med. 2014;2:41–59

Shindel AW, Xin ZC, Lin G, Fandel TM, Huang YC, Banie L, Breyer BN, Garcia MM, Lin CS, Lue TF Erectogenic and neurotrophic effects of icariin, a purified extract of horny goat weed (Epimedium spp.) in vitro and in vivo. J Sex Med. 2010 Apr; 7(4 Pt 1):1518-28.

Shiota A, Hotta Y, Kataoka T, Morita M, Maeda Y, Kimura K. Oral L-citrulline supplementation improves erectile function in rats with acute arteriogenic erectile dysfunction. J Sex Med. 2013 Oct;10(10):2423-9. doi: 10.1111/jsm.12260. Epub 2013 Jul 11.

Shirai M, Hiramatsu I, Aoki Y, Shimoyama H, Mizuno T, Nozaki T, Fukuhara S, Iwasa A, Kageyama S, Tsujimura A. Oral L-citrulline and Transresveratrol Supplementation Improves Erectile Function in Men With Phosphodiesterase 5 Inhibitors: A Randomized, Double-Blind, Placebo-Controlled Crossover Pilot Study. Sex Med. 2018 Dec;6(4):291-296. doi: 10.1016/j.esxm.2018.07.001. Epub 2018 Aug 24.

Suzuki T, Morita M, Hayashi T, Kamimura A. The effects on plasma L-arginine levels of combined oral L-citrulline and L-arginine supplementation in healthy males. Biosci Biotechnol Biochem. 2017 Feb;81(2):372-375. doi: 10.1080/09168451.2016.1230007. Epub 2016 Sep 26.

Ückert S, Bannowsky A, Albrecht K, Kuczyk MA (November 2014). "Melanocortin receptor agonists in the treatment of male and female sexual dysfunctions: results from basic research and clinical studies." Expert Opinion on Investigational Drugs. 23 (11): 1477–83. "FDA approves new treatment for hypoactive sexual desire disorder in premenopausal women." U.S. Food and Drug Administration (FDA) (Press release). 21 June 2019. Archived from the original on 20 November 2019. Retrieved 24 October 2019

Uckert S, Becker AJ, Ness BO, Stief CG, Scheller F, Knapp WH, Jonas U. Oxytocin plasma levels in the systemic and cavernous blood of healthy males during different penile conditions. World J Urol. 2003 May;20(6):323-6. Epub 2002 Oct 17.

Udani JK, George AA, Musthapa M, Pakdaman MN, Abas A. Effects of a proprietary freeze-dried water extract of Eurycoma longifolia (Physta) and Polygonum minus on sexual performance and well-being in men: a randomized, double-blind, placebo-controlled study evidence- based complementary and alternative medicine. eCAM. 2014:2014.

van de Poll MC, Ligthart-Melis GC, Boelens PG, Deutz NE, van Leeuwen PA, Dejong CH. Intestinal and hepatic metabolism of glutamine and citrulline in humans. J Physiol. 2007 Jun 1;581(Pt 2):819-27. Epub 2007 Mar 8

Vardi, Y., Appel, B., Jacob, G., Massarwi, O., & Gruenwald, I. (2010). Can Low-Intensity Extracorporeal Shockwave Therapy Improve Erectile Function? A 6-Month Follow-up Pilot Study in Patients with Organic Erectile Dysfunction. European Urology, 58(2), 243–248. doi:10.1016/j.eururo.2010.04.004

Vardi Y, Appel B, Kilchevsky A, et al. Does low intensity extracorporeal shock wave therapy have a physiological effect on erectile function? Short-term results of a randomized, double-blind, sham controlled study. J Urol 2012;187: 1769-1775.

Vardi Y., Appel B., Kilchevsky A., Gruenwald I. (2012). Does low-intensity extracorporeal shock wave therapy have a physiological effect on erectile function? Short-term results of a randomized, double-blind, sham-controlled study. Journal of Urology, 187(5), 1769–1775. doi:10.1016/j.juro.2011.12.117

Veronesi F, Borsari V, Contartese D, Xian J, Baldini N, Fini M. The clinical strategies for tendon repair with biomaterials: A review on rotator cuff and Achilles tendons. J Biomed Mater Res B Appl Biomater. 2019 Nov 30. doi: 10.1002/jbm.b.34525.

Vilchez-Cavazos F, Millán-Alanís JM, Blázquez-Saldaña J, Álvarez-Villalobos N, Peña-Martínez VM, Acosta-Olivo CA, Simental-Mendía M. Comparison of the Clinical Effectiveness of Single Versus Multiple Injections of Platelet-Rich Plasma in the Treatment of Knee Osteoarthritis: A Systematic Review and Meta-analysis. Orthop J Sports Med. 2019 Dec 16;7(12):2325967119887116.

Wang CJ, Wang FS, Yang KD, et al. Shock wave therapy induces neovascularization at the tendon-bone junction. A study in rabbits. J Orthop Res 2003;21:984-989.

Wang, R. Vacuum Erectile Device for Rehabilitation After Radical Prostatectomy. J Sex Med 2017;14:184-6

Wessells H, Dralnek D, Dorr R, Hruby C, Hadley M, Levine N. Effect of an alpha-melanocyte stimulating hormone analog on penile erection and sexual desire in men with organic erectile dysfunction. Urol. 200 56:4;641-646

Wessells H, Fuciarelli J Hanser, et al. Synthetic melanotropic peptide initiates erections in men with psychogenic erectile dysfunction: double-blind, placebo-controlled crossover study. J Urol. 1998 160:389-393

Wheatley D. Triple-blind, placebo-controlled trial of Ginko biloba in sexual dysfunction due to antidepressant drugs. Hum Psychopharmacol 2004 Dec:19(8):545-8

Witherington R Long term follow up (2–21 years) of users of external vacuum devices for treatment of impotence. Proceedings AUA New York Section Meeting. Oct 9–13   1995, Istanbul, Turkey

Wu Y.N., Wu C.C., Sheu M.T., Chen K.C., Ho H.O., Chiang H.S. Optimization of platelet-rich plasma and its effects on the recovery of erectile function after bilateral cavernous nerve injury in a rat model. J. Tissue Eng. Regen. Med. 2016;10:E294–E304

Xia JD, Han YF, Zhou LH, et al. Efficacy and safety of local anaesthetics for premature ejaculation: a systematic review and meta-analysis. Asian J Androl. 2013 Jul;15(4):497–502.

Yan X, Zeng B, Chai Y, et al. Improvement of blood flow, expression of nitric oxide, and vascular endothelial growth factor by low-energy shockwave therapy in random-pat

Yang J, Zhang Y, Zang G, Wang T, Yu Z, Wang S, Tang Z, Liu J. Adipose-derived stem cells improve erectile function partially through the secretion of IGF-1, bFGF, and VEGF in aged rats. Andrology. 2018 May; 6(3):498-509.

Yee C.-H., Chan E. S., Hou S.-S., Ng C.-F. (2014). Extracorporeal shockwave therapy in the treatment of erectile dysfunction: A prospective, randomized, double-blinded, placebo controlled study. International Journal of Urology, 21(10), 1041–1045. doi:10.1111/iju.12506

Yiou R, Hamidou L, Birebent B, et al. Intracavernous injections of bone marrow mononucleated cells for postradical prostatectomy erectile dysfunction: Final results of the INSTIN clinical trial. Eur Urol Focus 2017;3:643-645.

Zenico T, Cicero AF, Valmorri L, Mercuriali M, Bercovich E. Subjective effects of Lepidium meyenii (Maca) extract on well-being and sexual performances in patients with mild erectile dysfunction: a randomised, double-blind clinical trial. Andrologia. 2009;41(2):95–99. doi: 10.1111/j.1439-0272.2008.00892

KEY POINTS

- **As experts in the male genitalia,** urologists should reassert their leadership role in investigating and treating Erectile Dysfunction with these emerging technologies, especially as online pharmacies threaten patient referrals and eliminate urologists as the source of medical information.

- **Shock wave therapy** is a proven effective means of treatment Vasculogenic Erectile Dysfunction. However, many vital questions remain unanswered. Research is needed to standardize outcomes across the various treatment variables.

- **There have been few papers written on the utilization of Platelet Rich Plasma,** or PRP in the penis (aka, the P-shot®). It seems to be safe with no known side effects.

- **There are very few studies on the use of stem cells** in the penis, however, the completed small studies seem to show a beneficial effect with no observed side effects.

- **95% of men with ED** are able to obtain an erection using vacuum erection devices or VEDs, which are relatively inexpensive, easy to use, and have virtually no side effects.

- **Of the large number of sexual supplements available,** L-citrulline seems to have the best evidence for efficacy, while data is mixed for other compounds, including Tongkat Ali, Maca, Horny Goat weed, Yohimbine, DHEA, L-carnitine, and Ginkgo biloba.

- **A peptide called PT-141 (a Bremelanotide)** is administered as a subcutaneous injection and shown to be effective in improving erectile function and libido in men. The most common side effect is nausea.

- **There is some evidence that Oxytocin** is effective in improving libido, erection, and ejaculation.

- **Promising options for the treatment of Premature Ejaculation** include delay sprays, numbing creams, herbal supplements based on St. John's wort, and SSRI anti-depressants. Other agents that have been investigated with mixed results include Tramadol, Sildenafil, and Caffeine.

Judson Brandeis, MD

Dr. Judson Brandeis attended Brown University as an undergraduate and Vanderbilt Medical School. He trained in Urology at UCLA and currently practices sexual and rejuvenative medicine for men in San Ramon, California. He was a pioneer in Surgical Robotics, Greenlight Laser and MRI prostate biopsy.

Dr. Brandeis has appeared on The Doctors Show and dozens of Podcasts and Webcasts. He created the SWEET (Shock Wave Erectile Enhancement Trial) Study which is the largest study of Shock Wave therapy for ED ever done. His other clinical research studies include the SWAP Study (Shock Wave and Peyronie's) utilizing his special Peyronie's disease SWT protocol, the P-LONG study for minimally invasive penile elongation, the MenSella Study using HIFEM technology for improving the intensity and duration of orgasm and the SURGE study using a transdermal technology to deliver Nitric Oxide to the penis.

BrandeisMD in Northern California is at the leading edge of male rejuvenation and sexual medicine. Among the many cutting edge technologies, we use BioTE testosterone supplementation, Emsculpt and Emsella for muscular rejuvenation, and GAINSWave therapy and PRP for sexual rejuvenation. Dr. Brandeis also founded AFFIRM Science which creates supplements based on the most recent scientific data (**AFFIRMScience.com**).

CHAPTER

The Current Role of Telemedicine: Implications for the Large Urology Group Practice

Eugene Rhee, MD MBA
Matthew Gettman, MD
Eric Kirshenbaum, MD
Aaron Spitz, MD

When human spaceflight became a reality in 1961 and the world sent Yuri Gagarin, the first human into space, it answered a major answer to the question as to whether a human could survive without gravity. This was answered with the emergence of biometric data via a telemetric link that modern medicine would receive from various animals attached to medical monitors. This ability to transmit biometric data has led to an electronic revolution for physicians: telemedicine.

Today, information is available in ways that are changing how American medicine is practiced. Urology group practices will need to respond to how this information is used to deliver care strategically in a scalable fashion. This chapter aims to introduce telemedicine and understand a variety of encounters that might best suit a variety of large urology practices. Telemedicine and telehealth are terms that describe the interactive exchange of healthcare information electronically between patients, providers, and consultants for the purpose of education, evaluation, decision-making, and treatment. These interactions include text, audio, video, and audio-video communication. Platforms are increasing and include personal computers, pads, tablets, smart phones, wireless wearable sensors, and other emerging technologies.

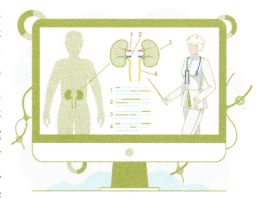

Telemedical applications have rapidly evolved to cover a wide array of chronic and emergent conditions. The emergence of the COVID-19 public health emergency (PHE) in early 2020 transformed the telemedicine landscape in a short period of time. For some specialties it had already become a routine way of delivering care, or others, such as urology it is only recently gaining adoption. Telemedicine had become a familiar tool for the psychiatrist, especially in the emergency room. Intensivists are running multiple ICUs simultaneously via telemedical platforms. Pediatric surgeons have been telemedically accessible to many hospitals that lack expertise on their staff. Consultations were increasingly provided telemedically by dermatologists,[6] orthopedists,[7] general surgeons,[8] and ophthalmologists.[9] In addition to hospital settings, telemedicine visits were conducted in satellite clinics,[1] retail minute clinics,[5] and elementary schools.[4] Additionally, patients may have telemedicine visits with their physicians or physician assistant from home.

Urologists had been trailblazing telemedicine successfully from academic pilots to standard operating procedures in the VA system.[16,17] Pediatric urologists were also early adopters.[10-12] Private practice urologists are now providing hospital consultations as well as postoperative follow up care through telemedical interfaces. Routine urology office visits are being conducted from the patient's home or workplace, and patients in skilled nursing facilities are seen by the urologist in their facility through a telemedical link.

During the COVID-19 public health emergency, legislation lifting many telemedicine restrictions was accomplished in weeks removing many of the restrictions that had plagued the progress of telemedicine. The combination of in-person office visit restrictions and the liberalization of telemedicine laws forced physicians across most specialties, including urologists, to integrate telemedicine into their practices in order to serve the needs of their patients and to ensure their practices financial stability. The early adoption of telemedicine by a minority of urologists facilitated a rapid dissemination of information and onboarding to the newly initiated majority.

"Telesurgery" is very new to telemedicine but is quickly evolving in a number of ways including teleconsults and teleproctoring/telementoring.[18,19] Surgery is an ancient craft that, unlike general medicine, relies on the human senses to deliver care. New technologies are being developed and implemented within the basic surgical tools that can enhance the ability of individual surgeons in the operating room. "IT-driven transformation" coupled with data storage, connectivity, and analysis will accelerate improvements in function, functionality, performance, and ultimately, the value of care delivery.[20]

Telemedicine may provide a high value solution for the workforce shortages in urology that have well been documented. The urology workforce will continue to be stressed with a progressive imbalance in available urologists and patients. It is estimated that by 2030, 20% of the population will be 65 or older with increasing surgical needs. By 2030 urology will face a 32% (3884 urologists) shortage for >350 million US citizens. According to the 2018 AUA census data, 30% of urologists are >65 years old, a clear concerning sign of a progressive urologist shortage. (Williams 2010, US Census Bureau 2000 - 2050). Urology is the second oldest specialty after thoracic surgery (Neuwahl et al 2012, AAMC Projections through 2025) and the reality that we could lose a quarter of our workforce in a short period of time is very real.

Telemedicine can alleviate some of the workforce concerns by providing efficient care to larger geographic areas and address the scarcity of urologists in rural areas.

> There are no urologists in **62.2%** of U.S. counties, limiting patient access to necessary care. Overall, the adoption of telehealth services in urology had been slow but on the rise. According to the 2018 AUA census data, **12%** of urologists utilized telemedicine in their practice, up from **8.6%** in 2016. A large majority **(83%)** of users expected services to continue to increase in their organization

Even large urology groups may be challenged to meet the demands of their contracted population in urban and suburban markets. Well after the COVID PHE, telemedicine can allow group practices to leverage their subspecialty expertise across a larger population and provide those patients the superior level of care that affords them a competitive advantage. Additionally, groups that adopt telemedicine for their patient's convenience will stay on par with rising patient expectations, as many patients will have been introduced to telemedicine during the PHE that otherwise would not have. Traditional sectors of our society have already incorporated and transformed a customer-centric focus, including travel, retail sales, and banking.

Prior to the PHE, health care reform with its emphasis on value was bringing more attention to the prospect of telemedicine. In many states, private payers were mandated to cover telemedicine services, often on par with office encounters. Medicaid covered telemedicine in almost all states. The department of Veterans Affairs had been a true trailblazer in the world of telehealth. In 2019 the VA reported >900,000 veterans utilized its telehealth services (235% jump from previous year). Furthermore, the VA announced a 17% increase in televisits, delivering >2.6 million telehealth episodes in 2019. (**https://www.va.gov/opa/pressrel/includes/viewPDF.cfm?id=5365**)

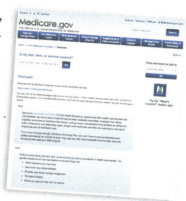

Medicare had been very restrictive prior to the PHE, limiting coverage to remote or certain chronic care scenarios but allowing some liberalization through alternative payment models such as Alternative Care Organizations or bundled payments. At the start of 2020, traditional Medicare and Medicare advantage plans expanded telehealth coverage, limiting restrictions on patient location requirements and expanding coverage for more diagnosis.(**https://www.medicare.gov/coverage/telehealth**) As of March 1, 2020, during the PHE, traditional Medicare has radically liberalized access to telemedicine across effectively all locations and all conditions. The extent to which this remains after the PHE has concluded is unknown but even with a significant retraction, large urology group practices can be well positioned to participate in alternative payment models which would compensate for telemedical services.

Regulations governing telemedicine vary by state. Prior to the PHE, the practice of telemedicine was limited to the state in which a physician was licensed, as it is with traditional medical practice. During the PHE, Medicare has suspended state-based licensure requirements for telemedicine allowing patients to be seen across state lines, but this allowance is subordinated to state law. The majority of states have cooperated in some fashion and details about state based licensure changes can be found on the Alliance for Connected Care Website (**http://connectwithcare.org/state-telehealth-and-licensure-expansion-covid-19-chart**/)

In practical terms, the implementation of telemedicine has become greatly simplified. Turnkey, HIPAA compliant software options are increasingly available which work on hardware platforms most physicians and patients already have at their disposal.

During the PHE HIPPA requirements for video visits have been lifted when they become onerous to patient access. The expectation, however, is that when the PHE is over the HIPPA waiver will expire and telemedicine platforms will have HIPPA compliance requirements. Additionally, telemedicine adoption became less restrictive with the signing of the 21st Century Cures Act as it deregulated telemedicine so that devices used for streaming are no longer regulated by FDA (**https://www.fda.gov/regulatory-information/selected-amendments-fdc-act/21st-century-cures-act**). Even as technology improves, the doctor-patient relationship must remain at the center of the encounter with all the constraints, courtesies, and compassion of traditional medicine.

Types of Telemedical Services

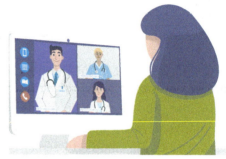

Video Visits: A video visit is a live face-to-face electronic audio-visual interaction between he provider and a patient. Prior to the PHE, the combination of both audio and video most all payers for reimbursement. Telephone encounters are reimbursed by Medicare during the PHE but the extent to which that will remain is uncertain. Other payers may or may not provide reimbursement for telephone calls. In spite of the limitations of an on-screen encounter, video visits are successfully providing alternatives to traditional visits in a variety of settings including clinic, office, urgent care, hospital, and skilled nursing facilities.

Online Services: Patients may access portions of their electronic medical record and communicate with their urology care team. Value added services also include online appointment scheduling, form submission such as history intake questionnaires, and online bill payment. Additionally, the practice can provide the patient alerts for preventative services as well as definitions of conditions and guidelines and reminders for care, such as urology cancer rechecks. These services were typically not billable, but they brought value to patients and helped satisfy government mandated meaningful use criteria for electronic health records.[24] During the PHE, Traditional Medicare is reimbursing these services.

eConsults: eConsults allow a urologist to asynchronously answer another provider's focused questions about the diagnosis or management of a specific patient. The urologist reviews the supporting material from the EHR and provides a formal response to the focused question. Consultations are most likely to be solicited from large academic centers but can also be solicited from large urology groups. eConsults can also be synchronous (involving real-time interactions similar to video visits) and in this context are also known as video consults. In contrast to video visits, the patient is typically not present during a video consult. eConsults are performed using electronic software and hardware specifically for electronic consultations. For example, a portal called WebSphere (Cisco) has been used for eConsults. The response is documented in the medical record of the provider completing the eConsult.

eConsults are convenient for requesting providers and patients alike because they provide timely access to specialty expertise without requiring the patient to actually travel to visit with another urologist. Thus, eConsults allow patient visits to be completed in a shorter timeframe and streamline the delivery of care. Scheduling is also more flexible with eConsults, especially asynchronous consults that can be completed outside of regular business hours. By using asynchronous eConsults particularly for more straightforward urologic problems, it is anticipated that more time would be allotted for synchronous eConsults or traditional face-to-face consults on more complex patients during regular business hours. The concepts used in synchronous eConsults have also been applied to virtual tumor boards. Studies assessing the benefit of eConsults have uniformly demonstrated a reduction in the number of required in person consults ranging from 62% to 92%, optimizing patient time and physician efficiency. (Modi et al. 2018)

With virtual tumor boards, detailed case presentations are made in the same way as traditional tumor boards. Radiologic studies and histologic findings are reviewed ahead of time with a radiologist and pathologist, respectively. Using this approach, a second opinion for the patient is obtained and the mechanism is a powerful means to keep high standards of clinical care and performance within the control of a private large group practice.

Teleintraoperative Consultation: The intraoperative consultation is perhaps the most innovative and valuable role in telemedicine. The urologist offers electronic consultations regarding intraoperative findings with other surgeons remotely. This type of encounter has implications as to assisting in the OR in ways that may very well prove to enhance productivity and surgical quality as this matures.

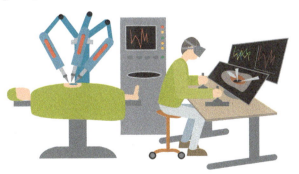

Hung and colleagues investigated the current utilization of telesurgery in minimally invasive procedures. They categorized currently available technologies into 4 categories: verbal guidance, telestration, guidance with tele-assist and telesurgery. Verbal guidance is simple a 2-way communication between surgeon and consultant with video monitoring. The benefit being it is easily implemented with low cost and minimal bandwidth requirements. Telestration allows the consultant or mentor to telestrate in 2D or 3D aiding the surgeon through various aspects of a procedure. Tele-assists allow for the mentor or consultant to reach into the patient remotely and physically aide in a procedure. Lastly, tele-surgery allows for the entire surgery to be completed remotely. (Hung et al. 2018) Sterbis et al, performed[4] porcine radical nephrectomies utilizing the DaVinci® robot from >1300 miles away. While the technology exists adoption is in its infancy. (Sterbis et al. 2008)

Telementoring and Teleproctoring:
A urologist can serve as a mentor and/or proctor during a telesurgical procedure creating telementoring and teleproctoriong services.[12] This has broad implications with licensure and credentialing in the practice of urology.

Telemedicine and robotic technology have addressed cumbersome and impractical physical mentoring to telementoring and teleproctoring. Hinat and colleagues in one of the first reported series of telementoring and teleproctoring in robotics used a telementoring system to promote surgical techniques associated with robotic-assisted radical prostatectomies. The group demonstrated proper function and acceptable latency with no differences in surgical outcomes, incline operative ties, complication rates, early continence status, and positive margin rates between the telementoring and direct mentoring group.[26]

Telesimulation and telesurgical rehearsal:
Simulators are now being used to learn minimally invasive surgical techniques as educational tools. Medical/surgical education can use a network of simulators to assist teaching and evaluating novice surgeons and those who need to improve. This would standardize teaching and as well allow for interactive proctoring during simulated procedures. A surgical "dress-rehearsal" may be possible before the actual operation. Currently urology patient-specific simulations are in development that could be rapidly and easily integrated into telemedicine.

Examples of Telemedicine in Urology

This section highlights the implementation of telemedicine by urologists across a wide spectrum of settings and patient types prior to the PHE. In many cases quality and satisfaction outcomes were examined. These implementations paved the way and provided reassurance for the wide-spread adoption of telemedicine by urologists that has been required by the PHE. The particulars of the various models may have changed with the liberalization of telemedicine in the PHE period, but the lessons demonstrated are useful to understand.

Outpatient Telemedicine

The VA is a national leader in the adoption of telemedicine, and they have committed billions of dollars to their effort of providing this access to over 700,000 veterans. A notable success has been the urology department at the Los Angeles VA where over 1000 new patients have been evaluated with video visits. These patients live sufficiently far that travel to the physical clinic is onerous, but Jeremy Shelton MD and his colleagues are conducting face to face audio-visual visits with these patients at satellite clinics that are closer to the patients' homes. All conditions are initially evaluated telemedically and in-office follow up and procedures are accomplished as needed. Lower urinary tract symptoms, elevated PSA and prostate cancer are the most common chief complaints. 95% of patients score satisfaction as very good to excellent and 80% of urologists score the encounters as excellent. In a study patients were spared on average 277 miles of travel and 200 dollars in expenses.[17] Similar outcomes were reported by the urology telemedicine program at the VA Medical Center in Omaha, Nebraska.[17] The economic benefit of televisits has been well established with a clear advantage in time saved and travel expenses for patients. Zholudev and colleagues sought to compare costs of teleurology visit vs conventional face-to-face encounters for the initial management of hematuria in a VA population. They assessed transportation cost, clinic operative expenses and patient time and compared the 2 cohorts. The average patient time was significantly greater in the face-to-face encounter (266 minutes vs 70 minutes, $p<0.001$). A similar advantage was shown for overall cost savings with a face-to-face encounter costing on average $135.02 compared to $10.95 for teleurology encounter. The primary drivers for cost savings were transportation cost ($83.47/encounter), patient time ($32.87/encounter) and clinic staff costs ($18.68/encounter). While this study was in a VA population, similar potential cost savings can be extrapolated in the private sector while improving a practices catchment area. In the same VA population, overall satisfaction with televisit was high with mean satisfaction scores exceeding 9 out of 10 for overall satisfaction, efficiency, convenience, friendliness, care quality, understandability, privacy and professionalism. (Safir et al. 2016) Assuming 1.5 million hematuria visits annually in the United States, there is a potential savings of $200 million per year on hematuria alone. (Zholudev et al. 2018)

Large urology group practices may expand their reach and provide larger catchments of patients access to their services with similar models of telemedical access. Dr. Paolo Andreassi and colleagues at University of California Davis Department of Urology provide telemedical initial consultations for urology consults for most adult and pediatric urological conditions. As with the VA model, the appointments are conducted at satellite clinics but in the presence of the primary care physician and after supporting records and results have been received. The appointments are conducted in the presence of the primary care physician at satellite clinics equipped with the telemedical audio-visual platform. Medical records and diagnostic studies are provided well ahead of the scheduled appointment.

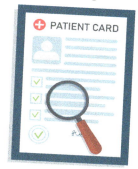

Many patients receiving care at the Mayo Clinic Department of Urology in Rochester Minnesota travel great distances and often across state lines. Matthew Gettman, MD and his colleagues provide telemedical visits for patients following prostatectomy saving them an average of 95 miles of travel and associated expenses. Many patients come from great distances (average 95 miles), including across state lines, for care. An earlier prospective study of When studied, this program demonstrated similar patient-to-provider facetime (14.5 minutes vs. 14.3 minutes), patient wait time (18.4 minutes vs. 13.0 minutes), and total time devoted to care (17.9 minutes vs. 17.8 minutes). Doctor satisfaction was nearly identical to in-office visits. However, the patient's time away from work was greatly reduced and travel expenses were eliminated. There was nearly identical satisfaction for urologists conducting the visits telemedically compared to in person.[27]

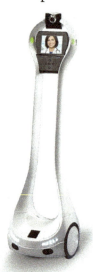

Dr. Robert Nguyen pioneered a postoperative telemedical program at Boston Children's Hospital where VGo remote-controlled telemedical robots were sent home with children who were discharged from the hospital after surgery. This enabled the urologist to closely monitor the children in their own homes during the critical post-operative period. This robotic presence was welcomed by the families, and children often did not want to return their new robotic "friend."[14]

As large private urology groups cultivate centers of excellence in subspecialty care, such as oncology, they may attract tertiary referrals and utilize telemedicine to facilitate follow up for patients referred from greater distances, but telemedicine can also be leveraged to enhance access to local patients as well.

Patients who are discharged from the hospital to a skilled nursing facility frequently require urological follow up or routine consultation. Even though a urologist may be located in close proximity, coordination of outpatient urological care for these patients can be cumbersome for the patient and family alike and may delay their discharge from the SNF. Dr Aaron Spitz, MD in collaboration with OptumHealth demonstrated the ability to provide telemedical urology care for patients at their bedside prior to discharge from the skilled nursing facility. This met with high patient and family satisfaction and instances of earlier discharge.

An easily adoptable use of telemedicine for large urology group practices is found in the practices of Eric Geisler, MD, in a large urology group in Austin, Texas as well as Aaron Spitz, MD, in a large urology group in Orange County, California. Both practitioners provide telemedical services to their local PPO or capitated patients in the form of follow-up visits for patients who would not require a hands-on physical exam or procedure at that particular visit. These encounters are conducted via an internet-based software utilizing the patient's iPhone, iPad, or a personal computer equipped with a camera. Physician assistants in the practice may conduct these visits as well. The patients report great satisfaction with the convenience of conducting these visits from their home, place of employment, or even while traveling out of town. These visits have augmented the practices while keeping the physical office space available for more complex patients requiring in-person evaluations.

An increasing number of studies have demonstrated the benefit of televisit for both patient and provider. A study out of the University of Michigan demonstrated a median level of interest of 72 (0 = interest, 100 = extremely interested) for outpatient televisits. With an aging urologic population, one concern is that patients do not have the necessary technology for virtual encounters. Andino et al, demonstrated that 94% of patients, in their academic practice, owned their own device sufficient for a televisit.(Andino et al. 2017)

With the emergence of teleurology, Glassman and colleagues sought to determine which urologic diagnosis were associated with highest patient satisfaction for televisits in an urban academic setting in order to better tailor the patient experience. They demonstrated very high patient satisfaction across all diagnosis (289 patients, satisfaction score 4.94/5). No differences were observed in satisfaction across primary diagnosis which ranged from urologic oncology encounters, stone disease, infertility, lower urinary tract disorders and cancer screening. (Glassman et al. 2018)

Driven by the scarcity of their services, some pediatric urologists have been early adopters of telemedicine Catherine Devries, MD, a pediatric urologist at the University of Utah, reaches remote pediatric patients in their homes. Dr. William Kennedy, a pediatric urologist at Lucile Packard Children's Hospital at Stanford, cares for numerous patients remote or hard to reach urban patients telemedically with the aid of practitioner's travel to rural clinics, as well as inner-city satellite hospitals. The majority of families prefer the telemedical visits and enjoy a 50% reduction in wait times.[10] Dr. Stephen Canon and associates at Arkansas Children's Hospital utilized telemedicine linked to local clinics to reduce travel and expense for preoperative consultations and postoperative follow-up for patients in remote rural areas. Travel was reduced from 335 km to 35 km. There was no increase in complications.[12]

Telemedicine: Systems and Procedures

As with traditional care delivery, telemedicine can be enhanced by following standard operating procedures. General and specialty medical societies are currently generating guidelines for telemedicine that include technical instructions and ethical considerations. Guidelines also increase the delivery of high-quality and safe patient care, key themes needed for telemedicine to be supported by legislators and payers.

Prior to the PHE, telemedicine was required to be delivered using secure internet-based videoconferencing technologies. During the PHE it is still encouraged but not required by Medicare when it creates a barrier to access. Non HIPPA compliant platforms such as Facetime are allowable but public facing platforms such as Facebook Live are not. Furthermore, during the PHE, telephone encounters may be conducted for reimbursement on par with video encounters. Nonetheless, after the PHE telephone only encounters may or may not continue to be reimbursed and HIPPA requirements for secure connections will likely return. It is advisable to select a secure video platform for a long term telemedical strategy. The network used for telemedicine is typically a secure VPN, with software that is typically licensed to a host institution.

Videoconferencing with encryption software can be downloaded to connect with patients directly in their own home or other non-institutional setting. Internet-based websites can also be used as an alternative portal for urologists and patients seeking telemedicine services. It is conceivable that urologists could sign up with one or more Internet-based companies that provide professional profiles that could be viewed online by prospective patients. In this model, patients would find such sites by searching online or by word-of-mouth. For practices considering implementation of video visits, it is important to consider urologic diagnoses for which video visits will be offered. The experience with many urologists during the PHE is that most, if not all diagnoses can be managed in part or in whole with telemedicine. Telemedicine need not be an either/or proposition such that a visit that is conducted telemedically does not preclude a rapid follow up in-person visit when deemed necessary. Next, it is important to verify the patient has required hardware and software capabilities for a video visit and sufficient broadband connectivity. The patient should be provided contact information for technical support in case troubleshooting is required. Rather than have the patient manage the requirements of the video visit, another option is for the patient to report to a telemedicine center where the hardware, software, and connectivity are provided and standardized for maximum reliability.

Informed consent is established prior to the start of the video visit. The consent is typically conducted in real time following laws within the patient's jurisdiction The provider should document the consent in the medical record.[2,11] The consent should include a discussion about the structure and timing of services, record keeping, scheduling, privacy, risks, confidentiality, mandatory reporting, and billing. Confidentiality and the limits of confidentiality in electronic communication should also be discussed. It is also important that the issue of video recordings be discussed. Specifics regarding technical failure of the video visit, protocols for contact between sessions, and conditions upon which the video visits will be terminated in lieu of a traditional visit also need to be established.

Video visits need to be carried out in an appropriate environment for both the provider and the patient to maximize privacy.[2,11] Video cameras and lighting should be optimized for both the patient and provider during a video visit. If the patient attempts to carry out a video visit in a public space, the provider should recommend that the consultation be delayed until a suitable private space is identified.

The consultation should start with identity verification of both the provider and patient. In many instances, a host clinic may perform the verification prior to starting the video visit. The location of the provider and the patient should also be established during the during the video visit. Contact information for both the provider and the patient should be verified during the video visit. Lastly, the expectations regarding the video visit and any subsequent visits should be discussed.

The urologist must make an entry in the medical record in a similar fashion as for traditional visits once the video visit is complete. The medical record entry should include an assessment and plan, patient information, contact information, history, informed consent, and information regarding fees and billing. As part of the documentation, it is also important to note that the patient was seen using telemedicine technologies.

In regard to connectivity, **audio-visual** telemedicine services can be provided through personal computers or mobile devices that use Internet-based videoconferencing software programs. A bandwidth of 384 kbps or higher in both the downlink and uplink directions is recommended.[2] Because different technologies provide different video quality results at the same bandwidth, each end-point should use bandwidth sufficient to achieve at least a minimum of 640 x 360 resolution at 30 frames per second. Each party should use the most reliable connection to the Internet during the video visit.

The increasing availability of 5G networks throughout the country will have a significant impact on telehealth availability as adequate IT infrastructure will be available to remote patients and clinicians. 5G wireless ecosystems will continue to grow given both regional and national initiatives from network and wireless providers. Compared to 4G, 5G can be expected to be 100x faster, with 25x lower lag times and 1 million devices supported in 1 square mile. The 5G systems will allow for reliable, faster connections resulting in high quality video connections and data transfer. (**https://datamakespossible.westerndigital.com/5g-vs-4g-side-by-side-comparison/**)

Efforts should be taken to make audio and video transmission secure by using point-to-point encryption that meets recognized standards. Currently, FIPS 140-2, known as the Federal Information Processing Standard, is the US Government security standard used to accredit software encryption and lists encryption types such as AES (advanced encryption standard) as providing acceptable levels of security. When patients or providers use a mobile device, special attention should be placed on the relative privacy of information being communicated over such technology. Mobile devices should require a passcode and should be configured to have an inactivity timeout function not exceeding 15 minutes.

Regulation

Prior to the PHE, State regulations of telemedicine practice varied more widely. During the PHE, there has been a significant liberalization of requirements following the lead of Medicare. Because the regulations are in flux, it is instructive to understand what the variables have been leading up to the PHE as there may be a reinstatement of some of the various regulations that have been lifted after the PHE is resolved. Key statutes have concerned the criteria for the doctor-patient relationship, the informed consent, the modality of communication, in-person support of the patient, and licensure of the doctor. In some states, consent had to be obtained in person. Some states allowed audio communication without video. Some states required a telepresenter which is a healthcare worker physically present with the patient during the telemedical visit. An excellent resource to track the various state regulatory and licensing requirements for practicing telehealth can be found on the Alliance for Connected Care Website **http://connectwithcare.org/state-telehealth-and-licensure-expansion-covid-19-chart/**.

MEDICARE

This section will review changes that have occurred specifically with Medicare as a result of the pandemic, with focus on reimbursement and regulatory considerations.

Prior to the COVID-19 pandemic, Medicare was particularly restrictive as they limited telemedicine coverage to those in counties outside of metropolitan areas or health professional shortage areas. Patients were often required to be present at a qualifying location, preventing patients from completing their visits at home. Evaluation and management (E&M) codes for telemedicine often reimbursed less for the same service as only face to face time was considered and physical exam requirements were difficult to accomplish.

Effective March 1st, 2020, numerous legislative changes have been passed to loosen telemedicine restrictions so as to and improve adherence to social distancing. While E&M codes prior to the COVID-19 PHE had history, physical exam and medical decision-making requirements, newly adopted laws allowed E&M codes to be based only on medical decision-making allowing providers to omit the physical exam. Additionally, coding time was expanded to pre-visit preparation, face to face time and post visit management which was a significant expansion from face to face time only.

Expansion of access

Telemedicine coverage is no longer restricted to rural or underserved populations with the CMS rule changes. Specifically, patients no longer have a specific site requirement, allowing all Medicare patients access to telemedicine in their homes. Additionally, coverage was expanded to new patient consultations in addition to return visits. Prior to the COVID-19 pandemic providers were required to register their homes with CMS, a restriction that was lifted by CMS.

Expansion of services

Prior to the COVID-19 epidemic permissible telehealth services were limited. The goal of many of CMS's new rules were to expand services offered to not only address the needs of COVID-19 patients but also limit exposure for non-COVID patients by promoting social distancing. The following is a list of legislative changes that expanded telehealth services to Medicare patients.

- Coverage for audio-only telephone evaluation and management visits for new and return patients. This allows patients without internet or video capabilities improved access to telehealth services.

- Significant expansion of allowable services able to be provided

- Removal of frequency limitations on telehealth utilization

- Expansion of providers covered in addition to physicians including physical and occupational therapist, nurse practitioners, physician's assistance, midwives, clinical nurse specialists, dietitians, nutritionist, social workers, psychologists, and speech pathologists.

Informed consent and privacy

CMS requires an annual consent for televisits and allows for verbal confirmation of consent. Amid the COVID-19 PHE HIPPA requirements for video visits were lifted and only public facing services were restricted. The expectation, however, is that when the PHE is over the HIPPA waiver will expire and telemedicine platforms will have HIPPA compliance requirements.

Billing visits

Billing televisits for Medicare fee for service is similar to billing for in-person visit with few modifications that have improved compensation for telemedicine visits. For those billing by time, the total billed time now includes pre-visit chart review, face to face time as well as post-visit management. Additionally, both new and established patient visits may be billed based on medical decision making (MDM) alone without the requirement of the key E&M elements (history, physical and medical decision). Similarly, for established patients billing may be based on medical decision making alone.

Telephone encounters

There has been significant expansion of reimbursement for telephone calls. Prior to the COVID-19 PHE reimbursement for telephone calls was significantly limited. Newly adopted CMS rules now cover E&M phone calls for both new and existing patients.

Restrictions include visits leading to an in-person visit within 24 hours and those visits related to a visit within the past 7 days. Documentation should be included to justify E&M codes. Furthermore, patient cost sharing can be waived for these visits. It is important to stay up to date on rule changes as these are subject to change as COVID-19 PHE evolves.

Inpatient Services

In an effort to limit face to face encounters, when clinically appropriate, Medicare liberalized rules surrounding telehealth inpatient services. While previously limited to follow up inpatient visits, CMS now allows for initial visits and ER visits with no limitation on the frequency of visits (daily visits permissible compared to every 3rd day limit).

Licensure:

During the COVID-19 public health emergency (PHE) new regulations by CMS suspended Medicare's state licensure requirements. States however can choose to enforce state licensure, but most have cooperated. It is unclear what licensure requirements will return after the PHE period. An excellent resource to track the various state regulatory and licensing requirements for practicing

Prior to the PHE, one of the greatest challenges facing the implementation of a telemedical practice was the issue of licensing across state lines. In most states, the provider had to be licensed where the patient is physically located at the point of care.[35] in addition to being licensed to practice in the originating site's state.(reference: Centers for Medicare & Medicaid Services. "Telemedicine") The Interstate Medical Licensure Compact (IMLC) was created to assure state regulation of medical practice while supporting telemedicine as a healthcare delivery model. At this present time, INLC is comprised of 29 states, the District of Columbia, the Territory of Guam and growing, aiming to streamline licensing requirements for interstate telemedical services. The average wait for a license is 19 days, with 51% taking seven days or fewer, according to the IMLC. This pace and ease of the application process is designed to encourage more physicians to care for patients across state lines. **https://imlcc.org/**

States issuing the most licenses through the compact are:

- Wisconsin 418
- Minnesota 387
- Arizona 331
- Iowa 320

During the PHE, many states have greatly liberalized access to their patients telemedically by providers from out of state but once the PHE has resolved there may be a retraction of some or all of these allowances telehealth can be found on the Alliance for Connected Care Website (**http://connectwithcare.org/state-telehealth-and-licensure-expansion-covid-19-chart/**)

Federal bills concerning the provision of telemedical services to Tricare, Medicare, and VA patients may obviate state licensure requirements for these patients. The National Defense Authorization Act for fiscal year 2017 contains a provision that allows a licensed physician to provide telemedicine services to Tricare patients in any state regardless of the physician's state of licensure. The Federation of State Medical Boards, the American Medical Association, and the American Osteopathic Association oppose this pending policy.36 The US Senate unanimously passed the Veterans eHealth and Telemedicine Support (VETS) Act of 2017 (S.925) following the House's unanimous approval of H.R. 2123. VETS would create an interstate medical license, giving physicians access to veterans across all state lines. Another piece of pending legislation, the TELE-MED Act of 2015, would authorize Medicare providers to reach patients in any state.[37] State lawmakers introduced more than 200 telemedicine bills in 2015. Large urology group practices may benefit from greater access to Tricare and Medicare patients across state lines as they provide attractive integrated care centers of excellence. Additionally, large urology groups may need to provide telemedical access to preserve access to their local patients who may otherwise be drawn to large institutional providers reaching them across state lines.

Prior to the PHE, the clearest indication of legislative movement in telemedicine has been the Creating Opportunities Now for Necessary and Effective Care Technologies (CONNECT) for Health Act of 2019. This is bipartisan legislation in both the House & Senate that aims to expand Medicare coverage for telehealth services. The CONNECT bill was first introduced in 2016 and was reintroduced in 2017 and several provisions of the CONNECT for Health Act of 2017 were enacted in the Bipartisan 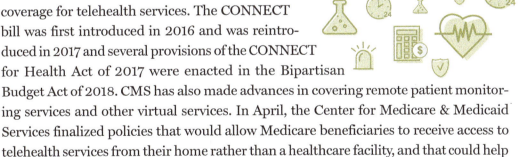 Budget Act of 2018. CMS has also made advances in covering remote patient monitoring services and other virtual services. In April, the Center for Medicare & Medicaid Services finalized policies that would allow Medicare beneficiaries to receive access to telehealth services from their home rather than a healthcare facility, and that could help drive more interest in telehealth tools.

In the event that the restrictions to telemedicine that have been lifted by CMS during the PHE are reinstated, CONNECT would allow for the Secretary of Health and Human Services to waive telehealth restrictions when necessary to promote telehealth services. The bill also improves the process of adding telehealth to approved services lists and adds rural health clinics and federally qualified health centers to the list of approved telehealth sites. CONNECT would have HHS study more ways to expand telehealth services so that more people can access health care services in their own homes.

Urology advocacy has strategically engaged with regulatory & legislative bodies to advocate for supportive telemedicine policies

Alternative Payment Models

Prior to the PHE, participation in an alternative payment models were a strategy to access more liberalized reimbursements for telemedicine to Medicare patients. The Connect for Health Act (S: Schwartz, R: Black) called for expanding telemedicine reimbursement to all Medicare patients within alternative payment models such as accountable care organizations as well as all Medicare Advantage patients. The Balanced Budget Act of 2018 waived Medicare's geographic and originating site limitations allowing patients enrolled in ACOs to receive care within their homes. The list of providers who could be reimbursed was also be expanded. The philosophy is that as long as the total costs of care are the same or less, telemedicine should be able to provide Medicare patients with the same or better quality and satisfaction at the same or reduced cost. Furthermore, the utilization of telemedicine is mandated in the Patient Protection and Affordable Care Act, which calls for ". . . timely communication of test results, timely exchange of clinical information to patients and other providers, and **use of remote monitoring or telehealth."**

Reimbursement

Medicare and other payers

The largest obstacle to the widespread adoption of telemedicine is not technology, rather it is reimbursement. Medicaid is the most ubiquitous of the payers. During the PHE Medicare telemedical services reimbursements and regulations have liberalized but vary from state to state. Requirements vary for eligible providers, qualifying distances to providers, settings such as in a clinic as opposed to one's home, and communication technologies.[38] Prior to the PHE, Store and forward was covered in 14 states including Alaska, Arizona, California, Connecticut, Georgia, Maryland, Minnesota, Nevada, New Mexico, New York, Tennessee, Texas, Virginia and Washington. An excellent resource to track the Medicaid policies by state can be found in the Center for Connected Health Policy. (**https://www.cchpca.org/telehealth-policy/current-state-laws-and-reimbursement-policies?keyword=medicaid**)

The majority of state employee plans cover some degree of telemedicine services. Prior to the PHE, Private payers were mandated in 36 states and Washington DC by "parity" laws to cover telemedical services on par with in-office services. The top payers include Blue Cross Blue Shield, Aetna, UnitedHealthcare, and Cigna[38] During the PHE, most PPOs are liberalizing services and reimbursement for telemedical services in conjunction with CMS, however the policies are not necessarily the same for each payor nor in each market so it is important to verify with a particular PPO what their policies for telemedicine are.

Retail providers of telemedicine utilize several strategies for reimbursement. They may privately contract patients, or they may be contracted with insurance companies on a fee-for-service basis. Teladoc, currently the nation's largest retailer of telemedical service, engages in capitation arrangements directly with private insurance payers and large employers while also requiring a copay. They are viewed as a value-added service of the plan for a modest out-of-pocket expense to the patient.

In highly integrated healthcare systems fee for service considerations do not influence the adoption of telemedicine. It is provided for efficiency, access, and patient and provider satisfaction which partly explains the more robust adoption of telemedicine by the VA, the Department of Defense, prisons,[27] and other commercial-capitated entities such as Kaiser Permanente. The VA spent $1.09 billion in 2019 and set its budget at $1.1 billion in 2020 with the hope to increase the percentage of veterans receiving some form of telemedicine from 13% to 20%. Hospitals themselves will provide reimbursement for telemedicine coverage when necessary to meet its obligation of provided services.

Discussion

Telemedicine promises to improve access to care while driving the value equation and maintaining high patient and provider satisfaction scores. Prior to the pandemic and the Public Health Emergency period, several studies had demonstrated that telemedicine can fulfill some or even all of these promises. Studies from the urologic literature demonstrated an unmet need and the potential benefits of telemedicine include expanding access for patients, improving time efficiency, reducing expense, improving patient satisfaction, improving provider satisfaction, and even improving quality of care. Postoperative in-patients reported higher satisfaction with telemedical robotic rounds in part because the urologist appeared to be less rushed and appeared to spend more time with the patient, even though the actual time spent was slightly less.[16] Tracked outcomes have so far have been equivalent or trending better than in-person encounters. The explosion of the utilization of telemedicine during the PHE has provided most urologists a profound demonstration of what was previously only a collection of niche demonstrations. Urologists and patients now have a working knowledge of the capability of telemedicine to provide care.

There are challenges and limitations to telemedicine that still must be addressed. Technical limitations include the limitations on the physical exam and the quality of the audio-visual information being exchanged.

The telemedical provider relies on two senses: sight and sound and may miss cues otherwise detectable by a keen observer in an in-person exam. The telemedical exam can be augmented by a medical assistant on the patient side, providing a surrogate physical exam under observation and sharing direct observations. Those new to telemedicine may initially engage in encounters in which the physical exam is not critical to evaluation and treatment planning as in a review of test results or evaluation of response to therapy. More experienced urologists can derive adequate information from the audio-visual encounter coupled with imaging and surrogate examinations which can lead to a proper evaluation of a broad array of presenting complaints. Inevitably many patients will require that follow up physical examination or procedures, but their treatment plan will still have been advanced by the telemedical provider. Once telemedical training has been incorporated into graduate medical education, the telemedical exam will become more routine. Technological advances may bring the telemedical experience closer to in-person as virtual reality including haptic feedback improves and becomes more widely available.

Another technical challenge is the disparity in access to the required technology that many patients face. Lower income rural and inner-city populations disproportionately lack high speed internet connectivity and mobile hardware platforms, yet this is the population which stands to derive the most benefit from telemedicine. During the PHE, reimbursement for telephone only encounters is helping to solve this disparity but the extent to which it remains is unknown. Another limitation is the technical literacy of the patients. At least 42% of patients over 65 years are not on line,[39] a population which comprises a large proportion of most urology practices. Even if technically literate, some patients in this age group may find the nature of the telemedicine encounter less satisfactory than younger patients whose work schedule provides greater incentive to avoid time spent traveling for health care and who are accustomed to electronic communication with colleagues, customers, friends, and family. Nonetheless, advanced aged patients are often facile with video formats they may use to communicate with their family members and many urologists are finding their older patients to be able to engage easily with a telemedical encounter and greatly enjoy its convenience.

Even with full access to current technologies, regulatory and reimbursement hurdles had traditionally presented the most immediate challenges to widespread adoption of telemedicine by urologists. HIPAA compliance had limited the options for connectivity and software. Urologists in states with fewer reimbursement mandates may have been unmotivated to make an investment in hardware and software as well as a change in practice patterns.

While "early adopter" physician satisfaction in surveys in urology had been high,[31, 33, 34] telemedicine can be logistically disruptive to a traditional schedule and can be technically frustrating for a urologist comfortable with traditional practice. While it is anticipated that the efficiency of telemedicine will offset the cost and disruption of getting started, the value of implementing telemedicine will need to be decided in the context of a specific urology group's needs and priorities. Although many urologists have been thrust into some degree of telemedicine by the pandemic PHE, Ideally, the incorporation of telemedicine should be organic and based on its realized merits. A "one size fits all" approach to telemedicine could doom telemedicine to suffer the same pushback that EHRs faced as a result of their premature mandate. Ultimately telemedical urology is the practice of urology, just with a different set of tools.

Conclusions

Urology telemedicine has developed in a variety of formats already and illustrates how the specialty has been recognizing an unmet need in American medicine. In addition to meeting the current demands for social distancing arising from the pandemic Telemedicine may specifically help address the needs of large urology group practices by addressing workforce shortages, clinical and surgical productivity, patient access to care, and data quality reporting, all mandates that will face urologists in the near future. Urologists, as telemedicine pioneers should continue to embrace new ideas in telemedicine. As the initial limitations have been radically removed and as new solutions are developed both in the technology and regulatory sides, it is possible that telemedicine will become completely integrated into urologic training and health care delivery to fulfill the proposition of access and quality urologic care for the large group practice.

REFERENCES

1. Brown, E.M. **The Ontario Telemedicine Network: a case report.** *Telemed J E Health.* 2013; 19: 373
2. Levine, S.R., Gorman, M. **"Telestroke": the application of telemedicine for stroke.** *Stroke.* 1999; 30: 464
3. Business Wire. **Specialists on Call oversees its 10,000th tPA administration to an acute stroke patient.** Business Wire Web site. Published 12/02/2015. http://www.businesswire.com/news/home/20151202006018/en/Specialists-Call-Oversees-10000th-tPA-Administration-Acute. Accessed 09-13-2016
4. McConnochie, K.M., Wood, N.E., Kitzman, H.J., Herendeen, N.E., Roy, J., Roghmann, K.J. **Telemedicine reduces absence resulting from illness in urban childcare: evaluation of an innovation.** *Pediatrics.* 2005; 115: 1273
5. Merritt Hawkins. **Physician appointment wait times and Medicaid and Medicare acceptance rates.** Merritt Hawkins Web site. Published 2014. http://www.merritthawkins.com/uploadedfiles/merritthawkings/surveys/mha2014waitsurvpdf.pdf. Accessed 09-13-2016
6. Watson, A.J., Bergman, H., Williams, C.M., Kvedar, J.C. **A randomized trial to evaluate the efficacy of online follow-up visits in the management of acne.** *Arch Dermatol.* 2010; 146: 406
7. Sathiyakumar, V., Apfeld, J.C., Obremskey, W.T., Thakore, R.V., Sethi, M.K. **Prospective randomized controlled trial using telemedicine for follow-ups in an orthopedic trauma population: a pilot study.** *J Orthop Trauma.* 2015; 29: e139
8. Hwa, K., Wren, S.M. **Telehealth follow-up in lieu of postoperative clinic visit for ambulatory surgery: results of a pilot program.** *JAMA Surg.* 2013; 148: 823
9. Matimba, A., Woodward, R., Tambo, E., Ramsay, M., Gwanzura, L., Guramatunhu, S. **Tele-ophthalmology: Opportunities for improving diabetes eye care in resource- and specialist-limited Sub-Saharan African countries.** *J Telemed Telecare.* 2016; 22: 311
10. Cook, J. **"There's my doctor from TV!"** Standford Children's Health Web site. Published 08-12-2015. http://healthier.stanfordchildrens.org/en/theres-doctor-tv/. Accessed 09-15-2016
11. Shivji, S., Metcalfe, P., Khan, A., Bratu, I. **Pediatric surgery telehealth: patient and clinician satisfaction.** *Pediatr Surg Int.* 2011; 27: 523
12. Canon, S., Shera, A., Patel, A., et al. **A pilot study of telemedicine for post-operative urological care in children.** *J Telemed Telecare.* 2014; 20: 427
13. Viers, B.R., Lightner, D.J., Rivera, M.E., et al. **Efficiency, satisfaction, and costs for remote video visits following radical prostatectomy: a randomized controlled trial.** *Eur Urol.* 2015; 68: 729
14. Nguyen, B. New telemedicine pilot program merges robotics and urology in Boston. YouTube Web site. Published 2012. https://www.youtube.com/watch?v=pjqX0E8KdaI. Accessed 09-15-2016
15. Darkins, A. **The growth of telehealth services in the Veterans Health Administration between 1994 and 2014: a study in the diffusion of innovation.** *Telemed J E Health.* 2014; 20: 761
16. Park, E.S., Boedeker, B.H., Hemstreet, J.L., Hemstreet, G.P. **The initiation of a preoperative and postoperative telemedicine urology clinic.** *Stud Health Technol Inform.* 2011; 163: 425
17. Chu, S., Boxer, R., Madison, P., et al. **Veterans Affairs telemedicine: bringing urologic care to remote clinics.** *Urology.* 2015; 86: 255
18. Himidan, S., Kim, P. **The evolving identity, capacity, and capability of the future surgeon.** *Semin Pediatr Surg.* 2015; 24: 145
19. Eadie, L.H., Seifalian, A.M., Davidson, B.R. **Telemedicine in surgery.** *Br J Surg.* 2003; 90: 647\
20. Porter, M.E., Heppelmann, J.E. **How smart, connected products are transforming competition.** Harvard Business Review Web site. Published 2014. https://hbr.org/2014/11/how-smart-connected-products-are-transforming-competition. Accessed 09-15-2016
21. American Urological Association. **2016 AUA Annual Census.** American Urological Association Web site. Published 2016. https://www.auanet.org/research/aua-census.cfm. Accessed 09-13-2016
22. US Department of Veterans Affairs. **VA telehealth services.** US Department of Veterans Affairs Web site. Updated 06-03-2015. http://www.telehealth.va.gov/. Accessed 09-13-2016
23. Interstate Medical Licensure Compact. **Interstate medical licensure compact.** Interstate Medical Licensure Compact Web site. Published 2016. http://www.licenseportability.org/wp-content/uploads/2016/01/Interstate-Medical-Licensure-Compact-FINAL.pdf. Accessed 09-13-2016

24. HealthIT.gov. **Meaningful use definition & objectives.** HealthIT.gov Web site. Updated 02-06-2015. https://www.healthit.gov/providers-professionals/meaningful-use-definition-objectives. Accessed 09-13-2016

25. Rhee, E., Baum, N. **The shared medical appointment: a proposed model of medical appointments.** *J Med Pract Manage.* 2013; 29: 172

26. Hinata, N., Miyake, H., Kurahashi, T., et al. **Novel telementoring system for robot-assisted radical prostatectomy: impact on the learning curve.** *Urology.* 2014; 83: 1088

27. Ellimoottil, C., Skolarus, T., Gettman M, et al. **Telemedicine in urology: state of the art.** *Urology.* 2016; 94: 10

28. Marescaux, J., Leroy, J., Gagner, M., et al. **Transatlantic robot-assisted telesurgery.** *Nature.* 2001; 413: 379

29. Hougen, H.Y., Lobo, J.M., Corey, T., et al. **Optimizing and validating the technical infrastructure of a novel tele-cystoscopy system.** *J Telemed Telecare.* 2015

30. TIMS Medical. **TIMS consultant.** TIMS Medical Web site. Publushed 2016. http://tims.com/timsconsultant/timsconsultant2/. Accessed 09-13-2016

31. Ellison, L.M., Nguyen, M., Fabrizio, MD, Soh, A., Permpongkosol, S., Kavoussi, L.R. **Postoperative robotic telerounding: a multicenter randomized assessment of patient outcomes and satisfaction.** *Arch Surg.* 2007; 142: 1177

32. Daniel, H.E. **2015-16 MMS President Peter N. Bretan Jr., MD.** *Marin Medicine.* 2015; 61: 21

33. Kau, E.L., Baranda, D.T., **Hain, P., et al. Video rounding system: a pilot study in patient care.** *J Endourol.* 2008; 22: 1179

34. Kaczmarek, B.F., Trinh, Q.D., Menon, M., Rogers, C.G. **Tablet telerounding.** *Urology.* 2012; 80: 1383

35. Center for Connected Health Policy. **Common legal barriers.** Center for Connected Health Policy Web site. Published 2016. http://cchpca.org/common-legal-barriers. Accessed 09-15-2016

36. American Urological Association Staff. **Letter to the Senate and House Committees on Armed Services from the American Medical Association, the American Osteopathic Association, and the Federation of State Medical Boards.**

37. 114th Congress. **H.R.3081 - TELE-MED Act of 2015.** Congress.gov Web site. Published 07-15-2015. Updated 07-21-2015. https://www.congress.gov/bill/114th-congress/house-bill/3081. Accessed 09-14-2016

38. Neufeld, J.D., Doarn, C.R. **Telemedicine spending by Medicare: a snapshot from 2012.** *Telemed J E Health.* 2015; 21: 686

39. Perrin A, Duggan M. **Americans' internet access: 2000-2015.** Washington, DC: Pew Research Center: Internet, Science & Tech. June 26, 2015 (http://www.pewinternet.org/2015/06/26/americans-internet-access-2000-2015/).

KEY POINTS

- **The emergence of he COVID-19** public health emergency in early 2020 transformed the telemedicine landscape in a short period of time.

- **Many formats of telemedicine** are readily reproducible and relevant to urology group practices, including video visits, online services, teleintraoperative consultation, and eConsults.

- **Telemedicine** may provide a high value solution for the workforce shortages in urology.

- **Medicaid** covers telemedicine in almost all states.

- **Regulations** governing telemedicine vary by state.

- **Medicare** has expanded coverage of telemedicine, as a result of the public health emergency; however, these changes may not continue into the future.

- **Alternative payment models** represent additional strategies to optimize the use of telemedicine in urology practice.

- **The biggest obstacle** to the widespread adoption of telemedicine is not technology, rather it is reimbursement for the services.

Eugene Y. Rhee, MD, MBA

Dr. Rhee is the Regional Coordinating Chief of Urology for Kaiser Permanente (KP) in Southern California and the National Chair of Urology for the Permanente Federation He also serves as Area Assistant Medical Director for the Business Line & Finance for KP in San Diego. Dr. Rhee serves as Chair of the Public Policy Council for the American Urologic Association (AUA). He was the 2013-2014 AUA Gallagher Health Policy Scholar. He served as the inaugural Section Editor for Health Policy for Urology Practice and as the inaugural Co-Chair of the AUA Telehealth Task Force.

Matthew Gettman, MD

Matthew Gettman, MD, is a Professor of Urology and Vice-Chair of Urology at Mayo Clinic College of Medicine in Rochester, Minnesota. He has authored greater than 150 scientific publications and has been an invited speaker nationally and internationally on the topic of robotic surgery, natural orifice surgery, and simulation training. He started the Robotic Surgery Program at Mayo Clinic in 2002. He is a member of numerous editorial boards including BJU International and European Urology.

Eric Kirshenbaum, MD

Dr. Eric Kirshenbaum completed his medical education at University of Illinois Chicago, residency in urology and fellowship in men's health and reconstructive urology at Loyola University Medical Center. He specializes in men's health and reconstructive urology with an emphasis on urethral stricture disease, erectile dysfunction, male incontinence, prosthetic surgery, benign prostatic enlargement (BPH), laser surgery, urologic cancers, telemedicine and robotic surgery. He is an active member of the American Urologic Association (AUA), and serves as a board member of the AUA telemedicine task force and has a particular interest in advancing the field of telemedicine.

Aaron Spitz, MD

Aaron Spitz, MD, is Co-chair of the American Urological Association Telemedicine Workgroup. He earned his MD from Cornell Medical College, completed his Urology residency at the University of Southern California, and obtained fellowship training in infertility at the Baylor College of Medicine. He is an assistant clinical professor in the U.C. Irvine Department of Urology, specializing in male reproductive medicine and surgery, and directs the Center for Male Reproductive Medicine and Surgery at Orange County Urology. He is also the President of the California Urologic Association and the Orange County District representative to the Western Section of the American Urologic Association.

CHAPTER

Building a Robust and Sustainable Research Program in the Tertiary Community Urology Setting

Neal D. Shore, MD, FACS, CPI
Raoul S. Concepcion, MD, FACS
Daniel R. Saltzstein, MD
Arletta van Breda, RN, MSN, CCRC, CIP
Thomas A. Paivanas, MHSA

There is great demand for high-quality clinical research in the United States, with the National Cancer Institute (NCI) noting that fewer than 4% of all eligible cancer patients are enrolled in clinical trials. The industry is desperate for tertiary community practice sites that are facile in research and can deliver high-quality, high-volume research.

Urology-related research in the tertiary community setting affords access to a more defined type and increased number of patients compared to those seen in academic practice. Patients seen include a greater variety of urology patients and those with pre- and early-stage disease. It is true that academic medical centers (AMCs) will continue to see later stage patients and those with rare diseases and conditions and will continue to be the crucibles for new technologies, medicine, and procedures. However, researchers who embrace conducting a robust clinical research program in the tertiary community practice setting will be the early adopters of these medical advances into broader clinical practice.

Academic researchers, and pharmaceutical and biotech sponsors now understand where most patients are truly being managed, especially in the world of urology. As such, these organizations are increasingly turning toward large independent groups that have a strong reputation and experience in clinical research, with a portfolio of successfully completed studies—as evidenced by abstract, article, and podium presentations.

The skills required to build and run a successful research program reflect the messy collision of the art, science, and business of medicine. It is not an endeavor for the practitioner who is faint of heart, whose priority is profit, suffers from hubris, or considers research as an intermittent or extracurricular activity. Clinician-scientists who embark on developing a research enterprise must be tenacious, evangelical, compulsive, and humble. They must embrace the fact that they are running a marathon, which is often personally and professional a lonely endeavor. They must be a politician, a CEO, a salesman, and a cheerleader, all while embracing the clinical role of a systemic therapist as opposed to that of urologic proceduralist. They must be prepared for any number of rational and irrational reasons to be loved and hated by their own practice's partners.

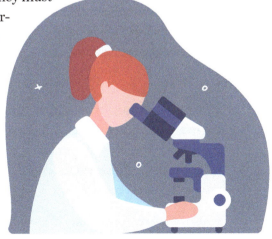

Once such a leader emerges, it is important to understand the geography and choreography of clinical practice vis-à-vis the research practice. Is there a clinical nexus within a clinical practice upon which to build research?

The following are ideal clinical practice characteristics to support a robust research program

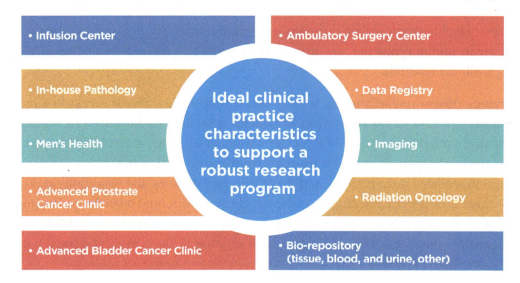

The strongest research programs have a close concordance of their mission and vision with the broader clinical practice's mission, vision, and operations.

THE BENEFITS OF CONDUCTING RESEARCH

Benefits for the Patient

The research program offers state-of-the-art therapeutic options at every stage of a patient's disease. Patients who participate in trials can obtain drugs at no cost before they are available on the market. The research program is also close to the patient's home, his or her established physician, and support services network. Additionally, the tertiary community research programs may provide an advantage over academic research programs in terms of availability, accessibility, continuity, cost of services and quality of individualized and personal care. Finally, a research protocol opens up options for care where there might otherwise be financial challenges impeding access to care (from managed care constraints, insurance status—underinsured or uninsured—and other coverage restrictions.)

Benefits for the Practice

Having a high-quality, well-structured research program that is closely integrated into the overall clinical practice will provide unique and significant benefits to that practice. From the perspective of the medical consumer marketplace, a vibrant research program will provide professional differentiation, not only for the group, but also for that sub-group of clinical researchers.

It also offers an opportunity to more clearly differentiate practice quality, thereby increasing attractiveness for inclusion by commercial insurer provider panels, Accountable Care Organizations (ACOs), and other collaborative endeavors. This, in turn, can provide the practice with leverage in direct payor negotiations and, potentially, with hospital collaborations. A robust research program also provides stronger professional differentiation to referring providers, not only within their primary service area (PSA), but also on a regional, state, or even national basis, if identified as a "destination service."

Perhaps, most importantly, research provides a forum for the evaluation and early adoption of new technologies, medicines, and procedures into the broader clinical group practice. This expands a practice's products and services offered to patients at every stage of their disease. Additionally, research underscores a practice environment that is uniquely attractive to newly minted urologists and urology fellows. Lastly, a successful research program can benefit a practice above and beyond direct and indirect costs of operating the program.

Benefits for the Clinician Scientist and Research Medical Director

Those who champion research are often driven to fulfill a relentless commitment to expanding therapeutic options at every stage of a patient's disease. This endeavor offers intellectual stimulation and excitement, as well as personal and professional reward. Without exception, research provides direct professional experience using new technologies, medicines, or procedures in a clinical practice setting. This, in turn, leads to the development of new skill sets, including business operations, business development, clinical management, etc. The camaraderie of extra-practice engagements with other like-minded clinical scientists and academic colleagues from across the United States, perhaps even internationally, can also be extremely satisfying and rewarding.

In addition, a well-defined research program provides an opportunity for a semi-autonomous practice within content of the larger clinical practice. This can offer variation from typical clinical practice, with a potential for modification of call and clinic hours. Finally, a successfully run research program can provide additional financial remuneration commensurate with meeting clinical and economic program objectives.

Carving out Research Time in a Practice

Without exception, several partners in a practice will view research activities as reducing the practice's overall productivity and profitability.

Partners should be continually reminded of the rewards of running a successful research practice. It is also important for leadership of a practice to overlap with leadership of medical research to ensure recognition and protected time for a research program within the practice.

While there is no perfect model in that each practice setting is different, typically, medical directors should have some amount of protected time one to two days a week to attend to research activities and manage operations. They can draw a modest flat salary, a salary based on productivity, or receive a percentage of net revenues from studies. Some practices allow carve out in terms of ownership, governance, and compensation. Often the practice is afforded shares, or sets up structured revenue sharing, but these agreements must be approached carefully and aided by professional consulting, accounting, and legal support.

Practice Allocation of Research Net Revenues

The allocation of research net revenues varies among practices. Options include sharing revenue equally across the practice, distributing it on a pro-rata basis, splitting it between the referring physician and the principal investigator, or a combination of these. It is important to note that remuneration to a referring physician should be based on the work-up completed to qualify the patient as a subject for a research study. When in doubt, seek legal advice.

TYPES OF RESEARCH

Clinical Research

Most research occurring in the clinical practice setting is typically latter stage clinical research, (e.g., Phase III or Phase IV), but there are many LUGPA research sites conducting Phase I and II trials as well. In urology, this focuses on genitourinary malignancies, overactive bladder, benign prostate diseases, erectile dysfunction, low testosterone, nocturia, and many other areas. A complete list of clinical trials offered worldwide can be found at **www.clinicaltrials.gov**.

Over the past three years, bio-marker studies for either diagnosis or disease progression—which usually require provision of tissue, blood, and/or urine plus clinical data—have been an area of intense interest and opportunity. These studies may be prospective or retrospective in nature. Urologists also often become involved in device studies. These are typically focused on improving diagnoses or therapeutic interventions and are often prospective in nature.

Drug-in-patient studies are prospective in nature and typically require a knowledgeable and experienced research staff. Note that the ability of a research site to perform pharmacokinetic/pharmacodynamic trials is very attractive to many sponsors conducting therapeutic trials.

Other Types of Research

In addition to clinical research, there are also options in econometrics. Examples include changing patterns of resource utilization and the resulting financial impact of new technologies, medicines, and procedures. Options exist in ethnographic research as well, which addresses practice issues affecting new product adoption and market diffusion. These often require custom data mining and focused practitioner interviews.

Determining the Optimal Mix of Studies

Several factors determine the optimal mix of studies to undertake, including the number of physicians interested in conducting research. Adding research to a busy practice requires overtime, extra commitment, and competent, interested staff. Staff qualifications (knowledge, experience, and credentials) must be considered as well as their work volume, interest, and burnout threshold.

Pursuing a mix of studies can optimize the utilization of research resources, provide opportunities to counter staff burnout, and ensure a strong return on investment. A staff's skill and capability mix can serve as a guide when deciding how many studies the practice can realistically handle—and how complex they can be. One's research reputation will quickly decline if the research program overpromises and under delivers in terms of quality and accrual.

Staffing

Each research program is required to conduct a myriad of functions to meet safety, regulatory, scientific, clinical, and operational objectives. These efforts require dedicated staff trained and experienced in research. In the early stages of program development, a small number of staff will wear many hats, but this is an untenable situation for larger active programs. Dedicated staff need to be recruited and assigned to specific functions to provide checks and balances as well as to ensure harmonious operations.

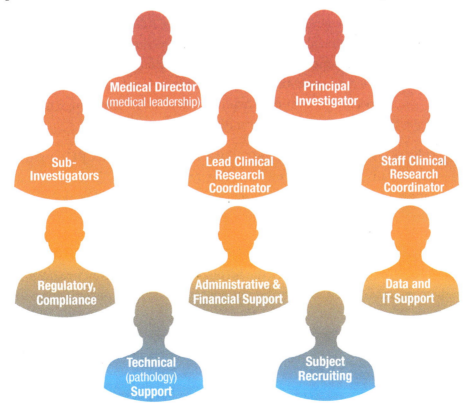

The Research Core

The number of clinical trials per staff varies according to study details. The program could be involved in one to 10 studies per staff member depending on the complexity of the trial(s).

Lead Clinical Research Coordinator

The nuts and bolts of the research program include staffing and infrastructure, clinical practice integration, enfranchising other practice clinicians, monitoring, feedback, and control. However, it cannot be stressed enough that second to the medical director, the quality of the lead Clinical Research Coordinator (CRC) is essential to the quality, volume, and success of the program. Several programs have broken down because the lead CRC was treated as having tenure within the organization. Never hire anyone who cannot be fired.

The primary responsibility of the CRC is to ensure the study's smooth progress from start-up to close-out, and through the day-to-day coordination of trial operations. Although the Principal Investigator (PI) delegates many duties to the CRC (and these delegated duties should be documented), the PI remains legally and ethically responsible and accountable for study operations and outcomes.

The CRC must comply with all regulations that apply to the PI, and ensure the PI is informed and up-to date on study subject and study-related issues. The role and general responsibilities of the CRC will depend on the allocation of responsibilities at the investigative site and the types of studies the site will conduct. For example, some facilities may allocate budget preparation and negotiation to another individual or department. There are no specified educational requirements for CRCs, although many have a clinical background and/or nursing degree.

The PI must be realistic about what expectations are placed on the CRC and hire the right person to fulfill those expectations. The more the CRC is qualified to do (e.g., phlebotomy, blood pressures, ECGs, etc.), the less he or she will be dependent on the investigator.

Staff Clinical Research Coordinator

Staff clinical research coordinators are the lifeblood of every research program. They provide the eyes, ears, and hands to the patient/subject who is participating in the research study. While semi-autonomous, they function under the direction of the lead CRC, completing all data gathering, subject clinical interface, reporting, and documentation. They are instrumental in ensuring communication among all key stakeholders in the research program.

Clearly, smaller programs will have the lead CRC wearing many of these hats. As the program expands, many of these functions can be supervised by the lead CRC and delegated to other CRCs or administrative staff. In this setting, the CRC should be considered a director or manager of the research and sit at the same table as the medical director.

The Cost of Doing Research

Research is a thin to modest margin endeavor. If the motivation is first to make money, it is best not to do research. That said, detailed cost accounting needs to occur on two levels: the research program level and the study level. Given the potential for financial loss, it is imperative that research leadership have a well-grounded understanding of its cost structure.

One should not hesitate to access internal practice and external business expertise to develop a continuous process to measure and monitor the following:

It is imperative to know how to develop a balance sheet, an operating statement, and a profit/loss statement for each study as well as the overall research program. To this end, it is strongly advised that the research program hire a dedicated financial analyst (either part or full time) to support study budget review, ongoing program financial analysis, and, most importantly, tenacious sponsor invoicing, and accounts reconciliation.

This responsibility cannot be simply added to a CRC or manager's plate at the end of a long list of other responsibilities. Site financial audits suggest that 5%-25% of study-related activities are simply not invoiced. Many busy, high-quality programs have been precluded from hiring or replacing staff because of a self-inflicted, weak bottom-line performance.

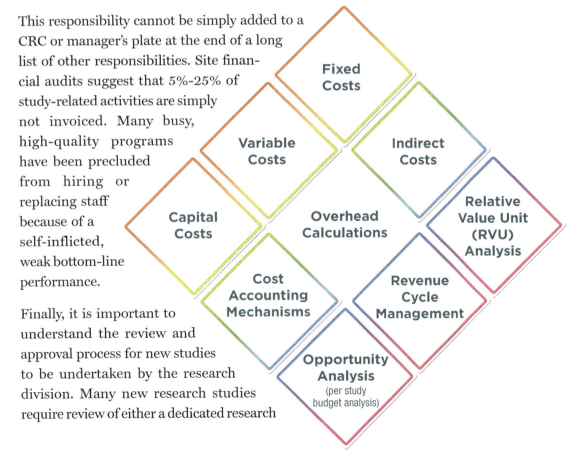

Finally, it is important to understand the review and approval process for new studies to be undertaken by the research division. Many new research studies require review of either a dedicated research committee or executive committee of the practice. Others allow medical directors the authority to unilaterally approve the undertaking of new research studies.

Developing Research Sponsors

Understanding the needs and demands of the market is essential for guiding the research program's development of scope of service. Different types and complexity of research require appropriate infrastructure and capacity to deliver high-quality product results (specimens and data) in a timely fashion. Achieving this level of quality requires approaching different types of research sponsors to fund practice research.

Industry (Drugs, Devices, Tests for Diagnoses or Progression)

These studies are typically developed by the sponsor and are designed to answer specific questions that address clinical efficacy or utility. A Clinical Research Organization or Trials Management Organization are often utilized to manage the study. An invitation to participate in such studies is based on research reputation as well as individual relationships with the sponsor at medical, clinical, and marketing levels. Budgets are negotiable but must go through the third-party study manager. However, remuneration often can be better aligned by direct interaction with the industry sponsor.

Cooperative Groups

The National Cancer Institute funds cooperative groups to study adult cancers. These groups are comprised of investigators from hospitals and academic research centers. Cooperative groups include the Society of Urological Oncology Clinical Trials Consortium, the Southwest Oncology Group, the Radiation Therapy Oncology Group, and the Comprehensive Unit-based Safety Program. Typically, active membership underscoring research qualifications is required. Usually these are funded by large pharmaceutical companies or foundations. Budget flexibility is generally narrow in these cases. Membership is often required to participate.

Foundations and Advocacy Groups

Foundations and advocacy groups, such as the Prostate Cancer Foundation, offer an increasing source of funding and referrals. Although funds are often provided to the industry developer, they are sometimes directly available to a research site for certain types of studies.

Academic Researchers with Grant Funding (Public and/or Private)

Often, academic researchers reach out to their community colleagues to collaborate on studies. The primary driver is that the community practitioner sees a much greater volume of patients and those at earlier stages of their disease. Participation and inclusion on subsequent publications can greatly contribute to the reputation of a research program. However, that funding is often limited and is typically at lower rates.

Investigator-Initiated Studies

These studies are not to be undertaken until the research program is very robust, with a deep clinical, financial, and legal bench. These types of studies take a long time to develop due to study design, statistical plan, budgeting negotiations, and contracting. The study PI has nearly all the responsibilities and accountabilities that usually are borne by an industry sponsor. While there exists a potentially high reward from several perspectives, it is also the type of research with the greatest operational, legal, and financial risk.

Subject Recruitment

The investigative site is responsible for recruiting and enrolling study subjects who meet the protocol's criteria for inclusion and exclusion.

Reasons sites do not meet enrollment goals:

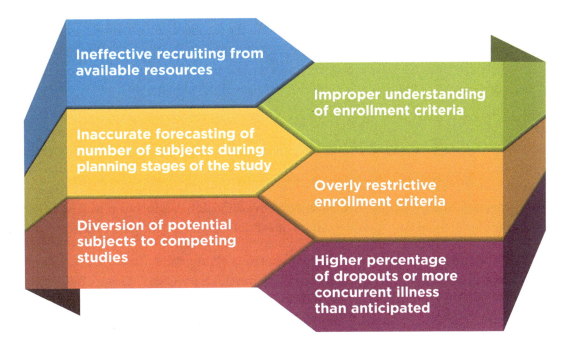

- Ineffective recruiting from available resources
- Improper understanding of enrollment criteria
- Inaccurate forecasting of number of subjects during planning stages of the study
- Overly restrictive enrollment criteria
- Diversion of potential subjects to competing studies
- Higher percentage of dropouts or more concurrent illness than anticipated

The secret to optimizing internal referrals is taking the physician out of the equation. It is helpful to build processes where clinical and administrative staff can identify patients entering the clinic that can be evaluated as appropriate subjects for specific research studies.

Empowering the CRC staff to work with the clinical staff to identify and screen potential patients is essential for robust subject recruitment. Often, this is accomplished with dedicated recruiters who can flow across different departments and access a variety of sources, both internal and external to the practice. Also, there is much interest and activity in utilizing clinical electronic medical records that are programmed to data mine for subjects based on inclusion/exclusion criteria. Using information technology to implement "forcing functions" prevents user mistakes. A forcing function initiates a "hard stop" so it is impossible to move forward in a program until the error is corrected. Programming forcing functions to identify potential subjects can expedite the CRC staff's process to approach them unless the clinician indicates otherwise.

Another critical component of success is the existence of a larger than average research core of clinician-scientists, for example, more than two to three sub-investigators typically driving a program. These factors combined with a strong commitment from physician partners to support research (>50% actively referring into the research program) can lead to significant rates of accrual over less structured community research programs.

An important distinction to underscore is that researchers do not treat patients; rather they study a subject. It is critical to understand that protocol drives diagnostic and treatment requirements apart from those involved in the standard of care. Both patient and researcher need to clearly understand the benefits and risks before the patient becomes a subject in a study. Deviation may very well remove a subject from the study or create false expectations of potential benefits on the part of the patient.

Regulation and the Regulatory Process

Conducting research is by definition pushing the boundaries of science and the practice of medicine. As such, for more than 50 years, research endeavors have become increasingly transparent and rigorous in terms of conduct and ensuring the safety of subjects. Research is no longer opportunistic as it is more difficult to begin a trial with all of the regulations that have been implemented, most notably during the past 15 years.

State and federal regulations, as well as other codes of professional conduct, have been put into place to guide all stakeholders in the research process. It is imperative that the community clinician-scientists fully understand the obligations and responsibilities placed on them, their staff, and their research and clinical practices. Once this is understood, it is not difficult to select a successful trial.

Good Clinical Practice (GCP): GCP describes the obligations of the sponsor, monitors, investigators, and Institutional Review Boards (IRB) to protect human subjects, both in the laws governing clinical research, and the ideals of research ethics and "good science." Although many of its precepts are not legally binding (e.g., guidelines and information sheets issued by the Food and Drug Administration (FDA)), GCP is widely accepted and expected in clinical research. Failure to meet GCP standards may result in sanctions and penalties.

Laws: All the government-approved rules of conduct are first codified by U.S. law and then regulation. An example would be HIPAA (Health Insurance Portability and

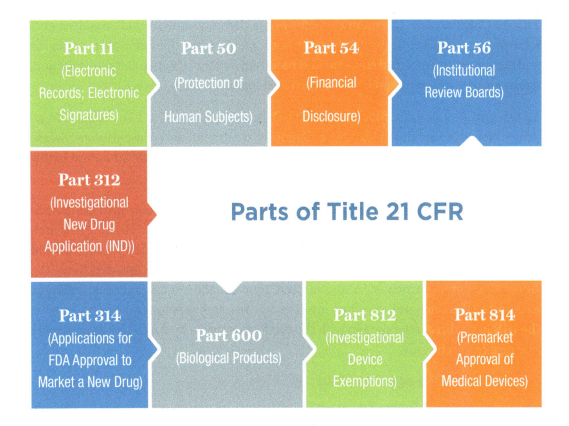

Accountability Act), **www.hhs.gov/ocr/hipaa**. It is important that the researcher keep apprised of changes in both federal and state law that may affect the conduct and/or reporting of research activities.

Code of Federal Regulations (CFR): Administrative agencies like the FDA, using authority delegated to them by Congress, create the rules and regulations to guide research practice activities and responsibilities. Often, regulations implement a statute or set procedures to allow an agency to exercise the authority delegated to it by Congress. New regulations are codified in the collection of all current regulations, called the Code of Federal Regulations (CFR). Although they are not laws, regulations have the force of law, since they are adopted under authority granted by statutes and often include penalties for violations.

Industry Guidance/Guidelines: Guidance documents for industry do not establish legally enforceable rights or responsibilities and are not legally binding. They provide assistance by explaining how a regulated industry may comply with those statutory and regulatory requirements.

Health and Human Services Department (HHS): The HHS oversees federally-funded studies (e.g., NIH grants) and is governed by the Federal Policy for the Protection of Human Subjects (also known as the "Common Rule," codified at subpart A of

Title 45 CFR Part 46). The main elements of the Common Rule include requirements for assuring compliance by research institutions; requirements for researchers obtaining and documenting informed consent; and requirements for IRB membership, function, operations, review of research, and record keeping.

Food and Drug Administration (FDA) Regulations: The FDA Regulates all drugs, biologics, and devices used for diagnosis, treatment, and prevention of disease in humans and animals. Investigational products under FDA jurisdiction are highly regulated and are subject to several parts of Title 21 CFR.

Institutional Research Board (IRB): IRBs are Academic or non-profit organizations that are given responsibility by the FDA and HHS (Office for Human Research Protection) for oversight of human subject research. Areas of review include ethical considerations, subject safety, protocol methodology (scientific consideration), the subjects' voluntary participation, and subjects' rights. In the tertiary community setting, a central IRB is often utilized when multi center research is being conducted. As such the IRB has a direct relationship with the site PI to approve and monitor their activity during a research study.

Insurance Coverage for Clinical Trials

It is important to understand that public and private insurance plans generally exclude covering what they deem experimental procedures, drugs, or devices. Unfortunately, this still results in denial of coverage for all related items and service provided as part of that research. However, given recent public attention and changes in regulation, routine patient care costs that occur when a patient is part of a clinical trial should be reimbursed.

For Medicare coverage, the research study itself must qualify by meeting certain requirements:

- Falls within a Medicare Benefit category

- The trial should have a therapeutic intent

- Patients must have a disease and not be healthy subjects; however, diagnostic trials may be exempted

- It is important that the category of trial fall under one of the major public funding bodies, such as the National Institutes of Health (NIH), Centers for Disease Control and Prevention, the Centers for Medicare and Medicaid Services, cooperative groups, FDA etc., to qualify for Medicare reimbursement for associated routine care costs.

For commercial or private insurance, there may be more variation in coverage. Note that coverage for clinical trials depends on whether a plan is regulated by state or federal law. (See **www.cancer.gov/clinicaltrials/learning/laws-about-clinical-trials-costs**.) A research practice participating in a multi-institutional study may have to confirm what is or is not covered with its state insurance regulatory agency.

Audits

An audit is a systematic and independent examination of trial-related activities and documents. The goal of an audit is to review, inspect, and verify the ethical conduct of human subject research, the integrity of previously reported data, adherence to the study protocol, and applicable institutional, state, and federal regulations and guidance.

Investigators have an obligation to take appropriate steps to protect both the integrity of science and human subjects who participate in research studies. It is important to always be audit ready, to know one's research protocol, and the standard operating procedure inside and out.

Audits can be study-related or routine research practice audits. There are also audits for studies submitted to the FDA, investigator-related audits, or for-cause and bioequivalence audits where one study is the sole basis for approval. Audits can be conducted by sponsors, the FDA or other federal agencies, the IRB, or by compliance departments.

The Research Program in Transition

All research programs ebb and flow, given changes in their staff composition. When a major or critical change occurs, the obligations of the research program, and by extension the practice, remain in effect. The practice must step in to insure the legal, financial, clinical, and safety obligations of the research practice. If a research practice closes, it is important to note that essential research documents must be preserved and stored for a minimum of seven years and possibly longer, depending on state and sponsor requirements. Immediate notification of subjects participating in ongoing trials and transference of their care must be organized and continuity insured. Again, the IRB must be notified as to any change in status of the PI and the research program vis-à-vis any active study.

In conclusion, conducting research can be an immensely intellectually rewarding endeavor that can bring significant benefits to patients and ultimately the clinical practice. It is important to reach out to other research practices for support. Endeavoring to make a difference as often as possible is the only way to advance the art, science, and business of the practice of urologic medicine in the tertiary community setting.

APPENDIX 1
Common Study Coordinator Tasks

- Administrative
- Marketing the site/securing studies
- Assessing the protocol
- Training study staff
- Preparing and negotiating study budget
- Preparing and submitting documents to the IRB
- Interacting with sponsor (Clinical Research Organization), IRB, office staff, niche providers, other department personnel
- Tracking study budget, payments
- Maintaining regulatory files
- Documenting communication and study progress
- Documenting subject study visits
- Resolving queries on study data
- Transcribing source information to the case report form
- Coordinating, preparing for, and participating in monitoring visits, audits, and inspections
- Ordering study supplies and drugs as needed
- Recruiting subjects
- Developing and coordinating advertising
- Screening subjects for eligibility
- Discussing study and conducting consent process
- Scheduling study assessments and visits
- Ensuring all visits, tests, and procedures are completed in required time intervals interviewing and evaluating subjects at appropriate intervals
- Reviewing laboratory and clinical information for signs of adverse events
- Identifying, documenting, reporting, and following up on adverse events
- Maintaining drug accountability
- Dispensing investigational product per protocol and under PI supervision
- Obtaining, preparing, and shipping biological specimens
- Coordinating study subject reimbursement

APPENDIX 2
Glossary of Terms and Acronyms

1. *AMC*—Academic medical center. Academic researchers often reach out to their community brethren to collaborate and improve accruals into cooperative and/or single institution trials.

2. *CRC*—Clinical research coordinator. This is the medical professional at the research site who is charged with implementing various duties and responsibilities defined by the protocol under the direction of the site PI.

3. *CRO*—Clinical research organization. An entity that is contracted by a sponsor to manage the execution of a specific protocol. Then the CRO is an agent of the sponsor and has proscribed standard operating procedures and protocols.

4. *GCP*—Good clinical practice is an international quality standard that is provided by the International Conference on Harmonization of Technical Requirements for Registration of Pharmaceuticals for Human Use (ICH), an international body that defines standards, which governments can transpose into regulations for clinical trials involving human subjects.

5. *PK/PD*—Pharmacokinetics/Pharmacodynamic studies.

6. *PRO*—Patient Reported Outcomes. Some studies require input from the patient and/or family to access quality of life changes, care burden, or symptom management.

7. *PSA*—Primary Service Area.

8. *PTS*—Patient-to-Subject consideration/conversion.

9. *QoL*—Quality of Life.

10. *Sponsor*—Funding entity supporting research; can be a foundation, public grant, industry partner, or self-funded.

11. *ROI*—Return on investment.

12. *RVU*—Relative value unit.

13. *SOC*—Standard of care.

14. *SOTA*—State-of-the-art. Referring to very contemporaneous technologies, medicines, and procedures; evidence-supported and have wide-spread practice.

15. *SSA*—Secondary service area.

16. *TMO*—Trials management organization. This type of organization is focused on developing and refining a study protocol to optimize its performance in a tertiary Uro-Oncology community setting. It is a provider-centric entity and often advocates for its member sites.

APPENDIX 3
Resources and Guidance for Research Programs

National Institutes of Health Protecting Personal Health Information in Research	http://privacyruleandresearch.nih.gov/pdf/HIPAA_Booklet_4-14-2003.pdf
Health Services Research and the HIPAA Privacy Rule	http://privacyruleandresearch.nih.gov/pdf/HealthServicesResearchHIPAAPrivacyRule.pdf
Research Repositories, Databases, and the HIPAA Privacy Rule	http://privacyruleandresearch.nih.gov/pdf/research_repositories_final.pdf
Clinical Research and the HIPAA Privacy Rule	http://privacyruleandresearch.nih.gov/pdf/clin_research.pdf
Institutional Review Boards and the HIPAA Privacy Rule	http://privacyruleandresearch.nih.gov/irbandprivacyrule.asp
Privacy Boards and the HIPAA Privacy Rule	http://privacyruleandresearch.nih.gov/privacy_boards_hipaa_privacy_rule.asp
HIPAA Authorization for Research	http://privacyruleandresearch.nih.gov/pdf/authorization.pdf
FDA regulation 21 CFR 11 Electronic Records; Electronic Signatures and the Federal Information Security Management Act (FISMA)	http://www.fda.gov/RegulatoryInformation/Guidances/ucm125067.htm

APPENDIX 4
Authoritative Bodies Providing Research Guidance and Regulation

Organization	Web page	Certification or Training	
		PI	CRC
CITI	www.citiprogram.org/ index.cfm?pageID=86	CMEs/CEUs	CEUs CEUs
CITI Biomedical Focus: an online course facilitated in CITI and offered by the University of Miami in collaboration with many institution's IRB. The course is web based. Offers CME and CEUs and is usually requested to be renewed every three years.			
CITI	www.citiprogram.org/index.cfm?pageID=90	CMEs/CEUs	CEUs CEUs
CITI Good Clinical Practice (GCP) and ICH: this online course is offered by the University of Miami in collaboration many institutions affiliations. The course is web based. Offers CME/CEU and is usually requested to be renewed as needed.			
SOCRA	www.socra.org		CCRP
The Society of Clinical Research Associates (SOCRA) is a non-profit, charitable, and educational membership organization committed to providing education, certification, and networking opportunities to all persons involved in clinical research activities. SOCRA, the premier educational organization for oncology site coordinators, has now emerged as a leading educational organization for clinical researchers in all therapeutic areas, supporting industry, government, and academia.			
ACRP	www.acrpnet.org	CPI	CCRC, CCRA
ACRP's vision is that clinical research is performed ethically, responsibly, and professionally everywhere in the world. ACRP's mission is to promote excellence in clinical research.			
EHSO	www.ehso.com/index.htm		
Environmental Health and Safety (EHSO): EHSO offers several courses to provide guidance for the use, storage, and disposal of the following materials used in research, clinical, academic, and operational activities: biological toxins, infectious agents, recombinant DNA agents, chemical, and radioactive materials.			
NIH	www.phrp.nihtraining.com/users/login.php	CERTIFICATE	CERTIFICATE
Protecting Human Research Participants			
	www.clinicaltrials.gov		
ClinicalTrials.gov is a registry and results database of publicly and privately supported clinical studies of human participants conducted around the world. Learn more about clinical studies and about this site, including relevant history, policies, and laws.			

APPENDIX 5
Principal Investigator Obligations/ Responsibilities and Regulation

- FDA regulated projects must sign a Form 1572: In signing the 1572, the investigator agrees to "... ensuring that an investigation is conducted according to the signed investigator statement, the investigational plan, and applicable regulation" (21 CFR 312.60).

- For devices: completes an Investigator Agreement instead of a 1572. Regulations 21 CFR 50, 54, and 56 still apply, but in addition, 21 CFR 803, 812 and 814 govern investigational device studies. Specifically, investigator obligations can be found in 21 CFR 812.

- Study Conduct. 21 CFR 312.53I: The investigator will personally conduct or supervise the investigations. This responsibility CANNOT be delegated.

- Human Subject Protection. 21 CFR 312.60: The investigator is responsible for protecting the rights, safety, and welfare of subjects under the investigator's care.

- Investigator's Brochure (IB). 21 CFR 312.53(f), ICH 4.1.2: The investigator will read the IB and understand the potential risks and side effects of the drug. Investigational Drug. 21 CFR 312.59, 21 CFR 312.61, 21 CFR 312.62(a), ICH 4.6:

- Subject Medical Records and Other Source Documents. 21 CFR 312.62 (b), 21 CFR 312.68: Prepare and maintain adequate and accurate case histories that record all observations and other pertinent data required by the sponsor. Make the records available for inspection to any properly authorized officer of FDA (21 CFR Part 312.68). FDA prefers to see the original source of documentation (i.e., where pen was first put to paper).

- Record Retention. 21 CFR 312.62I: Maintain records (study files) for the study for two years after study discontinuation, drug approval, or drug disapproval. Some studies conducted under ICH Guidelines may require storage for 15 years. ICH 4.9.5.

- Investigator Reports. 21 CFR 312.64, 21 CFR 54, ICH 4.10, 4.11, 4.13: Submit reports to sponsor at times required by regulations and the sponsor: a. Progress reports b. Safety Reports: adverse events (AE), and serious adverse events (SAE) c. Final Report at study end.

- Financial Disclosure Adverse Experiences. 21 CFR 312.64(b), ICH 4.11: Report adverse events (AEs) to the sponsor in accordance with 21 CFR Part 312.64. IRB. 21 CFR 56, 21 CFR 312.66, ICH 4.4: Financial
- Disclosure applies to the investigator and all those listed on the 1572. It also applies to spouses and dependent children of those disclosing.
- Assure that the IRB is in compliance with 21 CFR Part 56:
- Obtain IRB initial and continuing review and approval of the study.
- Promptly report all changes in the research activity and unexpected risks to subjects or others to IRB.

Do not make any changes in the research without IRB approval, except when necessary to eliminate a hazard to a subject.

- Protocol Compliance. 21 CFR 312.66, ICH 4.5: Changes to the protocol to be made only after receiving sponsor and IRB approval except to eliminate hazard to human subjects.
- Informed Consent and IRB Requirements. 21 CFR 50, 21 CFR 56, ICH 4.8:
- Obtain consent in compliance with 21 CFR 50 and 56.
- Obtain IRB approval of the informed consent prior to implementing the consent process with any subject.
- Obtain informed consent before enrolling subject in study.
- Provide subject with sufficient time to make decision about participating in study.
- Ensure subject understands language in the consent form and the consent contains all the required elements.
- Consent should not contain any language that is exculpatory or waives or appears to waive any of the subject's rights.
- Investigative Staff. 21 CFR 312.53(g), ICH 4.1.5: Ensure that staff are qualified, capable, and trained to perform their study-related responsibilities.
- Keep personnel informed of study-related information and changes. Maintain records documenting how staff members were trained to perform their duties (e.g., onsite training by team member, through their licensing, etc.). Maintain records on protocol-specific training.
- Investigator Disqualification. 21 CFR 312.70: Investigator may be disqualified for repeated or deliberate failure to comply with regulations or submitting false information to the sponsor.
- Code of Federal Regulations: https://www.gpo.gov/fdsys/browse/collection Cfr.action?collectionCode=CFR

APPENDIX 6
ADDITIONAL GUIDANCE DOCUMENTS

- The researcher must be knowledgeable and incorporate the following guidance documents into all studies to ensure the safety of the subjects and the project:

- ICH E6 Good Clinical Practices: http://www.fda.gov/downloads/Drugs/GuidanceCompliance-RegulatoryInformation/Guidances/UCM073122.pdf

- FDA 21 CFR 50 Protection of Human Subjects: http://www.accessdata.fda.gov/scripts/cdrh/cfdocs/cfcfr/CFRSearch.cfm?CFRPart=50

- HHS 45 CFR 46 Protection of Human Subjects: http://www.hhs.gov/ohrp/humansubjects/guidance

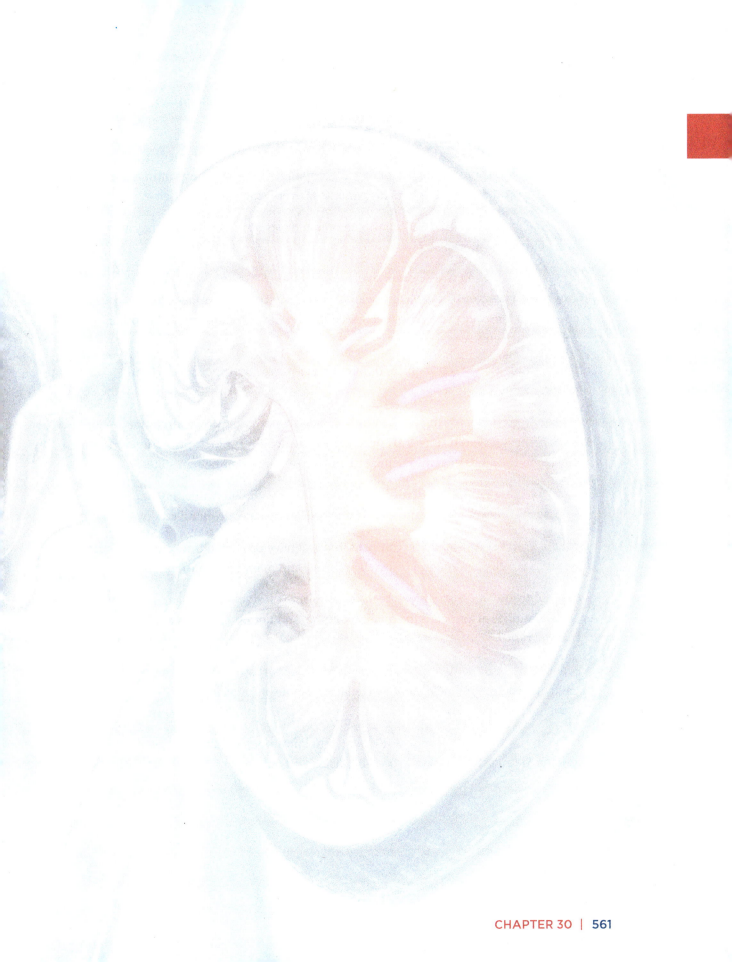

KEY POINTS

- **It can be difficult to begin a trial with state and federal regulations,** as well as other codes of professional conduct, that guide all stakeholders in the research process.

- **Research can lead to the early adoption of new technologies,** medicines, and procedures into the broader clinical group practice, thereby expanding the practice's product/service offers for patients at every stage of their disease.

- **Patients who participate in trials** can obtain drugs at no cost before they are available on the market.

- **A vibrant research program provides professional differentiation** for the group and sub-group of clinical researchers and is attractive for inclusion by commercial insurer provider panels, Accountable Care Organizations and other collaborative endeavors.

- **High-quality research** requires different types of research sponsors to fund practice research.

- **Most research occurring in the clinical practice setting** is typically latter stage clinical research (Phase III or Phase IV), which for urology, primarily focuses in the areas of genitourinary malignancies and other benign states.

- **Knowing one's staff's skill and capability** mix should determine the complexity and volume of studies the practice can realistically handle well.

- **Medical directors** should be compensated and have protected time one to two days a week to attend to research activities and manage operations.

- **Second to the medical director,** the quality of the lead clinical research coordination is essential to the quality, volume, and bottom-line success of the program.

- **A dedicated financial analyst** is beneficial to support study budget review, ongoing program financial analysis, tenacious sponsor invoicing, and accounts reconciliation.

- **It is important to always be audit ready,** to know one's research protocol, and the Standard Operating Procedure inside and out.

Neal D. Shore, MD, FACS, CPI

Neal D. Shore, MD, is the President of LUGPA and the Medical Director for the Carolina Urologic Research Center in Myrtle Beach, South Carolina, where he practices with Atlantic Urology Clinics. He has conducted more than 250 clinical trials, focusing mainly on Genitourinary Oncology. He is the Founding Director, CUSP, Clinical Research Consortium. He also serves on the executive boards of the Society of Urologic Oncology Board and the Society of Urologic Oncology-Clinical Trials Consortium.

Raoul S. Concepcion, MD, FACS

Raoul S. Concepcion, MD, FACS, is the Medical Director at The Comprehensive Prostate Center, in Nashville, Tennessee, and a Clinical Assistant Professor in the Department of Urology at the Vanderbilt School of Medicine. He is also Past President of LUGPA, and Founding Director of CUSP Clinical Research Consortium. He has more than 25 years experience in conducting research and clinical practice, and serves as an advisor or consultant for many pharmaceutical companies in the advanced prostate cancer world.

Daniel R. Saltzstein, MD

Daniel R. Saltzstein, MD, is the Medical Director at Urology San Antonio Research, and the Medical Advisor and Founding Director of CUSP Clinical Research Consortium. He has more than 25 years experience in conducting research and clinical practice.

Arletta van Breda, RN, MSN, CCRC, CIP

Arletta van Breda, RN, MSN, CCRC, is the Director of Clinical Research Operations of CUSP Clinical Research Consortium. She has more than 25 years of healthcare experience in research and clinical practice.

Thomas A. Paivanas, MHSA

Thomas A. Paivanas, MHSA, is the Executive Director of CUSP Clinical Research Consortium. He has more than 25 years of healthcare experience in conducting research as well as policy, strategic planning, and business development.

CHAPTER

The Future of Value-Based Payment in the U.S.

Alec S. Koo, MD, FACS

John McManus

The Medicare Access and CHIP Reauthorization Act (MACRA), which repealed the Sustainable Growth Rate (SGR) payment scheme, was intended to move physician payment from a system that rewarded volume to one that rewarded value. The law created two new approaches: alternative payment models (APMs) for providers entering risk arrangements and the Merit-Based Incentive Payment System (MIPS) for the vast majority remaining in fee-for-service.

Global Capitation and The Little-Known Secret of Medicare Advantage

The goal of MACRA is to end fee-for-service payments in healthcare by ushering healthcare providers into APMs and global capitation. MIPS was intended to be an intermediate step towards pushing physicians and healthcare systems to take financial risk for the total cost of care, or a return to global capitation.

From the payer's perspective, global capitation fixes the cost at a pre-determined level and assigns nearly all financial risks to providers. Global capitation has been in existence for more than 20 years. The Balanced Budget Act (BBA) of 1997 named Medicare's managed care program "Medicare+Choice," and the Medicare Modernization Act (MMA) of 2003 renamed it "Medicare Advantage." It is also known as Medicare Part C. Under Medicare Advantage(MA), private health plans, such as HMOs or PPOs receive capitated payments from Medicare to provide services to plan enrollees, while the payer, Medicare, has a fixed cost per beneficiary; thus, eliminating the financial risks Medicare bears.

Medicare Advantage is primed for growth as it appeals to two principal constituents of healthcare: health plans and government.

1. **Health plans:** MA plans yield higher nominal revenue and operating margin with per-member per-month (PMPM) revenue of $800-$1200 and operating margin of $30-$60 PMPM vs. $180-$220 and $10-$18 for Medicare Supplement plans.[1]

2. **Government:** MA plans enables an easily reachable budget target that derives its adherence to the fixed pay-out per capita of beneficiaries.[1]

Over the past decade, the number of beneficiaries enrolled in Medicare Advantage plans has nearly doubled from 11.1 million in 2010 to 22.0 million in 2019, a full 34% of the 64 million people covered by Medicare.[2] The Congressional Budget Office (CBO) projects that Medicare Advantage enrollment will continue to grow over the next decade, with plans including about 47 percent of beneficiaries by 2029.[2] Private-sector analysts project that by 2024 the majority of Medicare beneficiaries will be enrolled in Medicare Advantage plans and ultimately MA will enroll 70% of Medicare covered lives.[1] Even without the push towards global capitation provided by MACRA, Medicare has achieved effective cost control in a substantial portion of its covered lives.

The Early Failure of MIPS

Nearly five years since it was signed into law, progress on MACRA has been bumpy at best. Very few physicians are participating in APMs, and MIPS incentive payments are too insignificant to incentivize meaningful behavioral change.

The Centers for Medicare and Medicaid Services (CMS) initially excluded 60 percent of clinicians from the MIPS program using discretionary criteria, such as low volume and hardship. More troubling, CMS has diminished the reward of high performing physicians by watering down the standards. A provider need only score 45 out of 100 to avoid a penalty, which results in less than 2% of providers being subject to penalties.[3]

Because penalties fund bonuses, the exclusions and restricted incentive pool substantially limit resources available for high performing physicians. On a base of $70 billion of clinician spending, there is just $390 million available for bonuses.

Similarly, CMS also diminished the impact of the $500 million pool of annual bonuses intended for "exceptional physicians," which the statute reserved for the top 25% of performing physicians above the median. Unfortunately, CMS used its authority to instead designate 84% of physicians as "exceptional."[4] The result: a $6,600 expected bonus for a top performer plummets to about $1,100. If everyone is exceptional, then no one is exceptional.

What does this mean for the practices who invested substantial resources to get ready for the quality-improvement program? There is no economic payoff.

In its recent physician payment rule, CMS acknowledged problems with the MIPS program, such as "its burden and complexity, its inability to generate meaningful information that differentiates performance, and the difficulty of producing reliable measure data for clinicians with small panels of patients."[5]

But the Medicare Payment Advisory Commission (MedPAC) believes the problems are more fundamental and suggests scrapping the program entirely. MedPAC thereby concluded, "MIPS will not succeed in helping beneficiaries choose clinicians, help clinicians change practice patterns to improve value, or help Medicare reward clinicians based on value."[6]

APMs Offer Little Opportunity for Urologists

The other program under MACRA, APMs, is seen by policymakers as the future of healthcare because it encourages physician practices to accept capitated payments for value-based delivery arrangements. Yet it is fraught with even more problems. While an increasing number of physicians are participating in APMs, most do so through mostly hospital-led accountable care organizations (ACOs) or primary care models. The most recent information from CMS shows that just 88 urologists are enrolled in an APM.

Recognizing that not all good ideas come from government bureaucrats, Congress created a pathway for physicians to develop their own APM ideas for consideration. MACRA established the Physician-Focused Payment Model Technical Advisory Committee (PTAC) to review, vet, and recommend APMs submitted by physician organizations to the Center for Medicare and Medicaid Innovation (CMMI).

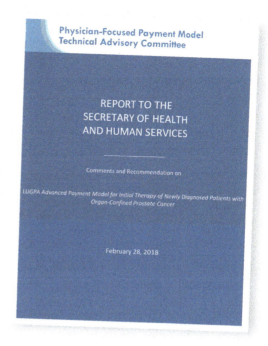

However, after four years of existence, CMMI has yet to approve a single APM of the 16 PTAC recommended for pilot testing or immediate implementation. In November 2019, two prominent Members of PTAC resigned in protest. In announcing his resignation, Harold Miller, CEO of the Center for Healthcare Quality and Payment Reform stated, "sadly not a single one of the models we have recommended is being implemented or tested by the Department of Health and Human Services, and the Secretary has stated none of them will be."[7]

This means Congress's vision of allowing a thousand flowers to bloom where physician-generated ideas for value-based delivery could be tested and experimented upon cannot succeed as they await CMMI approval of APMs that will never arrive.

Yet one type of APM is flourishing: accountable care organizations (ACOs), which were established by the 2010 Affordable Care Act (ACA). Today, there are more than 500 ACOs nationwide serving nearly 12 million Medicare beneficiaries.[8]

ACOs are mostly hospital-led and have provided a huge advantage to mega-hospital systems over independent physician practices. The Affordable Care Act empowered the Secretary of Health and Human Services to waive Stark, anti-kickback, and other Medicare regulations for ACOs and provide bonus payments to such organizations while adopting little risk.

A recent study by Avalere found hospital-employed physicians increased by more than 70 percent from July 2012 through January 2018. In just the last two years, an additional 8,000 physician practices were acquired by hospitals. From July 2012 through

January 2018, hospital acquisitions of physician practices more than doubled, with nearly one-third now owned by hospitals.[9] Why should this be of concern to policymakers? Hospitals cost a lot more than physician practices, even when delivering the identical items and services.

MedPAC's March 2018 report found that from 2011 to 2016, program spending and beneficiary cost-sharing on services covered under hospital outpatient departments increased by 51 percent, from $39.8 billion to $60 billion.[10] MedPAC noted, "A large source of growth in spending on services furnished in hospital outpatient departments (HOPDs) appears to be the result of the unnecessary shift of services from (lower-cost) physician offices to (higher-cost) HOPDs."

ACOs have been ineffective in controlling costs. Analysis by the Center for Healthcare Quality and Payment Reform found that ACOs have "yet to generate a net benefit to Medicare after five years of trying." Medicare bonuses exceed savings and penalties.

Hospitals have focused on acquiring physician practices because that strategy simultaneously quashes competition in the local market and creates downstream revenue through referrals on surgery and ancillary services. The revenue physicians generate far surpasses the cost of the employed physician's salary as documented in Merritt Hawkins' 2019 *Physician Inpatient/Outpatient Revenue Survey*.[11]

For example, the generated revenue per employed urologist was $2,161,458 while the average employed urologist's salary was just $386,000. The ratio is similar for other specialties and primary care.

Focus Turns to Revising Stark and Anti-Kickback Regulations

Amid these challenges comes a bold, new proposal from the Trump Administration to fundamentally modernize the Stark and Anti-kickback laws, which would enable independent practices to compete more fairly with large hospital systems.

The Stark law, written three decades ago in an era of fee-for-service, now serves as a barrier to coordinated and value-based care. It does not allow physicians practices to incentivize their doctors with resources from ancillary services, such as pathology, radiation therapy, and advanced imaging to promote treatment pathways. It does not allow sufficient integration among different physician practices working together to provide comprehensive care in a community, nor does it help facilitate coordination among practices and a hospital partner.

Recognizing these flaws, last year, CMS proposed comprehensive rules to fundamentally modernize regulations that implement the Stark and AKS laws. Central to the approach is providers' ability to enter value-based arrangements without needing an application or CMS approval. Providers do not have to await a CMMI-approved APM! Rather, providers need only retain documentation on how their activities further value-based purposes and the type, nature, and methodology of the remuneration.

The proposal gives flexibility for arrangements with varying degrees of risk-sharing, which is important because it does not presume that a one-size-fits-all approach can work for different specialties, regions, or size of practices.

> **Any value-based entity engaged in one of any of the four value-based purposes would qualify:**
>
> **1.** Coordinating and managing the care of a target population;
>
> **2.** Improving the quality of care for a target patient population;
>
> **3.** Appropriately reducing the costs to, or growth in expenditures of, payors without reducing the quality of care for a target patient population; **OR**
>
> **4.** Transitioning from healthcare delivery and payment mechanisms based on the volume of items and services to mechanisms based on the quality of care and control of costs of care.

Hundreds of stakeholders have welcomed the proposals as critical to modernizing these outdated laws. LUGPA submitted detailed comments to both the RFI and proposed rules that commended HHS for its bold steps, providing specific examples of value-based care activities that are prohibited under the current regulatory framework but could be provided under the proposed rules. In addition, LUGPA met with HHS Deputy Secretary Hargan several times and worked with GOP Doctors Caucus—comprised of retired physicians who are now Members of Congress—to support the proposal and urge its timely implementation.

However, the proposals have received a skeptical response from MedPAC, who argued that not enough risk is put on providers and too much is on the Medicare program.[13]

CMS will ultimately have to decide whether, how, and when it moves forward on these proposals. In the past, major regulatory revisions to the Stark law have taken years to finalize. The finalized rules will have vital importance on how well large urology groups can provide efficient care under the concept of a specialty driven APM.

What is certain is the growth of Medicare Advantage population. By 2029, essentially half of all Medicare beneficiaries will be covered by Medicare Advantage. As of 2019, 62% of Medicare Advantage enrollees are in HMO plans,[1] with the percentage certain to rise as plans struggle to control cost.

How Urology Groups Can Thrive in Value-Based Healthcare

Through growth of both Medicare Advantage plans and APMs under MACRA, Medicare is continuing its drive towards global capitation payment of healthcare. Given the anticipated growth of Medicare Advantage and ACO's, it is likely that urology groups will need to contract with these entities for majority of their Medicare patients. Private payers will certainly follow the lead of Medicare as global capitation payment model substantially eliminates financial risks for payers.

Typically, intermediary entities will accept global capitation from payers and then in turn contract with providers in downstream payment arrangements. Historically, health maintenance organizations (HMO) have been such entities and have paid physicians by a variety of methodology including: 1) discounted FFS, 2) managed FFS that place restriction in forms of authorization requirement for services or restrictions of site of service at preferred laboratories or imaging facilities, 3) sub-capitation where physicians are paid a pre-determined amount based on the numbers of "covered lives" under their care. More recently, other intermediary entities have embraced global capitation, and these entities may include: 1) various Medicare Advantage plans, 2) Provider sponsored plans (e.g. Geisinger in Pennsylvania or Providence in Oregon), 3) Medical groups driven by primary care (HealthCare Partners), 4) local or regional healthcare systems and ultimately, 5) ACO's. Invariably, unless these intermediary entities employ their own urologists, they will need to contract with existent urology groups. Integrated urology groups who offer the infrastructure and geographic coverage that mirror the needs of these entities are in a unique position to contract for professional urology services, as well as related ancillary services including possibly imaging facilities, ambulatory surgery centers, radiation oncology or anatomic pathology services.

The continued pressure from employers, government and payers will ensure wide adoption of price control in the form of global capitation. The changes will affect every provider regardless of location or readiness. Now is the time for integrated urology groups to adopt strategies and actions to ready themselves to thrive in a global capitation environment. The ultimate charge for urology groups is to take on the entirety of urologic care with a health plan and to manage the population efficiently. In other words, the urology group will take a set (capitated) dollar amount per beneficiary and efficiently care for the urologic needs of this group of patients. The prevalence and timeframe of such capitation implementation will vary widely across geographic regions. For the foreseeable future, most groups will face a mix of fee-for-service and capitated payer contracts.

While payer environment is in the transition phase urology groups can begin to develop internal infrastructure by engaging in activities that can generate current revenue while honing expertise to better prepare for a time when groups are expected to assume full risk capitation for managing urologic care of set populations. On the next page are examples that utilize some of the key principles of value-based care to both develop new business opportunities as well as internal processes and staffing that will ultimately facilitate population management of urologic diseases:

1. Develop clinical pathways and **care coordination** teams to manage certain urologic disease states. Clinical pathways allow for standardized care, and the outcome can then be measured. Only with metrics do improvements occur. Clinical pathways, run by efficient care coordinators, also reduce the cost of provision of care by enabling each level of personnel to practice at the highest level their training will allow.

   Many urology groups already have experience with advanced prostate clinics in managing care using pathways and coordination. Groups can take advantage of payment mechanisms such as Chronic Care Management (CCM) that provides payment for care coordination in the current fee-for-service environment to further develop infrastructure for care coordination.

   In addition to advanced prostate cancer care, pathways for disease states, such as chronic cystitis, kidney stone disease, and bladder cancer may be additional developmental targets. Several LUGPA groups have successfully implemented chronic cystitis virtual clinics where services are supported by Medicare CCM reimbursement (CCM are care-coordination CPT® codes, e.g., 99490, 99491, 99487, 99489, for non-face-to-face care provided by personnel under the supervision of physicians). Such care coordination infrastructure, once implemented, can also be used to navigate certain high-risk populations such as post-stone surgeries, post-prostate biopsies, or post-operative patients in general.

2. Work with health plans/healthcare systems to **gain-share**. Using care coordination infrastructure, urology groups can work on activities that reduce healthcare costs and negotiate with health plans to share in the savings (gain-share). Possible target areas to develop gain-share include:

   a. Reducing re-admission rates by proactively managing post-operative and post-discharge care of urology patients.

   b. Helping hospitals devise and implement programs to reduce catheter-related sepsis.

   c. Systematically transferring procedures into a lower cost environment, such as performance of TURP in ASCs.

3. Create **Integrated Practice Units** (IPU) with transparent pricing and outcome. An example would be a stone treatment center where the urology group can offer an all-inclusive case-rate treatment plan. The plan would include all professional physician and facility costs necessary to treat stones of a certain size and location,

with rapid scheduling of diagnostic and treatment procedures. Successful urology IPUs would also allow urologists to contract directly with health plans and consumers using bundled pricing of disease treatments. Examples of efficient IPUs are seen in other specialties, such as the COE programs Walmart utilized for its employees by negotiating **bundled pricing** for surgeries, such as organ transplant and joint replacements. Some urology procedures that may be suitable for bundled pricing include kidney stone treatment, robotic organ removal, and minimally invasive treatment of BPH.

 Manage high risk population. An example would be for urology groups to actively monitor and navigate certain populations, such as repeat stone formers or chronic cystitis patients to identify and treat disease onset early, and hence, reduce ER visits. Payers are targeting global capitation as the end-goal of value-based healthcare. The delivery of high-quality urology care at a lower cost point will require systemized care with good clinical pathways and efficient utilization of personnel. The main area of cost saving that urologists can impact are outside of the office setting.

Strategic actions such as these help healthcare systems reduce costs and improve quality, which are the basic tenets of value-based payment system. These activities also help urology groups develop processes and staffing that are necessary in becoming efficient in care coordination and population management activities. Urology groups should actively seek out, negotiate, and lead in such opportunities.

Given current market forces, global capitation will inevitably become the dominant payment strategy in US healthcare. Urologists can either be the driver or the passenger on the urology disease state management bus. To take on tasks(or contracts) of managing a population of beneficiaries with a set capitation payment, an efficient urology group will need to set up clinical pathways for multiple disease states, with care coordination to navigate patients through the diagnosis and treatment processes; thus utilize ancillary staffing to the highest level as allowed by training, and maximize the value of physician time. Successful urology groups will also negotiate for value-added payment in addition to the base capitation rate for activities that lead to overall savings for the payer as well as improved quality of care for patients.

Urologists are amongst the most resourceful and entrepreneurial physicians. By embracing the key tenets of care coordination and pathway-based care, urology groups will be well positioned to thrive in value-based healthcare.

1. Bill frack et al, "Why Medicare Advantage Is Marching Toward 70% Penetration of U.S. Healthcare Market," L.E.K. Consulting's Executive Insights 19, N0. 69 (2017), https://www.lek.com/sites/default/files/insights/pdf-attachments/1969_Medicare_AdvantageLEK_Executive_Inisghts_1.pdf.
2. https://www.kff.org/medicare/fact-sheet/medicare-advantage/
3. 2020 Physician Fee Schedule Rule (CMS-1715-F)
4. Ibid
5. Ibid
6. Medicare Payment Advisory Commission, "Moving Beyond the Merit-Based Incentive System" March 2018
7. "PTAC Members Resign, Say Congress Needs to Step in and Fix Process," Inside Health Policy, November 20, 2019.
8. Kaiser Family Foundation, "Medicare System Reform: The Evidence Link, 8 FAQs Medicare ACO Models"
9. Avalere analysis of SK&A hospital/health system ownership of practice locations data with Medicare
10. Medicare Payment Advisory Commission, March 2018
11. Merritt Hawkins 2019 Physician Inpatient/Outpatient Revenue Survey.
12. "Medicare Program; Modernizing and Clarifying the Physician Self-Referral Regulations," Federal Register, vol. 84 no. 201 (October 17, 2019)
13. Medicare Payment Advisory Commission, December 20, 2019 letter to CMS

KEY POINTS

- **The goal of MACRA is to end fee-for-service payments in healthcare** by ushering healthcare providers into APMs and global capitation.

- **MIPS was intended** to be an intermediate step towards physicians taking financial risk for the total cost of care.

- **Medicare Advantage (MA) plans** is an alternate pathway for Medicare to achieve global capitation. MA plans haven seen consistent growth and is projected to cover the majority of Medicare beneficiaries.

- **Progress on MACRA has been bumpy at best.** Very few physicians are participating in APMs, and MIPS incentive payments are too insignificant to incentivize meaningful behavioral change. There is no economic payoff from these programs.

- **Congress created a pathway for physicians** to develop their own APM ideas for consideration. The Center for Medicare and Medicaid Innovation (CMMI) was to recommend APMs for implementation. CMMI has yet to approve a single APM of the 16 PTAC recommended for pilot testing or immediate implementation.

- **Accountable care organizations (ACOs),** which were established by the 2010 Affordable Care Act (ACA). Today, there are more than 500 ACOs nationwide serving nearly 12 million Medicare beneficiaries. ACOs are mostly hospital-led and have provided a huge advantage to mega-hospital systems over independent physician practices.

- **The Stark law,** written three decades ago in an era of fee-for-service, now serves as a barrier to coordinated and value-based care. Recognizing these flaws, CMS proposed comprehensive rules to fundamentally modernize regulations that implement the Stark and AKS laws.

- **Urology groups** can begin to develop internal infrastructure by engaging in activities that can generate current revenue while honing expertise to better prepare for a time when groups are expected to assume full risk capitation for managing urologic care of set populations.

Alec S. Koo, MD, FACS

Dr. Alec S. Koo received his bachelor's Degree and MD from UCLA. He completed his residency in Surgery/Urology at UCLA in 1992 and is a Diplomate of the American Board of Urology. Dr. Koo is well known for his expertise in group management as well as value-based care and health economics outcomes. He is respected for his knowledge in areas including data integration and analytics in medicine, medical group dynamics and provider/pharmaceutical relations. Dr. Koo was the founding managing partner of Skyline Urology in Southern California. Dr. Koo is a former member of the LUGPA Board of Directors.

John McManus

John McManus is president and founder of The McManus Group LLC, a consulting firm specializing in strategic policy and political counsel and advocacy for health care clients with issues before Congress and the Administration. The McManus Group services clients who are leaders in their respective field across the health care spectrum from the pharmaceutical, biotechnology and medical device industries, to physician and other outpatient provider organizations. The McManus Group was founded in 2004 and has built a reputation of substantive policy expertise that is trusted by key policy makers in both legislative chambers and in the Administration. John has represented LUGPA since 2010.

Prior to founding The McManus Group, McManus served Chairman Bill Thomas as the Staff Director of the Ways and Means Health Subcommittee, where he led the policy development, negotiations and drafting of the Medicare Prescription Drug, Improvement and Modernization Act of 2003, which added the outpatient drug benefit.

CHAPTER

Medicare Quality Payment Program: Updates for Urology

Bob Dowling, MD
Alec S. Koo, MD, FACS

Information concerning the Medicare Program was current at the time of writing. Users should always verify the most recent program updates from **CMS.gov**

History

In 2015, the Medicare Access and CHIP Reauthorization Act (MACRA) was signed into law. This legislation significantly changed the way providers are reimbursed for professional services under Medicare and launched the modern era of value-based reimbursement in government health programs. Today MACRA is implemented as the Quality Payment Program (QPP) comprised of two mutually exclusive tracks: The Merit Based Incentive Payments System (MIPS), and Advanced Alternative Payment Models (APM). Success in either track depends upon performance on quality and cost measures, but the two tracks differ in terms of eligibility, reporting requirements, program incentives, rewards, and penalties. In 2020, the QPP entered its fourth year, and most urologists are eligible for and required to participate in MIPS; very few Advanced APMs are available for consideration by urologists today. This chapter will review these programs in the broader context of the shift from fee-for-service to value-based reimbursement.

Eligibility in the QPP

Each year, the Centers for Medicare and Medicaid Services (CMS) determines eligibility in the QPP by looking back at one or more eligibility periods. Providers who are associated with a CMS-endorsed Advanced Alternative Payment Model during the eligibility period and whose Medicare or All Payer collective participation in that APM exceeds a certain level of patients or payments are deemed a Qualifying Participant (QP) and are exempt from MIPS. (In 2020 to become a QP, at least 50% of the entity's Medicare Part B payments or at least 35% of Medicare patients must come through an Advanced APM at one of the determination periods). There is a slightly lower threshold to be eligible as a partial QP (in 2020, 40% of Medicare Part B payments or 25% of Medicare patients); partial QPs may elect to participate in MIPS but are not required to do so. Partial QPs who choose not to participate in MIPS will receive no fee schedule adjustment, and no bonus. Providers who are not QPs, are not in their first year of Medicare participation, and who exceed a [low] threshold of patients, payments, and services must participate in MIPS. From a practical perspective, the limited availability of advanced APMS and these thresholds are such that almost all urologists in clinical practice are subject to MIPS.

Payment Incentives in the QPP

In 2020, the fourth year following the implementation of MACRA, the Medicare Physician Fee Schedule conversion factor is no longer adjusted up or down each year. Instead, clinicians, individuals, or groups achieve a MIPS composite score each year (see below) that determines how their fees will be adjusted beginning two years after the participation period. The payment adjustments are applied at the claim line level, only to professional services (not drugs), and only to the Medicare payment amount—the patient responsibility is not affected by MIPS fee schedule adjustments. The amount of the net fee adjustment is determined by the individual/group performance relative to

TABLE 1

Payment Example	Year 1 QPP	Year 2 QPP	Year 3 QPP	Year 4 QPP
MIPS	0.5% fee schedule adjustment	0.5% fee schedule adjustment	0.25% fee schedule adjustment plus fee schedule adjustment determined by Year 1 MIPS Composite Score	fee schedule adjustment determined by Year 2 MIPS Composite Score
QP in an advanced APM (each year)	0.5% fee schedule adjustment	0.5% fee schedule adjustment	QP in Year 1 receives 0.25% adjustment + 5% of Year 2 qualifying payments (Lump sum)	QP in Year 2 receives 5% of Year 3 qualifying payments (Lump sum)
Partial QP in an advanced APM (each year)	0.5% fee schedule adjustment	0.5% fee schedule adjustment	No adjustment	No adjustment

all other MIPS clinicians' performance and a threshold set by law. Rulemaking in years one to five of the program has seen a gradually increasing threshold; in year six of QPP, that threshold will be the mean or median score of all participants. The impact of all the positive adjustments is required to equal the impact of all the negative adjustments to achieve budget neutrality. While the maximum fee schedule adjustments are defined by law, in the first few years of the program there have been few providers with negative adjustments, resulting in small amounts of dollars to distribute as positive fee schedule adjustments to everyone else. As a result, the maximum positive fee schedule adjustments have been much lower than the limits set in law: in year one of QPP, the limit was 4%, but the maximum adjustment was about 1.9%; in year two, the limit was 5% but the maximum adjustment was about 1.7%. Year three results are pending. On the other hand, negative adjustments are defined in the statute, and in year four of QPP include a maximum of 9%. Taken together, this means the upside in MIPS depends on relative performance and has turned out to be modest so far, but the impact of ignoring program requirements is known and a substantial penalty. As further incentive to perform well in MIPS, MACRA created a separate "exceptional" pool of $500M/year to be distributed pro rata to the top performers in the program. This incentive expires after year five of QPP.

QPs in an advanced APM are not subject to fee schedule adjustments and instead will receive a lump sum distribution of 5% of payments, in addition to whatever incentives are realized by participation in the APM. Like MIPS, this bonus is distributed two years following the year in which the QP designation is made. However, this 5% bonus structure—defined in MACRA and designed to jump start APM participation—expires in 2022.

Finally, in year eight of QPP (2024) MACRA calls for automatic baseline fee schedule increases of 0.25% for MIPS clinicians, and 0.75% for QPs in advanced APMs. (See **Table 1**)

TABLE 1

QUALITY PAYMENT PROGRAM YEAR	1	2	3	4	5	6	7	8
As of CY 2020	2017	2018	2019	2020	2021	2022	2023	2024
Baseline Fee schedule Adjustment	0.5%	0.5%	0.25%	0%	0%	0%	0%	0.25%
Quality Weight (%)	60	50	45	45	TBD	30	30	30
Cost Weight (%)	0	10	15	15	TBD	30	30	30
IA Weight (%)	15	15	15	15	15	15	15	15
PI Weight (%)	25	25	25	25	25	25	25	25
MIPS Composite Score Threshold (pts)	3	15	30	45	60	Mean Median	Mean Median	Mean Median
Exceptional Threshold (pts)	70	70	75	85	85	NA	NA	NA
Maximum Adjustment (+/- %)	4	5	7	9	9	9	9	9
Actual Scaled Maximum Positive adjustment (+/- %)	1.88	1.66	-	-	-	-	-	-

The MIPS Composite Score

The MIPS Composite Score (MCS) is a weighted average of performance in four separate categories: Quality, Cost, Promoting Interoperability, and Improvement Activities. Each category score has a set of required and/or optional objectives and measures, and the first transition years of QPP have seen significant changes to some of these measures (Table 1). In year six (2022) of QPP, the weight of each category will be: Quality 30%, Cost 30%, PI 25%, and IA 15%. A discussion of each category and success factors follows.

Quality Category

Quality measures are defined and endorsed by CMS, and can be reported via claims, electronic health record systems (called eCQMs), qualified data registries (called MIPS CQMs), and in a few cases by web interface. The reporting period is the entire 12 months of a performance year. The MIPS clinician/group must choose a minimum of six measures in this category, including one outcome measure (some exceptions apply). While there are hundreds of quality measures to choose from, the burdens of documentation and reporting are such that the electronic health record is usually the critical determinant in that choice. Not all EHRs are certified for all eCQMs, and it is not practical or cost efficient to extract data from many systems to take advantage of registry reporting. Consequently, many urology groups are limited by the capabilities of their EHR and forced to choose "generic" quality measures and use prebuilt reports. Success in the Quality category is dependent on understanding the general specifications of each measure, the workflow that optimizes performance, and the role of the clinical staff and/or physician in that workflow. High performers in this category will set goals, have a mechanism to track performance against goals, and apply continuous improvement. The availability of new, urology specific measures today outpaces their incorporation into EHRs for practical use, and the future of meaningful quality measures in the specialty will depend heavily on advances in health information technology.

Cost Category

The Cost Category requires no reporting from providers as the measures are calculated from Medicare claim information for a calendar year. This category has seen significant changes in year four (2020) that directly impact urologists. The first measure, Total per Capita Cost Measure (TPCC) is intended to standardize the overall risk-adjusted cost of care provided to Medicare patients, which is attributed to their primary care physician. In the early years of MIPS, this measure was configured in a way that urologists were often identified as primary providers and assigned beneficiaries. This measure has been changed to exclude certain specialties—including urology—from the attribution process; however, advanced practice providers who bill under their own NPI number could still be assigned costs under this measure if they exceed case minimums (20). The practical impact is that most urology clinicians/groups will not be subject to the TPCC measure, and the other measures will be proportionally weighted. The second measure, Medicare

What's New in MIPS COST Category Impacting Urologists:

> ▶ The Total per Capita Cost Category has been changed to exclude certain specialties—including urology—from the attribution process; as a result, urology providers/practices will not be subject to this measure and any other measures will be proportionally reweighted to the other cost category measures

> ▶ The Medicare Spending per Beneficiary Clinician (MSPB-C) has been refined to separate medical and surgical episodes; for surgical episodes, the core procedure of an inpatient stay will determine to whom costs are attributed during a window of 3 days pre admission, admission, and 30 days post discharge. Costs for inpatient urology episodes should be more appropriately assigned as a result

> ▶ A new episode based measure called Renal or Ureteral Stone Surgical Treatment has been implemented; with a case minimum of 10 this procedure based episode measure is expected to impact almost all practicing urologists who perform ureteroscopy, ESWL, or percutaneous procedures for stones.

Spending per Beneficiary Clinician (MSPB-C), has been refined to separate medical and surgical episodes. For surgical episodes, the core procedure of an inpatient stay will determine to whom costs are attributed during a window starting three days pre-admission, continuing through the inpatient stay period until 30 days post discharge.

Urologists who are primary surgeons of the core procedure will be attributed the cost measure. Medical episodes are attributed to the provider/group who bills the substantial share of evaluation and management codes during an inpatient admission. Examples of Medicare inpatient episodes that could be attributed to urologists include radical cystectomy, open nephrectomy, sepsis following prostate biopsy, or any patient requiring admission to the hospital for a primary urologic condition managed by the urologist. Costs for inpatient urology episodes should be more appropriately assigned as a result. The case minimum threshold for this measure is 35, so large practices will likely be scored on this measure. Third, a new episode-based measure called Renal or Ureteral Stone Surgical Treatment has been implemented; with a case minimum of 10 this procedure-based episode measure is expected to impact almost all practicing urologists who perform ureteroscopy, ESWL, or percutaneous procedures for stones. The cost of an episode triggered by one of these codes includes certain facility and Part B items determined by a set of "assignment" and timing rules, and will include procedures in all facility settings (inpatient, outpatient, ASC, even office). The score on MSPB-C and episode-based measures is based on average risk-adjusted cost of all episodes compared to a national average. The measures are weighted equally, so the category score for urologists in most cases will be the average of the MSPB-C score and the Renal or Ureteral Stone Surgical Treatment episode measure score; if cost is weighted at 30% of MIPS, then the episode-based stone procedures measure may be 15% of the MIPS score.

Success in this category will depend largely on controlling facility costs. Factors under a urologist's control include choosing a lower cost site of services (ASC instead of hospital outpatient) and keeping people out of the emergency room (which often leads to readmission). High performers in this category will have in place mechanisms to monitor surgical utilization, identify outliers, and navigate patients to minimize post-procedural ER visits and hospital stays. Large urology groups with control over ASCs, or lithotripsy services, and leverage with local hospitals are in the optimal position to perform well in this category.

Promoting Interoperability

Formerly known as Meaningful Use, then Advancing Care Information, this category has changed significantly to focus on and incentivize the use of EHR technology to communicate with patients and other providers. The measurement period is any 90 continuous days. The category score is calculated from performance on four objectives: electronic prescribing, health information exchange, provider to patient exchange, and public health/clinical data exchange. Success in this category will largely be determined by two best practices: enrolling patients in a portal (40% of the category score) and supporting the sending and receiving of health information (40% of the category score). Almost all states now have Prescription Drug Monitoring Programs, and the query of these databases is incentivized with bonus points in MIPS. High performers will understand the exact workflow that increments these measures; train all users in sending and receiving electronic health information; and use the embedded EHR reports to drive improvement. Urology groups with a single EHR and dedicated resources to standardize the EHR experience will be well positioned for success. Groups with multiple EHRs or a transition to a new EHR during a performance year will need to have a detailed understanding of reporting periods and exceptions in this category.

Improvement Activities

This category awards points for participation in best practices and activities known to improve patient outcomes, improve the health of populations, and lower the cost of care. Dozens of medium and high impact activities are available and reporting can be done electronically (EHR or registry) or by attestation. One important change in year four (2020) of QPP is that to receive credit for a category, at least 50% of a group's clinicians must perform that activity in a 90-day performance period. Success in this category is relatively straightforward, but high performers will look beyond the clerical aspects of MIPS for improvement opportunities in their clinical processes and workflows—especially in population health management and patient navigation. Value-based care models, such as the NCQA Patient Centered Specialty Practice designation incorporate many of these activities and exemplify the bridge between MIPS as a compulsory program and MIPS as a practice ground for value-based care.

Alternative Payment Models

CMS operates many alternative payment models (APMS), but two categories are of importance to urology groups: MIPS APMs and Advanced APMS. MIPS APMs are designated by CMS as models that hold their MIPS participants accountable for the cost and quality of care provided to Medicare beneficiaries. Scoring for clinicians who participate in MIPS APMs is modified to eliminate cost measures and redistribute that weight to the other three categories. In addition, the MIPS APM clinician or group gets credit in the improvement activities category for their APM participation. Finally, the APM may report the MIPS clinician/group's quality data to CMS on their behalf—relieving the urology group of a reporting burden (and assuming their quality score is at least what the group might have achieved on its own). In summary, MIPS clinicians who report through MIPS APMs, such as a Medicare Shared Savings Program track 1, have a lower reporting burden and the opportunity to participate as part of a larger group.

Some APMs are designated as Advanced APMS if they meet three criteria: (1) participants use certified electronic health record technology (CEHRT); (2) the APM provides payment for covered professional services based on quality measures comparable to those used in the quality performance category of MIPS; and (3) the APM is either: a Medical Home Model expanded under CMS Innovation Center authority; or requires participating entities to bear more than a nominal amount of financial risk (defined by CMS) for monetary losses. The most common advanced APMs of interest to urologists are Medicare Accountable Care Organizations with 2-sided risk, Next Generation ACO Model, and Oncology Care Model (OCM). There is an application, review, and approval process for new advanced APMs, but to date, no novel urology APM options have been approved. As a reminder, Qualifying Participants in Advanced APMs are exempt from MIPS and earn a 5% lump sum payment (until 2022). A list of 2020 MIPS and Advanced APMs is included in **Table 2**. Additional MIPS Alternate Payment Models are listed in **Table 3**.

TABLE 2

MIPS and Advanced Alternative Payment Models as of 2020

Bundled Payments for Care Improvement (BPCI) Advanced

Comprehensive ESRD Care (CEC) – Two-Sided Risk

Comprehensive Primary Care Plus (CPC+)

Medicare Accountable Care Organization (ACO) Track 1+ Mode

Medicare Shared Savings Program – Track 2, Track 3, Level E of the BASIC track, the ENHANCED track

Next Generation ACO Model

Oncology Care Model (OCM) – Two-Sided Risk

Comprehensive Care for Joint Replacement (CJR) Payment Model (Track 1-CEHRT)

Vermont Medicare ACO Initiative (as part of the Vermont All-Payer ACO Model)

Comprehensive ESRD Care (CEC) Model

Maryland All-Payer Model (Care Redesign Program)*

Maryland Total Cost of Care Model (Maryland Primary Care Program)

Maryland Total Cost of Care Model (Care Redesign Program)*

*Not MIPS APM

MIPS Reporting Options

One choice that a large urology group may consider is whether to report MIPS data at the individual level, or at the group level (unless they are reporting under MIPS APM). Bearing in mind that the Cost category score is usually assigned at the organization (tax ID) level, the principal differences in individual versus group scoring will probably occur in the Quality category and the Promoting Interoperability category. In recent rulemaking,

TABLE 3

Additional MIPS Alternative Payment Models

Comprehensive ESRD Care (CEC) Model (LDO arrangement)

Comprehensive ESRD Care (CEC) Model (non-LDO one-sided risk arrangement)

Medicare Shared Savings Program – Track 1, BASIC Levels A, B, C, D

Oncology Care Model (OCM) (one-sided Risk Arrangement)

Independence at Home Demonstration

CMS clarified that it will apply the higher of an individual's MIPS composite score or its group score. This has two implications for the group practice. First, the quality data must be reported in a way that allows any aggregation of data to still be identifiable at the clinician level. Second, in large groups this may result in very different MIPS scores for clinicians, and thus, very different fee schedule adjustments to track and manage in the revenue collection and adjudication of claims. Large groups will need to develop compensation strategies that align with both the group culture and the reality that providers may receive different amounts from Medicare for the same service.

The Future of MIPS

In year four (2020) of QPP, CMS announced the concept of MIPS Value Pathways (MVP), further clarifying the agency's desire to move clinicians along into advanced alternative payment models. The framework for MVPs calls for streamlining the quality measures, cost measures, and improvement activities by specialty, so providers are all working on the same broader goals. MVPs also promise to shift more reporting burden away from participants and onto CMS for collection and analysis. The details are pending, but MVPs incorporate some of the same characteristics as alternative payment models and look to be another preparatory step in that direction.

KEY POINTS

- **The QPP is currently complex,** compulsory for most urologists, and still largely based on fee-for-service reimbursement.

- **Participation in MIPS is an opportunity for large urology groups** to refine work processes and build culture in preparation for alternate models that compensate physicians for quality and financial outcomes rather than volume.

- **While the upside in early years of MIPS has been modest**, and the cost of participation may be substantial, most groups cannot afford the penalties (negative fee schedule adjustments up to 9%) associated with limited or no efforts at participation.

- **Success in the QPP may signal preparedness** for value-based care in the future.

Bob Dowling, MD

Bob Dowling is the President of Dowling Medical Director Services, a health care consultancy specializing in clinical quality improvement, Medicare Part B policy issues, adoption and optimization of health information technology, and the practical application of clinical and business analytics in today's challenging health care environment.

Bob completed his medical education and residency at the University of Texas Medical School and Affiliated Hospitals (Hermann Hospital and MD Anderson Cancer Center) in 1987. He has been continuously certified as a diplomate of the American Board of Urology since 1989 and was board certified in Clinical Informatics in 2015. He opened a private urology practice in 1990 in Ft. Worth, Texas, and was a founding leader, Medical Director, and Chief Medical Information Officer of Urology Associates of North Texas (now USMD Health System).

Alec S. Koo, MD

Dr. Alec S. Koo received his bachelor's Degree and MD from UCLA. He completed his residency in Surgery/Urology at UCLA in 1992 and is a Diplomate of the American Board of Urology. Dr. Koo is well known for his expertise in group management as well as value-based care and health economics outcomes. He is respected for his knowledge in areas including data integration and analytics in medicine, medical group dynamics and provider/pharmaceutical relations. Dr. Koo was the founding managing partner of Skyline Urology in Southern California. Dr. Koo is a former member of the LUGPA Board of Directors.

CHAPTER
Political Advocacy

Deepak A. Kapoor, MD

Political advocacy is a constellation of different activities, all which dovetail to advance LUGPA's membership's interest. Advocacy promotes helpful legislation and regulation, while simultaneously thwarting adverse legislative and regulatory activities. These efforts include but are not limited to:

- Lobbying

- Civic engagement, such as "grassroots" communication involving many stakeholders, or "grass tops" engagement, which involves a smaller number of key individuals. Communications, including advertising, earned media, and public affairs; and

- Fundraising/political contributions.

Political advocacy is not new—the Greek democratic system was predicated on citizens influencing each other through public oratory. Advocacy as we know it in this country likely developed in the early 19th century. As legend has it, the term "lobbyist" may have originated in the Willard Hotel in Washington, DC. President Ulysses S. Grant would often visit this establishment in the evening to enjoy a cigar and brandy. Political advocates frequented the hotel's lobby to gain access to the President to voice their interests and concerns.

While changing campaign finance laws and new ethics rules have transformed the ways in which we engage in political advocacy in recent years, the core components are largely unchanged. Lobbying, fundraising, communications, and civic engagement continue to be the essential components to advocacy. While many groups use the above techniques, what is unique to the healthcare market is that we not only advocate for our own interests, but also for the patients who are under our care.

While LUGPA has utilized all these components to protect its independent practice business model and the patients that rely on its urological care, we are far from the only voice speaking on these issues. It is important to remember that healthcare comprises nearly one-sixth of our nation's gross domestic product. There is an enormous amount of money spent to influence decision-making in our field; consequently, LUGPA has adopted several political advocacy strategies. Whether proactive or responsive, widespread or targeted, LUGPA's advocacy efforts will always have one element in common: to ensure that the voice of independent and integrated physician practices is considered when national policies are drafted that directly or indirectly impact patient care.

To have and maintain that voice, LUGPA builds relationships with key policy makers. These relationships are predicated on leveraging data that support the critical role independent physicians play as a competitive counterbalance to more expensive and less convenient institutional-based care. Over time, this strategy has resulted in LUGPA's voice being trusted as a resource in policy debates; this has benefitted both independent physician practices, and most importantly, enhanced patient care.

According to the Center for Responsive Politics, these Sectors spent the most on lobbying in 2019.

♥	Health	$603,290,786
📊	Finance	$503,072,659
👥	Business	$500,737,207

One important point regarding political advocacy is that, while the support and vote of every member of Congress is important, legislation must move through key committees of jurisdiction before being considered by Congress as a whole. With respect to healthcare, there are three such committees of jurisdiction: The Senate Finance Committee, the House Energy and Commerce Committee, and the House Ways and Means Committee. The policies of greatest impact to LUGPA members all flow through these key committees. Consequently, LUGPA's efforts on Capitol Hill over the years have focused on the development of political champions by working closely with members of Congress on these three key committees of jurisdiction. These efforts, which heavily rely on objective data to support our Association's positions, have resulted in long-term bipartisan relationships with both members and key staffers; LUGPA is often called upon as a resource when healthcare legislation is being crafted.

Also, critically important to LUGPA's advocacy has been engagement with physician members of Congress; most are part of the Doctors Caucuses in their respective chamber. This caucus is open to not only physicians, but other healthcare professionals as well. Although bipartisan, most healthcare professionals are currently members of the Republican party. Engagement with these members is critical as other members rely on their medical expertise to help shape healthcare policy.

But LUGPA's advocacy extends beyond "preaching to the choir." While it makes great sense to align ourselves with legislators who are like-minded and have significant knowledge of LUGPA's issues, it is equally important to branch out and share our views with members of Congress who may be more skeptical or less familiar with our specialty and the policies that impact it.

LUGPA has devoted significant time and resources to working with certain members who may not always align with its policies, in efforts to educate them on its perspectives. The importance of engaging with key leaders who may not align with any member's individual political views cannot be overstated. Connecting these members with LUGPA leadership and physician leaders in their districts has proven effective in helping these representatives and senators understand and even support LUGPA issues.

I. WHAT LUGPA HAS ACCOMPLISHED

A. Reform of Physician Self-Referral Law

The Physician Self-Referral Law (known as the Stark law), allows group medical practices to offer ancillary services, such as advanced imaging, radiation therapy, and pathology within their practices—collectively, these are known as designated health services (DHS). The ability to provide capital intensive DHS is important to many LUGPA practices' ability to serve patients, provide integrated and comprehensive care, and compete against conglomerated hospital systems.

- Reform of Physician Self Referral Law
- Protetcting Reimbursement for Physician Services
- MACRA
- Site Neutrality
- Pharmaceutical Reimbursement

Moreover, Medicare and beneficiaries save substantial money when they receive DHS in our physician offices and procedures in our ambulatory surgery centers. Naturally, patients migrate to the most convenient and cost-effective site of service. This has led to a continuous drumbeat from interest groups that stand to benefit if our practices were barred from providing these important services through legislative fiat. In fact, these historical monopoly specialists have banded together to develop government champions of their own.

Historically, LUGPA's efforts centered around preservation of a specific component of Stark Law known as the "in-office ancillary service exception" or IOASE. Through LUGPA's leadership in working with physician colleagues, more than 30 physician specialty organizations and the American Medical Association joined to demand that the IOASE be preserved in order to promote competition and deliver superior, coordinated care. These efforts united virtually the entire house of medicine and isolated those specialists who sought to restore their therapeutic monopolies. The support of the united medical community was instrumental in helping LUGPA successfully secure several sign-on letters from both the House and Senate Doctors Caucus, underscoring those points and admonishing Congressional leadership not to use IOASE as a potential offset. Because of these efforts, other than a handful of highly partisan co-sponsors, legislation to curb the IOASE has not gained broad traction in the United States House of Representatives and has never been introduced in the Senate.

As we move to value-based paradigms, the ability to provide ancillary services is integral to LUGPA's member practices' ability to serve patients, provide integrated and comprehensive care, and compete with large hospital systems. Furthermore, ancillary services performed at physicians' offices are far more cost effective than when done at the facility setting, greatly reducing expense to both patients and third-party payors. For years, Stark has been viewed in some areas of healthcare policy as a "third rail" that cannot be touched without creating a "wild west" scenario that leads to inappropriate utilization by physicians seeking to generate more revenue at the expense of patients and the Medicare program. But the law was written three decades ago in an era of fee-for-service. Stark now serves as a barrier to coordinated and value-based care.

Therefore, we spent months developing consensus with bipartisan Members of committees of jurisdiction and the same coalition of physician organizations on legislation that would modernize the antiquated fraud and abuse laws. Getting the House of Medicine to speak with one voice on targeted reforms amplified LUGPA's voice and advocacy prowess. And securing bipartisan introduction of the bill by highly regarded members from both parties on committees of jurisdiction conveyed our clear message that for value-based care delivery to succeed, Stark and other fraud and abuse laws must be modernized.

We were able to secure introduction of bipartisan and bicameral legislation that would provide the same protections for physicians engaged in Alternative Payment Models (APMs) as providers participating in Accountable Care Organizations, and also repeal the "volume and value" prohibitions for physicians and other providers wishing to test or operate APMs. The Medicare Care Coordination Improvement Act (S. 966/H.R.2282) was introduced by Senators Portman (R-OH) and Bennet (D-CO) and Reps. Ruiz (D-CA) and Bucshon (R-IN).

That bill would allow greater collaboration among physicians within our practices as well as with other providers in the community by allowing them to share resources from designated healthcare services (such as pathology and radiation therapy) to incentivize adherence to clinical guidelines and treatment pathways. This means physicians can be rewarded or penalized based on certain volume or value metrics.

In addition to submitting comments in response to the Center for Medicare & Medicaid Services (CMS) and Office of Inspector General's (OIG's) respective Requests for Information (RFI) regarding the Stark law and Anti-Kickback Statute (AKS), we testified alongside HHS Deputy Secretary Hargan before the House Ways & Means Subcommittee on Health. There, we noted the critical importance of modernizing fraud and abuse laws to promote the transition to value-based care in the Medicare program and in our healthcare system more broadly.

Perhaps even more significant is a complete overhaul of the regulatory interpretation of Stark law by CMS. After soliciting ideas through an RFI, CMS issued comprehensive proposed rules to Stark and AKS in 2019. Central to the approach is providers' ability to enter into value-based arrangements without needing an application or CMS approval. Providers need only to retain documentation on how their activities further value-based purposes and the type, nature, and methodology of the remuneration.

The proposal gives flexibility for arrangements with varying degrees of risk-sharing, which is important because it does not presume that a one-size-fits-all approach can work for different specialties, regions, or size of practices.

Any value-based entity engaged in one of the four value-based purposes would qualify:

1. Coordinating and managing the care of a target population;

2. Improving the quality of care for a target patient population;

3. Appropriately reducing the costs to, or growth in expenditures of, payors without reducing the quality of care for a target patient population; **OR**

4. Transitioning from healthcare delivery and payment mechanisms based on the volume of items and services to mechanisms based on the quality of care and control of costs of care.

LUGPA submitted detailed comments to both the RFI and proposed rules commending the Department of Health and Human Services (HHS) for its bold steps, providing specific examples of value-based care activities that are prohibited under the current regulatory framework. While still pending finalization, these changes broadly expand the ability of independent physician practices to engage in value-based initiatives by expanding the exceptions to Stark law. These exceptions will allow for the development and operation of innovative care delivery systems—across medical specialties and sites of service—that will improve outcomes and decrease cost.

B. Protecting Reimbursement for Physician Services

Another aspect of LUGPA's regulatory advocacy efforts is directed towards agencies who create reimbursement policies that impact LUGPA member groups. Such has been the case every summer when the HHS promulgates its annual regulations known as the Medicare Physician Fee Schedule (MPFS) and Outpatient Prospective Payment System (OPPS), which updates payment policies and payment rates for physicians and ambulatory surgery centers (ASCs). LUGPA performs detailed analysis of these rules and when appropriate, comments in a substantive fashion. In fact, LUGPA's comments have been specifically cited several times in the rulemaking process, suggesting that our Association is viewed as a valuable resource to regulatory bodies.

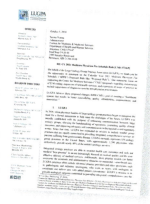

Radiation Therapy

Over the past decade, CMS sought to dramatically reduce payments for radiation therapy provided in the physician office while simultaneously increasing payments for the identical services in hospitals. LUGPA and allied stakeholders generated data that served to avert draconian cuts repeatedly proposed since 2008 that would have effectively ended non-institutional radiation services.

These efforts continued for years, when LUGPA, working with allies in the Radiation Therapy Alliance and others, were able to block cuts entirely for 2015 and substantially mitigated proposed cuts of more than 30% to prostate cancer in 2016.

Subsequently, LUPGA worked with Congress to pass legislation that imposed a two-year freeze on reimbursement for radiation therapy at existing levels, providing important stability after years of volatility. That same legislation also included a provision that LUGPA worked on to allow physicians to obtain hardship exemptions from meaningful use penalties.

More recently, LUGPA has been actively engaged with CMS and CMS Innovation Center (CMMI) regarding its proposed, mandatory Medicare payment model for the delivery of radiation oncology services (the "RO Model"). While there are aspects of the proposal that LUGPA strongly supports, in particular provisions with respect to true site neutral payments between hospitals and physicians' offices, LUGPA opposed implementation of the rule as written. In summary, LUGPA expressed concerns that the proposed RO Model—particularly as applied to treatment of prostate cancer—fails to deliver on the Innovation Center's statutory charge of testing innovative payment and service delivery models for the purpose of decreasing Medicare program expenditures, but to do so "while preserving or enhancing the quality of care furnished" to Medicare beneficiaries. LUGPA expressed concerns regarding CMS's intent to subject the entire country to a mandatory, untested demonstration project that threatens to undertreat men with prostate cancer and deprive beneficiaries to choose where they receive radiation therapy services, when the driver of utilization and cost is confined to the hospital outpatient department setting.

Pathology

An important service provided to our patients by LUGPA members is anatomic pathology data on the management of our patients. Surgeons recognize that the ability to control quality and interact with professionals who provide data critical to management of our patients is invaluable. Despite this, the ability to provide these services in the physicians' office setting has come under continued attack by professional organizations that seek to restore silo-based models of healthcare. LUGPA's analytics have refuted shoddy publications and resulted in preserving the ability to provide integrated pathology services within our practices.

LUGPA has also provided detailed commentary on prostate histology, fluorescent in-situ hybridization (FISH), cytology, and immunohistochemistry. These comments served as the basis for CMS substantively altering its payment policy on urinary FISH and cytology testing, and we continue to present data to modify reimbursement for the interpretation of prostate biopsies.

Ambulatory and Professional Services

LUGPA's commentary goes far beyond supporting members in their ability to continue to perform DHS in their offices. LUGPA has provided extensive commentary on a variety of Current Procedural Terminology (CPT)® codes performed in the hospital, ASCs, and the office setting. LUGPA has provided substantive data on items ranging from support of professional services for laparoscopic radical prostatectomies, to ensuring that reimbursement for services, such as greenlight laser and lithotripsy in the ASC setting is appropriate, to defending reimbursement for commonly performed services in our offices. These comments have resulted in tangible changes in HHS payment policy—changes that directly benefit LUGPA member groups.

C. Medicare Access and CHIP Reauthorization Act

LUGPA took a leadership role in lobbying Congress to repeal the deeply flawed sustainable growth rate (SGR) payment formula and move to value-based payments outlined in the Medicare Access and CHIP Reauthorization Act (MACRA). Across the country, LUGPA's member practices generated thousands of emails, telephone calls, and other contacts with their Congressional representatives in support of the bill that eliminated the unconscionable pending cuts to physicians. MACRA passed with more than 90% support of Congress, a rare bipartisan achievement. In fact, LUGPA's grassroots efforts were specifically and publicly recognized and appreciated by the bipartisan leadership in the House and Senate—one of but a handful of physician organizations to be acknowledged.

LUGPA is now focused on MACRA implementation to ensure that all our practices can succeed in the new payment framework of the Merit-based Incentive Payment System (MIPS) and Alternative Payment Models (APMs). LUGPA submitted extensive comments to CMS on how CMS can use its current authority to modernize the Stark law and permit greater coordination demanded by the statute.

As stated earlier, the critical barrier to independent practices' ability to succeed under MACRA is related to the regulatory burden under Stark law. LUGPA has again aligned with other physician groups we have worked with on IOASE to form a coalition to support Stark reform. Continued advocacy by the physician community has resulted in CMS and OIG working with one another to develop the complementary proposed rules designed to modernize the Stark law and AKS. MACRA demands care coordination across sites of service and the development of value-based care delivery models; yet, our fraud and abuse laws were not updated in MACRA or since its passage. Given how critical these issues are to the continued viability of independent urology (and other specialty) practices, LUGPA submitted comment to OIG in response to the AKS Proposed Rule at the same time we also submitted these comments in response to the Stark Proposed Rule.

An important component of MACRA was the development of physician-focused payment models. This was Congress's vision to allow a "thousand flowers to bloom" where physician-generated ideas for value-based delivery could be tested and experimented upon. Although not specifically part of legislative advocacy, LUGPA was an early proponent of developing alternative payment models and other value-based payment structures for use in treating patients with cancer, and in fact submitted one of the earliest (and as of yet, still only urology specific) models to be submitted for review. Regrettably, the APM approval process at CMMI has been dysfunctional: in the past three years, CMMI has not approved a single APM recommended for pilot testing or immediate implementation. That said, while CMS has yet to implement LUGPA's proposal, the early submission established LUGPA as a serious voice in the nation's transition to value-based care.

D. Site Neutrality

For years, one of the major adverse market trends affecting independent specialty groups has been the hospital systems' ability to systematically dominate market share with the acquisition of physician practices. LUGPA has continuously made the case to policymakers that independent physician practices can deliver high-quality care more efficiently than hospitals. LUGPA has supported this argument by providing lawmakers academic literature that clearly shows that this conglomeration of services has not only failed to deliver on the promise of enhancing care coordination but serves to reduce access and increase costs.

These efforts have produced tangible results. Congress enacted a provision in the Bipartisan Budget Act of 2015 to prevent windfalls in future hospital acquisitions of physician practices and ambulatory surgery centers. This provision prohibits hospitals from charging hospital rates for off-campus physician and ambulatory services at sites acquired after passage of the bill (November 2015); these payments must be made at the prevailing MPFS and ASC rates rather than the higher rates specified in the Outpatient Prospective Payment System (OPPS). In addition to leveling the playing field between independent practices and hospitals, this legislation will save taxpayers nearly $8 billion over 10 years. In the 2017 final OPPS rule, HHS created regulatory guidelines to implement this legislation that were broadly favorable to independent physicians; LUGPA's detailed commentary supported this approach and provided recommendations for future modifications to further strengthen the rule.

As expected, advocates for the American Hospital Association and its allies strongly opposed these efforts, which resulted in a court decision vacating the portions of the 2019 OPPS Final Rule that had reduced reimbursements to off-campus provider-based departments (PBDs) based on the finding that CMS had exceeded its statutory authority. More recently, there has been a significant (albeit, anticipated) development in the hospitals' lawsuits challenging Secretary Azar's implementation of the OPPS site-neutral payment policy. In December 2019, HHS filed notices of appeal challenging the D.C. District Court's grant of summary judgment to the hospital-plaintiffs. Secretary Azar's filing of the notices of appeal starts the process for the U.S. Court of Appeals for the D.C. Circuit—the appellate court right below the US Supreme Court—to evaluate the Secretary's authority to implement the site-neutral payment policy. This is a critical step because, given that the Supreme Court takes so few cases, most law is decided in the intermediate federal appellate courts.

At the time of this writing, LUGPA has taken the extraordinary step of filing an amicus curiae brief on behalf of HHS in its appeal. The government has focused its argument on the high bar the hospitals must overcome to sustain an ultra vires challenge (i.e., their claim that the Secretary was without authority to cap payment rates for clinic visit services furnished in excepted, off-campus outpatient departments). LUGPA, as a non-party, was able to provide a voice to those factual arguments. In late July 2020, the U.S. Court of Appeals for the District of Columbia Circuit overturned a federal district judge's ruling that CMS exceeded its statutory authority by reducing Medicare Part B drug reimbursement for 340B hospitals in 2018 and 2019. This effort is a unique and tangible indicator of LUGPA's commitment to protecting the independent practice of urology.

E. Pharmaceutical Reimbursement

At the time of this writing, there is bipartisan consensus that the skyrocketing costs of medication, both prescription (Medicare Part D) and physician administered ("buy-and-bill", Medicare Part B) needs to be addressed. That is where the consensus ends. There are at least three proposals being contemplated, one by the Administration, and one by the House and Senate, respectively. While substantially different in detail, all these proposals include potentially substantial cuts to reimbursement for lifesaving medications, including those used to treat patients with advanced prostate, bladder, and renal cancer. Some introduce profit-driven middlemen into clinical decision making that must remain between patient and provider. While LUGPA is committed to the responsible stewardship of the nation's healthcare resources, we joined other stakeholders to share our deep concerns about the impact the various proposals will have on our ability to provide care to our most gravely ill patients. We urged both CMS and Congress to defer making changes until it addresses stakeholder input regarding the serious clinical, operational, and legal challenges with the various reforms as currently framed.

II. GETTING INVOLVED

There are many ways for LUGPA practices—physicians, administrators, and employees—to get involved in the political process. One of the most effective advocacy tools is introducing members of Congress to one's practice. It can be helpful to invite Congressional representatives to visit physician offices, take tours, and see firsthand how an integrated and independent urology practice serves its patients—their constituents! It is important to remind them of the group's role as an employer in their district to share how many employees work in the offices, how many patients are served, what procedures are performed, and which medical conditions are treated. Members of Congress also benefit from viewing the equipment required to perform all these services being used in a cost-effective and high-quality manner.

LUGPA members also may wish to schedule a meeting in their district offices with the member of Congress and/or their staff. Most members have several offices located strategically throughout their districts. It is equally important to get to know the Congress person's staff since that is where much of the policy making begins! One can also offer to be a resource to members and their staff when they are grappling with policy matters or simply in need of medical assistance.

These meetings and visits will allow LUGPA members to develop a relationship with members of Congress and their staff. And most importantly, one does not need to wait for a problem or issue to arise. Communicating with staff—via telephone or email—has proven helpful when Congress is in the heat of debating a policy matter, but that should not be the first time they hear from LUGPA member. Relationships take time to build, and it is important to initially introduce oneself and one's practice to begin laying the groundwork for communication whenever the next policy matter arises.

Finally, it is important for our physicians to fully engage in the political process. LUGPA is very active in supporting members of Congress who share our views and are focused on healthcare policy. This is a vital way to get our message out and raise the profile of independent urology and the value that our groups provide to patients and the healthcare system. Physicians can help LUGPA help their practices and patients by supporting friendly members of Congress when LUGPA calls upon them to do so!

There is an old saying in Washington D.C.: "You are either at the table or on the menu." LUGPA knows that consolidated hospital systems and other specialties that stand to gain from monopolizing care are active politically. Our Association must be just as active so that we can be part of the process to ensure that our views and perspectives are considered when legislation and regulations are crafted.

III. CONCLUSION

Clearly, there is no shortage of work to be done. The nation's healthcare agenda is robust, and there are a significant number of issues impacting LUGPA practices. For every battle LUGPA has engaged in to date—be it battles to protect the IOASE or to prevent and reverse reimbursement cuts for ancillary and professional services in the MPFS or OPPS rules—advocacy has played a critical role. LUGPA's lobbying, combined with its grassroots actions, communications, and fundraising activities has proven vital in each of these successful efforts.

As lawmakers and regulatory agencies seek to shift payments from volume-to-value-based models, LUGPA's advocacy efforts will become even more critical. Without question, LUGPA has laid a very solid foundation in an impressively short period of time; we need to build on that foundation to ensure that our voice continues to be heard. But LUGPA as an organization cannot advocate effectively without the support and help of its membership—our voice, our commitment, our advocacy, and yes, our financial commitment is vital to the future of independent urology groups.

We are at the cusp of very exciting changes, but we must keep the pressure on policymakers to follow through and finalize these proposals. That will require continued engagement with congressional champions, political leaders, and line staff at HHS as well as our physician brethren. These changes will invigorate independent practice of medicine and allow us to provide better, more efficient care to our patients.

KEY POINTS

- **Political advocacy** promotes helpful legislation and regulation, while simultaneously thwarting adverse legislative and regulatory activities.

- **Political advocacy** includes lobbying, civic engagement, communications, and fundraising.

- **LUGPA's political advocacy** strategies ensure that physician practices are considered when national policies are drafted that will directly impact their ability to treat patients.

- **The policies of greatest impact to LUGPA** all flow through the Senate Finance Committee, the House Energy and Commerce Committee, and the House Ways and Means Committee.

- **It is important to align** with legislators who have significant knowledge of our issues and to share our views with members of Congress who may be more skeptical or less familiar with policies that impact urology.

- **LUGPA** is often called upon as a resource when healthcare legislation is being crafted.

- **LUGPA lobbied Congress** to repeal the flawed sustainable growth rate payment formula and move to value-based payments outlined in the Medicare Access and CHIP Reauthorization Act (MACRA). LUGPA is now focused on ensuring that all of our practices can succeed in the new the Merit-based Incentive Payment System (MIPS) and Alternative Payment Models (APMs), and has submitted comments to CMS urging CMS to modernize the Stark law and permit greater coordination demanded by the statute.

- **LUGPA successfully prompted Congress** to enact a provision in the Bipartisan Budget Act of 2015 that prohibits hospitals from charging hospital rates for off-campus physician and ambulatory services at sites acquired after passage of the bill (November 2015). This legislation will save taxpayers nearly $8 billion over 10 years.

- **LUGPA is currently urging both CMS and Congress** to defer making changes to proposals that will reduce reimbursement for lifesaving medications until they address stakeholder input regarding the serious clinical, operational, and legal challenges with the various reforms as currently framed.

- **Physicians, administrators, and employees** can get involved in the political process by inviting Congressional Representatives to their practices to take tours and see first-hand how an integrated and independent urology practice serves its patients.

Deepak A. Kapoor, MD

Dr. Deepak A. Kapoor is Chairman and Chief Ecosystem Officer of Solaris Health Holdings, LLC, Market President for Integrated Medical Professionals, PLLC (IMP) and President of Advanced Urology Centers of New York. His expertise includes basic science research in molecular biology, as well as extensive experience in oncologic and reconstructive surgery.

Dr. Kapoor is Clinical Professor of Urology at the Icahn School of Medicine at Mount Sinai, Chair of the LUGPA Health Policy Committee, Past President of LUGPA, and Chairman of SCRUBS RRG. He has also served as a Director of UroPAC and Chairman of Access to Integrated Cancer Care. Dr. Kapoor was founder of the New York Urology Trade Association and Integrated Medical Foundation. In addition, he is a Fellow of the American College of Physician Executives.

Dr. Kapoor has published and lectured extensively on clinical, business and health policy issues and is Associate Editor of the journal Urology Practice. He serves on several medical advisory boards, including the New York State Governor's Prostate Cancer Advisory Panel. Dr. Kapoor has received numerous accolades, including the 2011 AUA Ambrose-Reed socioeconomic essay award, the 2014 New York Section AUA Russell W. Lavengood distinguished service award and was recognized in 2018 by LUGPA for outstanding contributions to health policy and the preservation of independent medicine.

EDITORS' DISCLOSURE

David Chaikin, MD
COR Medspa, Owner; Symptelligence, advisor

Evan R. Goldfischer, MD, MBA
AbbVie, speaker/consultant, research; Astellas, speaker/consultant, research; Bayer, speaker/research/consultant, research; Janssen, speaker/research/consultant; Bristol Meyers, speaker/research/consultant; Pfizer, speaker/research/consultant, research, Altor, research; Onco Cell MDx, research; Solace, research; AWCT, research; Siemens, research; Urovant, research; Clovis Oncology, research

Jonathan Henderson, MD
Janssen, speaker/consultant; Clovis, consultant; AstraZeneca, consultant

Alec Koo, MD
AbbVie, speaker/advisor; Astellas, speaker/advisor; Bayer, advisor; Dashko, shareholder; Dendreon, advisor; EMD Serono, advisor; Integra, advisor; Janssen, speaker/advisor; Merck, advisor; Symptelligence, shareholder; UroGPO, shareholder

Bryan Mehlhaff, MD
Amgen, speaker/consultant; Astellas, speaker/consultant, research; AstraZeneka, speaker/consultant; Bayer, speaker/consultant, research; CUSP, research; Dendreon, speaker/consultant, research, Janssen, speaker/consultant, research; Merck, speaker/consultant; Pfizer, speaker/consultant; Myovant, research; UroGPO, advisor

Scott Sellinger, MD
Amgen, speaker; Astellas, speaker; Bayer, speaker; Ferring, speaker; Genomic Health, speaker/consultant; Pfizer, speaker; Janssen, speaker/consultant; Tolmar, speaker

Alan Winkler, MHSA, FACMPE
Nautic Partners, LLC, shareholder

Unless listed here, contributing authors have no relevant financial disclosures for the chapters they authored. Authors reporting disclosures are listed alphabetically.

David C. Chaikin, MD
COR Medspa, Owner; Symptelligence, advisor

Raul S. Concepcion, MD, FACS
CUSP, Medical Advisor

Robert Di Loreto, MD
CMIO Vxtra Health – a Value Based Health Insurance Company

Michael Ingber, MD
InMode, consultant/speaker; Allergan, proctor/speaker; Hologic: speaker

Bryan A. Mehlhaff, MD
Amgen, speaker/consultant; Astellas, speaker/consultant, research; AstraZeneka, speaker/consultant; Bayer, speaker/consultant, research; CUSP, research; Dendreon, speaker/consultant, research, Janssen, speaker/consultant, research; Merck, speaker/consultant; Pfizer, speaker/consultant; Myovant, research; UroGPO, advisor

M. Ray Painter, MD
PRS (Physician Reimbursement Systems) Officer, Employee, stock ownership

Mark Painter
PRS (Physician Reimbursement Systems) Consultant fees, stock ownership

Christopher Pieczonka, MD
Astellas, speaker/consultant, research; Janssen, speaker/consultant, research; Bayer, speaker/consultant, research; Pfizer, speaker/consultant, research; Dendreon, speaker/consultant, research; AstraZeneca, speaker/consultant, research; Veru, research; Merck, speaker/consultant, research; Myovan, research; Invitae, research; Myriad, research

Daniel Saltzstein, MD
CUSP, Consultant and Advisor

Neal D. Shore, MD, FACS
CUSP, Ownership interest, Advisor

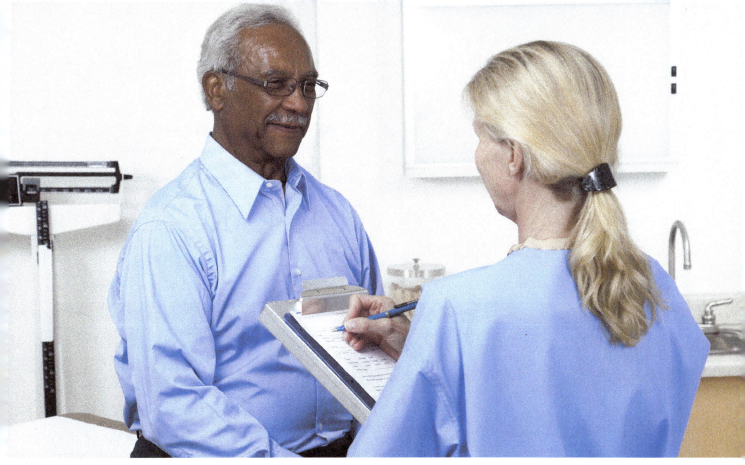

Gene Chutka - Getty Images
The image depicted contains models and is being used for illustrative purposes only.

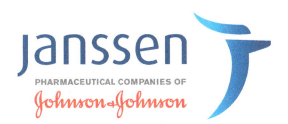

wants to thank you all for the incredibly important work you do each day.

Janssen Biotech, Inc.

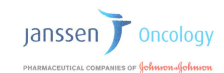

© Janssen Biotech, Inc. 2019   02/19   cp-54411v2

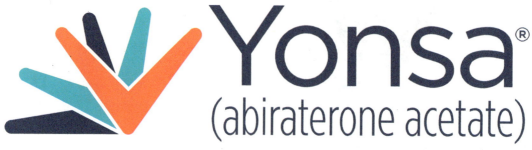

Yonsa®
(abiraterone acetate)
125 mg tablets

HOW MIGHT YONSA® BE A TREATMENT OPTION FOR YOUR PATIENT?

To learn more —
visit **www.YonsaRx.com**

Yonsa is a registered trademark of Sun Pharma Global FZE.
©2020 Sun Pharmaceutical Industries, Inc.

SUN PHARMA

PM-US-YON-0372